Children's Medicine
and Surgery

Children's Medicine and Surgery

Forrester Cockburn MD, FRCP, DCH

*Samson Gemmell Professor of Child Health at the University
of Glasgow and Honorary Consultant Paediatrician at
the Royal Hospital for Sick Children, Glasgow, UK*

Robert Carachi MD, PhD, FRCS

*Senior Lecturer of Paediatric Surgery at the
University of Glasgow and
Honorary Consultant Paediatric Surgeon
at the Royal Hospital for Sick Children, Glasgow, UK*

Krishna N Goel MD, FRCP, DCH

*Honorary Senior Lecturer of Child Health,
University of Glasgow and Consultant Paediatrician at
the Royal Hospital for Sick Children, Glasgow, UK*

Daniel G Young MBChB, FRCS, DTM&H

*Professor of Paediatric Surgery at the University of Glasgow
and Honorary Consultant Surgeon at the
Royal Hospital for Sick Children, Glasgow, UK*

ARNOLD

A member of the Hodder Headline Group
LONDON • SYDNEY • AUCKLAND
Co-published in the USA by Oxford University Press, Inc., New York

First published in Great Britain 1996 by
Arnold, a member of the Hodder Headline Group,
338 Euston Road, London NW1 3BH

Co-published in the United States of America by
Oxford University Press, Inc.,
198 Madison Avenue, New York, NY10016
Oxford is a registered trademark of Oxford University Press

Whilst the advice and information in this book is believed to be true and
accurate at the date of going to press, neither the authors nor the publisher
can accept legal responsibility or liability for any errors or omissions
that may be made. In particular (but without limiting the generality of the
preceding disclaimer) every effort has been made to check drug dosages;
however it is still possible that errors have been missed. Furthermore,
dosage schedules are constantly being revised and new side-effects
recognized. For these reasons the reader is strongly urged to consult the
drug companies' printed instructions before administering any of the drugs
recommended in this book.

British Library Cataloguing in Publication Data
A catalogue record for this book is available from the British Library

Library of Congress Cataloging-in-Publication Data
A catalog record for this book is available from the Library of Congress

ISBN 0 340 55143 7 (pb)

1 2 3 4 5   96 97 98 99

Typeset in 9/11pt Sabon by
Scribe Design, Gillingham, Kent
Printed and bound in Hong Kong

Contents

Preface

The origins of physical and mental health and disease lie predominantly in the early development of the child. Most of the abnormalities affecting the health and behaviour of children are determined prenatally or in the first few years of life by genetic and environmental factors. In this book the authors have summarised the current knowledge of causation and have indicated where health education and prevention might reduce the burden of childhood ill health. They have given practical advice about the diagnosis, investigation and management of the full spectrum of childhood disorders, both medical and surgical.

Professor James Holmes Hutchison, author of *Practical Paediatric Problems* died in 1988 and when Forrester Cockburn was approached by the publisher to consider a 7th edition of the book he consulted his medical students, professional colleagues and friends and asked them to join in the creation of a new book. This new book also supersedes in a sense the late Wallace Dennison's *Surgery of Infancy and Childhood*, which was the companion to the textbook *Practical Paediatric Problems*. A new combined medical and surgical text is in keeping with the Glasgow tradition; in the second half of the nineteenth century the St Mungo's College had a lecturer in the surgical and medical diseases of children. This holistic approach to the child is, the authors believe, fundamental to good health care.

The four authors acknowledge their debt to clinical colleagues and teachers past and present who have contributed to the creation of this new text. It is intended in a true apprenticeship fashion of pedagogy to provide a manageable, readable and practical account of clinical paediatrics for medical undergraduates, for postgraduates specialising in paediatrics and for general practitioners whose daily work is concerned with the care of children in health and in sickness.

Particular thanks must go to Dr David S James who contributed the chapter on Child Psychiatry. Mr Derek Attwood, Dr T James Beattie, Mrs Brenda Clark, Dr William B Doig, Dr Malcolm DC Donaldson, Dr John Dudgeon, Professor MS Elbualy (Oman), Dr Brenda Gibson, Dr R Hague, Dr Alan B Houston, Dr A Howatson, Dr Ruth J MacKenzie, Dr Neil W Morley, Dr A Patrick, Mr Michael GH Smith and Professor John BP Stephenson gave unstintingly of their time and expertise to provide ideas and illustrations for the book. The secretarial and organisational skills of Mrs Myra Fergusson were a key element in the creation of this text and we gratefully acknowledge her support and help. Miss Sylvia McCulloch and Mrs Lynda McCarroll assisted with the typing and preparation of the drafting for the book. Mr Alastair Irwin and his staff prepared the photographs and special thanks are due to Miss Jean Hyslop, Medical Artist who created the line drawings and artwork and helped to integrate the text with the illustrations.

The authors had to be selective in deciding what to exclude in order to keep the book manageable and practical. We have also had to be selective in our expressions of gratitude to individual colleagues in the many different professions which make up the complex hospital and community services which care for our children. Our thanks go to our wives and families and to the many children and their families who contributed to our knowledge and understanding of Children's Medicine and Surgery.

Forrester Cockburn
Robert Carachi
Krishna M Goel
Daniel G Young
1996

1

Early Development of the Child

INTRODUCTION

Given a normal genetic endowment, a healthy well nourished mother, a normal pregnancy and delivery, the provision of appropriate nutrition and a supportive home and community environment a child will grow and develop normally. It is not possible to separate the reproductive health needs of women and the health of the newborn human infant. Adverse genetic and environmental factors can compromise the health of an individual from the time of conception. Processes of cell division within the individual organs of the developing embryo, fetus, infant and child are dependent on adequate nutrition and freedom from environmental insult. The healthy child is one who shows no evidence of defective organ function and has normal growth and development. The Director General of the WHO reported that 12.9 million deaths occurred in 1990 of children under the age of 5 years. He estimated that one-third occurred during the first month of life, one-third during the period from 1 month up to 12 months and the remaining third among those from 1 to 5 years of age. Approximately 500 000 women die each year during pregnancy or childbirth and these deaths are particularly common in countries where there is unequal access to health care and a balanced diet. Excessive work during pregnancy, denial of equal opportunity for education, and obstacles to reproductive health leave the women physically, socially and mentally unable to exercise their full rights for personal and social development. They are unable to protect themselves from unwanted pregnancies or sexually transmitted diseases. The majority of conditions affecting women during pregnancy and delivery which increase the risk of death or severe morbidity also have adverse affects on the fetus and newborn. Traditional beliefs and birth practices in some circumstances increase the risks of mortality for mother and infant. Delays in seeking skilled attention and failure to ensure cleanliness of those involved in the delivery increase the risk of the woman rupturing her uterus, developing sepsis and the subsequent long-term risks of chronic pelvic inflammatory disease, infertility and ectopic pregnancy. WHO estimates that only 55% of all births in the world are attended by trained personnel. Interventions aimed at lowering perinatal or neonatal mortality must address maternal health, the social position of women and the provisions for ensuring maternal health during pregnancy and delivery.

FETAL MEDICINE

Embryonic development and genes

Embryonic development commences from the time of conception and lasts for 8 weeks. Adverse genetic and environmental factors can result in disordered embryonic development with the production of congenital malformations and inherited metabolic disorders. Major congenital malformations are apparent at birth in approximately one in 40 and in half a genetic factor can be identified.

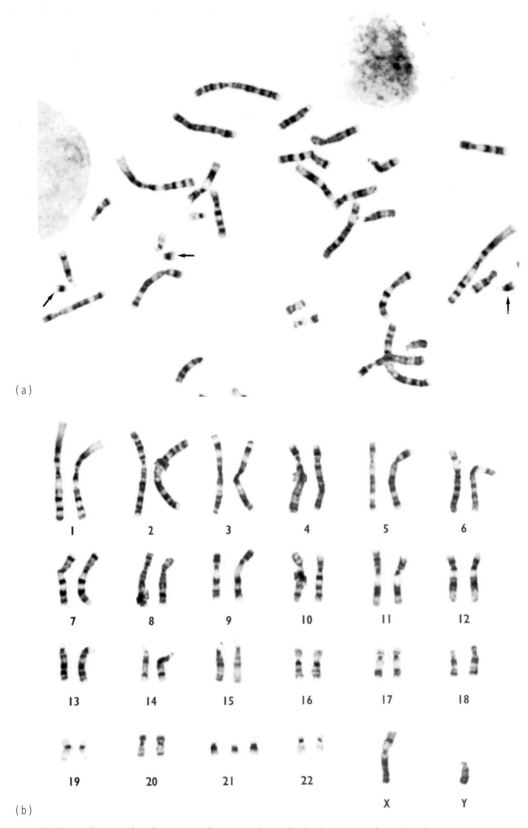

FIGURE 1.1 Photographs of (a) a metaphase spread and (b) the karyotype of a male infant with trisomy 21.

Chromosomes and chromosome abnormalities

Normally each fertilised ovum contains 46 chromosomes comprising 22 pairs of autosomes and a single pair of sex chromosomes, XY in the male and XX in the female. Subsequent divisions of the original fertilised ovum, given a nutritious and "safe" environment in which to develop, will result within 8 weeks in a recognisably human embryo with all major organs identifiable. More than 15% of all conceptions end in spontaneous miscarriage and in about 40% of these there is a chromosomal abnormality. In developed countries the perinatal mortality rates are 10 per 1000 or less and approximately a quarter of these babies die as a result of a serious congenital malformation and 5% will have a chromosomal abnormality.

Most chromosome abnormalities arise from errors in the meiotic cell divisions in gametogenesis. Occasionally one or other parent may have an autosomal imbalance which usually will result in infertility but if the autosomal translocation or inversion exists in a balanced form there may be a high risk of transmitting the rearrangement in an unbalanced form to their child. Any loss or gain of autosomal material will predispose to congenital abnormality including abnormal brain development. Chromosomal abnormalities account for about one-third of all cases of moderate and severe learning difficulties with Down syndrome (trisomy 21) and the fragile X syndrome as the most common causes.

Chromosomal abnormalities

Figure 1.1(a) shows a photograph of a metaphase spread of chromosomes from a peripheral blood lymphocyte arrested during metaphase at the stage of maximum chromosome condensation. Figure 1.1(b) is the karyotype derived from Figure 1.1(a) and it shows the chromosomes are from a male infant with Down syndrome due to an additional number 21 chromosome (T21). This additional 21 chromosome is derived from the mother in over 90% of cases and the recurrence risk of a straightforward trisomy 21 is approximately 1%. If a female with Down syndrome due to trisomy 21 conceives, there is a 50% risk that her infant will also have trisomy 21. Mosaicism (e.g. 46XX, /47XX, + 21) can occur in 2% of Down syndrome and the children are usually less severely affected. Indeed, if a small proportion of the cells are trisomic then these individuals may lead normal lives. In 3% of cases of Down syndrome there may be unbalanced translocation (e.g. 46XX, – 15, + t (15q 21q)). Approximately three-quarters of children with Down syndrome as a result of an unbalanced translocation are due to *de novo* chromosomal changes and have a low recurrence risk.

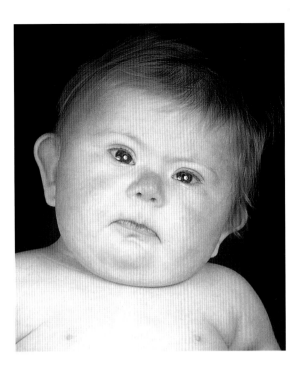

FIGURE 1.2 Down syndrome.

However, in the remaining 25% one of the parents will carry the translocation in a balanced form. This will increase the risk of further affected children to up to 5% for a carrier male and 15% for a carrier female. Very rarely there may be a balanced 21q 21q translocation in a parent and in this case the risk of Down syndrome for subsequent infants is 100%.

Down syndrome affects approximately 1 in 700 live births but there is an association with advancing maternal age. Thus, a women under 25 has a 1 in 2000 likelihood of an affected child but a women over 40 years has a more than 1 in 50 chance. There is no independent paternal age affect.

Clinical features

Figure 1.2 shows typical facial features with upwards sloping palpebral fissures and marked inner angle epicanthic folds. The nose tends to be small with a flat bridge and the tongue, which is normally shaped and pointed, frequently protrudes from the unduly small mouth; this is quite different from the large, fleshy myxoedematous tongue of a hypothyroid infant. The Down infant tongue becomes deeply fissured and enlarged in later life. The ears are often abnormally simple or shell shaped and the skull brachycephalic with a flat occiput. Hands tend to be broad with short fingers and in particular the little finger is excessively short due to hypoplasia of the second phalanx and is curved towards the ring finger (clinodactyly). There is frequently only a single palmar (simian) crease and there are characteristic abnormalities of dermatoglyphic patterns. There is an excessively wide gap between the large and second toes and on the soles there is a longitudinal skin crease at this point. Hair is usually straight and rather sparse and a most characteristic feature is the marked muscular hypotonia and laxity of ligaments. There may be cataracts, squints or a speckled iris (Brushfield spots) and blepharoconjunctivitis is common.

The children are of small stature due to a reduced total number of cell divisions during early development and frequently other major developmental anomalies such as duodenal atresia, Hirschsprung disease, or imperforate anus may be found. The most common involve the heart, e.g. tetralogy of Fallot, ventricular septal defect or ostium primum defects. Death may occur in childhood from congenital cardiac defects and from respiratory infections to which they are particularly susceptible. IQ scores are usually between 20 and 70 but unlike other severe learning disorders they develop good social skills and can function better in the community than those who fail to develop such skills. Development of the genitalia and secondary sex characteristics is delayed and hypothyroidism is more common. There is also an increased incidence of leukaemia in these children and by the age of 40 years almost all will have developed Alzheimer disease. This may be as a result of a disorder of amyloid protein, the gene for which is located on chromosome 21.

After trisomy 21 the next most common autosomal trisomies in live-born children are trisomy 18 (Edward syndrome) and trisomy 13 (Patau syndrome). Trisomy 18 affects approximately 1 in 3000 infants with increased risk in mothers aged over 35 years. Low birthweight due to intrauterine growth retardation with an elongated skull and prominent occiput are common features. The ears are low set and dysplastic. There is axial deviation and overlapping of the index and ring fingers. The hallux tends to be short and dorsiflexed and there may be talipes calcaneovalgus. The calcaneus may be unduly prominent posteriorly, "rocker-bottom feet" and the nails of hands and feet are frequently small. The neck may show webbing or redundancy of skin on the nape. The chest is short and unduly broad and the nipples often hypoplastic. Cleft lip or palate occur in a minority when clinical differentiation from Patau syndrome may be difficult. Cardiovascular anomalies are almost universal and there are characteristic dermatoglyphic findings. Spina bifida, tracheo-oesophageal fistula, oesophageal atresia and fixed flexion deformities of the limbs have also been reported.

Patau syndrome (T13) is also associated with advanced maternal age and occurs in approximately 1 in 5000 live births. There tend to be major craniofacial abnormalities in this syndrome with holoprosencephaly due to failure of development and migration of the frontonasal process to fuse with the maxillary process during branchial arch development. In the most severe defects there may be absent nose, single nostril (cebocephalus), or because of the failure of descent of the frontonasal process the eyes which develop from the central nervous system may fuse (cyclops) and a proboscis may appear above the single eye (ethmocephalus). Less severe defects cause a variety of cleft lip and palate anomalies with microcephalus, scalp defects and colobomata. Cardiac malformations occur in about 80% and polycystic kidneys in one-third. As in all the other trisomies birthweight is small for the length of gestation, and (fibular) polydactyly is a feature of most affected infants. Abnormal dermatoglyphics are present. Exomphalos with cryptorchidism and hypospadias may be found and survival beyond a few weeks is most unusual. As with the other trisomies recorded in those who do survive for any length of time they have severe developmental retardation, failure to thrive and frequently deafness and seizures. Although 80% of affected children have T13, about 20% have an unbalanced translocation with one of the parents occasionally found to carry the defect in a balanced form. Mosaicism has been reported and can result in less severe features.

In addition to the trisomies there are autosomal deletion defects such as the *cri-du-chat* syndrome where there is partial deletion of the short arm of chromosome 5. About two-thirds of the patients have been female and the birth frequency is around 1 in 50 000 or less. The name of this syndrome derives from the characteristic mewing-like cry which is present from the neonatal period. Birthweight is low and there is often an antimongoloid slant to the eyes (epicanthic folds), some degree of hypertelorism and microcephaly with a rounded face. Congenital heart defects may be present and both physical and mental development are markedly delayed. It is important that parental chromosome studies for a balanced rearrangement are undertaken. In Wolf syndrome many features similar to *cri-du-chat* syndrome occur although the cat-like cry is often absent. It is due to partial deletion of the short arm of chromosome 4. Differentiating features included broad root of nose and prominent glabella, marked hypertelorism, coloboma of iris, pre-auricular dimples, midline defects of the scalp, hypospadias and low set ears. Various other chromosome deletions and abnormalities have been associated with less well defined clinical manifestations which include severe learning disorder.

Abnormalities of sex chromosomes

Abnormalities of sex chromosomes also cause severe developmental delay but usually of a less severe degree than that found in the trisomies. The common chromosomal abnormalities are Klinefelter syndrome

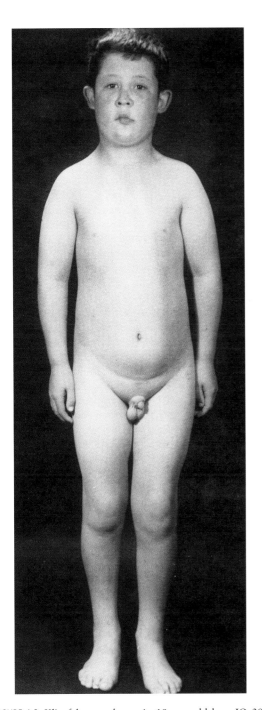

FIGURE 1.3 Klinefelter syndrome in 10-year-old boy. IQ 30. Chromosome type XXXXY.

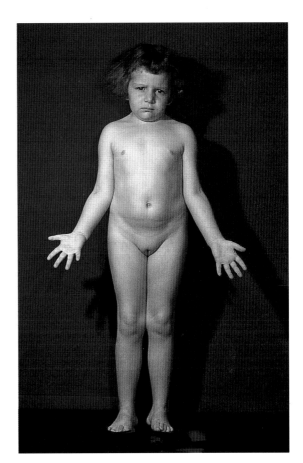

FIGURE 1.4 Turner syndrome.

for non-specific learning difficulties. The frequency of X-linked mental retardation is reported as 1.83/1000 males and of carriers 2.44/1000 females. This makes mental retardation due to X-linked genes at least as common among males as mental retardation due to Down syndrome. In many of the affected males a marker X chromosome has been identified. The marker in this "fragile X syndrome" is a "fragile site" occurring at band q27 or q28 towards the end of the long arm of the X chromosome. One-third of female carriers show mild mental retardation. Affected males usually have a long face with large ears and a prominent jaw. When affected males reach puberty they develop large testes and in earlier childhood autistic behaviour and convulsions may occur. It is also associated with an increased frequency of Wilms tumours and liver tumours. Recognition before treatment with chemotherapy and/or radiotherapy is important as these therapies are poorly tolerated.

Single gene (Mendelian) inheritance

Gregor Mendel working in the gardens of a monastery first recognised the inherited characteristic

with a chromosome status of XXY, XXXY or even XXXXY (Fig. 1.3) and Turner syndrome XO (Fig. 1.4). A sex chromosome configuration of XXX also called the "triple-X state" or (inaccurately) the "super-female" is associated with learning difficulties. X-linked gene defects are quite frequently responsible

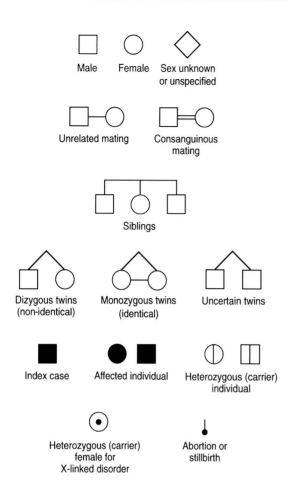

FIGURE 1.5 Conventional notation of family tree.

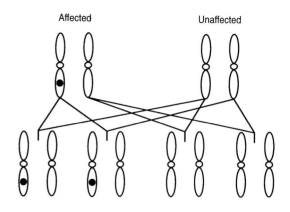

FIGURE 1.6 Dominant inheritance.

or trait in round and wrinkled peas. From his observations he delineated the principles of single gene inheritance long before DNA, genes and chromosomes were understood. Figure 1.5 gives the conventional notation for building up a family tree to designate individuals affected by gene defects and those with heterozygous or carrier potential. Inheritance of a disorder can occur as a result of an autosomal dominant, an autosomal recessive, an X- or sex-linked recessive disorder, a sex-linked dominant disorder, and there have recently been recognised disorders of mitochondrial inheritance. Apparently identical genes inherited from the father or mother may sometimes differ in their expression in the child. This genomic imprinting is probably due to different patterns of DNA methylation during meiosis. The effect of this maternal or paternal imprinting persists throughout the life of the child but can be altered during the gametogenesis of the child depending on whether transmission is occurring in the ova or sperm. Congenital myotonic dystrophy occurs only in the offspring of affected females and never in the children of affected males. The age of

onset of Huntington chorea is earlier in general if the transmitting parent is male rather than female. If a new deletion occurs on the long arm of chromosome 15 inherited from the father, Prader–Willi syndrome results whereas an apparently identical deletion on the maternal chromosome 15 results in Angelman syndrome. Over 3000 autosomal dominant conditions or traits have been identified in which conditions there is transmission from generation to generation. There is a one in two chance that the child of an individual with an autosomal dominant disorder will inherit that disorder (Fig. 1.6). Males and females are equally affected and can transmit the disorder to offspring of either sex. When both parents have the same autosomal dominant disorder there is a one in four chance that the child will inherit both copies (alleles) of the mutant gene, a one in two chance of inheriting one allele and a one in four chance of inheriting neither. Children who receive two copies of the mutant gene (homozygote) usually show a severe form of the disorder. There may be variable expressivity or penetrance of a gene in which case the child may show no obvious clinical abnormality. This can give rise to an autosomal dominant disorder apparently skipping generations. In general autosomal dominant disorders are associated with structural abnormalities such as achondroplasia, neurofibromatosis, Marfan syndrome, osteogenesis imperfecta, adult onset polycystic renal disease and tuberous sclerosis.

Figure 1.7 shows the pattern of autosomal recessive inheritance. An autosomal recessively inherited disorder occurs when the individual inherits two copies of an abnormal autosomal gene, one from each parent. The gene defect in the two heterozygous (carrier) parents does not have to be identical but the severity of the disorder reflects the qualities of the gene defect inherited from both parents. There is a one in four risk of subsequent offspring being affected after the birth of the initial index affected child. In

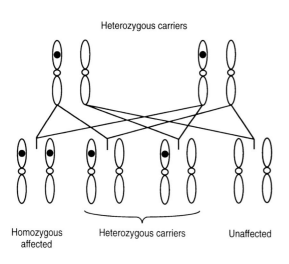

FIGURE 1.7 Autosomal recessive inheritance.

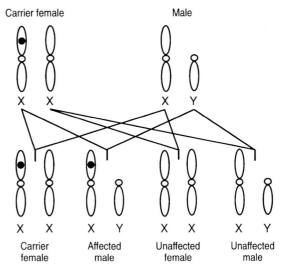

FIGURE 1.8 X-linked recessive inheritance.

communities where there is a preference for consanguineous mating there is an increased incidence of recessively inherited disorders. The closer the family relationship the greater the risk of both parents carrying the same abnormal gene defect. Certain recessively inherited conditions tend to occur more commonly in certain ethnic groupings. Thus congenital adrenal hyperplasia is common in Eskimos, cystic fibrosis and phenylketonuria in those of Celtic origin in the UK, Tay–Sachs disease in Ashkenazi Jews and alpha-1-antitrypsin deficiency in Scandinavians. It may be that there is heterozygote advantage for some conditions. Carriers of some autosomal recessive conditions such as sickle cell disease may render them more resistant to malarial infection. Cystic fibrosis and phenylketonuria are examples of recessively inherited conditions where a variety of gene defects have been identified. Different varieties of gene defect seem to have arisen by spontaneous mutation in different world communities. The movement of ethnic groups in the various world migrations are clearly seen from the movement of specific gene defects.

Sex (X)-linked disorders are those which are caused by gene defects on the X chromosome. When women who have only a single copy of the abnormal gene do not manifest the disorder then the disorder is said to be an X-linked recessive disorder. The carrier of an X-linked recessive disorder has a one in two chance of transmitting the abnormal gene so that for each daughter there is a one in two chance of being a carrier or for each son a one in two chance of being affected. When an affected male has children all of his daughters will be carriers and none of his sons will be affected (Fig. 1.8). Occasionally a woman may be affected with an X-linked recessive disorder because she has inherited two copies of the abnormal

gene from a carrier mother and affected father or she has Turner syndrome (45 XO) with her single X chromosome showing the gene defect or because X chromosome inactivation (lyonisation) has inactivated her X chromosome containing the normal gene. Occasionally a woman may transmit an X-linked recessive disorder to more than one child when lymphocyte DNA shows no mutation. This is probably due to the presence of a mutant gene-bearing cell line in her ovaries (gonadal mosaicism). Examples of X-linked disorders include Duchenne muscular dystrophy, haemophilia A, haemophilia B, glucose 6 phosphate dehydrogenase deficiency, Lesch–Nyhan syndrome, red/green colour blindness and agammaglobulinaemia (Bruton's type).

Vitamin D resistant rickets, pseudo hypoparathyroidism and incontinentia pigmenti are examples of X-linked dominant disorders.

It is thought that some time during evolutionary development bacterial-like organisms migrated into the cells of primitive animals and established themselves as the mitochondria. The DNA which codes for 13 proteins involved in the mitochondrial respiratory chain accounts for some 20% of the DNA in the mitochondrion and is unrelated to the genomic DNA. Disorders of mitochondrial DNA result in the rare disorders of mitochondrial function such as mitochondrial encephalomyelopathy associated with lactic acidosis and stroke-like episodes (MELAS), MERRF in which there is myoclonus, epilepsy and ragged red muscle fibres and the Kearns–Sayer syndrome in which there are various endocrinopathies in children of short stature who develop pigmentary retinopathy, ragged red fibre myopathy, heart block and severe neurological signs related to spongy degeneration of the brain.

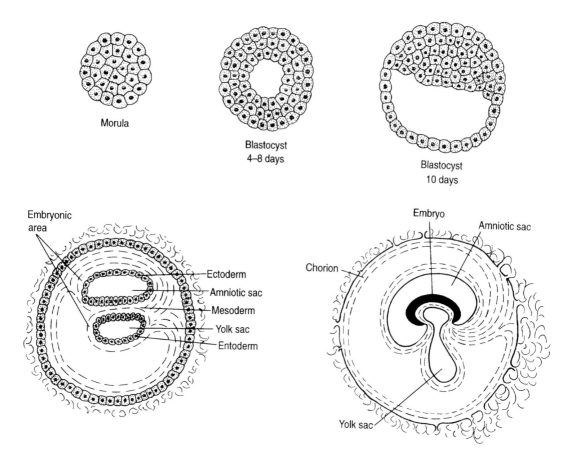

FIGURE 1.9 Trophoblastic cells and the placenta.

Multifactorial or polygenic inheritance is a concept used to explain a number of disorders such as cleft lip and palate, coeliac disease, congenital dislocation of the hip, neural tube defects and pyloric stenosis. It may be that the concept is incorrect and that there are mutations which will only become evident given specific environmental circumstances. This would certainly seem to be true for neural tube defects, asthma, insulin dependent diabetes mellitus and schizophrenia.

The apparently healthy child may carry many genetic abnormalities which may be manifest only when faced with a specific environmental insult or trigger or when one of their children or grandchildren manifests a disorder.

EMBRYONIC DEVELOPMENT

The ovum is fertilised by the sperm usually in the ampulla of the fallopian tube. After fertilisation the ovum is propelled along the tube to the uterus and at the same time undergoes repeated cell division. The resulting ball of cells (morula) develops a cavity (blastocoele) at which stage the ovum is known as a blastocyst. Thereafter the multiplying cells of blastocyst gather together to form what is called the inner cell mass whilst cells nearer to the surface develop into trophoblast. For a time the trophoblast and the inner cell mass remain connected by a stalk of cells known as the body stalk. The trophoblastic cells begin then to erode into the uterine endometrium eventually to form the placenta (Fig. 1.9).

The ovum or blastocyst penetrates and eventually becomes completely embedded in the endometrium which is then known as the decidua. Two cavities develop in the inner cell mass of the blastocyst. One is the amniotic sac and the other yolk sac. Between them is a cellular area called the embryonic plate because it is from this area that the embryo grows. In the embryonic plate area the cells become grouped into three primitive layers known as the ectoderm, the mesoderm and the endoderm. Subsequently the skin, certain mucous membranes and the central nervous system develop from the ectoderm; the blood, muscle, bones and certain organs from the mesoderm; and the lungs, alimentary mucosa, bladder, pancreas and

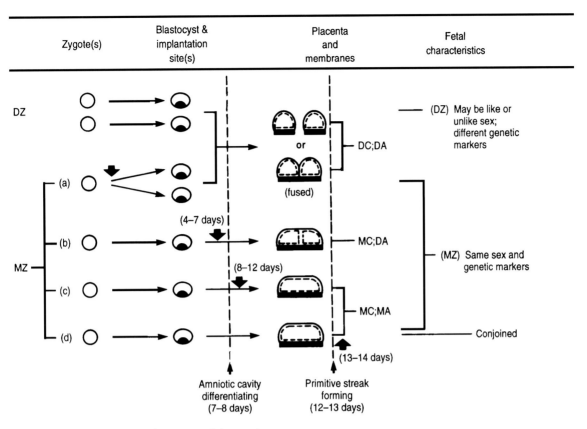

FIGURE 1.10 Twins, zygosity and structure of the membranes.

parts of the liver from the endoderm. Amniotic fluid which fills the amniotic sac serves to protect and encourage the growth of the embryo which derives its nutrient from the yolk sac pending the development of a rudimentary placenta. The yolk sac is connected by a duct (vitelline duct) with the embryonic gut. The amniotic cavity gradually envelopes the embryo and at the same time brings the yolk sac and the vitelline duct into contact with the body stalk to form the umbilical cord. Development of the cord is usually complete by the sixth week.

PLACENTAL DEVELOPMENT

Buds of multiplying cells sprout out from the trophoblast where it comes into contact with the decidua and form the villi. These multiply in number to cover the entire ovum. Some of the villi become attached to the deep layer of the decidua (decidua basalis) and anchor the ovum to the decidua. Other villi penetrate decidual blood vessels around the third week after fertilisation. The villi develop to contain a central core of fetal mesoderm and embryonic vessels in which fetal blood circulates and two cellular layers:

an inner Langhan's layer or cytotrophoblast and an outer, the syncytium or syncytiotrophoblast. Trophoblast is responsible for the absorption of nutrients from maternal blood into the fetal circulation and for the return of waste products through the arterial vessels of the developing umbilical cord. By the end of the third month the placenta acquires a discoidal shape consisting of some 15–20 clumps (cotyledons) of chorionic villi anchored to the decidua basalis.

TWINNING

In most instances twin pregnancy results from fertilisation of a single ovum (monozygote). There is one placenta, one chorion and two amniotic sacs. Exceptionally, however, two placentae may develop. Where in a twin pregnancy fertilisation of two ova has taken place (dizygote), there are two placentae which may, however, fuse and have the appearance of a single placenta. Dizygotic twins may be born with separate placentae or with an apparently single placenta with two separate amniotic sacs (diamniotic) and two chorionic membranes (dichorionic).

Monozygotic twins may be born with (1) separate placentae and membranes, (2) one placenta and dichorionic, diamniotic membranes, (3) one placenta with monochorionic membranes. Monozygotic twins originate from the division of one fertilised egg and are identical. Splitting can occur at different stages of development. Early splitting (2–3 days) after conception will result in a different outcome from intermediate splitting (4–7 days) and late splitting (8–12 days), see Fig. 1.10. When the splitting is delayed beyond 13 days the twins may be fused (conjoined or "Siamese"). Twins of different sex must be dizygotic. In Europe, approximately 33% of monozygous twins are dichorial, 66% monochorial-diamniotic and 1% monochorionic-monoamniotic. Decisions as to whether twins are identical or not cannot always be made by examination of the placentae and membranes and it may require blood grouping and DNA fingerprinting analyses to make the final determination.

PLACENTAL FUNCTION

The placenta transfers CO_2 from fetal tissues to the maternal circulation and obtains oxygen and other nutrients from the maternal blood in the intervillous spaces. Chorionic villi are capable of selective absorption of substances necessary for embryonic and fetal growth. In addition to the transfer of all nutrient materials necessary for the formation of the embryo and fetus, the waste products of fetal metabolism such as urea and heat are transferred back across the placenta to maternal blood. The placenta acts as a protective barrier preventing the passage of some, but by no means all, potentially harmful substances from the maternal circulation. Viruses such as those of rubella, cytomegalovirus, HIV and parvovirus can pass the barrier as can the spirochaete of syphilis, the bacillus of tuberculosis and the protozoon of toxoplasmosis.

Temporary passive immunity to many infections is acquired from the mother through placental transfer of IgG antibodies to infections previously experienced by the mother. Transfer of fetal antigens in a reverse direction can take place. Rhesus positive cells from a fetus may enter the circulation of the rhesus negative mother and stimulate the formation of antibodies. Other substances which can penetrate the placental barrier include alcohol, nicotine and sedative, anaesthetic, antibiotic and other drugs.

The placenta functions as an endocrine organ for the production of oestrogens and other hormones. Maternal hormones can also transfer to the fetus to a varying degree.

Disturbance to normal placental growth and function can result in abnormalities of embryonic and fetal development. Abnormalities of placental structure and size, degenerative change and premature separation of the placental cotyledons can result in damage to the developing fetus.

THE EMBRYO

Embryonic development takes place during the first 8 weeks after conception. Rudimentary eyes, ears, and the projecting buds representing the beginnings of limb formation are recognisable about 4 weeks after conception. At this stage the embryo consists of a large head and a rather tapering body and weighs approximately 1–1.3 grams and measures 9–12 mm in length. By the 8th week the hands and feet are recognisable, the external genitalia are developing and the head has assumed a recognisable shape. Although the name embryo has been used by custom until the end of the 8th week, and the name fetus is used thereafter, this distinction is arbitrary. At 12 weeks the placenta is well developed, the umbilical cord begins to show normal spiral characteristics and fingers and toes are identifiable. By 12 weeks the fetus measures 9 cm in length and weighs about 30 g. Centres of ossification are present in many bones. By 24 weeks after conception hair appears on the head and the deposition of subcutaneous fat begins. As subcutaneous fat is laid down in increasing amount the skin acquires a smooth texture and pink colour and the body develops a more rotund appearance. At 40 weeks the fetus measures approximately 51 cm in length and weighs about 3200 g with the male being slightly larger and heavier than the female. During fetal development various organ systems differentiate anatomically and progressively through a series of cell divisions which are genetically determined in number and type. If intrauterine development of one or more organ systems does not progress normally, this may result in fetal death or the delivery of an infant with anatomical and functional abnormalities. The introduction of embryonic and fetal ultrasound by Ian Donald in Glasgow in 1957 brought about a revolution in our ability to assess fetal growth and development of individual organs. Gestational age, that is the age from conception, is generally calculated by reference to the date of the first day of the last menstrual cycle which gives menstrual age. The mean interval between conception and delivery (gestational age) is around 265 days. More usually the duration of pregnancy, dated from the last menstrual period gives an average duration for a term pregnancy of 280 days. The first day of the last menstrual period is generally accepted as the date from which the gestational age is calculated to the nearest week. Since the introduction of ultrasonic techniques accurate assessments of fetal age can be obtained.

Measurement of crown–rump length in early pregnancy (12 weeks) gives a very accurate assessment of fetal maturity. In later pregnancy, measurements of trunk area in relation to skull area can give accurate assessment of fetal growth and development. Doppler ultrasound is used to assess fetal and placental blood flow and can give an early indication of placental failure or fetal circulatory anomalies. Measurement of fetal growth rate can be determined as can the presence of fetal anomalies, some of which may be treated before delivery.

The introduction of ultrasound has allowed the development of techniques such as amniocentesis, chorionic villus biopsy and fetal blood and tissue sampling to be developed and to allow prenatal diagnosis of a wide range of inherited metabolic disorders and chromosomal defects. Fetal monitoring techniques using fetal electrocardiograms, heart rates and the determination of fetal pH by obstetricians has helped reduce the number of infants damaged by prenatal and intranatal disorders.

BIRTH

Adaptation from the fetal intrauterine state to the infant extrauterine state is not without its problems. The move from complete dependence on placenta and maternal tissues for succour to a dependence on the individual organs of the infant is complex. The infant systems principally involved in the initial stages are the respiratory, cardiovascular and nervous systems. Later, digestive, renal and hepatic, skin and musculoskeletal function become of more importance.

RESPIRATION

Respiratory patterns of the human fetus *in utero* determined by fetal ultrasound show that fetal breathing movements are necessary for normal lung development and can be affected by extrinsic factors such as maternal smoking. The breathing pattern is related to the sleep state of the fetus. The fetal lung produces a fluid which is normally swallowed although some may be expelled into the amniotic sac by fetal movement. Fetal blood gas exchange is dependent on a good blood flow on both the maternal and fetal sides of the placenta. Fetal tissues *in utero* are relatively hypoxaemic (20–30 mmHg/ 3–4 kPa). This is partly due to the large requirement of the placental tissues for oxygen and partly to the relative imbalance of fetal and maternal blood flow with uneven blood gas exchange in the cotyledons. There is, however, a large margin of safety in placental gas exchange to compensate for small rapid changes in maternal blood gas status. Larger changes in fetal blood gas status may be reflected in fetal tachycardia which is the first true sign of fetal distress and which may be sufficient to compensate for a temporary period of difficulty such as that which occurs during a uterine contraction. Progressive hypoxaemia of the fetus is manifest as bradycardia with associated fetal tissue acidaemia. The introduction of continuous recording of fetal heart rate in relation to the state of uterine contraction and the use of fetal scalp blood for measurement of hydrogen ion concentrations has allowed fairly exact measurement of fetal tissue hypoxia. Measurements of beat-to-beat variation in fetal heart rate give a sensitive indication of impending fetal hypoxaemia. The fetus is able to regulate blood distribution and in states of hypoxaemia can vasoconstrict the vessels supplying skin, limbs, lungs and abdominal organs. This allows more oxygen to be made available to the heart and brain. Some of the metabolic acid (lactic acid) produced in the underperfused tissue areas where anaerobic glycolysis is taking place, returns to the central circulation and is evident as a metabolic acidosis.

INITIATION OF RESPIRATION

Normal vaginally delivered infants make their first respiratory movement within a few seconds of complete delivery. The time interval between the appearance of the nose and first breath is usually between 20 and 30 seconds. Within 90 seconds of complete delivery most infants have started rhythmic respirations. The strong initial respiratory efforts and the subsequent rhythmic activities of respiratory muscles are largely dependent upon brain stem respiratory centres. Table 1.1 summarises factors which can initiate or influence the patterns of neonatal respirations. There are a number of factors which influence respiratory centres to respond to each or any of these various stimuli, e.g. maternal anaesthetic and analgesic drugs, both high and low environmental temperatures, gestational age, pre- and perinatal asphyxia, intracranial or brain stem haemorrhage, vascular thrombosis, cerebral oedema and increased intracranial pressure. Once breathing is established the pattern of respiration is primarily determined in the medulla. Ventilation is regulated by the P_{CO_2} and hydrogen ion concentration [H⁺] perfusing chemoreceptors in the medulla. Breathing may also be stimulated by decrease in P_{O_2} acting on chemoreceptors in the carotid bodies. This hypoxic drive may assume great importance if the medullary centres have been depressed by hypoxia or maternal anaesthesia or analgesia. In the healthy newborn infant at delivery the sensory stimuli and blood gas alterations are sufficient to arouse in the brain motor impulses which

TABLE 1.1 Factors which can initiate or influence the patterns of neonatal respirations

Thermal	Chilling through loss of heat at about 2.5 kJ/min
Pain	Skin, muscle and tendon receptors
Pressure	Gravity (departure from liquid environment)
	Increased intrathoracic pressures during delivery
	Increased intracranial pressures during delivery
	Changes in intratracheal and intrathoracic pressure
Tactile	Trigeminal area particularly important
Receptors in lungs and pleura	Hering–Breuer reflex
Receptors in muscle, tendon and joints of limbs, spine and chest wall	Stimulated by alterations in posture during and after delivery
Auditory	
Visual	
Olfactory	
Cord clamping:	
Increased arterial pressure	Carotid baroreceptors
Decreased arterial P_{O_2}	Aortic and carotid body receptors
Increased arterial P_{CO_2}	Direct effect on respiratory centre
Increased arterial $[H^+]$	

produce the initial muscle movements in the diaphragm and intercostal muscles required to create the intermittent negative intrathoracic presssures which allow air to enter and leave the alveoli. Although a falling oxygen tension and increase in CO_2 tension at first stimulate the respiratory centres persistence of hypoxia and hypercapnia will depress these functions. An infant who has been chronically hypoxic during labour may have a non-responsive respiratory centre.

FETAL CIRCULATION

A variable proportion of oxygenated fetal blood from the placenta travels from the umbilical vein where the P_{O_2} is 4.0 kPa (30 mmHg) directly to the inferior vena cava via the ductus venosus. A smaller proportion enters the left lobe of the liver where there is admixture with portal venous blood (Fig. 1.11). Most inferior vena caval blood is directed through the foramen ovale into the left atrium where, after mixture with pulmonary venous blood, it enters the left ventricle and is pumped towards the head and upper limbs. A smaller flow of inferior vena caval blood enters the right atrium, mixes with poorly oxygenated blood returning from the superior vena cava and enters the right ventricle. From the right ventricle this blood mainly enters the ductus arterio-

sus, bypassing the lungs and entering the descending aorta. This relatively less oxygenated blood supplies the trunk, abdominal organs and lower limbs and also the lungs through the bronchial arteries. Blood from the abdominal aorta returns through the umbilical arteries to the placenta. This pattern of circulation is maintained through cardiac contractility and muscle tone in the fetal vessel walls. Pulmonary arterial pressure is higher than left ventricular and aortic pressure because of a higher resistance in the pulmonary arterioles than in the ductus arteriosus and aorta. Muscle tone in fetal blood vessels depends largely on the oxygen content of the blood perfusing them, mediated locally through prostaglandins and also on autonomic activity and NO predominantly affecting the small vessels.

CIRCULATORY CHANGES AT BIRTH

The vascular changes associated with gas exchange being transferred from placenta to lungs take place abruptly with cessation of umbilical arterial and venous flow with the removal of the low resistance placental circuit. Pulmonary arterial blood flow increases dramatically when the infant lungs expand and is the result of a reduced pulmonary arteriolar resistance and functional closure of the ductus arteriosus, ductus venosus, foramen ovale and umbilical vessels. The foramen ovale and ductus venosus close mainly as a result of mechanical pressure changes, but the constriction of the ductus arteriosus and dilation of the pulmonary arterioles is mediated through the increased oxygen content of blood perfusing these vessels and vasoactive substances. In studies of the isolated ductus arteriosus, prostaglandin ($PGF_{2\alpha}$), thromboxane A_2 (TXA_2), acetylcholine, bradykinin, angiotensin, adrenaline and noradrenaline produce constriction. Inhibition of the dilator prostaglandins, PGE_2 and PGI_2, which maintain ductal patency during fetal life, might also contribute to ductal closure. The balance between vasodilatation and ductus arteriosus constriction determines the effectiveness of vascular adaptation to birth. Asphyxia of the infant during or after birth maintains a patent ductus arteriosus and increases the pulmonary vascular resistance, thus maintaining the fetal situation and causing profound hypoxia.

THE FIRST BREATH

Within the intra-alveolar spaces and tracheobronchial tree of the fetus there is a substantial volume of fluid, some of which is expressed during the normal birth process but most of which is absorbed into

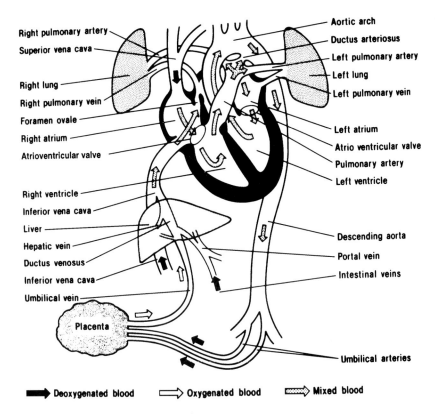

FIGURE 1.11 Schematic representation of the fetal circulation.

pulmonary lymphatics. In the normal infant sensory stimuli initiate a first breath of some 30–40 ml air, and this requires the creation of a negative intrathoracic pressure of between –4 and –10 kPa (–40 and –100 cmH$_2$O). This negative pressure opens the terminal airways and expands the stiff (low-compliance) fluid filled lungs. Lung compliance (volume for unit pressure change) increases from about 1.5 ml/cmH$_2$O to about 6 ml/cmH$_2$O, whilst the negative intrathoracic pressures required fall to –5 cmH$_2$O. Infants born at term have an average tidal volume of 20 ml and a breathing frequency of about 30 breaths/min, creating a minute ventilation of about 600 ml/min. Preterm infants may have tidal volumes as low as 5–10 ml. During the first few days of life there may be minor degrees of right-to-left shunting through the foramen ovale and ductus arteriosus. Because of an inadequate ventilation/perfusion balance some blood is not fully oxygenated during passage through the lungs. This ventilation/perfusion balance can be aggravated by an absence or deficiency of alveolar surfactant material produced by type 2 alveolar lining cells or pneumonocytes. The lipoprotein–surfactant complex lowers surface tension in the fluid film lining the alveolus. This film lowers surface tension further as alveolar surface area falls during expiration and increases it as alveolar surface area increases during inspiration. Prematurely born infants develop the respiratory distress syndrome when surfactant production is inadequate.

At term the fetal blood haemoglobin concentration is between 16 and 18 g/dl and is predominantly (60–80%) fetal haemoglobin (HbF). The PO$_2$ at which blood is 50% saturated with oxygen in the term fetus is only about 2.6 kPa (20 mmHg) but in the mother about 4.0 kPa (30 mmHg). This difference enables the fetal blood to take up oxygen readily from maternal blood and is due to the greater affinity of HbF for oxygen. Although fetal red cells are avid for oxygen, fetal tissues have a very low PO$_2$ (approximately 2.0 kPa). The fetus is able to unload more of this oxygen to the fetal tissues because of a higher level of 2,3–diphosphoglycerate in the fetal blood.

ASPHYXIA

Asphyxia means without pulse but it is defined as a combination of hypoxaemia, hypercapnia and metabolic acidaemia. Fetal responses to asphyxia and haemorrhage during delivery are prompted by chemoreceptor and baroreceptor activity causing release of catecholamines. This catecholamine surge which occurs during normal delivery improves breathing by increasing lung surfactant, lung liquid absorption, lung compliance and bronchiolar dilatation. It mobilises energy from fat and glycogen reserves, stimulates gluconeogenesis by liver and increases blood flow to brain and heart. Significant asphyxia produces, after an initial period of tachycardia, a vagal bradycardia so that there is a combined autonomic response when hypoxaemia is severe, similar to those responses found in submerging mammals. In the "diving reflex" there is a sympathetic discharge with noradrenaline release causing a redistribution of blood flow to increase cardiac, cerebral and adrenal flow and to diminish flow to the skin of the trunk and limbs, skeletal muscle, liver, kidneys and intestine. There is also a vagally mediated bradycardia. During delivery fetal noradrenaline values exceed maternal and this ratio is markedly increased in asphyxial states. In the acutely asphyxiated newborn monkey immediately after birth there is an initial period of rapid breathing (hyperpnoea) followed by a period of initial or primary apnoea. Regular gasping follows the initial apnoea and after a terminal acceleration in rate but diminution in depth, gasping ceases about 8 minutes after birth. The apnoeic period which follows the last spontaneous gasp is called secondary or terminal apnoea and death will ensue unless resuscitation is successfully instituted. Acute asphyxia of the fetus may occur with sudden complete placental separation or umbilical cord obstruction but the more common hypoxic insults are intermittent or subacute and are detected with fetal heart monitoring and blood sampling.

RESUSCITATION

Inadequate or delayed resuscitation of an asphyxiated infant may lead to permanent brain damage and death. It is best to have someone skilled in tracheal intubation present at all high-risk deliveries. Most normal newborn infants (75%) breathe within 1 minute of delivery and most of the remainder have breathed before 3 minutes. Only 5% of normal infants take longer than 3 minutes before their first breath.

ASSESSMENT AND EARLY PROGNOSIS

When possible a time clock with a clearly visible second hand should be commenced at the time of infant's delivery. It is customary to aspirate the nasal and oral passages carefully immediately after delivery using a sterile, plastic tipped catheter. This removes amniotic and lung fluid from the oropharynx and stops the aspiration of blood, meconium and other debris into the upper airway. Excess fluid is normally dried from the infant's skin with a warm towel and the infant checked briefly for the presence of severe congenital anomalies such as spina bifida and microcephalus. The Apgar score (Table 1.2) is assessed at 1 minute and if the infant is apnoeic gentle sensory stimuli such as the blowing of cold air/oxygen over the infant's face through a face mask should be tried. If such stimuli fail to initiate breathing movements tracheal intubation should commence at 2 minutes. A heart rate of less than 80 per minute would be an indication for intubation and ventilation before 2 minutes of age. Virginia Apgar's clinical score based on heart rate, respiratory effort, muscle tone, responses to stimuli and skin colour has been found valuable in the assessment of the newborn. The score is usually made at 1 minute after birth and repeated at 5 minutes. A time interval of 1 minute was chosen by Apgar because at this time most infants in her large series had achieved their lowest scores. The 5-minute score has been shown to have some correlation with subsequent brain damage whereas the 1-minute score gives some index of the need for active resuscitation, correlates well with biochemical assessment of acidosis and is inversely proportional to the neonatal death rate.

TABLE 1.2 Clinical evaluation of the newborn infant (Apgar scoring method). Sixty seconds after complete birth of the infant (disregarding the cord and placenta) the five objective signs are evaluated and each given a score of 0, 1 or 2. A score of 10 indicates an infant in the best possible condition

SIGN	0	1	2
Heart rate	Absent	Slow (below 100)	Over 100
Respiratory effort	Absent	Weak cry; hypoventilation	Good: strong cry
Muscle tone	Limp	Some flexion of extremities	Active motion: extremities well flexed
Reflex irritability (response to stimulation of sole of foot)	No response	Grimace	Cry
Colour	Blue; pale	Body pink; extremities blue	Completely pink

VENTILATION

Figure 1.12 demonstrates the technique of tracheal intubation and the appearance of the larynx. Lung inflation at a rate of 20–30 times per minute, maintaining inflation for approximately 1 second, at inflation pressures limited to 30 cmH_2O should be instituted. Chest movement should be observed and the chest auscultated to ensure adequate air entry on both sides of the chest. If there is no entry, the tube is likely to be in the oesophagus and it should be withdrawn and the infant reintubated. Air entry to the right lung alone indicates that the endotracheal tube has entered the right main bronchus and air entry to the left lung usually improves if the endotracheal tube is withdrawn slowly whilst listening over the unventilated lung. Occasionally a pneumothorax or a diaphragmatic hernia can confuse the picture. Should the heart rate fail to increase in spite of adequate ventilation it is likely that the infant has a

severe metabolic acidaemia and the injection of sodium bicarbonate 8.4% intravenously over 3–5 minutes, 10 ml to a normal term infant and 5 ml to a preterm infant, should be given. If the heart rate remains less than 100 external cardiac massage at 100–120 beats per minute should be instituted. Seven to ten cardiac compressions should be alternated with three to four ventilations. If opiates have been given to the mother in the 6 hours prior to delivery and the infant fails to establish respiratory efforts, naloxone 0.01 mg/kg can be given by intravenous or intramuscular injection. Even when respiratory depression is thought to be due to maternal opiates the same indications for intubation and intermittent positive pressure ventilation (IPPV) should be used. The infant should be extubated as soon as regular respiration and good colour are achieved. When the infant is born without pulsation or heart sounds (Apgar 0–1) but a fetal heart is recorded up to 20 minutes before delivery, intubation, external cardiac massage, intravenous sodium bicarbonate and intracardiac or intrapulmonary adrenaline 1 ml of 1:10 000 IU should be given. If there is no respiratory effort by 30 minutes after institution of resuscitation these attempts should be abandoned. If intermittent but inadequate respiratory movements occur then it is reasonable to ventilate the infant for 24 hours, assess the neurological status and make a decision whether to withdraw or continue support. Resuscitation units with overhead heating, a time clock, an oxygen supply and a 30 cmH_2O pressure valve should be available in all areas where at-risk infants are to be delivered. It is most important to maintain the infant's temperature and prevent cooling during resuscitation. Much of the heat loss is from the head of the infant and this must be covered and the infant warmed with an appropriate heating unit. The majority of infants who require resuscitation can be extubated within 1 to 2 minutes and are probably not at significant risk and should be returned to their mothers for nursing supervision. Those requiring longer resuscitation may require admission to a special or intensive care nursery for subsequent observation for apnoea, convulsions and neurological status. Such infants require a check of their haemoglobin, blood glucose and blood gas determinations at intervals determined by the clinical status of the infant. If the term infant has no convulsions and is feeding normally within 48 hours the long-term prognosis is usually good.

Initial resuscitation may be carried out using a bag and face mask (Fig. 1.13). After the airway has been adequately cleared with gentle suction (–5 cmH_2O) the mask is positioned to ensure an adequate face seal and the bag with a 30 cmH_2O leak-valve inflated at a rate of 20–30 per minute. A complication can be gaseous distension of the stomach. When prolonged bag and mask ventilation is necessary the insertion of a nasogastric tube may help.

(a)

(b)

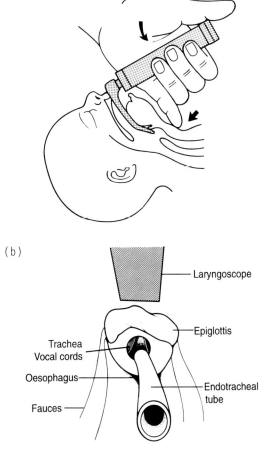

FIGURE 1.12a,b Tracheal intubation technique.

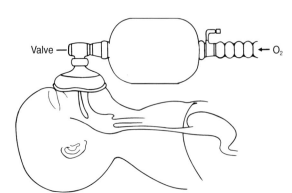

FIGURE 1.13 Bag and mask ventilation.

More effective ventilation may be obtained with a system which allows for a more prolonged inspiratory phase and the ability to increase the inspiratory pressures to 40 or 50 cmH$_2$O pressure.

BIRTH-RELATED DISORDERS

PERINATAL HEALTH SERVICES

In many countries obstetrics has developed in relation to the surgery of women (gynaecology) and neonatal medicine has developed as a branch of paediatrics and neonatal surgery as a branch of surgery. Midwife training has developed in the care of the mother during pregnancy and of her infant after delivery. Fortunately the disadvantages and even dangers of such artificial divisions of interest and responsibility are being recognised and the strict training schemes which tended to perpetuate professional differences are now being adapted to meet the needs of mother and child. Particularly in Australia and the USA the concept of perinatal medicine and health services which are required to improve standards of care in the perinatal period are being adopted. Improved standards of care have resulted in a very marked reduction in maternal mortality due to childbirth during the past century from over 500 maternal deaths per 100 000 deliveries at the beginning of the century in the UK to levels where maternal mortality rate is no longer a useful measure by which to assess the success of maternity services. The current maternal mortality rate in most developed countries is 1 per 10 000 births or less. Attention is now focused on infant mortality and morbidity. Many infant deaths in the first year of life are due to causes directly or closely related to factors occurring during fetal life or delivery.

DEFINITIONS

The following definitions are those of the Standing Joint Committee of the British Paediatric Association and Royal College of Obstetricians and Gynaecologists and are based on current World Health Organization definitions. Those involved in collecting and disseminating perinatal statistics whether at national, regional, area, district, or local hospital level should adhere to standard definitions. It is appreciated that gestational age often cannot be determined by reference to the last menstrual period. None the less, whichever method of gestational age assessment is used the definitions of various gestational age categories are still appropriate. The definitions highlight the need for all live births and fetal deaths to be accurately weighed as soon as possible after birth.

Live birth

"Live birth is the complete expulsion or extraction from its mother of a product of conception, irrespective of the duration of the pregnancy, which, after such separation, breathes or shows any other evidence of life, such as beating of the heart, pulsation of the umbilical cord, or definite movement of voluntary muscles, whether or not the umbilical cord has been cut or the placenta is attached; each product of such a birth is considered live born."

Fetal death

"Fetal death is death prior to the complete expulsion or extraction from its mother of a product of conception irrespective of the duration of the pregnancy; the death is indicated by the fact that after such separation the fetus does not breathe or show any other evidence of life, such as beating of the heart, pulsation of the umbilical cord, or definite movement of voluntary muscles."

Birthweight

"The first weight of the fetus or newborn obtained after birth. This weight should be measured preferably within the first hour of life before significant postnatal weight loss has occurred."

Low birthweight

"Less than 2500 g (up to, and including, 2499 g)."

Gestational age

"The duration of gestation is measured from the first day of the last normal menstrual period. Gestational age is expressed in completed days or completed weeks (e.g. events occurring 280 to 286 days after the onset of the last normal menstrual period are considered to have occurred at 40 weeks of gestation). Measurements of fetal growth, as they represent continuous variables, are expressed in relation to a specific week of gestational age (e.g. the mean birthweight for 40 weeks is that obtained at 280–286 days of gestation on a weight-for-gestational age curve)."

Preterm

"Less than 37 completed weeks." (Up to and including the 258th day of gestation.)

Term

"From 37 to less than 42 completed weeks" (259 days up to and including 293 days).

Post-term

"42 completed weeks or more" (294 completed days or more).

PERINATAL MORTALITY STATISTICS

National perinatal statistics should include all fetuses and infants delivered weighing at least 500 g or, when birthweight is unavailable the corresponding gestational age (22 weeks) or body length (25 cm crown–heel), whether alive or dead. It is recognised that legal requirements in many countries may set different criteria for registration purposes, but it is hoped that countries will arrange the registration or reporting procedures in such a way that the events required for inclusion in the statistics can be identified easily. In the United Kingdom the "fetal death" component of perinatal mortality includes only those fetuses which have completed 24 weeks (168 days) in the uterus. Fetuses below this age, whether stillborn or live born, are classified as abortions. There is much sense in defining perinatal mortality as "fetal deaths weighing 500 g or more plus deaths occurring less than 7 completed days after birth in babies weighing 500 g or more". The inclusion of extremely low birthweight babies within the definition of perinatal mortality underlines the need for all fetal deaths and live births to be accurately weighed. In this way perinatal mortal-

ity can be analysed within specific birthweight groups and when comparing perinatal mortality rates, allowances can be made for differences in birthweight distributions between populations:

1 Early neonatal death (included in perinatal mortality): death less than 7 completed days from birth
2 Late neonatal death (not included in perinatal mortality): death from 7 completed days to less than 28 days from birth
3 Post neonatal death: death from 28 completed days to less than 1 year from birth (i.e. up to and including 364 days).

Early neonatal death may be further subdivided:

1 Under 1 hour, 1–23 hours, 24–167 hours;
2 Birthweight classification for perinatal mortality statistics by birthweight intervals of 500 g, i.e. 500–999 g, 1000–1499 g, 1500–1999g etc;
3 Gestational age classification for perinatal mortality statistics under 28 weeks (under 168 days), 24–28 weeks (168–195 days), 28–31 weeks (196–223 days), 32–36 weeks (224–258 days), 37–41 weeks (259–293 days), 42 weeks and over (294 days and over).

Birth rate is the number of births live and still (registered per 1000 of the population). *Stillbirth rate* is the number of still births registered per 1000 live and stillbirths. *Neonatal mortality rate* is the number of deaths registered of infants dying under the age of 28 days per 1000 registered live births in the same year. *Perinatal mortality rate* is the number of stillbirths and early neonatal births per 1000 live and stillbirths. *Infant mortality rate* is the number of deaths registered of infants dying under 1 year of age per 1000 registered live births in the same year. *Post-perinatal infant mortality rate* is the number of deaths between the 8th day and end of the first year of life per 1000 live births. Crude perinatal mortality rates vary with factors such as social background and environment which are not directly under medical or nursing control. Attempts have therefore been made to use "adjusted perinatal mortality rates" which allows for birthweight and major malformations which are incompatible with extended postnatal life. Such adjusted figures give better indications of the standard of perinatal care than crude perinatal mortality rates. The most satisfactory index of perinatal health is the subsequent growth and development of the infant into a healthy, happy child and subsequently a healthy adult able to fulfil his/her genetic potential.

PERINATAL MORTALITY

In most countries where population growth has not out-stripped the economic growth there has been a

TABLE 1.3 Stillbirth rates and death rates in the first year of life

	STILLBIRTHS[1] a	EARLY NEONATAL[2] b	PERINATAL[1] a+b	LATE NEONATAL[2] c	NEONATAL[2] b+c	POST NEONATAL[2] d	INFANT b+c+d
1983	5.8	4.8	10.6	1.0	5.8	4.1	9.9
1984	5.8	5.2	11.0	1.2	6.4	3.9	10.3
1985	5.5	4.3	9.8	1.2	5.5	3.9	9.4
1986	5.8	4.4	10.2	0.8	5.2	3.6	8.8
1987	5.1	3.8	8.9	0.9	4.7	3.8	8.5
1988	5.4	3.5	8.9	1.0	4.5	3.7	8.2
1989	5.0	3.3	8.3	1.4	4.7	4.0	8.7
1990	5.3	3.4	8.7	1.0	4.4	3.3	7.7
1991	5.4	3.2	8.6	1.2	4.4	2.7	7.1
1992*	5.4	3.6	9.0	1.0	4.6	2.2	6.8

[1] Per 1000 total births. Source: Registrar General Scotland.
[2] Per 1000 live births.
* Provisional.

steady fall in perinatal mortality. Since 1940 the perinatal mortality rate in Scotland has fallen from 65 per 1000 total births to less than 9 per 1000 in 1992. This change is largely due to improvement in living standards and in particular to higher standards of nutrition and hygiene. Improved antenatal care, a reduction in family size and improved perinatal care are other major factors in the improved outcome for all birthweight and gestational age categories during this time. There is still room for improvement when Scottish data are compared with those, for example, of Japan and closer examination of population subgroups within Scotland and within the major cities such as Glasgow indicate that perinatal mortality rates in some city areas, for example, are up to five times those found in more advantaged parts of the city. This continuing discrepancy in perinatal mortality between social classes and between supported and unsupported mothers presents a continuing challenge to our social, educational and medical services. Table 1.3 shows the stillbirth and death rates in the first year of life from the General Register Office (Scotland) data. It shows a fall in the infant mortality rate from 10 to 6.8 per l000 live births during the

TABLE 1.4 Birthweight and gestation: specific neonatal mortality rates per 1000 total births – Scotland 1992 (total registered births 66 145)

BIRTHWEIGHT (g)		GESTATION (weeks)	
< 1000	531.1	< 26	684.2
1000–1499	80.8	26–27	401.6
1500–1999	33.5	28–31	61.1
2000–2499	11.8	32–36	14.5
2500–2999	2.6	37–41	1.7
3000–3499	1.4	42 or more	0.9
3500–3999	0.9	Not known	4.1
4000 and over	1.7		
Not known	5.5		

10-year period. The sustained improvement in infant mortality stemmed from a reduction in deaths in the first week of life. Over the last 3 years there has been a reduction in the post-neonatal mortality rate (deaths after the first 28 days) which is largely attributed to a reduction in sudden unexplained infant deaths. In October 1992 the law in the United Kingdom was changed so that stillbirths had to be registered from a gestational age of 24 weeks and not 28 weeks as before. Table 1.4 shows the birthweight and gestational age specific neonatal mortality rates for Scotland during 1992. It is evident that the lower the birthweight and gestational age the higher the neonatal mortality rates. Table 1.5 shows the known and unknown causes of stillbirths and neonatal deaths by obstetric and paediatric classifications for 1992. Information about the same classifications in relation to time of death is also available. Once it is possible to collect this type of information within national populations it becomes possible to identify preventable factors. By the study of such data for individual hospitals or individual urban and rural areas much can be learned of the success or failure of the methods of care and prevention. Many of the environmental factors such as maternal nutrition, hygiene, housing conditions, smoking, alcohol intake, maternal age and family size are known to influence stillbirth, neonatal and perinatal death rates and probably also the quality of survival. From the data shown it can be seen that a reduction in preterm and low birthweight deliveries could significantly improve the outcome with prevention of congenital malformation likely to have a major effect on the quality of survival of the larger infants. Measurements of the quality of life of those who survive are not easily obtained. The Scottish low birthweight 1984 cohort study has started to identify some factors related to life quality for the higher risk low birthweight infants. Table 1.6 gives some outcome measures for this group of high risk infants. Table 1.7 shows that low

TABLE 1.5 Known and unknown causes of stillbirths and neonatal deaths by obstetric and paediatric practices

OBSTETRIC CLASSIFICATION	TOTAL SINGLETON	MULTIPLE	PAEDIATRIC CLASSIFICATION	TOTAL SINGLETON	MULTIPLE
Total	**597**	**63**	**Total**	**597**	**63**
CNS	16	1	CNS	16	1
CVS	26	1	CVS	26	1
Renal	18	1	Renal	18	1
Alimentary	1	–	Alimentary	1	–
Chromosomal	20	–	Chromosomal	20	–
Biochemical	2	–	Biochemical	2	–
Other	47	2	Other	47	2
Rhesus incompatibility	3	–	Rhesus incompatibility	3	–
Non-rhesus incompatibility	1	–	Non-rhesus incompatibility	1	–
Severe toxaemia	17	–	Antepartum anoxia	253	11
Other toxaemia	2	–	Intrapartum anoxia	69	5
Abruptio placentae	59	–	Birth trauma	2	–
Placenta praevia	4	1			
Other APH	12	–	Lung immaturity	40	17
			HMD with IVH	18	6
Breech	5	–	HMD without IVH	11	4
Cord prolapse	1	–	IVH with mild HMD	–	–
Other mechanical	12	1	IVH with no HMD	1	–
			Subarachnoid haemorrhage	–	–
Maternal trauma	2	–	Subdural haemorrhage	–	–
Essential hypertension	5	2	Intracerebral haemorrhage	–	–
Diabetes	10				
Abdominal operations in pregnancy	–	–	NEC	5	–
Other (incl. infection)	24	–	Antenatal infection	9	3
			Intranatal infection	9	–
Miscellaneous	23	5	Other postnatal infection	5	–
			DIC	–	–
Unexplained 2500 g and over	111	–			
Unexplained <2500 g	168	49	Pulmonary haemorrhage	1	3
Postnatal cause only	8	–	Other haemorrhage	5	–
Not known	–	–	Other paediatric factors	13	9
			Unexplained	22	–
			Not known	–	–

birthweight is now a major factor in the aetiology of cerebral palsy in Scottish children. This contrasts greatly with data from 1940 where a majority of cerebral palsy infants were of normal birthweight. Improvements in obstetric and neonatal practice have significantly reduced the number of term asphyxiated infants and this has reduced the numbers of children with cerebral palsy in this mature group. The collection of such data is essential, not only to audit outcome for the population but also to detect potential harmful practices in perinatal care. One example of a harmful effect was the delayed feeding of preterm infants practised during the 1950s which led to impaired school performance and cerebral palsy in many of the children so treated. The association of retrolental fibroplasia with oxygen therapy is another example. Good record keeping is an absolute requisite for the accurate collection of basic information about an infant's pre- and postnatal condition and this information can act as a basis of an ongoing lifelong record of health for that individual.

ORGANISATION OF SERVICES FOR THE NEWBORN

Each country must assess how best to meet the needs of mothers and their infants in relation to the individual cultural and financial resources of that country. Even with very limited resources considerable improvements can be achieved through improvement of the hygiene and nutrition of mothers. In countries with a high socio-economical standard outcomes depend more on effective organisation of services and the supply of well trained nursing, medical and paramedical staff combined with a willingness of mothers to use the available facilities and their confidence in the staff and in the methods employed. Ease of access to clinics and methods of delivery which satisfy maternal instincts and needs can achieve an economically efficient and good quality outcome and be acceptable to the local populations. In most

TABLE 1.6 The number (%) of Scottish children born in 1984 with neuromotor and sensory impairment and scoring <10th centile on British ability scales by birthweight group at age 4.5 years

	BIRTHWEIGHT			
	<1000 g	1000–1499 g	1500–1749 g	TOTAL
No. of children assessed	60	298	253	611
Neuromotor impairment	13 (21.6)	42 (14.1)	27 (10.7)	82 (13.4)
Abnormal signs only	5 (8.3)	16 (5.4)	14 (5.5)	35 (5.7)
Impairment with disability				
Severe	4 (6.7)	10 (3.4)	9 (3.6)	23 (3.8)
Moderate	4 (6.7)	16 (5.4)	4 (1.6)	24 (3.9)
Rate of neuromotor disability/1000 live births	39.2	65.3	44.2	52.5
95% CI	17.1–75.8	43.1–94.3	23.8–74.4	37.9–67.1
Visual impairment				
Blind	3 (5.0)	1 (0.3)	3 (1.2)	7 (1.1)
Squints	12 (20.0)	35 (11.8)	23 (9.2)	70 (11.6)
Nystagmus	5 (8.8)	2 (0.7)	5 (2.0)	12 (2.0)
Visual acuity <6/18	5 (9.4)	10 (4.4)	7 (3.6)	22 (4.6)
Rate of blindness/1000 live births	14.7	2.5	10.2	7.8
95% CI	3.0–42.4	0.0–13.9	2.1–29.6	3.1–16.0
Hearing impairment				
Deaf with aids	2 (3.0)	4 (1.4)	5 (2.0)	11 (1.8)
Hearing loss >40 dB	0	2 (0.6)	2 (0.7)	4 (0.6)
Rate of deafness/100 live births	9.8	10.0	17.1	12.3
95% CI	1.2–34.9	2.7–25.5	5.6–39.4	4.6–17.5
British ability scales				
Verbal comprehension	15 (27.8)	66 (22.7)	47 (19.1)	128 (21.7)
Visual recognition	12 (22.6)	96 (26.8)	66 (26.8)	174 (29.5)
Naming vocabulary	6 (11.3)	33 (11.4)	33 (13.4)	72 (12.2)
Digit recall	6 (11.3)	39 (13.8)	23 (9.8)	68 (11.9)
Basic number skills	12 (24.0)	49 (18.4)	30 (13.5)	91 (16.9)

countries a high level of intensive care provision for the newborn human infant is available on a regional basis with the provision of safe transport for mother and infant to these specialised facilities.

THE PARENTS

The most important factors determining the outcome for an individual infant are the parents. In the traditional family the birth or impending birth of a new infant is a major family and life event. Parents may seek advice before embarking on a pregnancy and this attitude to planned parenthood is in part related to improved education and increased knowledge of hereditary factors and an ability to examine the embryo and fetus *in utero* as well as to control fertility. Parents are mainly concerned about possible abnormal development of their child before birth. Apart from this concern parents are also anxious to make sure that they will be able to look after their new infant properly. Problems may arise because of inadequate housing, low income, ill health and family size. About one in seven of all partnerships have problems with infertility and the introduction of

methods for investigation of endocrine and anatomical disorder has helped many previously infertile couples. Many legal and ethical dilemmas are now being faced by society as they come to terms with technologies of *in vitro* fertilisation and prenatal screening and diagnostic tests for a variety of inherited metabolic and other abnormalities. Preparation for parenthood begins in childhood when children watch their own parents' and relatives' methods of

TABLE 1.7 Cerebral palsy in Scottish children aged <7 years by birthweight and type

	<2500 g No. (%)	>2500 g No. (%)	TOTAL
Quadriplegia	57 (51.4)	54 (48.6)	111
Diplegia	56 (68.3)	26 (31.7)	82
Hemiplegia	23 (31.1)	51 (68.9)	74
Monoplegia	4 (66.7)	2 (33.3)	6
Ataxic	5 (22.7)	17 (77.3)	22
Athetoid	1 (12.5)	7 (87.5)	8
Cerebellar ataxia	4 (50.0)	4 (50.0)	8
Mixed	19 (50.0)	19 (50.0)	38
Total	169 (48.4)	180 (51.6)	349
Population (%)	7%	93%	

child rearing. Educational programmes within schools should be encouraged to add instruction in parentcraft to lessons on home management and sex education and education authorities should ensure that teachers have appropriate knowledge and understanding of the importance of these matters. Of major importance is the need in many so-called developed countries to encourage young women to breast feed their infants. The role of the father in the support of the mother and child is crucial and the joint responsibilities of the two parents in the creation of a healthy child and healthy community cannot be overemphasised.

CONGENITAL ABNORMALITIES

Congenital means present at birth and malformations evident at birth represent only a small proportion of the seriously malformed products of gestation. Most cause embryonic and fetal death at an early stage of pregnancy and are generally unrecognised when they are aborted. The remaining abnormal fetuses, whether live-born or stillborn, have congenital abnormalities caused by a wide variety of genetic and environmental factors, some known and others as yet unrecognised. As birth trauma, infection and other causes of perinatal death come under control congenital abnormalities are now of greater relative importance as a cause of perinatal mortality and morbidity. Potentially remedial developmental anomalies are present in more than 2 per 1000 live-born infants. Many abnormalities are now diagnosed antenatally through alpha-fetoprotein screening and detailed ultrasound. Prompt and effective management of these malformations is one of the most important aspects of neonatal surgery.

AETIOLOGY

Of the many factors responsible for congenital malformations some are clearly defined. These include genetic and environmental factors including malnutrition, infections, drugs, smoking, alcohol, vascular incidents, the effects of chemotherapy, radiotherapy, ultrasound and second generation malformations. There are clusters and trends in the incidence of congenital malformations, e.g. spina bifida in the west of Scotland as in many other countries has shown a decline in recent years. The interaction of genetic predisposition and environmental factors is well described in relation to the genesis of tumours (oncogenesis) but can also be applied to the causes of congenital malformations (teratogenesis). There are congenital malformations which predispose to malignancy such as those skin abnormalities related to chromosome fragility syndromes and the Beckwith–Wiedemann syndrome which is associated with Wilms tumours. Table 1.8 shows some of the drugs or other agents which may cause fetal abnormalities if taken by the mother and the relative teratogenicity of these drugs. From Table 1.8 it can be seen that many drugs are a potential danger to the unborn child but thalidomide was the first to create international alarm with its clearly defined effects. Introduced as a mild sedative and hypnotic, it proved to be teratogenic when taken in early pregnancy, affecting principally the limbs (amelia, phocomelia, etc.) and to a lesser extent the bowel and other organs. After the introduction of thalidomide in Western Germany in 1957 thousands of children throughout the world were born with severe limb defects. Thalidomide (under 49 different names) given to women in early pregnancy caused congenital malformations in about 20% of the infants. The drug was withdrawn from the European market in 1961 and from Japan in 1962. Subsequent siblings born to affected mothers have been normal. It has been postulated that part at least of the teratogenic action of thalidomide is due to its immunosuppressive properties allowing survival to term of deformed embryos which would otherwise have aborted. The firm responsible for its manufacture and distribution funded specialist treatment centres which allowed the development of powered prostheses of the Heidelberg type. The information gained from these centres has found application in the treatment of infants with similar limb abnormalities due to teratogens other than thalidomide.

When clinical examination of the newborn infant reveals a congenital malformation it is important to look for other abnormalities since there are sometimes more than one abnormality present. Where there are a series of abnormalities present then this may allow the identification of a syndrome. There are now a number of databases available for the categorisation of such malformation groupings. Many malformations are now detected prenatally but some may only become evident in later childhood or indeed in adult life.

DEVELOPMENTAL ANOMALIES AND THE PARENTS

Parents whose child is born with a defect are always concerned to know the cause. The two most common questions they ask are: "Is the defect due to any fault in the father or mother?" and "Will a second child be likely to have a similar or other defect?" Unfortunately a satisfactory answer to these questions is not always

TABLE 1.8 The effect of drugs taken by the mother on the embryo and fetus *in utero*

DRUG/AGENT	ORGANS AFFECTED
Alcohol	Eyes, cranium, face, skeleton, brain; stunted
Aminopterin	Cranium, face, skin, ears; death
Amphetamines	Heart, lip, skeleton, urogenital
Anaesthetics	Skeletal and face suggested – very rare: affects theatre staff
Androgens and synthetic progestagens	Masculinised females
Anti-emetics	All probably harmless save diphenylhydramine
Antithyroid drugs	Thyroid, brain
Atropine	Tachycardia
Aspirin	Probably nil
Beta-blockers	Diminished adaptive response to asphyxia
Busulphan	Eyes, palate; stunted
Chlorambucil	Urogenital
Chloroquine	Deafness and choroidretinitis possible
Cigarette smoking	Reduced birthweight
Corticosteroids	Probably nil
Cyclophosphamide	Palate
Diazepam	Cleft lip and palate possible + respiratory depression
Diethylstilboestrol	In first trimester predisposes to vaginal carcinoma and adenosis (after 15 years)
Diuretics	Reduced birthweight
Folic acid deficiency	Brain, neural tube
Hydralazine	Hypotension
Iodine excess or deficiency	Goitre, hypothyroidism, brain
Lithium	Heart great vessels
Methotrexate	Skeletal
Paramethadione	Heart, palate, face, brain
Phenytoin and barbiturates	Lips, skull, skeleton, ear, heart
Progestagens	Virilization
Quinine	Hypoplasia of optic nerve and deafness in high doses
Radiation	Neural tube, skeleton; microcephaly
Ritodrine	Hypoglycaemia
Streptomycin	Deafness
Tetracycline	Teeth discoloured and enamel hypoplasia
Thalidomide	Skeleton, heart, ears, eyes
Troxidone (trimethadione)	Heart, palate, face, brain
Vitamin A deficiency	Brain, eyes, palate, skeleton
Vitamin D excess	Infantile hypercalcaemia possible
Valproate	Face and neural tube
Warfarin	Nose, skeleton, eyes, brain; nasal hypoplasia, chondrodysplasia punctata in first trimester; optic atrophy, microcephaly, mental retardation in second and third trimesters

possible. It is, however, important that someone with understanding of the psychological impact of the birth of a deformed child on the family should interview the parents on at least two occasions within the first few days after the birth. A simple and honest appraisal is given by the doctor who must attempt to dispel the shame or guilt felt by the parents. Facial deformities such as cleft lip and extensive facial haemangiomata are particularly distressing to parents.

Where there is a gene abnormality responsible for the transmission of anatomical, physiological or biochemical defects the parents must have explained to them the relative risk for future pregnancies. Many such defects are caused by spontaneous mutations and are unlikely to recur. Probably less than 20% of malformations are determined by mutant genes, and less than 10% by viral infection. Thus, more than

60% are from as yet undetermined causes. Maternal rubella can be prevented through protective immunisation of children. Pregnant women should take no drugs without good reason during their pregnancy and non-urgent abdominal X-rays in women of child-bearing age should be avoided. In families with a known high risk of abnormal offspring genetic counselling may help the family to decide whether they wish to have further children. If they do not, contraceptive advice should be given. Where there has been proven exposure to harmful factors in early pregnancy or where there is high risk of hereditary abnormality, consideration has to be given to the justification for therapeutic termination of pregnancy. In some situations examination of chorionic villus biopsy material, the amniotic fluid, ultrasonography or direct inspection of the fetus using an endoscope passed into the amniotic cavity may be necessary before a decision can be reached.

ABNORMAL DEVELOPMENT

Because in 60% of the cases of congenital abnormality there is no identifiable cause and therefore no ability to take preventive action the paediatrician and paediatric surgeon continue to be faced with the management of such infants. Most of the abnormalities have resulted from a disturbance in the embryological development. In general terms these abnormalities arise because of:

- failure of development, e.g. amelia, microcephaly
- failure to unite, e.g. cleft lip, spina bifida
- failure to divide e.g. syndactyly, conjoined twins
- failure to canalize, e.g. intestinal atresias
- failure to migrate, e.g. malrotation of bowel, Hirschsprung disease
- failure to atrophy, e.g. branchial clefts, thyroglossal cyst
- excess division, e.g. polydactyly, duplex renal systems.

The medical and surgical management of such abnormalities are dealt with in the various organ chapters.

FETAL SURGERY

Some fetal and neonatal surgical centres have attempted correction of malformation of the fetus *in utero*, e.g. draining of hydrocephalus, drainage of an obstructive uropathy and repair of congenital diaphragmatic defect. A team of ultrasonographers, obstetricians, paediatricians and paediatric surgeons, together with specialist midwives/nurses should meet regularly to discuss individual prenatally diagnosed problems. It is now recognised that in the past before such expertise and consultation was available infants with abdominal wall defects and those with sacrococcygeal teratomas who might otherwise have had corrective surgery have been terminated. In some instances of prenatally detected obstruction of the urinary system there can be apparent spontaneous resolution later in the pregnancy. These and other as yet unexplained phenomena require a cautious approach to surgical intervention in the antenatal period.

PERINATAL INJURIES

During the last two to three decades there has been a gratifying decline in the incidence of "mechanical"

birth injuries. Trauma is at times an inevitable accompaniment of the mechanics of birth even when delivery is spontaneous and uncomplicated. The nature of the injury varies greatly and depending upon the site and severity may be of minor or major significance.

ANTENATAL INJURY

During induction of labour superficial trauma generally of a minor degree can result from the rupturing of membranes, the application of scalp electrodes or the taking of fetal blood samples. Occasionally during Caesarean section fetal skin may be incised. Mechanical injury during delivery may be precipitated when there is disproportion between the size of the fetal head and the maternal pelvis, excessive uterine contractions (augmented labour), abnormal presentations, low birthweight and instrumental delivery.

INJURY TO SUPERFICIAL TISSUES

A caput succedaneum consists of oedematous swelling and bruising in the superficial tissues of the presenting part of the fetus. In vertex presentations the caput is not sharply defined and may extend across suture lines. If presentation is abnormal the caput will be formed elsewhere. The affected tissue "pits" on pressure, is present at birth and disappears within 48 hours. Abrasions are sometimes present in the skin overlying the caput and unless particular care is taken may allow entry of organisms, leading to sepsis. Bruising and minor abrasions of the scalp not infrequently result from the application of a vacuum extractor.

CEPHALHAEMATOMATA (SUBPERIOSTEAL HAEMATOMA)

This is a swelling resulting from bleeding deep between the periosteum and underlying skull bone and is therefore restricted to the limits of that bone (usually parietal). The swelling is not usually present at birth but becomes evident on the second or third day. Thereafter it may increase in bulk and in extent for a few days. It is well defined, may persist for a number of weeks or even months but invariably disappears completely. The swelling is at first fluctuant but becomes firmer as absorption of fluid takes place. A firm ring may be felt surrounding the swelling and is evidence of commencing calcification which sometimes extends to form a localised hard elevation around the site of the original swelling. Occasionally there may be bilateral swelling. In general neither a caput succedaneum nor a cephalhaematoma need cause concern. It is important that infants with cephalhaematomata should have been given vitamin K_1.

Subaponeurotic haemorrhage (subgaleal haemorrhage) occasionally results from the application of a vacuum extractor. The swelling of this haemorrhage extends across the lines of the sutures and is a potentially dangerous complication. There can be excessive blood loss and vitamin K prophylaxis must be ensured. Other neonatal injuries are described in Chapter 17.

LOW BIRTHWEIGHT INFANTS (LBW)

Low birthweight infants (LBW) is a phrase used to describe all infants weighing less than 2500 g (up to and including 2499 g). These infants are at a major disadvantage when compared with those weighing more than 2500 g. Very low birthweight (VLBW) is a phrase used to describe infants weighing less than 1500 g (up to and including 1499 g). The effects of preterm and low birthweight on survival are shown in Table 1.4. It is evident that the mortality increases with reducing maturity and birthweight. Such infants require the facilities available in neonatal intensive care units and where these are available survival rates of 90% can be achieved for infants weighing between 1001 g and 1500 g. VLBW infants account for about 10% of the number of LBW infants but for about 60% of the perinatal deaths in LBW infants. Management of these infants poses a most important challenge for those responsible for the care of the newly born infant.

TABLE 1.9 Outline of causes of low birthweight

Preterm delivery
Maternal ill health
Complications of pregnancy
Fetal abnormality
Slow fetal growth
Malnutrition *in utero*
Poor placental function
Fetal poisoning (alcohol and smoking)
Hypoplasia
Constitutional
Chromosome abnormality
Fetal poisoning (alcohol and smoking)
Combination of above

There were 908 infants with birthweight less than 1.75 kg born alive in Scotland in 1985. Twenty-nine per cent did not survive and of the survivors 16% were disabled; 47 had cerebral palsy, 7 were blind and 11 deaf. Amongst those not overtly disabled the prevalence of poor neuromotor competence was high and related to birthweight at the age of 4.5 years.

PRETERM INFANTS

A birth is preterm if it occurs up to and including the 258th day of gestation. Most preterm infants are of low birthweight and weigh less than 2500 g at birth. LBW may be caused by preterm delivery or slow fetal growth (Table 1.9). Infants weighing less than the 10th percentile of the weight distribution for their gestational age are termed light for dates and infants over the 90th centile heavy for dates (Fig. 1.14). Some infants who are born light for dates have a normal birth length but others have a combination of low

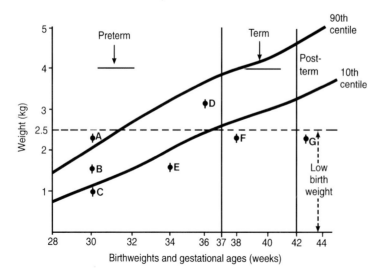

FIGURE 1.14 Classification of low birthweight infants: A, preterm, heavy for dates; B & D, preterm, appropriate for dates; C & E, preterm, light for dates; F, term, light for dates; G, post-term, light for dates.

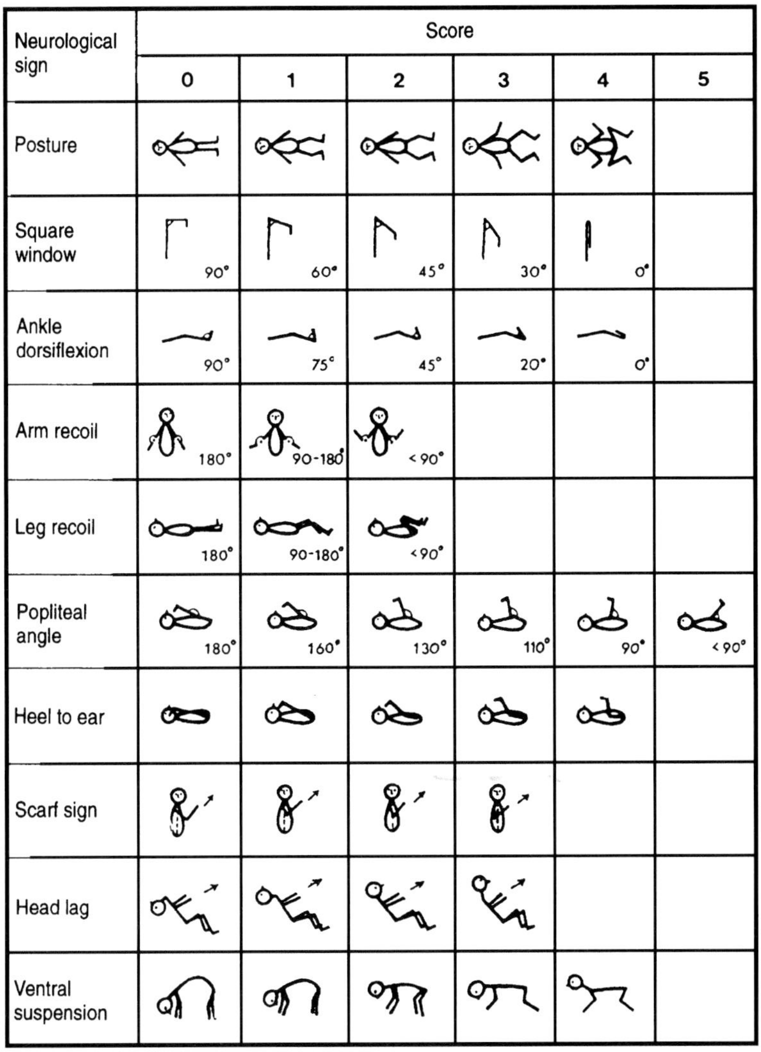

FIGURE 1.15 Scoring system for neurological signs. (Reproduced by kind permission of the authors and CV Mosby Co. from Dubowitz LMS, Dubowitz V and Goldberg C (1970). Clinical assessment of gestational age in the newborn infant, *Journal of Pediatrics*, 77, 1–10.)

birthweight and low birth length and are termed small for dates or small for gestational age. Frequently the chest and head circumference in these small infants are below the 10th centile. This growth failure may be detected prenatally. It is important to recognise infants who have failed to grow adequately *in utero* as they have different problems from those LBW infants who are adequately nourished but delivered preterm.

POSTNATAL ASSESSMENT OF MATURITY

Assessment can be based on a series of external characteristics and a number of neurological signs affecting posture and primitive reflexes. Each sign is given a score. It can be carried out at any time during the first 5 days of life provided that there is no evidence of intrapartum asphyxia or birth injury.

The external signs and scoring system used are shown in Table 1.10 and Fig. 1.15. The final score is plotted on a graph in Fig. 1.16 which correlates the (Dubowitz) score with gestational age.

THE PRETERM INFANT

Preterm delivery is the major cause of low birthweight and is associated with a greatly increased risk of mortality and morbidity. The degree of risk increases progressively in the more preterm infant. Although improved methods of management have increased the chance of survival and its quality the risk of complications remains sufficiently high to justify every effort being taken to prevent preterm delivery.

TABLE 1.10 Scoring system for external criteria of maturation

| EXTERNAL SIGN | SCORE* | | | | |
	0	1	2	3	4
Oedema	Obvious oedema of hands and feet; pitting over tibia	No obvious oedema of hands and feet; pitting over tibia	No oedema		
Skin texture	Very thin gelatinous	Thin and smooth	Smooth; medium thickness. Rash or superficial peeling	Slight thickening. Superficial cracking and peeling especially of hands and feet	Thick and parchment-like; superficial or deep cracking
Skin colour	Dark red	Uniformly pink	Pale pink; variable over body	Pale; only pink over ears, lips, palms, or soles	
Skin opacity (trunk)	Numerous veins and venules clearly seen, especially over abdomen	Veins and tributaries seen	A few large vessels clearly seen over abdomen	A few large vessels seen indistinctly over abdomen	No blood vessels seen
Lanugo (over back)	No lanugo	Abundant; long and thick over whole back	Hair thinning especially over lower back	Small amount of lanugo and bald area	At least half of back devoid of laguno
Plantar creases	No skin creases	Faint red marks over anterior half of sole	Definite red marks over > anterior ½; indentations over < anterior ⅓	Indentations over > anterior ⅓	Definite deep indentations over > anterior ⅓
Nipple formation	Nipple barely visible; no areola	Nipple well defined; areola smooth and flat, diameter <0.75 cm	Areola stippled, edge not raised, diameter < 0.75 cm	Areola stippled, edge raised, diameter > 0.75 cm	
Breast size	No breast tissue palpable	Breast tissue on one or both sides, <0.5 cm diameter	Breast tissue both sides; one or both 0.5–1.0 cm	Breast tissue both sides; one or both > 1 cm	
Ear form	Pinna flat and shapeless, little or no incurving of edge	Incurving of part of edge of pinna	Partial incurving whole of upper pinna	Well defined incurving whole of upper pinna	
Ear firmness	Pinna soft, easily folded, no recoil	Pinna soft, easily folded, slow recoil	Cartilage to edge of pinna, but soft in places, ready recoil	Pinna firm, cartilage to edge; instant recoil	
Genitals Male	Neither testis in scrotum	At least one testis high in scrotum	At least one testis right down		
Female (with hips half abducted)	Labia majora widely separated, labia minora protruding	Labia majora alomst cover labia minora	Labia majora completely cover labia minora		

*If score differs on two sides, take the mean.
From Dubowitz LMS, Dubowitz V, Goldberg C (1970). Clinical assessment of gestational age in the newborn infant. *Journal of Pediatrics* **77**, 1–10; adapted from Farr V, Mitchell RG, Neligan GA, Parkin JM (1966). The definition of some external characteristics used in the assessment of gestational age in the newborn infant. *Developmental Medicine* **8**, 507–11.

Some factors which are recognised as carrying a high risk of inducing preterm labour are listed in Table 1.11. Raising the general standard of living in a community with parallel improvements in the quality of the nutrition of young women before and during pregnancy will have a bigger impact in affect-

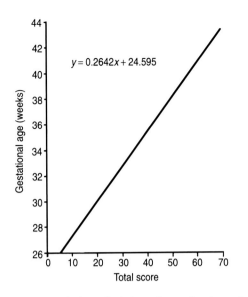

$y = 0.2642x + 24.595$

FIGURE 1.16 Graph for calculation of gestational age from total score.

TABLE 1.11 Factors carrying a high risk of preterm delivery

MATERNAL
  General
    Age: below 20 years
    Height: less than 155 cm
    Poor socio-economic status
    Heavy workload
    Poor nutrition
    Unmarried
  Obstetric
    Primiparity
    Pre-eclampsia
    Antepartum haemorrhage
    Chronic ill health
    Smoking
    Previous history of preterm delivery
FETAL
  Multiple pregnancy
  Congenital abnormalities
  Slow intrauterine growth

ing a reduction in preterm delivery than advances in medical knowledge. It requires an improved political and economic effort to achieve this end. Regular and careful supervision during the antenatal period will improve the chance of early recognition and treatment of complications of pregnancy which may lead to preterm delivery. Education of the mother in general health care and in the early recognition of warning signs will all help to reduce preterm delivery.

When the mother goes into preterm delivery every effort should be made to admit her promptly to a maternity unit with tertiary intensive care for her newborn. The mother's uterus is the ideal transport incubator for transferring the infant to such a unit. The use of beta-agonists such as ritodrine which act as uterine relaxants may delay delivery long enough to allow the institution of maternal dexamethasone therapy to achieve improved lung function in the infant.

CLINICAL FEATURES

The preterm infant's head and abdomen appear relatively large whilst the skin is soft in texture and pink in colour. A generalised lack of subcutaneous tissue results in prominence of the body skeleton, with a thin, lined face, loose skin over the limbs and the frequent appearance of intestinal peristalsis visible through the abdominal wall. The infant sleeps more or less continuously, the cry is infrequent and feeble and respiratory movements may be rhythmic with periodic spells of apnoea not uncommon. Muscular hypotonicity results in the characteristic posture in which the limbs are widely abducted, knees and ankles flexed, head lolling to one side. The ability to suck and to co-ordinate sucking and swallowing is not well developed in the VLBW infant. Oedema may be present at birth or become marked during the first 24–48 hours. Severe oedema is an unfavourable omen and may be associated with maternal antepartum haemorrhage, pre-eclampsia or diabetes mellitus. The heart rate in preterm infants averages 140 per minute. The respiratory rate is 40–50 per minute in the first 24 hours, thereafter decreasing to 35–45. A continued rapid rate should arouse suspicion of the respiratory distress syndrome or pneumonia. Preterm infants have high surface area to body weight ratios and little reserve of subcutaneous or brown adipose tissue. During the first few days they lose water rapidly through their skin and these physical characteristics make it difficult for them to maintain their temperatures. Cold exposure greatly jeopardises their survival and particular attention must be paid to ensuring the correct ambient temperatures. Liver immaturity will predispose to "physiological" jaundice but early establishment of feeding and phototherapy has reduced the risk of neurological damage from hyperbilirubinaemia.

The skin and mucous membrane surfaces are easily damaged in preterm infants and such breaches of these protective layers, together with a limited immunological competence, predisposes preterm infants to infections. They fail to show the signs found in older infants with sepsis; therefore a very high degree of suspicion of infection must be maintained. Any infant suspected of having an infection requires culture of urine, blood and sometimes cerebrospinal fluid and the commencement of therapy with an appropriate broad spectrum antibiotic.

A combination of septicaemia, hyperbilirubinaemia and hypoxia with metabolic acidaemia predisposes the infant to central nervous system damage. Intraventricular haemorrhage from the fragile, poorly supported vessels in the germinal matrix of the brain results from a combination of hypoxia, hypotension and disordered cerebral blood flow. The commonest clinical signs of intraventricular haemorrhage are apnoeic episodes, convulsions or unexplained deterioration in clinical state. Mortality from intraventricular haemorrhage is high and in those who survive there may be an obstructive hydrocephalus signalled by a rapid increase in head size, vomiting and convulsions.

As more and more immature infants survive it is important to maintain longer-term follow-up to assess the effectiveness of medical interventions in the management of these infants. Children born too soon do show impairment of performance at school age which may be related not only to the preterm delivery but also to early postnatal management particularly the provision of adequate nutrition.

MANAGEMENT

It is likely that most infants with birthweights of under 2 kg will be managed in hospital.

Maintenance of body temperature

As a general rule infants weighing less than 2 kg will require incubator care for safe temperature control. The nursery temperature should be maintained between 27 and 29 °C (80 and 85 °F) and it is an advantage when humidity can be controlled at 40–50%. When incubators are situated in cold nurseries infants can suffer considerable radiant heat loss and will only maintain body temperature by an undesirable increase in oxygen consumption. Maintenance of the infant within the neutral range of thermal environment when oxygen consumption is minimum at rest while the body temperature remains normal is the ideal. The neutral thermal environment will vary according to the design of the incubator, temperature of the nursery, humidity and other factors. Optimal operative temperatures of the incubator for infants of different birthweights and ages have been calculated but in general an incubator temperature between 32 and 35 °C (90 to 95 °F) is satisfactory. The humidity within the incubator should be about 50%. If there are difficulties in maintaining the infant temperature between 36 and 37 °C (96.8 and 98.6 °F) a perspex "heat shield" or

"bubble blanket" placed over the infant within the incubator will significantly diminish heat loss. Most incubators are equipped with a temperature sensor (thermistor probe) which is attached to the infant's skin and by means of a servo mechanism controls the incubator's heater so that the infant's skin temperature will be maintained at the pre-set level. Current practice is to dress most preterm infants in bonnets and mittens but the VLBW and those who are sick may require to be nursed naked in order that observations can be readily made. The presence of cyanosis is an indication to check the blood gases and to increase the oxygen concentration in the incubator. Normally the oxygen concentration is limited to 40% unless blood gas determinations indicate that higher oxygen concentrations are required. The LBW infant's scalp constitutes a large part of the total surface area and body heat loss can be diminished by the application of a cotton or wool and cotton bonnet.

NUTRITION AND THE PRETERM INFANT

In the normal term human infant there is a continuum of growth which, given a normal labour and delivery, together with satisfactory establishment of breast feeding, proceeds uninterrupted during the change from the intrauterine to extrauterine existence. In the first few days, whilst breast feeding is established, some infant nutrient reserves are mobilised to maintain cell division and growth in most major organs. For the infant born preterm it is almost impossible to prevent disruption of genetically predetermined programmes of cellular divisions, growth, maturation and activities. The more immature the infant at birth, the greater the difficulty of ensuring adequate nutrition and the more likely the infant is to suffer the consequences of impaired tissue growth, development and function. Nutritional deficits may result in disordered central nervous system function in childhood and in disordered cardiovascular and cerebrovascular function in later life. The infant born preterm has two major problems. The first is lack of nutritional reserve and the second is immaturity of organ function.

NUTRITIONAL RESERVES

Table 1.12 gives some relative compositions of infants born at 22, 26 and 29 weeks gestation weighing 500–1500 g and a 3.5 kg infant born at 40 weeks gestation. Virtually all of the fat, carbohydrate and protein in the preterm infant is structural whereas in

TABLE 1.12 Relative body compositions of human infants born preterm and at term

Gestational age (weeks)	22	26	29	40
Weight (g)	500	1000	1500	3500
Water (g)	433	850	1240	2380
Fat (g)	6	23	60	525
Carbohydrate (g)	2	5	15	34
Protein (g)	36	85	125	390

Adapted from Widdowson EM, Dickerson JWT (1964). Mineral metabolism. In: *Chemical Composition of the Body*, vol. 2A (Connor CL, Bronner F, eds). Academic Press, New York: 1–247.

TABLE 1.13 Mineral content of preterm infants born at 26 and 34 weeks gestation compared with that of a 40-week infant

MINERALS*	GESTATION (WEEKS)		
	26	34	40
Sodium (mmol)	94	200	286
Potassium (mmol)	42	108	185
Chloride (mmol)	68	139	192
Calcium (g)	6.3	19	33.6
Phosphorus (g)	3.9	11.9	19.6
Magnesium (g)	0.2	0.58	0.91
Iron (mg)	65	200	229
Copper (mg)	3.4	8.8	16.4
Zinc (mg)	20	40	70

*Minerals are expressed in terms of fat-free body tissue.
Adapted from Widdowson EM, Dickerson JWT (1964). Mineral metabolism. In: *Chemical Composition of the Body*, vol. 2A (Connor CL, Bronner F, eds). Academic Press, New York: 1–247.

the term infant there are reserves of glycogen, fat and other nutrients. After oxygen requirements have been met the next immediate need for survival in the preterm infant is an adequate water supply. It has been calculated that a VLBW infant might survive 3–4 days, a term infant 30 days and an adult 90 days if supplied with water alone. In starvation states a minimal energy expenditure of about 76 kcal/kg per 24 hours (0.32 MJ) is necessary to maintain life. If new functional peptides and proteins such as hormones and enzymes are to be manufactured by the preterm infant they can only be obtained by the destruction of structural proteins in organs such as muscle and liver if there is any failure to supply exogenous protein or amino acid. A relative excess of water, particularly extracellular water, in the preterm infant confers no protection against dehydration since the obligatory daily turnover of water is equal to 15–20% of the total body water pool. Table 1.13 shows the mineral content of a 26-week infant expressed in terms of fat free body tissue compared with the composition at term. Water-soluble vitamins B and C transfer readily from mother to fetus so that at term fetal tissue concentrations of these vitamins exceed maternal. Fetal concentrations of the fat-soluble vitamins A, D, E and K are not as high as adult values and, because of their high rate of utilisation and low initial values, preterm infants quickly run into deficit unless an early adequate intake is assured.

IMMATURITY OF ORGAN FUNCTION

Lung immaturity results in many preterm infants requiring ventilatory assistance. Renal immaturity reduces water tolerance and can be aggravated by exogenous osmotic loads in the form of glucose, amino acids and electrolytes or endogenous from urea production. A preterm infant has virtually no response to a water load in the first 3–5 days of life but thereafter can dilute to about 50 mosmol/kg unless hypoxia or hypotension reduces renal function. By 1 month of postnatal age the preterm infant can concentrate urine to approximately 400 mosmol/kg and by 3 months of postnatal age this can reach 750 mosmol/kg. Both kidneys and lungs are important in the maintenance of acid–base balance. Lung immaturity may cause hypercapnia with respiratory acidosis and hypoxia with metabolic acidosis, both of which interfere with cell membrane and tissue function. Renal threshold for bicarbonate is lower in the preterm newborn who relies on the reclamation of bicarbonate at the proximal tubules as the ability to excrete hydrogen ions in combination with ammonia as ammonium ions is limited. The principal urinary buffer is the phosphate buffer disodium, monohydrogen phosphate (Na_2HPO_4) and unless phosphate intake is adequate the preterm infant has a limited capacity to excrete titratable acid. Renal mechanisms largely under the influence of ADH and aldosterone are mainly responsible for electrolyte balance and extracellular fluid volume control. In preterm infants presented with large or imbalanced quantities of electrolyte, either parenterally or from tissue breakdown, or with kidneys poorly perfused or poorly oxygenated, gross distortion of fluid and electrolyte occur readily. Maintenance of good renal perfusion and oxygenation is a key factor in promoting anabolism. Hyperoxygenation will decrease renal blood flow as much as hypoxia and aggravate a catabolic state. Preterm birth creates stress which imposes increased demands on endocrine function at a time when particular endocrine responses may be absent, poor or even inappropriate. Immaturity of function of the gastrointestinal tract, the liver and exocrine pancreas make difficult the maintenance of the anabolic state. Structural development of the fetal gut is well in advance of functional capacity and there is a progressively changing pattern of enzyme differentiation during fetal life. With preterm delivery the later developing enzymes responsible for amino acid metabolism and gluconeogenesis may not yet be "switched on". Preterm infants are at particular risk of damaging hypoglycaemia as a result of the combination of a limited reserve of glycogen and reduced ability to synthesise glucose. An infant born preterm is an unphysiological creature who is unable to root, suck and swallow in a co-ordinated fashion because of central nervous system immaturity. Immaturity of other organs which subserve normal gastrointestinal function and waste product excretion means that even the ingestion of human milk is an "unphysiological" process for the very low birthweight preterm infant.

FEEDING

Infants of less than 34 weeks gestation require specialised feeding methods. Enteral feeding is usually by a nasogastric or orogastric feeding tube although on occasion transpyloric feeding (into the duodenum or jejunum) may reduce the frequency of vomiting and inhalation of stomach content. This method of feeding, however, is much less popular than previously as it may lead to complications including intestinal perforation, necrotising enterocolitis and diarrhoea. There is also some evidence that weight gain and growth is less satisfactory in infants fed nasojejunally. Continuous or bolus intragastric feeds may be given. Feeding with human milk should commence at about 2 hours of age to reduce the risk of hypoglycaemia and at a rate of about 60 ml/kg in the first day, increasing to 150 ml/kg/day by the 4th day of life. Most infants weighing more than 1500 g will tolerate 3-hourly feeds but smaller infants will require to be fed hourly or even continuously. Preterm infants may reach an intake of 200 ml/kg/day by the end of the 2nd week of life. Very immature infants of 24–26 weeks gestation frequently require total parenteral nutrition with slower introduction of enteral feeding. The currently available foods recommended for preterm infants are mother's own "preterm milk", banked donor milk, human milk fortified with special preterm formulae or with concentrated extracts of human milk, standard infant cow milk or soya based formulae, special "preterm" infant formulae and parenteral nutrition, either total or combined with enteral feeding. There is evidence that the use of fresh human milk with its protective effect against infection will provide important protection for the vulnerable preterm infant and reduce the incidence of necrotising enterocolitis. There is also a possibility that the use of human milk might protect against future allergic disease in preterm infants. At present it is probably wise to recommend the use of mother's own fresh milk complemented with a special preterm formula which contains increased concentrations of protein, energy, sodium, calcium, phosphorus, magnesium, copper, zinc, vitamins, essential and long-chain polyunsaturated fatty acids.

It is important to ensure that there is little or no separation of mother and infant as this may have adverse effects on the relationship between mother and infant. There are many strategies now developed to help mothers overcome the enormous difficulties of achieving successful feeding and an intimate relationship in the intensive care situation. There are now findings to suggest that preterm infants who do not receive human milk and do not grow well in the first months of life are subsequently less intelligent, have poorer visual function and have a greater risk of ischaemic heart disease, chronic bronchitis, hypertension, stroke and non-insulin dependent diabetes.

RESPIRATORY DISORDERS

Prolonged respiratory pauses (greater than 20 seconds) in preterm infants may be associated with cyanosis and bradycardia. These are called apnoeic attacks and may be a sign of septicaemia, meningitis or intracranial haemorrhage but in the majority of instances are unassociated with any obvious metabolic problem or illness. Neonatal convulsions may present as apnoeic episodes. Careful investigation for infection, hypoglycaemia, hypocalcaemia and intracranial haemorrhage should be undertaken and oxygen administered if the infant is hypoxic. When no trigger for apnoea is found, oral theophylline given in an initial dose of 5 mg/kg and thereafter maintained on the basis of blood concentration measurements (8–15 µg/ml) with a dose of theophylline between 1 and 2 mg/kg 12-hourly may reduce the frequency of apnoeic episodes.

RESPIRATORY DISTRESS

Respiratory difficulties may result from perinatal asphyxia which may cause primary atelectasis or aspiration of meconium and meconium-stained amniotic fluid into the lungs. Postnatal aspiration of gastric contents particularly in the tube-fed preterm infant may give rise to respiratory problems. Aspiration of foreign materials, such as meconium or gastric content, leads to severe lung congestion, oedema and haemorrhage with radiological evidence of patchy emphysema, secondary atelectasis and pulmonary oedema. Tachypnoea, costal recession and crepitations on auscultation are the clinical features. Severe meconium aspiration is more common in the more vigorous term infants who develop pneumomediastinum and/or pneumothorax. If there is persistent fetal circulation and standard techniques of ventilation prove inadequate, treatment with nitric oxide (NO) and/or extracorporeal membrane oxygenation (ECMO) and high frequency ventilation may prove life saving. At present ECMO is not a feasible proposition for infants weighing less than 2 kg but as technology improves treatment of smaller infants may become feasible.

Transient tachypnoea of the newborn is a condition in which there is a moderate degree of intercostal retraction and respiratory difficulty related to poor or delayed clearing of normal lung fluid. Chest X-ray shows a slightly enlarged heart with streaky infiltrates radiating from the hilum of the lung. Treatment with supplemental oxygen is required for those infants whose arterial oxygen tensions fall below 50–60 mmHg (6.7–8.0 kPa). Arterial PO_2 should be maintained at 70 mmHg (9.3 kPa). Measurements of transcutaneous oxygen tension ($TcPO_2$) and oxygen saturation (SaO_2) are helpful in ensuring adequate oxygenation. Because of the shape of the haemoglobin dissociation curve, saturation monitors may increase the risk of hyperoxia. An increase in SaO_2 from 90 to 98% may represent an increase in PaO_2 of more than 50 mmHg. Measurement of transcutaneous PO_2 ($TcPO_2$) is safer in the care of the acute phase of respiratory support whereas measurement of transcutaneous SaO_2 is of greater value in older infants with, for example, bronchopulmonary dysplasia (BPD).

THE IDIOPATHIC RESPIRATORY DISTRESS SYNDROME (RDS)

This condition is characterised by pulmonary resorption atelectasis associated with intense congestion, the presence of an eosinophilic hyaline membrane within dilated alveolar ducts and sometimes intrapulmonary haemorrhage. The hyaline material is not invariably present and is probably the result of a transudate of fibrinous material. It is only found in infants who have lived for at least 1 hour and the condition is rarely found in mature infants. Predisposing factors are antepartum haemorrhage, Caesarean section, maternal diabetes mellitus and severe rhesus immunisation. The aetiology is not fully understood but a most important factor is a deficiency of surfactant which reduces surface tension within the alveoli, facilitates expansion during inspiration and prevents atelectasis during expiration. It is synthesised in cells known as type II pneumonocytes and stored in osmiophilic lamellar bodies within these cells. Surfactant synthesis is inhibited by acidosis, hypothermia and hypoxia. There is a marked increase in surfactant production in the fetal lung at 32–43 weeks gestation although the stimulus for this is unclear. Its release from the pneumonocytes comes about by the fusion of the lamellar bodies' membranes within the cell membrane. Surfactant production may be expedited in the fetal lung by administration of betamethasone to the mother before delivery.

Clinical features

The infant who develops RDS has usually been in poor condition at birth with a low Apgar score. Tachypnoea (over 50 per minute) which persists for longer than 2 hours after birth is a simple and significant observation which almost invariably heralds some form of pulmonary insufficiency. Within a few hours there is inspiratory retraction of the subcostal margin, sternum and intercostal spaces. Expiratory grunting is associated with violent inspiratory efforts, but breath sounds are greatly diminished. The respiratory rate increases to 75 per minute or greater. Muscle hypotonicity causes the infant to lie with thighs widely abducted and knees flexed while the arms are flexed at the elbows and the hands are held in supination alongside the head. Greyish cyanosis may be present and oedema often becomes severe during the first 12 hours. Spells of apnoea occur with increasing frequency in deteriorating infants. Radiographs show a characteristic granular mottling. As this becomes more confluent the bronchial tree stands out clearly as an "air bronchogram" (Fig. 1.17). Severe respiratory acidosis and metabolic acidosis may result and the arterial PO_2 is reduced. Serum potassium concentrations increase and may be associated with ECG changes such as widening of P-R and QRS, prolongation of Q-T and left ventricular preponderance. The kidneys, unable to conserve base because of an inability to excrete phosphate, permit the bicarbonate concentrations in the plasma to decrease. Increased catabolism releases excess potassium, nitrogen, and phosphorus from damaged cells.

Treatment

The aim of treatment is to maintain the infant's tissue oxygenation until spontaneous recovery takes place and the type II alveolus cells begin to synthesise surfactant. The best outcome for infants with RDS is obtained in regional intensive care units with a major expertise in neonatal medicine. The problems of treatment may be considered under several categories:

1 temperature control;
2 feeding with fluid and electrolyte balance;
3 acid-base homeostasis;
4 oxygenation and respiratory support;
5 drug therapy.

It is also necessary to stress that in these very ill infants handling and intervention procedures must be kept to a minimum.

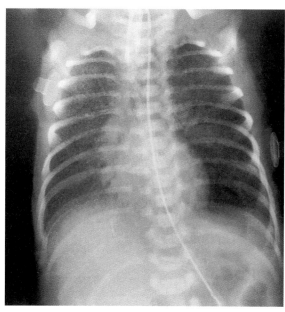
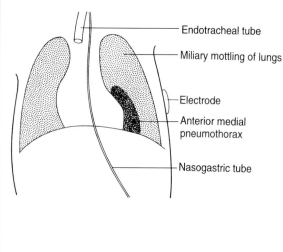

- Endotracheal tube
- Miliary mottling of lungs
- Electrode
- Anterior medial pneumothorax
- Nasogastric tube

FIGURE 1.17 Idiopathic respiratory distress syndrome. Preterm baby showing miliary mottling of the lung fields with an air bronchogram. An endotracheal tube is *in situ* and there is a small anterior pneumothorax immediately adjacent to the left heart border.

Temperature control

Temperature control should be achieved by placing the infant in an incubator, preferably equipped with servo control. Skin temperature should be kept within 36–37 °C. Accurate temperature control is imperative to conserve the infant's utilisation of oxygen.

Feeding

Feeding is a major concern because of the dangers of aspiration, the frequent development of paralytic ileus, and the fact that any handling, such as the passing of a nasogastric tube, is liable to cause sudden hypoxia. Calories can be supplied by parenteral nutrients given through peripheral veins or umbilical arterial catheters. It is important to avoid overhydration which may encourage persistence of the ductus arteriosus or the development of necrotising enterocolitis. A degree of intravenous fluid restriction may be necessary in the first few days but a balance between this and the damage caused by undernutrition must be weighed. When necessary, surgical closure of the ductus will allow adequate nutrition and fluid intake to be given. Plasma electrolytes should be assessed daily and any electrolyte disorders corrected with appropriate supplements. Provided there is no abdominal distension and meconium has been passed, nasogastric or nasojejunal milk feeding may be introduced after the

first 24 hours. When the infant cannot tolerate enteral feeding, total or partial parenteral feeding with amino acids, glucose, lipids, minerals and vitamins may be given although this procedure carries its own risks.

Acid–base homoeostasis

Occasionally intravenous sodium bicarbonate may be required to correct base deficits. The quantity given may be calculated from the formula: base excess in mmol/l × body weight in kg × 0.35. It can be administered as 8.4% solution (1 ml = 1 mmol) into a central vein at a rate not to exceed 0.5 mmol/min.

Oxygenation and respiratory support

Oxygenation and respiratory support constitute a top priority of treatment. Periodic sampling of aortic blood through an umbilical artery catheter for measurement of Pao_2 may not reflect the Pao_2 in vessels supplying the brain and retinae if there is right-to-left shunting through a patent ductus arteriosus. Samples obtained by puncture of a radial artery will obviate this problem but the necessary handling of the infant may result in undesirable fluctuations in the Pao_2. $TcPo_2$ can be measured but the electrode has to be repositioned every 6 hours. The problems of transcutaneous saturation measurements have already been considered.

The objective in treatment is to maintain the PaO_2 above 50 mmHg (7.0 kPa) and below 90 mmHg (12.0 kPa). Swings above 120 mmHg (16.0 kPa) are associated with an increased risk of retrolental fibroplasia but they can be extremely difficult to prevent. In addition to monitoring PaO_2 it is, of course, essential that the oxygen concentration in the incubator is measured with a suitable, preferably continuous recording, analyser. While a satisfactory PaO_2 concentration can be achieved in mild cases with an oxygen concentration of 35–40%, in severe cases much greater oxygen concentrations are required. This will necessitate enclosure of the infant's head in a plastic hood when the oxygen flow should pass through a nebuliser and be warmed to 30–33 °C. In the most severely affected infants, particularly those below 1500 g, the regimen described above proves inadequate. They are characterized by PaO_2 values < 50 mmHg (7.0 kPa) in 90% oxygen, $PaCO_2$ values which increase to 70 mmHg (9.3 kPa) or higher and attacks of apnoea with marked bradycardia. In such infants intermittent positive-pressure ventilation (IPPV) is life saving. It is, however, not free from risks such as pneumothorax and pneumomediastinum, pulmonary interstitial emphysema, lung sepsis and the later development of chronic pulmonary disease (bronchopulmonary dysplasia). There are a variety of techniques of IPPV and different types of ventilators have their protagonists. Peak inspiratory pressures should be kept as low as possible consistent with satisfactory PaO_2 values. Peak inspiratory pressures rarely should exceed 26 cmH_2O or the rate 30 per minute. It is an advantage if the ventilator has the facility for providing intermittent mandatory ventilation (IMV) whereby inspiratory pulses are superimposed 5–20 times/min on a continuous gas flow and 2–5 cmH_2O of positive airways pressure. This technique is helpful in weaning infants off IPPV by allowing them to start some spontaneous respiration for themselves. Continuing positive airways pressure (CPAP) may be delivered to the infant airways through a face mask or by placing the infant in a negative pressure chamber, or by the use of nasal prongs. While CPAP has not been proved to increase the survival rate, it does increase the PaO_2 and reduce the need for IPPV. It has its greatest application in infants less than 1500 g but to be effective it must be instituted early in the course of the illness. Suitable indication for use is where the inspired oxygen concentration has to be increased above 60% to achieve a PaO_2 of 60 mmHg (8.0 kPa). Transpulmonary pressures of about 6 cmH_2O should be used initially, and sufficient oxygen administered in the inspired air to give a PaO_2 above 60 mmHg (8.0 kPa). As in the case of IPPV, CPAP is not without its hazards, such as pneumothorax and even with its use IPPV will still be unavoidable in at least half of the infants.

Drugs

Surfactant materials extracted from animal lungs and from human amniotic fluid or synthesised in the laboratory have been found of value in prophylaxis and in the treatment of RDS. Surfactant is instilled into the lungs via the endotracheal tube. It has been shown to benefit infants of less than 30 weeks gestation when used prophylactally and has significantly improved the outcome when used therapeutically. Trials are still ongoing to determine the most cost-effective material and dosage. Current evidence suggests that calf lung surfactant (CLSE), human surfactant, artificial lung expanding compound (ALEC-pumactant; Britannia Pharmaceuticals and Exosurf; Wellcome) are the best prophylactic materials and that porcine surfactant (Curosurf; Chiesi) is the most effective in the rescue or therapeutic situation.

Apart from surfactant, drug therapies have limited but controversial roles in RDS. This applies, for example, to the routine prophylactic use of antibiotics. In view of the difficulty which may be experienced in differentiating early onset Group B streptococcal sepsis from RDS the routine administration of penicillin is probably justified. Furthermore, as Gram-negative bacteria and penicillin-resistant staphylococci may also produce rapidly fatal illness, in these immature preterm infants we recommend the addition of an aminoglycoside or third generation cephalosporin. Tolazoline has been used because of its ability to dilate pulmonary arteries but a careful watch much be kept for systemic hypotension. It has been recommended in cases of RDS where there is persistence of the fetal circulation with right-to-left shunting through the ductus arteriosus and foramen ovale due to severe pulmonary hypertension. It has been said that tolazoline is most effective where the PaO_2 is low despite IPPV and high oxygen concentrations whilst the $PaCO_2$ remains normal or low. However, the role of tolazoline and other drugs such as sodium nitroprusside, prostacyclin (PGI_2) and nitric oxide (NO) has yet to be established in RDS. Pancuronium bromide, a non-polarising muscle paralysant, has been shown to improve oxygenation in mechanically ventilated infants but does add additional risks to the treatment regimen and predisposes to limb and trunk oedema which may produce further respiratory and circulatory embarrassment.

PATENT DUCTUS ARTERIOSUS (PDA)

There is often delay in spontaneous closure of the ductus in preterm infants, particularly VLBW infants. This is more likely in the presence of RDS in the presence of fluid overload. Patent ductus becomes clinically obvious, usually in the second week, when the peripheral pulses become collapsing in type and a systolic or continuous murmur can be heard at the base of the heart. Cardiac failure commonly develops with radiographic signs of cardiomegaly and pulmonary oedema. The size of the shunt can best be assessed by echocardiography.

In addition to restricting fluid intake to less than 100 ml/kg per 24 hours frusemide 2 mg/kg may be given intravenously. Indomethacin, which is an inhibitor of prostaglandin synthetase, has been used to close the ductus. Its use is based upon the finding that prostaglandin E_1 relaxes the ductus arteriosus, tending to keep it open. It should not be prescribed if there is any evidence of a bleeding tendency, thrombocytopenia or if the plasma bilirubin concentration is > 180 μmol/l (10.5 mg/100 ml). Indomethacin dissolved in phosphate buffer (0.2 M) at pH 7.2 in a concentration of 1 mg/ml may be given either orally or rectally. Closure rates with intravenous administration are, however, consistently greater. Dosage varies from 0.2 to 0.3 mg/kg given on up to three occasions at intervals of 12 hours. There is some evidence that the earlier indomethacin is commenced the better the chance of closure of the ductus and it is seldom effective if used later than 2 weeks after birth. If this treatment fails and cardiac failure persists the ductus should be closed surgically.

INTRAVENTRICULAR HAEMORRHAGE (IVH)

Spontaneous bleeding into one or both lateral ventricles is a not infrequent complication of the preterm infant, particularly the infant who develops RDS. The development of computer-assisted axial tomography (CAT scanning) and scanning by real-time ultrasound have made accurate diagnosis of IVH possible during life. In infants < 1500 g more than 40% suffer a degree of IVH. Whilst large IV haemorrhages are likely to prove fatal, real-time ultrasound has shown that smaller haemorrhages into the germinal layer or ventricles are frequently compatible with survival. Some survivors develop post-haemorrhagic hydrocephalus, porencephalic cysts or neurodevelopmental handicaps but others appear to progress quite normally.

In an infant less than 33 weeks gestation, bleeding may start in the germinal layer which lies just under the ependyma in the roof of the lateral ventricles. Haemorrhage may be confined to the germinal layer (GLH) or it may rupture into the ventricle (IVH). In some infants the haemorrhage disrupts the substance of the brain. The microvasculature of the germinal layer consists of an extensive arrangement of fine capillaries and also of large, irregular thin-walled vessels which form short connecting channels between the arterial and venous trees. These vessels readily rupture when exposed to sudden surges in pressure which can be provoked by hypoxaemia and hypercapnia. On the other hand, hyperoxaemia and hypocapnia can cause abrupt falls in cerebral blood flow so that in some instances ischaemia in the subependymal layer results in infarction and cerebral atrophy. The germinal layer involutes from 32 weeks gestation and it is presumed that IVH in older infants of > 2000 g then arises in the choroid plexus. CAT scanning and real-time ultrasound reveals the frequency with which GLH and IVH develop in preterm infants and shows that survival in 30–50% of affected children is possible. These techniques have also confirmed that IVH may occur within 6 hours of birth.

Clinical features

GLH and IVH can apparently remain asymptomatic and even when attacks of apnoea or convulsions occur they do not necessarily reflect the presence of haemorrhage. Deviant neurological signs have been shown to correlate with the appearance of GLH and IVH on sequential real-time ultrasound scans. A useful sign from 30 weeks gestation is inability to fix and follow (horizontally and vertically) a small red woollen ball at a distance of 6 inches. Another significant sign is an unduly tight popliteal angle for the length of gestation. Abnormal results would be a popliteal angle of $< 130°$ up to 31 weeks and $< 110°$ at 32–35 weeks. About 2 weeks after the onset of haemorrhage the presence of roving eye movements is strongly suggestive of cerebral damage. In the infant of 32–35 weeks gestation the development of hypotonia is significant, but this is less of a concern in the infant of < 32 weeks. The degree of haemorrhage observed on ultrasound scanning can be graded as follows: Grade 1, GLH; Grade 2, intraventricular haemorrhage; Grade 3, intraventricular haemorrhage with ventricular distension; Grade 4, haemorrhage into brain substance (Fig. 1.18).

RETINOPATHY OF PREMATURITY (ROP)

This name is now preferred to *retrolental fibroplasia* because it takes account of the important fact that some cases are arrested early, before advancing to blindness. The disease first appeared in the USA in 1942 and in the UK in 1946. These dates coincided with the widespread use of incubators in both countries and this aroused early suspicion that oxygen therapy might have aetiological importance. Experimental proof of the role of oxygen came from

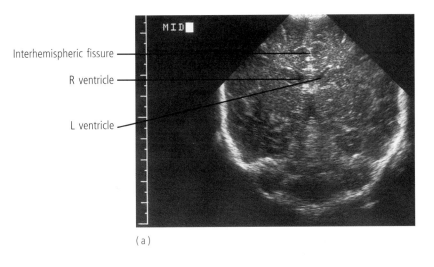

Interhemispheric fissure

R ventricle

L ventricle

(a)

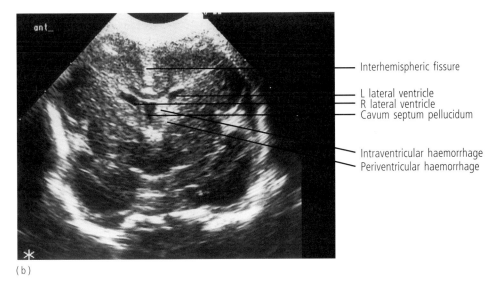

Interhemispheric fissure

L lateral ventricle
R lateral ventricle
Cavum septum pellucidum

Intraventricular haemorrhage
Periventricular haemorrhage

(b)

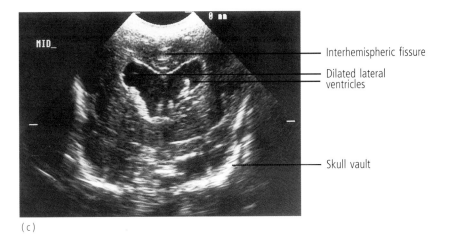

Interhemispheric fissure

Dilated lateral
ventricles

Skull vault

(c)

FIGURE 1.18 Cranial ultrasound. (a) Normal coronal scan. (b) Coronal scan showing increased echoes in floor of left lateral ventricle due to intracranial haemorrhage. (c) Coronal scan 2 weeks later showing dilatation of both lateral ventricles and resolving thrombus in the left ventricle.

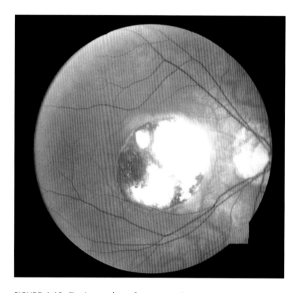

FIGURE 1.19 Retinopathy of prematurity.

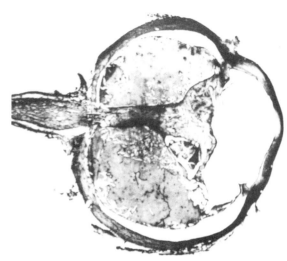

FIGURE 1.20 Fully established retrolental fibroplasia showing complete retinal detachment.

a series of observations on newborn kittens. While the kittens were exposed to high concentrations of oxygen the retinal vessels underwent intense vasoconstriction. On subsequent transfer to air these vessels showed gross vasodilatation followed by the proliferation of new vessels in a completely disordered fashion. In the human infant the same sequence of events is directly related to the degree of immaturity, the arterial oxygen tension and the duration of exposure.

Clinical features

This disorder is seen only in preterm infants. The acute stage is first seen between the ages of 3 and 6 weeks in the form of dilatation of retinal veins and arteries. This is followed by the growth, in a disorderly pattern, of new capillaries. Clusters of new capillaries may simulate haemorrhages. Subsequently, some of the new vessels begin to grow forwards into the vitreous towards the lens. Retinal oedema occurs and is followed by peripheral retinal detachment when the condition becomes irreversible (Fig. 1.19). In the cicatricial stage there may be complete retinal detachment, leaving only a stalk of rolled-up retina connected posteriorly around the optic disc (Fig. 1.20). Finally, there is a retrolental mass of fibrous tissue visible behind a clear lens with the naked eye. In severe cases the condition is bilateral with microphthalmos, a narrow anterior chamber, irregular small pupil and gross loss of vision. Squint is common and glaucoma frequent. There is also an increased incidence of learning disorder and cerebral palsy in these children.

Prevention

It is essential to prevent factors which predispose to ROP:

1 Oxygen concentrations in incubators must not be allowed to increase above 40% unless there is carefully monitoring of the arterial P_{O_2} at frequent intervals;
2 Oxygen should never be given in the absence of respiratory distress or cyanosis;
3 Administration of oxygen should not be continued a minute longer than necessary.

There is evidence that ROP which rapidly declined in incidence after discovery of the causal role of oxygen is again increasing. It is occurring particularly in infants weighing between 501 and 1500 g. It would seem that at present some degree of ROP is unavoidable in VLBW survivors. It is reasonable to examine routinely all infants weighing less than 1500 g or 34 weeks gestational age. Larger infants who have required prolonged oxygen therapy may also be worth careful examination. Proper examination by an ophthalmologist skilled in the examination after pupil dilatation is required. Results are recorded using an international classification. Those found to have significant ROP are reviewed every 1–2 weeks until regression occurs or the threshold for treatment is reached. Cryotherapy of peripheral avascular retina has been shown to be effective in reducing the progression of the retinopathy. This ablation of the ischaemic retina is thought to reduce the concentrations of angiogenic factors. Severe visual impairment in early infancy may also be due to damage to the visual cortex. Electrophysiological testing in such infants shows a normal electroretinogram but absent or abnormal visual evoked responses.

THE EARLY ANAEMIA OF PREMATURITY

This condition must be clearly differentiated from the hypochromic anaemia of iron deficiency to which the preterm infant is susceptible after the age of 4 months. The latter condition may be thought of as the "late anaemia of prematurity". Unlike the early anaemia of prematurity it can be prevented or cured with iron.

The Hb level at birth in venous blood of both term and preterm infants is high by adult standards (19–21 g/100 ml). In all infants there is a fairly rapid decrease during the early weeks of life. This is because the oxygen saturation of blood increases at birth from a fetal level of 65% to the normal adult value of 95%, when the lungs take over the supply of oxygen from the placenta. There is, in consequence, a decrease in the need for circulating haemoglobin and the bone marrow goes into a resting phase with relative erythropoietic inactivity. The decrease in red cell mass and circulating haemoglobin depends also on the infant's rate of growth. As preterm infants grow more rapidly than term in relative terms there is an exaggerated rate of fall in red cell mass and haemoglobin concentration. A value of 8 g/l00 ml is not uncommon at the age of 6–8 weeks. This early anaemia of prematurity is normochromic. Recovery tends to take place as the bone marrow responds to the low level of oxygenation in the tissues. However, as rapid growth also continues this spontaneous increase in haemoglobin concentration may be slow. It will be ill sustained unless adequate supplies of iron are made available from the age of 6–8 weeks.

Treatment

When the early anaemia of prematurity is aggravated by infection or haemorrhage blood transfusion is indicated. Treatment with erythropoietin has been shown to stimulate the marrow of preterm infants to produce more red cells and a higher haemoglobin concentration. Clinical trials are currently underway to assess the necessity and/or effectiveness of such therapy.

JAUNDICE OF PREMATURITY

There is an increased incidence of non-obstructive jaundice in preterm infants, particularly those who develop RDS. The pathogenesis of jaundice and its management are discussed subsequently.

INTRAUTERINE GROWTH RETARDATION

Approximately 30% of all infants weighing 2.5 kg or less at birth are light for dates. As has already been suggested there are many important causes of infants being light for gestation and small for gestation. Small for gestation infants include those with congenital abnormalities such as the trisomies, microcephaly, single umbilical artery, "bird-headed dwarfs" and congenital heart disease as well as infants who have acquired intrauterine infections such as rubella, cytomegalic inclusion disease, toxoplasmosis and syphilis. It is a feature of this group of infants that they have smaller head circumferences than other light for dates infants.

AETIOLOGY

Causes of slow intrauterine growth are shown in Table 1.14. When fetal growth retardation is detected from before 28 weeks by fetal ultrasound it is likely that at birth the infant's weight and body size (length and OFC) will be small for dates. Such small for dates (SFD) infants may have congenital abnormalities. The contrasting features of preterm appropriate for dates and light for dates malnourished infants are shown in Table 1.12. It has been suggested that if smoking, hypertension and pre-eclampsia could be eliminated the number of light for dates infants could be halved. The high levels of light for dates infants

TABLE 1.14 Causes of intrauterine growth failure

MATERNAL
  General
    Poor socio-economic conditions
      Malnutrition
      Heavy workload
      Unmarried
    Height: less than 155 cm
    Living at high altitudes
    Racial and constitutional
    History of previous light for dates infants
    Maternal metabolic disorder
  Obstetric
    Complications of pregnancy (e.g. pre-eclampsia)
    Poor placental function
    Alcohol consumption
    Smoking
    Poor antenatal care
    Parity first or third onwards
FETAL
    Multiple pregnancy
    Congenital abnormalities
    Chromosomal abnormality
    Congenital infection

in socially deprived inner city areas highlights a point for the introduction of preventive strategies.

Whatever may be the precise aetiology, the light for dates infant has poor energy reserves of glycogen in liver, heart and skeletal muscle whilst the growth of the brain and mature lungs contrast with the shrunken liver. In the normal newborn infant the brain is about three times heavier than the liver whereas in the light for dates infant the brain may be seven or eight times the weight of the liver. Pulmonary haemorrhage is a not uncommon postmortem finding in the severe growth restricted infant.

CLINICAL FEATURES

In intrauterine growth retardation the infant may be born term or preterm and the growth retardation in length and head circumference may be less than indicated by body weight. The infant looks thin and wasted; the skin is dry and desquamating and often shows transverse cracks over the lower chest and abdomen and at the ankles and wrists; meconium staining of nails and cord may be present; and there is commonly a characteristic wide-awake expression which is not seen in the preterm low birthweight infant. Appearances in general reflect a fairly long period of malnutrition or undernutrition *in utero*.

MANAGEMENT

The light for dates infant is usually eager to feed and oral feeds should be commenced between 2 and 4 hours after birth to reduce the dangers of hypoglycaemia. Blood glucose concentrations should be determined every few hours by testing capillary blood with an indicator stix test, e.g. Dextrostix (Ames & Co). True blood glucose measurements should be performed if a reading of < 2.5 mmol/l (45 mg/100 ml) is obtained on the stix test. Continued tachypnoea 1 or 2 hours after birth may indicate the presence of meconium aspiration and deep body temperatures should be carefully recorded and precautions taken to avoid hypothermia.

COMPLICATIONS OF INTRAUTERINE GROWTH RETARDATION

Meconium aspiration syndrome

Whereas RDS is common in the preterm infant the usual cause of respiratory difficulties in the light for dates infant is meconium aspiration. Meconium is intensely irritating to the bronchiolar epithelium. Radiographic appearances of the lung fields are quite different to those of RDS with more coarse streaking with varying degrees of collapse and emphysema. Treatment, however, is similar to that for RDS.

Transient symptomatic hypoglycaemia of the newborn

It is now clear that this dangerous condition occurs predominantly in male light for dates infants. If not promptly recognised and vigorously treated, permanent brain damage is a common sequel. The only complication of pregnancy known to increase the risk of spontaneous hypoglycaemia in the infant is preeclamptic toxaemia present in about half the cases. The pathogenesis is not yet clear although the extremely poor glycogen stores of the light for dates infant is an important factor. There may be an insufficiency of glucose available for the relatively large glucose-dependent brain and the metabolically active mature body.

Clinical features

The infant usually appears well for a period which may vary from 6 hours to 7 days after birth. Then various signs manifest themselves, such as jitteriness or twitchings, attacks of apnoea and cyanosis, pallor, reluctance to feed, limpness, apathy or generalised convulsions. When these manifestations occur in an infant showing the signs of intrauterine growth retardation the diagnosis of hypoglycaemia should be suspected and true blood glucose estimations arranged immediately. The diagnosis is confirmed when a blood glucose value of less than 1.1 mmol/l (20 mg/100 ml) is detected. Values below 2.2 mmol/l (40 mg/100 ml) should be used as the indication for increased glucose intake.

Treatment

An intravenous injection of 15% glucose in water, 2 ml/kg body weight, should be given immediately followed thereafter by continuous infusion of 10% glucose in water, 60–75 ml/kg/day. Oral feeds where tolerated should be increased to tolerance. If the intravenous 10% dextrose has to be given for longer than 24 hours then it should be combined in quarter-strength physiological saline to prevent hyponatraemia. Occasionally it may be necessary to use cortico-steroids such as oral hydrocortisone (5 mg/kg/day) or ACTH (4 units/kg/day) in resistant cases. In some instances plasma calcium concentrations below 2 mmol/l (8 mg/100 ml) may be found in which case the intravenous infusion of 3–5 ml of 10% calcium gluconate should be given by slow intravenous injection. Long-term follow-up of such infants to assess development is essential.

It is common practice to monitor blood glucose values of all post-term and light for dates infants at 6-hourly intervals with one of the glucose test strip methods. This regimen will reveal a number of infants with blood glucose values below 1.1 mmol/l (20 mg/100 ml) who are asymptomatic. It is important as stated earlier to increase glucose intake in any infant with blood glucose valuess below 2.2 mmol/l (40 mg/100 ml). Glucose test strip screening of newborn infants may also reveal some pre-symptomatic cases of hypoglycaemia in infants with severe perinatal asphyxia, intracranial haemorrhage, haemolytic disease of the newborn and in the infants of diabetic mothers. Such infants are managed in the same way.

Temporary neonatal diabetes mellitus

This is a rare but fascinating complication of intrauterine growth retardation. It has also been called "transient idiopathic hyperglycaemia of the newborn".

NEONATAL INFECTIONS

Infections may be acquired prenatally, perinatally or postnatally. Development of intensive anti-infection measures has greatly reduced both mortality and morbidity from neonatal infections in developed countries during recent years. None the less there are still significant numbers of deaths and handicaps resulting from such infections. Antibiotic resistance has assumed major importance and a more critical approach to their use is necessary.

PRENATAL INFECTIONS

During pregnancy infecting organisms pass from the maternal circulation to the intervillous spaces of the placenta and penetrate the fetal circulation. Viruses known to cross the placenta include rubella, poliomyelitis, Coxsackie, variola, herpes, varicella zoster, human immunodeficiency virus and cytomegalovirus. Some of these such as rubella produce early damage to the developing embryo, others such as cytomegalovirus or Coxsackie produce late effects such as hepatitis or myocarditis in the newborn infant. Fetal damage from maternal viral infection during very early pregnancy can be severe. Many pregnancies abort but other fetuses survive with a continuing viraemia which may indeed persist for 2 years or more after birth. It is recommended that all children, boys and girls are immunised against rubella at the age of 15 months with a combined mumps, measles, rubella immunisation in an attempt to eradicate the severe damage of congenital rubella. A surviving fetus may have congenital heart defects, deafness, cataracts and where the maternal infection is contracted later in pregnancy may present with purpura (mulberry muffin spots), thrombocytopenia, hepatosplenomegaly and have radiological evidence of an osteitis. Damage to the brain may result in severe learning difficulties. Eighty-five per cent of infants affected during the first 8 weeks of pregnancy will have multiple defects whereas 15% of infants affected in mid-pregnancy may present with sensorineural deafness alone. Infections in later pregnancy appear to carry less risk of damage to the fetus.

Suspected rubella in a mother during pregnancy is an indication for testing maternal serum for haemaglutinin inhibition antibodies (HI). If the antibody concentration is increased within the incubation period of rubella the mother can be considered protected by previous infection or immunisation. If low titres are obtained a repeat serum sample should be obtained 2–3 weeks after first exposure. An increased titre confirms primary infection and a high risk of fetal damage which may be an indication for termination of pregnancy. After birth the finding of specific rubella IgM antibody in the blood or rubella virus in the urine will confirm the diagnosis.

Cytomegalovirus (CMV) is now the commonest congenital infection in the UK. Approximately 50% of pregnant women have antibodies to CMV and it is estimated that between 1 and 5% of pregnant women contract CMV infections with fetal involvement in about 50% of infected pregnancies. Mothers are usually asymptomatic and in most instances the infant appears normal. In severe infections the infant may be acutely ill, small for gestational age, have signs of meningoencephalitis, jaundice, petechiae, hepatosplenomegaly and feeding difficulties. The virus may be cultured from urine, upper respiratory tract secretions and cerebrospinal fluid. In milder cases in which there may be no clinical evidence of the disease there can be late sequelae such as mental handicap, epilepsy and nerve deafness. Approximately 5% of infected infants have clinical signs at birth and most of these infants will have long-term sequelae. A further 5% will develop severe handicaps particularly deafness later in life. Presence of virus in the urine with raised CMV-specific IgM antibody in the blood confirms the diagnosis. There is no value in routine screening for CMV in pregnancy. Termination cannot be justified on the basis of fetal infection as 90% of infants will be unaffected. Also fetal infections can occur after primary or secondary CMV infections in pregnancy and fetal damage can occur from infection occurring at any time in pregnancy.

Human immunodeficiency virus (HIV) may be transmitted to the infant before, during or after birth. Maternal antibodies may persist in the infant for up to 18 months of age and neonatal diagnosis is difficult in asymptomatic infants. There are varying estimates of the percentage of infected infants born to HIV positive mothers and these vary between 15 and 35%. Non-attributable screening programmes on Guthrie cards for the presence of HIV antibodies puts the prevalence in Scotland at 0.3 per 1000 deliveries. With the spread of the virus into the heterosexual population a high index of suspicion and care in handling blood from mothers and newborn infants is necessary. Some infants progress rapidly to full blown AIDS and develop serious opportunistic infections during the first year of life whilst others may show features such as persistent lymphadenopathy, hepatosplenomegaly, chronic diarrhoea, unexplained fevers and failure to thrive. Postnatal infection may occur via the breast milk and in developed countries it is probably best to persuade known HIV positive mothers to avoid breast feeding. In developing countries the other risks associated with artificial feeding probably outweigh the risks of the infant acquiring HIV infection from the mother.

Maternal herpes varicella zoster infection in early pregnancy rarely affects the fetus but when it does there can be extensive scarring skin lesions, choroidoretinitis, cataracts and damage to the brain. When the mother develops the chicken pox between 4 days before and 4 days after delivery neonatal mortality from pneumonia can be high. This is because there is no time for protective transplacental antibodies to be acquired by the fetus. Infants born to a mother who develops chicken pox at this late stage should be given passive immunisation with zoster immune globulin as soon as possible after birth. Acyclovir may be given to infants showing clinical features of infection and any mother developing a perinatal rash should be isolated with barrier nursing of the infant and avoidance of breast feeding until skin lesions have resolved.

Other viral infections such as coxsackie, ECHO, myxo, parvo, and hepatitis B are amongst the viruses to be considered when meningoencephalitis, hepatitis, myocarditis, fetal oedema or hydrops, pneumonias, diarrhoea, jaundice and cataract are unexplained. Neonatal hepatitis B (HB) infections are more common in some populations than others, but world wide they are a major public health problem. Neonatal liver disease due to HB viraemia is very variable and can present as fulminant hepatic necrosis, chronic persistent hepatitis, mild focal necrosis or

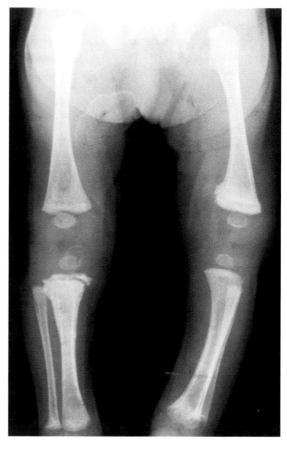

FIGURE 1.21 Radiograph of legs of syphilitic infant showing osteitis, osteochondritis and periostitis.

may be asymptomatic. Portal hypertension and primary liver cancers are later complications. The infant is most at risk when the mother has acute HB hepatitis during the third trimester and at delivery. Chronic HB surface antigen (HBsAg) positive carrier mothers, particularly if they are also HBeAg positive, HBe antibody negative or have high serum HBcAb values are highly infective to their infants. In endemic areas, infants act as carriers and excreters of the virus. Protective immunisation of susceptible women of childbearing age and of infants within 48 hours of birth, particularly infants born to carrier mothers, should be instituted in populations or sub-populations with high rates of HB virus infection.

Congenital syphilis can present in the newborn with hepatomyaly, splenomegaly, anaemia, thrombocytopenia, jaundice and oedema. There may be characteristic bone changes on X-ray (Fig. 1.21). After 3–4 weeks a maculopapular skin rash with mucocutaneous lesions, snuffles and pseudo-paralysis may develop. Most newborn infants with congenital syphilis remain well and there may be no manifestation of disease for several weeks when jaundice,

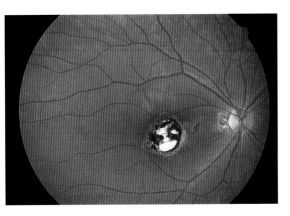

FIGURE 1.22 Toxoplasma – choroidoretinitis.

anaemia, hepatosplenomegaly, oedema and signs of meningitis may develop. Adequate treatment of mothers with secondary syphilis detected by routine serological testing should reduce the incidence of congenital syphilis. Prompt treatment of affected infants with penicillin is indicated if there is clinical or radiological evidence of the disease or if cord blood serology is positive and the mother has not been adequately treated. If there is uncertainty about the presence of infection the infant should be given protective penicillin therapy and quantitive serological measurements and physical examinations made at monthly intervals. Infants with congenital syphilis require lumbar puncture and abnormal CSF is an indication to give crystalline penicillin G 50 000 units/kg by intramuscular or intravenous injection daily in two divided doses for a minimum of 10 days. Infants with normal cerebrospinal fluid should be given benzathine penicillin G 50 000 units/kg by intramuscular injection in a single dose.

Toxoplasma gondii is a protozoan transmitted to the fetus from the placenta *in utero* and is associated with intrauterine growth retardation, cerebral haemorrhage and microcephaly or hydrocephaly, intracranial calcification, choroidoretinitis (Fig. 1.22), microphthalmia, thrombocytopenia and jaundice (see Chapter 7). A combination of pyrimethamine given orally in a dose of 0.5 mg/kg twice daily and sulphadiazine given orally in a dose of 100 mg/kg/day is recommended for 3–4 weeks. Spiramycin is also reported to be effective. The organism may be cultured and the diagnosis confirmed by the indirect fluorescent antibody test in the maternal and infant serum. In the UK about 20% of women have toxoplasma antibodies and only a small percentage of women contract infection during the first trimester. The infection may be contracted by the ingestion of undercooked meat or from cat faeces. Pregnant women should avoid dealing with cat excreta.

The malarial protozoan plasmodium in many parts of the world is a major cause of fetal damage. Congenital malaria is rare except in non-immune mothers who during pregnancy have received inadequate protection or none. The degree of immunity to malaria possessed by an infant at birth is directly related to that of the mother, so that in spite of heavy or passive parasitisation of the placenta found in highly immune indigenous dwellers of endemic areas, the incidence of congenital malaria is rare. When it does occur fever, convulsions and severe haemolytic anaemia with jaundice, hepatosplenomegaly and brain damage with a high mortality are the result. In the partially immune child less severe infections occur and present with signs similar to that of bacterial septicaemia. In endemic areas transfused blood may be an important source of acquired infection in the newborn, which should be treated with a full therapeutic course of chloroquine or other relevant antimalarial drug for that area. Treatment of the infected newborn is usually with chloroquine 5 ml/kg by injection or 75 mg chloroquine base orally followed by 37.5 mg twice daily for 2 days (see Chapter 20).

Maternal infections with *Listeria monocytogenes*, a Gram-positive bacteria, may cause preterm labour or transplacental fetal infection. This organism has flourished in undercooked chicken and "cook-chill" foods, unpasteurised milk and soft cheeses, causing a mild flu-like illness in the mother. After birth the infant may present with pneumonia, meningitis, septicaemia and a skin rash. The amniotic fluid has characteristically an offensive smell and there is a 30% mortality. Infection can be acquired during delivery and there may be a later presentation with septicaemia and meningitis. Treatment with ampicillin and gentamicin of the mother and affected newborn is indicated.

PERINATAL INFECTIONS

Infection acquired during the birth process or after rupture of the membranes is not uncommon. Premature membrane rupture before or during labour together with a long interval before delivery are important predisposing factors to the development of placentitis and infection of the amniotic fluid. Infection may also occur with intact membranes during prolonged labours especially when there has been excessive manipulation or sources of contamination. The fetus may inhale infected amniotic fluid, resulting in a congenital pneumonia. Alternatively infection may spread from an infected placenta to the fetal circulation, causing septicaemia. Infection of the eyes, for example, by gonococcus during delivery was once a major cause of blindness in childhood in the UK but is now rare. Unfortunately it persists in many parts of the world as a major cause of blindness. Frequent irrigation of the conjunctivae with antibiotic eye drops, together with a course of systemic penicillin is recommended. Some organisms are resistant to penicillin and a broad spectrum antibiotic is required. The maternal vulva and cervix may be infected with *Chlamydia trachomatis* and this may be a cause of conjunctivitis and, more rarely, neonatal pneumonia in the newborn. Chlamydial pneumonitis may present 4–6 weeks after birth and is best treated with systemic erythromycin.

One of the most worrying organisms presently affecting newborn infants is the Group B streptococcus which can produce severe fulminating pneumonia and septicaemia, resulting in the death of infants within hours of birth. The clinical presentation is similar to that of the idiopathic respiratory distress syndrome, and as it is more common in preterm low birthweight infants, a high index of suspicion for infection should be maintained. If there is any doubt the infant and mother should have bacteriological cultures of blood and vulva respectively taken and the infant treated with high dosage penicillin.

Herpesvirus type II infection may be transmitted to the fetus from a maternal cervicitis. The fetus may be aborted or there may be preterm delivery of the infant. The risk to the fetus is greatest if the maternal cervical lesion is primary rather than a reactivation lesion. Neonatal disease does not usually present until about a week after birth when there may be vesicular skin lesions, hepatosplenomegaly, jaundice, petechia, encephalopathy and seizures associated with the generalised viraemia. Choroidoretinitis or cataract may be found at a later stage. Herpesvirus antigen may be detected in fluid from blisters and treatment with intravenous acyclovir should be commenced immediately.

POSTNATAL INFECTIONS

Whilst intrapartum infection is an important cause of perinatal mortality most fatal infections occur after birth. There has been a considerable change in the relative importance of different types of infection in hospital nurseries over the past 50 years. Puerperal fever with Group A β-haemolytic streptococcus caused severe morbidity in both mothers and infants together with epidemics of gastroenteritis probably mainly bacterial in origin were major problems in the 1940s. Infections with the coagulase-positive *Staphylococcus aureus* resistant to antibiotics such as benzylpenicillin, tetracycline, streptomycin and erythromycin then made their appearance. The staphylococcus could cause sudden outbreaks of severe sepsis and particular phage types e.g. 80/81 caused major problems of pneumonia, osteitis and

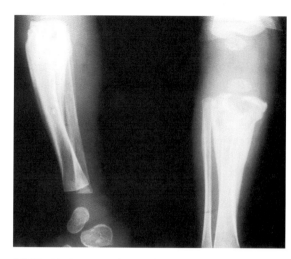

FIGURE 1.23 Osteitis in femur of young infant showing extensive destruction of bone and periostitis.

pyaemia (Fig. 1.23). In addition there were problems of septic spots, paronychiae, conjunctivitis and umbilical sepsis. The marked fall in the incidence of staphylcoccal lesions in newborn nurseries from the mid 1960s was related to improved standards of hand care and the introduction of hexachlorophane for skin cleansing. Although this seemed to help control the problems of the *Staphylococcus aureus* the Gram-negative bacilli, particularly *Escherichia coli*, *Proteus* and *Klebsiella* entered the arena. More recently the Group B streptococcus has colonised mothers and infants, causing severe problems in the preterm.

DIAGNOSIS

The diagnosis of infection during the neonatal period can be extremely difficult. Localising signs are frequently absent and the primary portal of entry is often not obvious. In fact the infection may so quickly become a generalised septicaemia or pyaemia as a result of the poor local resistance of the newborn tissues to micro-organisms that a "local diagnosis" has little relevance. Often the first indication in the term infant is a reluctance to finish feeds, vomiting, undue drowsiness sometimes alternating with excessive irritibility, or a rise in the respiratory rate which may rapidly progress to dyspnoea. A sudden weight loss in an infant who has been progressing satisfactorily is significant. The infant may develop a characteristic greyish pallor and anxious face. Diarrhoea is not uncommon. Oedema, jaundice, purpura and other haemorrhages, together with convulsions indicate severe sepsis. Hepatosplenomegaly is common in septicaemias. Fever may or may not be present. In preterm infants hypothermia and sclerema are frequent concomitants of an infective process. The appearance of any of these manifestations should indicate the need for careful physical examination and relevant laboratory investigations. These may include urine analysis, blood culture, white cell count, C-reactive protein, lumbar puncture and radiography. They should precede treatment and there should be no delay in instituting the investigations and giving "best guess" therapy.

MAJOR INFECTIONS

PNEUMONIA IN THE NEWBORN

In many parts of the world pneumonia is the most commonly fatal infection of the newborn period.

Congenital (intrauterine) pneumonia

Congenital (intrauterine) pneumonia is often mistaken for asphyxia, respiratory distress syndrome or intracranial haemorrhage. Accurate diagnosis may be difficult because the affected infant is often apnoeic at birth and later shows the same type of grunting respiration with subcostal and sternal recession, and cyanosis as seen in IRDS. Pneumonia, however, is equally common in mature and preterm infants and should always be suspected when more than 24 hours have elapsed between rupture of the membranes and delivery, particularly if the mother is febrile. The chest radiograph shows softer and more confluent opacities than in IRDS. Clinical signs over the lungs are usually few and unhelpful. Air entry may be poor and crepitations may be heard.

Treatment

Treatment with oxygen and intravenous antibiotics appropriate to the knowledge of the maternal microbiology and to the currently problematic microorganisms in the nursery environment should be given. One combination which gives wide spectral cover is benzylpenicillin 100 000 units 6-hourly with gentamicin (7.5 mg/kg/day) in two 12-hourly doses. In other nurseries the introduction of a third generation cephalosporin would be appropriate. This treatment will cover Group B haemolytic streptococci but occasionally organisms such as the *Enterobacter cloacae* resistant to cephalosporins emerge so that regular microbiological determination of organism sensitivities in each neonatal nursery must be performed.

Staphylococcal pneumonia

Staphylococcal pneumonia is common in many neonatal nurseries throughout the world and may follow minor staphylococcal lesions such as paronychiae. The staphylococcus produces massive lung consolidation in many infants and this may proceed to abscess formation, empyema or pyopneumothorax. The onset is sudden with listlessness, dyspnoea, reluctance to feed and sometimes cyanosis. Coughing may be a feature but, when spasmodic and distressing, the possibility of cystic fibrosis should be considered. Physical signs with dullness to percussion, diminished or bronchial breath sounds and numerous crepitations may be found in staphylococcal pneumonia. Empyema produces marked dullness and displacement of heart to the opposite side. Tension pneumothorax associated with severe respiratory difficulties may need emergency thoracocentesis. The initial X-rays may show a homogeneous opacity and subsequently emphysematous bullae (pneumatoceles) can be visualised, an appearance which is almost diagnostic of staphylococcal pneumonia (see Fig. 6.11). Metastatic abscesses may develop in brain, kidneys, liver and bones. Methicillin-resistant *Staphylococcus aureus* (MRSA) strains have come about through indiscriminate antibiotic therapy and occasionally neonatal wards have had to be closed because of an epidemic.

Treatment

In addition to oxygen, intravenous infusion of flucloxacillin 25 mg/kg initially reducing to 12.5 mg/kg four times daily should be given.

Streptococcal pneumonia

Streptococcal pneumonia due to the Group B streptococcus has already been discussed. In addition to the characteristic features of respiratory distress, cyanosis and lethargy there may be either fever or hypothermia. In some infants there are signs of disseminated intravascular coagulation with thrombocytopenia, diminished plasma fibrinogen and raised serum fibrin degradation products. Both clinical features and radiographic appearance may closely mimic IRDS although in most cases the lung fields show coarser mottlings. Blood cultures will usually yield a positive result.

Treatment

The drug of choice is benzylpenicillin given intravenously but until culture results confirm the streptococcal origin of the respiratory problem it is wise to add gentamicin.

Other pneumonias

Other pneumonias which occur less commonly are caused by organisms including pneumococci, Group A β-haemolytic streptococci or *Haemophilus influenzae* as in older infants, but in the newborn, organisms not usually associated with pneumonia may infect lung tissue, e.g. *Escherichia coli*, enterococci, *Enterobacter*, *Proteus*, *Pseudomonas* and *Chlamydia*.

EPIDEMIC DIARRHOEA OF THE NEWBORN

This name for infantile gastroenteritis stresses the fact that in neonatal nurseries the disease tends to occur in explosive epidemics which may have considerable mortality. Such outbreaks are reported less frequently in the UK in recent years and may reflect improved standards of care in newborn nurseries. It is important, however, to safeguard against the introduction of the *E. coli* with specific serotypes classified by their somatic (O) antigens. The most common are *E. coli* O.111; O.55; O.26; O.119; and O.128. Outbreaks due to *Salmonella* group organisms are still seen. However, the most common aetiological agent in most neonatal nurseries today is the rotavirus.

Clinical features

The illness may vary from a mild upset with lethargy, anorexia, slight loss of weight and loose stools to a fulminating outburst of severe diarrhoea and vomiting. In cases due to rotavirus there may be associated respiratory signs such as nasal discharge or inflamed tympanic membranes. The stools are large, fluid, green or orange coloured and losses of body water and electrolytes may be massive with resultant diminution in plasma volume. A severe metabolic acidosis may arise from the considerable losses of sodium and potassium, with renal failure due to the diminished blood flow through the kidneys. Within a few hours of the onset the infant may have developed the classical picture of severe dehydration with sunken eyes, depressed fontanelle, overriding sutures, scaphoid abdomen, glazed corneae and semi-coma. The extremities, lips and ears may be cold and cyanosed due to peripheral circulatory failure.

Treatment

Oral feeds should be discontinued and replaced with an oral rehydration fluid, although there is room for controversy as to its composition. Suitable solutions are the BPC sodium chloride and dextrose oral powder compound, small size, to be dissolved in 200 ml of water (per litre: Na 35 mmol, K 20 mmol, HCO3, 18 mmol, dextrose 200 mmol); or Dextrolyte® (ready-to-feed) (per litre: Na 35 mmol, K 13 mmol, lactate 18 mmol, dextrose 200 mmol). The rehydration fluid should be given in small quantities every 1–2 hours (180 ml/kg/day). However, if the dehydration or vomiting is severe, fluid and electrolytes must be given by continuous intravenous infusion for 24–72 hours. A suitable fluid is 4% dextrose in sodium chloride 0.18% (120–150 ml/kg/day). If there is evidence of peripheral circulatory collapse, plasma diluted with equal parts of 10% dextrose in water can be given directly by syringe (30 ml/kg). Severe acidosis may require correction by slow intravenous infusion of 8.4% sodium bicarbonate under careful biochemical control. This is not often required and it is safer to restore the pH to no greater than 7.25 in the first instance. After 24–48 hours, milk feeds are re-started and gradually increased, the electrolyte fluids being correspondingly reduced. If potassium deficit is revealed by hypokalaemia after dehydration has been corrected potassium chloride may be given orally (1 g twice daily) or intravenously (20 mmol/l). Antibiotics are of no value, even when the cause is bacterial, and drugs of all kinds should be avoided.

PYOGENIC MENINGITIS

This grave infection of the newborn is most commonly due to Group B streptococcus or *E. coli*. Other organisms which might be involved include *Salmonella*, *Listeria*, pneumococci and staphylococci.

Clinical features

The onset is insidious with loss of weight, drowsiness, reluctance to feed and vomiting. Convulsive twitchings are frequently seen. Significant signs are a bulging anterior fontanelle and head retraction. Nuchal rigidity and Kernig's sign do not occur in the newborn. The most important aid to diagnosis is a marked degree of suspicion when a newborn develops the general signs of severe infection and becomes excessively drowsy. Diagnosis must be confirmed by lumbar puncture. The cerebrospinal fluid is turbid due to large numbers of pus cells. Culture is required to determine antibiotic sensitivities.

Treatment

The mortality is high and many of the survivors suffer permanent brain damage and/or deafness. Early diagnosis is therefore essential and various antibiotics are available for *E. coli* and the other organisms involved (see Chapter 9).

PYELONEPHRITIS

Gram-negative infections in the newborn seem to have a preference for settling in renal tissue when there has been a bacteraemia or septicaemia.

Clinical features

The infant becomes ill with fever, and there is reluctance to feed, vomiting, greyish pallor and loss of weight. Diagnosis will be missed unless urine is obtained and subjected to microscopy and culture. In the newborn a urinary white cell count is likely to be significant if it exceeds 15 per mm^3 in boys or 50 per mm^3 in girls. Urine for culture is much more reliably obtained by suprapubic bladder aspiration than by plastic bag. Pyuria may also be part of the clinical picture in a jaundiced baby suffering from Gram-negative septicaemia. In this event the pyelonephritis arises from the blood stream and sometimes there is also present a pyogenic meningitis. In such cases blood culture and sometimes lumbar puncture should be performed in addition to urine culture.

Treatment

When the infant is not severely ill the choice of antibacterial drug can await the results of bacterial sensitivities. In septicaemic cases a combination of ampicillin and gentamicin or third generation cephalosporin is likely to be effective and must not be delayed.

ACUTE OSTEITIS

Osteitis in the newborn is a metastatic lesion which is usually due to a penicillin-resistant *Staph. aureus* but may occasionally be due to the *Haemophilus* organism.

Clinical features

In most cases the infant is seriously ill although fever is inconstant. Localising signs are sometimes slow to appear and should be diligently sought in every ill infant. These are: local swelling with or without discoloration; extreme irritability on handling the affected part or limb; or immobility of the affected limb (pseudoparesis). In the newborn, osteitis is not infrequently multiple and sites of predilection are the superior maxilla and pelvis. When the maxilla is involved, retro-orbital cellulitis causes proptosis as a presenting sign. If diagnosis is delayed, extensive bone destruction and disorganisation of the neighbouring joint (see Fig. 4.23) may lead to permanent crippling. In some infants general systemic illness is remarkably slight, when the dangers of late diagnosis are even greater.

Treatment

An attempt should be made to isolate the causal organism by blood culture. Aspiration of pus through a wide-bore needle from the affected bone site may be possible. An intravenous infusion of flucloxacillin 25 mg/kg four times a day may be required as the initial antibiotic treatment.

TETANUS NEONATORUM

Neonatal tetanus is still an important cause of death in many parts of the world where the umbilical cord may be cut with a dirty knife or other implement and may be tied with a makeshift ligature or even dressed with animal dung.

Clinical features

The onset of the disease occurs between the 3rd and 10th day of life with difficulty in sucking due to masseteric spasm followed by tetanic spasms which result in risus sardonicus and opisthotonus. Between spasms there is continuous muscle rigidity with clenched jaw, risus sardonicus and stiff back, neck, abdominal wall and limbs. Death can result from arrest of breathing during a spasm or from intercurrent pneumonia.

Treatment

The mortality is high and most infants die within a few days. Antitetanus immunoglobulin of human origin (HTIG) has replaced tetanus antitoxin. An intramuscular injection of 1250 units of HTIG may be combined with another 250 units infiltrated locally around the umbilicus. A broad spectrum antibiotic should be given intramuscularly. Sedation can be achieved by intramuscular sodium phenobarbitone 15 mg, chlorpromazine hydrochloride 5 mg, or diazepam

2 mg. In situations with intensive care units anaesthesia and the use of muscle relaxants with carefully controlled intermittent positive-pressure ventilation may improve the high mortality rates otherwise found. Feeds should be given through a nasogastric tube. Neonatal tetanus can be reduced by the active immunisation of mothers during pregnancy by means of two injections of tetanus toxoid, thus ensuring a degree of passive immunity in the infant during the neonatal period (see Chapter 20).

SYSTEMIC CANDIDIASIS

Infants can acquire cutaneous and oral candida (thrush) colonisation and infections during delivery, from skin contact with adult carriers or from contaminated bottles and teats (see page 316). Systemic candidiasis is particularly common in very low birthweight infants receiving antibiotic therapy and intensive care with indwelling vascular catheters. Signs of infection are the same as those of bacterial septicaemia and localised signs may be found in affected organs including the kidney, heart valves, joints, brain and meninges.

Renal, brain and cardiac ultrasound studies may reveal fungal lesions and the yeasts or hyphae may be identified in blood and urine.

Treatment

If possible all central lines and indwelling catheters should be removed and intravenous amphotericin B 0.25 mg/kg/day initially diluted to 1.0 mg/10 ml in 5% dextrose/water given slowly, then increased on alternate days by 0.25 mg/kg/day to reach a maximum of 1.0 mg/kg/day. This dosage should be continued for 4–6 weeks (total dosage of 30 mg/kg). Amphotericin therapy can be combined with 5 flucytosine given intravenously in a dose of 200 mg/kg/day when the candida is sensitive. Plasma 5-flucytosine concentrations should be maintained between 200 and 400 µmol/l and not exceed 600 µmol/l. Amphotericin and flucytosine therapy can be toxic to kidneys, liver and blood so that regular checks of haematology and liver and renal function are required. Amphotericin is now available for intravenous use encapsulated in liposomes which is reported to make it less toxic. The initial daily dose is 1 mg/kg/day and may be increased in the absence of evidence of toxicity, gradually to 3 mg/kg/day.

Fluconazole has been used orally to treat mucosal candidiasis and as a prophylactic measure in neutropenic older children. Its value in systemic candidiasis and cryptococcal infection when used intravenously is currently being tested.

JAUNDICE

In order to understand the investigation and management of a jaundiced infant it is useful to have some knowledge of the metabolism of the pigment bilirubin which is the cause of the yellow discoloration of tissue known as jaundice. Bilirubin is a breakdown product of haem (ferroprotoporphyrin IX). The degradation of l gram of haemoglobin releases 600 µmol (35 mg) of bilirubin. The normal newborn infant during the first 2–3 weeks of life releases 135–137 µmol (8–10 mg) of bilirubin per kg body weight per day. This is more than twice the adult output and probably reflects the relatively larger red cell mass, shorter red cell lifespan and possibly an increased turnover of hepatic haem. The bilirubin load to the liver is further increased by intestinal reabsorption of the excreted pigment from the small intestine. Prolonged jaundice occurring in some breast fed infants may be mediated by facilitation of intestinal absorption of bilirubin.

Hepatic conjugation

Haem is oxidised by microsomal enzyme found in liver, spleen and macrophages. The bilirubin product (tetrapyrrole biliverdin) is transported in the plasma attached to albumin and is transported across the hepatocyte membrane via a specific membrane receptor. In the liver the bilirubin is transported by ligandin and is subsequently conjugated by the microsomal enzyme uridyl diphosphate (UDP) glucuronyl transferase using UDP-glucuronic acid as substrate. This glucuronation effectively converts the bilirubin from a fat soluble toxic substance to a non-toxic water soluble substance which can be excreted via the bile and kidney. Glucuronyl transferase activity as well as ligandin concentration can be increased by the use of microsomal enzyme-inducing drugs such as phenobarbitone and traditional Chinese medicine yin zhi huang. The former is used in Western countries and the later in Asian countries to treat neonatal jaundice. Several other substances important in medicine, including steroids, salicylates, aniline and chloramphenicol, are excreted by the same bilirubin conjugating system. The availability of glucose is of importance in bilirubin excretion. Other pathways of bilirubin excretion exist in addition to glucuronation and one of these is by conjugation to sulphate. In the newborn this pathway does not seem to be available and cannot compensate for defective glucuronation. The excretion of conjugated bilirubin from the hepatocyte into bile is a process which can be inhibited by organic ions and suggests a carrier-mediated system. Obstructive jaundice occurs when the liver is unable to excrete conjugated bilirubin into the gastrointestinal tract by the bile duct system. It may be caused by hepatic cell disorder or from obstruction of the intrahepatic or extrahepatic biliary ducts.

TABLE 1.15 Causes of non-obstructive jaundice

IMMATURITY OF LIVER FUNCTION
Jaundice of immaturity
Physiological jaundice
INHIBITION OF LIVER FUNCTION
Breast milk jaundice
HAEMOLYTIC ANAEMIAS
ABO incompatibility
Rh incompatibility
Glucose-6-phosphate-dehydrogenase (G-6-PD) deficiency
Spherocytosis
Haemoglobinopathies
Severe infections
Drug sensitivity
Extravasated blood
OTHER RARE CAUSES
Hypothyroidism
Crigler–Najjar syndrome
Pyloric stenosis
Malrotation of the intestine
Cystic fibrosis

NON-OBSTRUCTIVE JAUNDICE

Causes of non-obstructive jaundice are shown in Table 1.15.

"Physiological" jaundice

The serum "indirect" (unconjugated) bilirubin value is increased above the adult concentration (13.6 µmol/l; 0.8 mg/100 ml) in most newborn infants. Some develop the yellow skin discoloration on the second or third day of life, are not unwell, show no evidence of excessive haemolysis and the jaundice fades some 7–10 days later. This has long been known as "physiological" jaundice although it is better regarded as a functional immaturity of the glucuronyl transferase enzyme system. Preterm infants have a higher maximum bilirubin peaking on the 5th or 6th day with a prolonged period, sometimes lasting weeks, of relative hyperbilirubinaemia. There is some difficulty in deciding when non-physiological becomes pathological but in general any infant whose plasma bilirubin concentration exceeds 210 µmol/l (12 mg/100 ml) by the 3rd day of life should be considered to have a non-physiological jaundice.

BILIRUBIN ENCEPHALOPATHY

Unconjugated bilirubin can produce transient encephalopathy or irreversible brain stem damage. As brain damage increases twitching, convulsions and episodes of cyanosis occur. Kernicterus literally means nuclear jaundice and refers to damage to the basal nuclei. It can occur when the unconjugated bilirubin concentration exceeds 340 µmol/l (20 mg/100 ml) from whatever cause. The affected brain is stained yellow but certain structures, the corpus striatum, thalamus, subthalamic nuclei, hippocampus, nucleus of the third nerve, mammillary bodies, red nucleus and nuclei on the floor of the fourth ventricle are intensely coloured. In older infants who survive the acute stage there is a marked loss of nerve cells and replacement gliosis. There are many factors which predispose an infant to kernicterus and these include hypoglycaemia, hypoproteinaemia, high plasma free fatty acid composition and the use of drugs which compete for albumin binding sites together with acidosis whether metabolic or respiratory. In the acute stage of kernicterus there may be rolling of the eyes, marked lethargy, convulsions, refusal to suck, increased muscle tone, head retraction or opisthotonos and coma. If the infant survives the period of intense jaundice, later in the first year he develops spasms of muscular rigidity, opisthotonus and sometimes convulsive seizures. After the age of 2 years the surviving infant may show the typical picture of athetosis with increased muscle tone. There may be pyramidal signs but extrapyramidal rigidity is more common. High-tone deafness is present and this leads to interference with the acquisition of speech and language. This in turn aggravates the learning difficulties of such children. In addition to brain damage hyperbilirubinaemia affects the growing tooth buds so that the first dentition may show an unwelcome green staining and sometimes a visible line of hypoplasia of the enamel and dentine between the antenatal and postnatal parts. It is likely that the bilirubin damage to neurones is related to the vulnerability of these cells which in turn depend on metabolic state, the lipid composition of the neuronal membrane and the ability of the neurone to detoxify bilirubin with mitochondrial bilirubin oxidase. The only means of preventing kernicterus, of proved effectiveness, is exchange transfusion. This removes bilirubin not only from the plasma but also from the tissue cells.

BILIRUBIN PHOTOCHEMISTRY

When the skin of jaundiced infants is exposed to light in the spectrum of blue to green (420–450 nm) bilirubin can be transformed into pigments which can be excreted without conjugation. The water soluble isomers of bilirubin produced in human infants undergoing phototherapy are bound to albumin before being excreted in bile or urine. In human infants lumirubin appears to be the major photodegradation product of the pyrrole rings which make up the original porphyrin of the haem molecule.

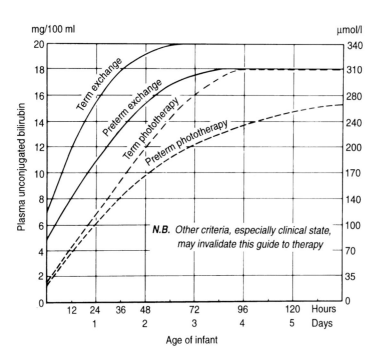

FIGURE 1.24 Neonatal jaundice. Criteria for exchange transfusion and phototherapy.

In the treatment of mild to moderate hyperbilirubinaemia, the standard method of reducing bilirubin concentrations in serum and tissues is by replacement (exchange) transfusion. The value of this technique in haemolytic disease of the newborn is proven but the indications for its use in the hyperbilirubinaemia of prematurity are less clearly defined. The not inconsiderable risks of the procedure in the preterm infant with poor coagulation function must be weighed against the risk of developing kernicterus. Infants with IRDS, relative hypoxaemia, acidosis or hypoglycaemia with lower levels of plasma albumin are at risk of kernicterus at lower values of plasma bilirubin than in the mature infant. Figure 1.24 gives a guideline to the criteria for exchange transfusion and phototherapy in preterm and term infants. Phototherapy is most readily carried out in an incubator with the infant fully exposed apart from the eyes which should be covered by a mask made from non-irritant material. It is, however, possible to provide phototherapy in a cot provided the naked infant is kept in a sufficiently heated environment. Phototherapy units providing an artificial source of light at the appropriate wavelength (425–475 nm) are most effective in reducing plasma bilirubin concentrations. Phototherapy is more effective in the prevention of an increase in bilirubin rather than reducing a high value. Treatment should be given to infants as soon as their unconjugated plasma bilirubin reaches 250 μmol/l (15 mg/100 ml) in term infants and 170 μmol/l (10 mg/l00 ml) in preterm infants. Phototherapy is most suitable for the treatment of jaundice due to immaturity of liver function but may also be used prophylactically in infants with haemolytic anaemias. When haemolytic anaemias are treated in this way it is important to remember that the therapy has no effect on the underlying anaemia and a careful record of haemoglobin concentrations as well as unconjugated bilirubin must be kept. Infants treated with phototherapy lose an increased amount of water both through the skin and in the loose stools which frequently develop. Fluid intake therefore should be well maintained during phototherapy. Early feeding with adequate fluid and carbohydrate intake will help reduce the risk of metabolic acidaemia and increase in free fatty acids which compete with bilirubin for albumin binding sites.

HAEMOLYTIC ANAEMIAS

The earlier that jaundice appears and the longer it persists the greater is the risk to the infant. Jaundice appearing on the first day of life should never be accepted as physiological and is highly suggestive of a haemolytic anaemia or of severe liver dysfunction. Similarly any jaundice which persists for more than 10–14 days after birth must be investigated thoroughly with particular reference to signs of obstructive jaundice and hypothyroidism. In European countries Rh incompatibility was until recently the most frequent cause of severe haemolytic anaemia. On a world wide scale incompatibility of the fetus and mother for the ABO blood groups is the most frequent potential cause of haemolytic anaemia but fortunately it seldom results in severe degrees of jaundice. In Mediterranean peoples, black African and Far Eastern races deficiency of the enzyme glucose-6–phosphate dehydrogenase (G-6-PD) is a more common cause of haemolytic anaemia than Rh incompatibility. Red cell membrane abnormalities such as thalassaemia associated with unusual haemoglobins are a cause of haemolysis in certain racial groups. Antenatal detection of such haemolytic anaemias is now possible by the examination of fetal blood.

BLOOD GROUP INCOMPATIBILITY

These occur when the fetus inherits from the father a blood group such as the Rh factor which is not present in the mother. If fetal cells should pass across the placenta into the mother in sufficient numbers she may develop antibodies to these "foreign" red cells which will destroy them within her circulation. Should the immunoglobulin (antibody) pass back to the fetus across the placenta it will cause haemolysis of fetal cells thus releasing haemoglobin and rendering the fetus anaemic. The bilirubin produced in this process will be transferred back across the placenta into the maternal circulation for conjugation by the maternal hepatic enzyme systems. Where extreme fetal haemolysis occurs the fetal anaemia can produce cardiac failure and severe fetal oedema (hydrops fetalis).

RHESUS INCOMPATIBILITY

About 83% of northern Europeans carry the rhesus antigen in their red cells (Rh positive). The remaining 17% do not possess this antigen and are referred to as Rh negative. When during pregnancy fetal red cells cross the placenta to sensitise the mother or if mother has been previously sensitised to the Rh antigen by a transfusion of Rh incompatible blood or the miscarriage of a Rh positive fetus, any subsequent pregnancy with a Rh positive fetus is at risk of developing haemolytic anaemia. Although it is rare it is now recognised that a mother can be sensitised by her first rhesus positive fetus and that this fetus may develop a haemolytic disease (usually mild) during the first pregnancy. The rhesus factor was first identified in 1940 and it has been shown to include at least six antigens (Cc, Dd, Ee which are determined by three allelomorphic pairs of genes similarly labelled). A mother may therefore be sensitised by any of these antigens which she herself does not possess. The most important of these is the D antigen and those who possess it are Rh(D) positive, whereas those who do not are Rh(D) negative. The three genes Cc, Dd and Ee are carried close together on the same chromosome and there are eight possible combinations of genes in descending order of frequency, CDe, cde, cDE, cDe, cdE, Cde, CDE and CdE. In somatic cells there are two autosomes carrying these genes and the commonest types in the UK are CDe/cde, CDe/CDe, cde/cde, CDe/cDE and cDE/cde. If the father is homozygous (D/D) with two D genes all his children must receive a D gene so that once haemolytic disease has made its appearance all subsequent children of the marriage will be similarly affected. When, however, the father is heterozygous Rh positive (D/d) half his children will inherit d. As they will also have inherited d from their Rh negative (d/d) mother they will be Rh(D) negative and so unaffected by the disease. The majority of cases of Rh sensitisation involve D antigen but in some the other antigens (e.g. c) are involved. These explain cases of haemolytic disease which occur in the offspring of some Rh(D) positive women.

CLINICAL FEATURES

Fetus affected

The disease develops severely during fetal life in only a minority of cases. It may then result in stillbirth, intrauterine death and the subsequent delivery of a macerated fetus, or in the birth of a living infant with hydrops fetalis.

The hydropic infant is grossly oedematous with marked enlargement of liver and spleen which are the sites of extensive extramedullary erythropoieses. The placenta is large, pale and oedematous and the amniotic fluid a deep yellow colour. The presence of hydrops fetalis may be recognised antenatally by ultrasonography.

Infant affected

In the majority of cases the infant is born apparently normal but subsequently develops signs of the disease. In its most severe form (icterus gravis) jaundice appears within minutes or hours of birth. It gradually deepens and develops a characteristic golden yellow colour. Purpura and haemorrhages may appear in the skin and liver and spleen become grossly enlarged. The peripheral blood shows anaemia, reticulocytosis, many erythroblasts and normoblasts and immature white cells of the granular series. If the condition remains untreated the unconjugated bilirubin concentration increases and there may develop in the later stages an increase in conjugated bilirubin with an obstructive element previously designated the inspissated bile syndrome.

This term in fact is a misnomer and this obstructive type of jaundice reflects immaturity of the excretory function of the liver rather than blockage of the intercellular canaliculi by "inspissated" bile.

DIAGNOSIS

In most instances it is possible to predict the appearance of haemolytic disease during pregnancy and by timely treatment to prevent most of the serious manifestations. The rhesus and ABO blood groups of every pregnant women should be determined early in pregnancy. In the case of Rh(D) negative women the serum should be tested for Rh antibodies then and periodically throughout the pregnancy. The finding of antibody is a strong indication that the infant may be affected and the mother should be delivered in a hospital with neonatal intensive care facilities. In women who have had previously affected infants the husband's Rh genotype must also be determined to help in more accurate prediction. The history of previous pregnancies gives an indication of the probable severity of the disease. In some families the disease pattern tends to be similar in each pregnancy; in others, succeeding infants show a worsening severity.

ANTENATAL MANAGEMENT

Spectrophotometric examination of amniotic fluid obtained by amniocentesis can be used to predict the probable severity of the disease. The method gives an accuracy of prediction above 95% so permitting infants seriously at risk to be delivered before they are hydropic or moribund. The technique of amniocentesis and amniotic fluid optical density measurements is still used for "missed" third trimester problems. Improved methods of fetal monitoring have made this a less common necessity. Maternal Rh antibody concentrations are measured from 18 weeks gestation and rising values suggest increasing severity of haemolysis. Ultrasound measurements of placental thickness, umbilical vein diameter and fetal intraperitoneal volume and measures of cardiac output have proved unreliable in predicting the degree of anaemia. However, if fetal ascites appears this indicates a severe anaemia (Hb less than 4 g/100 ml). These methods are not entirely satisfactory as ascites is found in less than two-thirds of fetuses with such a low haemoglobin and at this level of haemoglobin the fetus may already be suffering from relative hypoxaemia. Fetal blood sampling allows direct assessment of the fetal haematocrit and haemoglobin concentration and will permit transfusion to be performed at the same procedure when anaemia is identified. Fresh

rhesus negative packed cells compatible with the mother are infused in a volume determined by the estimated fetal placental volume and the fetal and donor haematocrits. Transfusions are performed at between 2- and 4-weekly intervals thereafter based on the rates of fall of fetal haematocrit between the procedures. Survival rates of 80–90% have been achieved in severely affected fetuses by these methods.

POSTNATAL MANAGEMENT

A replacement blood transfusion is indicated in the infant where a cord haemoglobin is below 12 g/100 ml and/or the cord unconjugated bilirubin concentration about 85 μmol/l (5 mg/100 ml). Clinical judgement will be required and lower criteria may be accepted in a preterm infant or where there has been a history of a previously severely affected infant or stillbirth. Confirmation of the diagnosis is seldom required but the Coombs' direct anti-human globulin test which detects antibody bound to the infant's red cells may be performed. Early exchange transfusion will correct anaemia, remove damaged and antibody-coated red cells from the circulation and remove unfixed antibodies. Donor blood should be Rh negative, preferably of the same ABO group as the infant's, and should also be compatible with the mother's serum by the indirect anti-globulin technique. The total volume of blood exchanged usually amounts to 175 ml/kg. Subsequent exchange transfusions may be required if the unconjugated bilirubin concentration increases above the values shown in Fig. 1.24. Phototherapy can be used to help control the degree of hyperbilirubinaemia. It is important that the infant's haemoglobin be checked regularly for at least 6 weeks after birth as after these procedures the infant's red cell production may be suppressed for some time and quite severe anaemia may develop.

PREVENTION OF Rh HAEMOLYTIC DISEASE

The incidence of haemolytic disease has been reduced from 6 per thousand in the UK to less than 1 per thousand by the introduction of a preventive programme. The programme is based on the fact that the "bleed" from the Rh(D) positive fetus which sensitises the Rh(D) negative mother usually occurs at the end of pregnancy or during labour and Rh antibodies take some weeks to develop. A very high degree of prevention of haemolytic disease is achieved by the intramuscular administration of anti-D immunoglobulin to the Rh negative mother soon after the birth of her Rh positive infant. Any fetal red cells which have entered her circulation are thus destroyed. The principal supply of anti-D immunoglobulin has been from naturally sensitised Rh(D) individuals. Mothers at greatest risk are those Rh(D) negative mothers who give birth to Rh(D) positive infants who are ABO compatible with their mothers. When the fetal cells are incompatible with the mothers in the ABO system, Rh sensitisation only rarely occurs, because AB antibodies are already present in the blood of the mother, and if ABO incompatible fetal cells enter her circulation they are unlikely to survive for long enough to initiate the production of Rh antibodies. A protective dose of 100 μg anti-D immunoglobulin is now offered to all non-sensitised Rh(D) negative women delivered of Rh(D) positive infants irrespective of whether they are ABO compatible or incompatible. A smaller dose (50 μg) is offered to Rh(D) negative women having a pregnancy terminated, an amniocentesis, chorionic villus sample or fetal blood sampling procedure or a spontaneous abortion. These measures have proved highly effective and there remain only a few women who develop antibodies during their first Rh(D) positive pregnancy. Antenatal prevention has been used in some communities where anti-D immunoglobulin (100 μg) is given to all Rh negative primigravidae at 28 and 34 weeks, a further dose being given after delivery if the infant is Rh(D) positive.

ABO INCOMPATIBILITY

Cases of ABO incompatibility are probably more common than any other form of blood group incompatibility between mother and infant. Many are so mild that they are mistaken for "physiological" jaundice. The condition rarely leads to severe jaundice and anaemia but many cases produce sufficient jaundice to require phototherapy. Usually ABO antibodies are of the IgM variety rather than IgG (Rh antibodies are predominantly IgG) and therefore do not cross the placenta. Mothers of blood group O are more likely than those of Groups A or B to have IgG antibodies. In any infant developing jaundice within 24 hours of birth blood groups of both infant and mother should be determined and if they are potentially incompatible (e.g. mother O, infant A or B) the mother's serum must be examined for immune type antibodies specific for A and B antigens. In ABO incompatibility the direct Coombs' test in the infant is usually negative. Replacement transfusion is only required if the infant's unconjugated bilirubin increases above 340 μmol/l (20 mg/100 ml). Group O blood of homologous rhesus group should be used.

GLUCOSE-6-PHOSPHATE DEHYDROGENASE (G-6-PD) DEFICIENCY

Glucose-6-phosphate dehydrogenase catalyses the oxidation of glucose-6-phosphate to 6-phosphogluconate. Deficiency of this enzyme results in a block in the first stage of the pentose shunt pathway. Many different variants of G-6-PD have now been identified and all are determined by mutant alleles at a locus on the X chromosome. They differ from normal enzyme in electrophoretic mobility and it is likely that each is related to a single amino acid substitution on the enzyme protein. The different alleles have been designated Gd^B, Gd^{A-}, Gd^A, $Gd^{Mediterranean}$, Gd^{Athens}, Gd^{Canton} and so forth. Some result in more severe deficiencies of enzyme activities than others.

In some parts of the world G-6-PD deficiency can cause a degree of haemolysis after the ingestion of drugs such as primaquine, sulphonamides and nitrofurantoin. It has long been recognised in Mediterranean countries that acute haemolytic anaemia can occur in some families following the ingestion of fava beans (favism). In some infants G-6-PD deficiency can cause a degree of haemolysis in the newborn sufficient to increase the unconjugated bilirubin to a level requiring exchange transfusion without obvious drug ingestion. This has been reported from Greece, Singapore and Hong Kong. In these neonatal cases jaundice has not been confined to hemizygous males or to hemizygous females and the X-linked gene seems to show great variability of expression in the heterozygous female. This variability in enzyme activities may be related to the Lyon hypothesis in which it is presumed that only one X chromosome is genetically active in any cell during interphase.

ACHOLURIC JAUNDICE (CONGENITAL SPHEROCYTOSIS)

It is uncommon for this hereditary disease, which is transmitted as a Mendelian dominant trait, to manifest itself during the neonatal period. When it does it may require splenectomy during early infancy because of persistent jaundice and anaemia. Whenever possible, however, splenectomy should be avoided during the first year of life because of the subsequent increased susceptibility to bacterial infections. Rarely, exchange transfusion is necessary in the neonatal period to prevent kernicterus. The spleen is enlarged, the blood shows anaemia with a reticulocytosis, some erythroblasts, increased fragility of the red cells and microspherocytosis. The plasma unconjugated bilirubin is increased and there is urobilinogenuria.

NEONATAL HAEMORRHAGE

The newborn infant is peculiarily liable to bleed under a variety of circumstances. These include anoxia, birth trauma, hypothermia, haemolytic anaemia, infections of bacterial, viral or protozoal origin and inadequacies of the blood clotting mechanisms.

FETAL HAEMORRHAGE

Whereas haemorrhage in the newborn infant is usually visible and when severe accompanied by signs of shock and haemorrhage, in the fetus it is usually unheralded and undetected but may cause severe fetal damage. A variety of intracranial haemorrhages have been detected early in fetal development with ultrasonic examination. These may be subdural or intracerebral and may be associated with major CNS anomalies. Bleeding from the fetus may also occur when the placenta is accidentally incised during lower segment Caesarean section for anterior placenta praevia. Rupture of a velamentous vessel overlying the cervix or a blood vessel on the fetal aspect of the placenta or, indeed, haemorrhage into the placenta itself may occur. Artificial rupture of the membranes may precipitate fetal placental haemorrhage, fetal placental blood loss and should be suspected whenever blood is obtained at this procedure.

The fetus may bleed across the placenta into the maternal circulation (fetomaternal transfusion). The factors which predispose to transplacental bleeding are unclear and although it has been associated with high rupture of the membranes, and in one case with a choriocarcinoma, in most instances no abnormality of the placenta is obvious.

An intriguing situation arises when one monovular twin bleeds into the other so that one is anaemic and the other polycythaemic whilst one portion of the monochorionic placenta is pale and bloodless and the other purple and engorged. A monochorionic placenta is found in approximately 70% of twin pregnancies and a significant twin-to-twin transfusion occurs in at least 15%.

Clinical features

Fetal haemorrhage during labour should be suspected if there is a sudden flow of bright red blood from the introitus. The same applies to the appearance of blood during the artificial rupture of membranes. The fetal origin of the blood can be quickly confirmed by testing it for fetal haemoglobin which is alkali-resistant. Early delivery and ligation of the umbilical cord should be instituted. The infant may be delivered in a state of oligaemic shock with severe pallor, but there will rarely be apnoea and the heart rate will be rapid in contrast to the bradycardia which is usual in severe asphyxia. When bleeding has been less severe or has been taking place some time before birth, as in cases of fetomaternal transfusion, the presenting sign is pallor alone. Indeed, this may not become manifest for some hours after birth. The infant will have a hypochromic anaemia, reticulocytosis and increased numbers of erythroblasts and normoblasts.

Diagnosis

Fetomaternal transfusion can be confirmed by differential agglutination provided there is a major blood group difference between mother and her infant but more usually the diagnosis of fetomaternal transfusion is made by the treatment of methanol-fixed blood films of the maternal blood with an acid buffer at pH 3.4. Fetal erythrocytes resist lysis by the buffer solution so that they react subsequently with ordinary haemoglobin stains whereas the adult maternal cells appear as ghosts. This test is known as the Kleihauer test.

Treatment

Blood transfusion can be life-saving. When the haemorrhage has taken place shortly before birth the infant haemoglobin concentration may not be much reduced, but as restoration of the blood volume takes place over the next few hours serial determinations will reveal a reducing haemoglobin concentration. Values of haemoglobin below 14 g/100 ml are an indication for top-up transfusion. In the emergency situation Group O rhesus negative blood should be given. In twin-to-twin transfusion the anaemic twin may require blood transfusion. The recipient twin may suffer from respiratory distress and cerebral signs if polycythaemia is marked. In some instances the haemoglobin concentration is in the region of 30 g/100 ml and the haematocrit 75%. The relevant treatment in these circumstances is partial replacement transfusion with plasma, 30 ml/kg body weight.

HAEMORRHAGIC DISORDERS OF THE NEWBORN

Haemorrhagic disorders of the newborn may be associated with vitamin K_1 deficiency, disseminated intravascular coagulation, deficiencies of other clotting factors or thrombocytopenia. The laws of Moses recognised that newborn infants were prone to bleed excessively during the first week of life and made allowance for this in their ordinance in relation to circumcision which is deferred until the 8th day. The term haemorrhagic disease of the newborn was first used in the 19th century and was thought to be entirely explicable by deficiency of vitamin K_1. The disorder is somewhat more complex and the term haemorrhagic disease of the newborn should be confined to infants in which there is a temporary coagulation defect associated with spontaneous haemorrhage.

Vitamin K_1 deficiency

Vitamin K_1 is essential for the synthesis of four of the factors involved in the clotting process – factors II (prothrombin), VII, IX and X. These factors are present in the newborn but at lower concentrations than in the adult reaching a nadir on the 3rd day. The subsequent rise depends upon the provision of vitamin K_1 in the diet or as a result of bacterial action in the bowel producing vitamin K_1. Breast milk contains low concentrations of vitamin K_1. "Haemorrhagic disease of the newborn" due to lack of dietary vitamin K_1 is virtually confined to infants who have been breast fed or who have had no oral feeds. Maternal anticonvulsant therapy may also lower the maternal breast milk supply of vitamin K.

Clinical features

The presenting feature is bleeding of varying severity. Most commonly it appears as melaena stools and in severe cases frank blood is passed per rectum and the infant may look shocked and pale. Haematemesis, haematuria, vaginal bleeding and haemorrhage from the umbilicus or into the skin may also occur. Visceral haemorrhages are uncommon but occasionally retroperitoneal haemorrhage, subcapsular haematoma of the liver and intracranial bleeding can occur. Diagnosis is confirmed by finding the infant's prothrombin time prolonged (normal 14–16 seconds) or the thrombotest low (normal 40–60%).

Treatment and prevention

Treatment with blood transfusion or fresh frozen plasma may be required if the bleeding has been severe. Otherwise treatment is with parenteral vitamin K_1 1 mg by intramuscular injection. Haemorrhagic disease of the newborn can be prevented by providing all infants with vitamin K_1 500 µg by intramuscular injection soon after birth. Preterm infants should be given 250 µg by intramuscular injection. Oral therapy with vitamin K is presently undergoing evaluation and may prove an acceptable means of prophylaxis.

Disseminated intravascular coagulation (DIC; secondary haemorrhagic disease)

The process of DIC or consumptive coagulopathy results in a decrease in platelets, fibrinogen, factor V and factor VIII. There is often purpura or multiple bruising, intracranial haemorrhage, bleeding from mucous membranes or into internal organs. However, DIC is likely only to develop in a baby already unwell from, e.g. Gram-negative septicaemia, severe asphyxia, hypothermia, renal vein thrombosis. Diagnosis is based on the finding of thrombocytopenia, reduced plasma fibrinogen levels and raised values for fibrin degradation products (FDP). The blood film contains fragmented red blood cells.

Treatment

The treatment of haemorrhagic disorders in the newborn period must be related to diagnosis of the specific cause of the bleeding tendency. Where bleeding is occurring and a haemorrhagic disorder suspected a prothrombin time or thrombotest and platelet count are essential investigations. When specimens have been taken 1 mg of vitamin K_1 by slow intravenous injection should be given. This will prove effective only in haemorrhagic disease of the newborn but will do no harm in other conditions and will not obscure the diagnosis. Where the platelet count is below $40 \times 10^9/l$ a platelet transfusion may be indicated especially if there is bleeding. The use of heparin and exchange transfusion in the treatment of DIC has not been established but there are reports in favour of the controlled use of heparin (see Chapter 13).

Thrombocytopenia

When the platelet count is less than $100 \times 10^9/l$ there is significant thrombocytopenia and the range of causes shown in Table 1.16 must be considered (see Chapter 13).

TABLE 1.16 Causes of thrombocytopenia in the newborn

MATERNAL FACTORS INVOLVED
Maternal idiopathic thrombocytopenic purpura
Isoimmune thrombocytopenia
Transplacental infection
Severe rhesus incompatibility
Thiazide diuretics given to mother
Inherited thrombocytopenia
OTHER CAUSES
Infection acquired postnatally
Disseminated intravascular coagulation
Marrow hypoplasia
Giant haemangioma

Maternal idiopathic thrombocytopenic purpura (ITP)

Purpura in the newborn may be produced by thrombocytopenia or by capillary damage related to venous obstruction or hypoxia. In about half the infants of mothers with ITP there is a purpura which may be temporary and is apparently due to transplacental transfusion of maternal platelet IgG antibodies. It may occur even when the mother's platelet count has returned to normal. It is usual to deliver such infants by Caesarean section because of the high risks of intracranial haemorrhage.

Isoimmune thrombocytopenia

This is due to the transplacental passage of platelet antibody from a platelet antigen negative mother, who has been immunised either by blood from her platelet antigen positive fetus or previous blood transfusion, to a platelet antigen positive fetus. The outcome is similar to that found in rhesus immunisation. Ninety-eight per cent of all individuals are platelet antigen positive, only 2% antigen negative. The mother will have a normal platelet count. Other causes of thrombocytopenia are antenatal infections with syphilis, toxoplasmosis, rubella, cytomegalovirus and herpesvirus. Thrombocytopenia has also been described in a number of infants born to mothers on prolonged courses of thiazide diuretics. Inherited thrombocytopenias are rarely manifest in the newborn. Severe postnatal infection, bacterial or viral, may be accompanied by purpura due to platelet deficiency and the thrombocytopenia may be a manifestation of DIC. Marrow depression from any cause such as drugs, congenital leukaemia and bone disorders may present as purpura due to thrombocytopenia. The platelet consumption which occurs in giant haemangiomas may rarely be a cause of purpura in the newborn period.

Treatment

A platelet count of less than $40 \times 10^9/l$ is an indication in a bleeding infant for platelet transfusion. Where the cause is maternal ITP platelets will be consumed rapidly by the antibody and may require to be given frequently. Where there is isoimmune thrombocytopenia the platelets transfused must be platelet antigen negative. These can be obtained from the mother and "washed" prior to transfusion, or from other family members who are antigen negative. Steroid therapy is controversial.

INFANT NUTRITION

The mother provides a continuum of nutrition throughout pregnancy and the first year of life. The initial phase is intrauterine from yolk sac and placenta whilst the secondary phase is via breast milk. In order to maintain this continuum of nutrition the infant feeding reflexes must be established and undamaged by toxins or trauma. Knowledge of the anatomical, physiological, biochemical and psychosocial aspects of the feeding of infants is not essential to a mother feeding her infant but is necessary for those to whom she may turn for advice and reassurance.

ROOTING

The rooting reflexes are initiated by contact of the infant's cheek with mother's nipple. This reflex, mediated by the trigeminal nerve, ensures that the infant's head turns towards the stimulus and the mouth opens to accept the nipple. When the infant is hungry this reflex is enhanced so that a stimulus applied anywhere on the face supplied by the trigeminal nerve will elicit the response. It is important that the infant is not confused by stimulating one cheek with the nipple while pushing or stroking the other cheek.

SUCKLING

The infant draws the nipple well into the mouth so that the areola of the nipple lies at the level of his gums. By closing the gums (fixing) and by a rolling movement of the tongue, milk is squeezed from the areolar milk ducts which are compressed against the infant's palate. Milk enters the pharynx and passes by co-ordinated muscle action into the oesophagus and stomach. The gums and tongue are relaxed while the milk ducts refill and a further cycle commences. During each cycle the mouth is sealed anteriorly by the closure of the lips and the nasopharynx is closed off by the soft palate. If the nose is completely or partially obstructed nasal breathing may be difficult and the infant will have to stop feeding in order to breathe through the mouth. Nasal obstruction is a common cause of feeding difficulty. Normal sucking and swallowing requires a co-ordination of several movements mediated through brain stem reflexes which are not fully developed in the immature infant and which may be inhibited by sedative drugs and intrapartum hypoxia or injury.

THE BREAST

The lactating breast has 18–20 segments each consisting of large numbers of secretory alveoli. These drain by small ducts which join others to form a large duct in each segment. Each large duct has a separate opening in the nipple. The walls of the duct contain smooth muscle which can propel milk towards the nipples. Proximal to the nipple the lactiferous sinus, a distensible segment of the main duct, acts as a small temporary reservoir for milk. When the infant fixes at the breast the sinuses lie under the areola between the infant's gums. Pressure by the gums helps to eject milk.

Growth and development of breast and the production of milk are controlled by hormones, predominantly oestrogens and prolactin. Maternal plasma concentration of oestrogens diminishes after delivery and this fall, together with higher plasma concentrations of prolactin produced during labour, are the factors primarily responsible for the initiation of lactation. Suckling is the strongest stimulant to further milk production. Milk secretion takes place in the alveoli continuously but muscle sphincters at the nipple prevent leakage between feeds. A variety of stimuli, principally placing the infant to the breast, produces a reflex propulsion of milk from the alveoli and relaxation of the nipple sphincters (draught reflex). Once the draught reflex has been initiated milk may continue to flow from both breasts even when the infant is not suckling. If the mother cannot relax during infant feeding the draft reflex may be delayed and the infant becomes frustrated. The mother can be greatly helped in the successful establishment of breast feeding by the help of those around her during delivery and the immediate postnatal period. If antenatal instruction has prepared her well and her birth attendants are confident and sympathetic, the mother will be more relaxed and confident of her own ability to feed the infant.

HUMAN MILK

An infant fed at its own mother's breast benefits not only from the nutritional properties of the milk but also from the immunological protection against infection which mothers provide specifically for their own babies. Hormonal changes induced in the mother by regular suckling at the breast inhibits ovulation and thus constitutes a form of contraception and contributes to better spacing of pregnancies.

During the first 2–3 days the breast secretes colostrum which increases progressively in volume and alters in composition until by the 3rd or 4th day milk is being produced together with colostrum which declines in volume thereafter. Colostrum has a high protein content but less sugar and fat than milk. The large globulin fraction includes immunoglobulins, some of which may be absorbed by the infant. IgA is one of the most important globulins and can act in a protective manner in the bowel against viruses and bacteria. Colostrum contains about 2000 cells/ml and most of these are macrophages. Some have the ability to synthesise lysozyme, lactoferrin and complement. Some lymphocytes synthesise the IgAs specific to infections to which the mother has been previously exposed. Bifido bacteria and lactobacilli are the principal organisms found in the alimentary tract of breast fed infants and these organisms reduce the risk of colonisation by other more potentially harmful bacteria. The bifido bacillus is a normal commensal organism of the lactiferous sinuses of the breast and is very sensitive to antibiotics. It may be absent when a mother has been given antibiotics prenatally and unavailable to colonise the infant's gut. There are also a variety of stimulators and regulators of growth (growth factors) present in colostrum and milk. These substances are low molecular weight proteins which stimulate cells to grow and divide and also stimulate protein synthesis. In human colostrum and milk, epidermal growth factor (EGF), insulin-like growth factor (IGF) and a number of other factors capable of stimulating growth in a wide range of different body organs have been identified. Human milk feeding may reduce and probably delays the subsequent incidence of allergic disorders such as eczema and asthma in infants born into families with atopic predisposition.

Human breast milk varies in its composition between the commencement and end of a feed. The initial part of the feed (first course) contains relatively more water whilst the hind milk produced at the end of the feed (third course) has a high fat content. The intermediate part of the feed contains the bulk of the protein requirement for the infant. It can be seen that if the infant feeds predominantly from one breast at each feed, the requirement of water to satisfy thirst and the finishing of the feed with a high fat content satisfying energy requirement will produce a satisfied, well nourished and contented infant. It may take from 4 to 6 weeks to achieve complete balance of maternal milk output and a satisfied infant. For a singleton infant the breast milk output is about 700–750 ml/day whilst with twins this figure can double. By the end of the first week of life an average daily intake for a term infant would be 150 ml/kg body weight but this may increase to 190 ml/kg by the end of the first month. Thereafter, there is a fall to 150 ml/kg by the 4th month. It is important to realise that there is a considerable range of normality in infant requirement and that measurement of the infant's progress in terms of growth and development is the best short-term measure of the adequacy of diet.

DIGESTION

The infant's gastric contents are normally passed on to the intestine via the pylorus. A term infant can digest and absorb 90% of the fat present in human milk when pancreatic lipase activities are low and bile salt production poor. There are at least three lipase enzymes in human milk: a lipoprotein lipase, a bile-salt stimulated esterase, and a non-activated lipase. These ensure that human milk fat is completely digested. Heat treatment of human milk can diminish these lipase activities. Milk fat globules are resistant to the action of pancreatic lipase and of milk bile-salt stimulated lipase, but are readily hydrolysed by lingual lipase, which penetrates into the core of fat particles and hydrolyses triglyceride. Lingual lipase is synthesised and secreted by the serous glands of the tongue from before 25 weeks gestation and acts in the acidic environment of the stomach. Infants fed intragastrically rather than intrajejunally are better able to digest and absorb fat, probably as a result of lingual lipase activities. In the newborn, including the preterm, gastric digestion by this means has been estimated to contribute 60–70% of the hydrolysis of ingested fats. The combined action of intragastric lipolysis by lingual and gastric lipases and intestinal hydrolysis of fat by the bile-salt stimulated lipase of human milk effectively substitutes for low pancreatic lipase activity and low concentrations of bile salts.

Starches and glucose polymers are hydrolysed by salivary amylase, small intestinal brush-border glucoamylase and mammary amylase. Salivary amylase is active in the gastric fluid of preterm infants. Human milk amylase is stable in the gastric and duodenal content of the newborn infant. The physiological role of these amylases is at present uncertain but may act to digest the polysaccharide walls of invading bacteria. The preterm infant can utilise glucose polymers because of the presence of these amylases and this is an effective way of increasing the preterm infant's energy intake.

There are no protein digestive enzymes in human milk and upper gastrointestinal tract. This may be a mechanism which allows the passage to the jejunum and ileum of undamaged immunoglobulins and growth promoting factors.

ESTABLISHING BREAST FEEDING

Placing the infant at the breast immediately after delivery is an excellent way of beginning mother–child bonding. Oxytocin is released from the mother's posterior pituitary gland in response to the cry of her infant and to a direct reflex stimulation from the infant suckling her nipple which hastens the contraction of the uterus and expulsion of the placenta. If not put to the breast at this early stage the first feed should be offered within 2–3 hours after delivery. Around the 3rd or 4th day after delivery some

mothers, particularly primiparae, may develop a degree of breast engorgement. Accumulation of milk causes parts of the breast to become tense and tender and there may be oedema of the overlying skin. This can be helped by manual expression or by the use of a hand pump or mechanical breast pump. The pain of severe engorgement and poor subsequent lactation may discourage the mother and it is during this period that she needs expert and sympathetic help.

It is now evident that the quality of fetal nutrition and postnatal nutrition affect the health of the adult to a considerable degree. The introduction of milk formulae to infant feeding during the past 130 years has created many hazardous situations for newborn human infants (convulsions from pyridoxine deficiency, convulsions from high phosphate intake with hypocalcaemia and hypomagnesaemia and iron deficiency anaemia). Excessive intakes of sugar, salt and saturated fatty acids during infancy may predispose to obesity, hypertension and atheroma in adult life. Deficiencies of specific essential fatty acids (docosahexaenoic acid) are now known to affect the visual acuity and visual function as well as the intellect of preterm and probably of term human infants. There are also emotional factors related to the close bonding of a satisfactorily breast fed infant. For these reasons it is most important that mothers are encouraged to satisfy their infants and their own needs through breast feeding their infants.

ALTERNATIVE INFANT FEEDING

Alternative methods of feeding when breast feeding is not possible can satisfy the requirements for growth. Cows' milk is readily available in most parts of the world and usually forms the basis for milk formulae. Cows' milk has many biochemical differences from human milk and requires considerable modification to make it suitable for infants. Modified milks have much of the casein removed and replaced by whey milk protein which contains a higher content of lactalbumin. Part of the milk fat is replaced by vegetable fat in an attempt to approximate the composition of human milk. The mineral content in terms of sodium and phosphorus is reduced but iron salts are added and the energy value restored by the addition of lactose. Vitamins A, D and C are usually added. The final chemical composition of such milks is as closely approximated to human milk as possible. It is evident that such milks cannot contain the anti-infective properties nor the active living cells and enzymes contained within human milk. These milks must be reconstituted as directed on the packet. Other formulae are prepared from soya and are sometimes used when there is a cow milk protein allergy or when there is a religious objection to the

TABLE 1.17 Nutritional comparison of baby milks available in the United Kingdom

Composition per 100 ml		Mature human milk		Whey-based infant milks				Casein-based infant milks			
		DHSS[s]	Macy[b] et al.	Farley's first milk	Cow & Gate Premium	SMA Gold	Milupa Aptamil with Milupan	Farley's second milk	Cow & Gate plus	SMA White	Milupa Milumil
Energy	kcal	70	68	68	66	67	67	66	66	67	69
	kJ	293	285	284	277	280	281	277	277	280	290
Protein†	g	1.34	1.45	1.45	1.4	1.5	1.5	1.7	1.7	1.6	1.9
Casein	%	–	32	39	40	40	40	77	77	80	80
Whey	%	–	68	61	60	60	60	23	23	20	20
Carbohydrate‡											
Lactose	g	7.0	7.0	7.0	7.1	7.2	7.2	2.8	7.2	7.0	6.0
Maltodextrin	g	–	–	–	–	–	–	5.5	–	–	2.4
Total	g	7.0	7.0	7.0	7.1	7.2	7.2	8.3	7.2	7.0	8.4
Fat	g	4.2	3.8	3.82 (veg oils)	3.6 (veg oils + milk fat)	3.6 (veg oils)	3.6 (veg oils + milk fat + egg lipid)	2.9 (veg oils)	3.4 (veg oils + milk fat)	3.6 (veg oils)	3.1 (veg oils + milk fat)
Saturated	%	50.1	52	36.6	42	42.9	53	36.6	38	42.9	53.3
Unsaturated	%	48.5	48	63.4	58	57.1	47	63.4	62	57.1	46.7
Minerals											
Calcium	mg	35	33	39	54	46	51	61	80	56	71
Cloride	mg	43	43	45	40	43	39	55	56	55	44
Magnesium	mg	2.8	4	5.2	5	6.7	5.7	6	5.4	5.3	6.0
Phosphorus	mg	15	15	27	27	33	31	48	47	44	55
Potassium	mg	60	55	57	65	65	74	86	90	80	85
Sodium	mg	15	15	17	18	16	20	25	25	22	24
Trace elements											
Copper	μg	39	40	42	40	33	40	40	40	33	27
Iodine	μg	7	7	4.5	10	10	5.9	10	10	10	2.1
Iron	μg	76	150	650	500	800	700	660	500	800	430
Manganese	μg	ND	0.7	3.4	7	10	5.0	3.3	7	10	13
Zinc	μg	295	530	340	400	600	400	330	400	600	400
Potential renal solute load*	mosm/l	88	91	93	92	96	99	116	118	110	121
Vitamins											
A (retinol)	μg	60	53	100	80	76	60	97	80	75	57
Thiamin (B₁)	μg	16	16	42	40	100	40	39	40	100	32
Riboflavin (B₂)	μg	31	42.6	55	100	150	50	53	100	150	49
B₆	μg	6	11	35	40	60	40	33	40	60	42
B₁₂	μg	0.01	trace	0.14	0.2	0.2	0.15	0.13	0.2	0.2	0.2
Biotin	μg	0.76	0.4	1.0	1.5	2.0	1.0	1.0	1.5	2.0	1.1
Folic acid	μg	5.2	0.18	3.4	10	8.0	10.1	3.3	10	8.0	5.0
Niacin	μg	230	172	690	400	900	700	660	400	900	240
Pantothenic acid	μg	260	196	230	300	300	370	220	300	300	220
C	mg	3.8	4.3	6.9	8	9.0	6.0	6.6	8	9.0	7.6
D	μg	0.01	0.01	1.0	1.1	1.1	1.0	1.0	1.1	1.1	1.0
E (d-alpha-tocopherol)	mg	0.35	0.56	0.48	0.8	0.74	0.6	0.46	0.8	0.74	0.8
K	μg	ND	1.7	2.7	5	6.7	3.0	2.6	5	6.7	4.0

*Method of Ziegler and Fomon, 1971: Calculated values.
†Total nitrogen × 6.38.
‡Figures declared as disaccharide.
ND, not determined.
[a]DHSS Reports on Health and Social Subjects Nos. 12 (1977), 18 (1980), 20 (1980).
[b]Macy IG, Kelly HJ, Sloan RE. The composition of milks: A compilation of the comparative composition and properties of human, cow, and goat milk, colostrum and transitional milk. Washington DC, Pub No. 254, National Academy of Science–National Research Council, 1953; Mettler AE. Infant milk powder feeds compared on a common basis. *Postgrad Med J* 1976l **52** (Suppl 8): 3–20.
Literature made available by Farley Health Products Ltd, Lenton Lane, Nottingham NG7 2LJ.

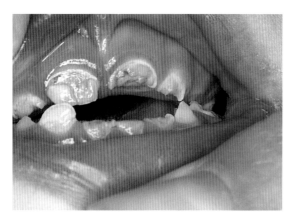

FIGURE 1.25 "Bottle" caries. Characteristic pattern of caries caused by sugary feeds and dummies.

ingestion of cow milk protein. Feeding with these milks involves the use of a delivery system which will be accepted by the infant and which protects the infant from the danger of aspiration of food or of infection from a contaminated bottle or teat. The design of bottles and teats has changed over the years and now disposable systems have been made available by the milk manufacturers.

Table 1.17 gives a nutritional comparison of infant formulae available in the UK.

FEEDING

It is important that the processes of sterilisation and cleaning of reusable bottles and teats is as per the manufacturer's instructions. Although in most areas of the UK tap water taken directly from the mains supply is virtually sterile and it is unnecessary to boil it before use, it is recommended that where water is obtained from a tank it should be boiled before being used for mixing feeds. It is convenient to prepare a 24 hour requirement of feeds if adequate refrigeration is available. This requires that a bottle is removed from the refrigerator ahead of time in order to allow the feed to reach room temperature. The technique of feeding a baby requires that the mother be relaxed and the bottle held so that the teat is always full of milk. As with breast feeding it is important that the teat be allowed to pass well into the baby's mouth. The rate of flow from a well worn teat may be too fast for the baby's comfort, whereas if it is too small the infant may swallow air and develop feeding difficulties. Most infants will finish their feed within 15 minutes and there is a time honoured custom of "breaking wind". Positioning of the infant so that air rises to the fundus of the stomach makes it less likely that milk will be "brought up" when

wind is broken. Manoeuvres commonly applied, such as rubbing or patting of the infant's back, seem to be aimed at giving the mother something to do and therefore may serve some purpose. It is important that midwives and mothers appreciate that a good burp by the infant is an indication of excess air swallowing rather than a source of pride to whoever is feeding the infant. Air swallowing is also encouraged by offering the infant a "dummy" or "comforter" to suck between feeds. Poor artificial feeding and the use of such comforters encourages air swallowing and the consequent colic.

The use of non-milk extrinsic sugars to sweeten a dummy or in bottle feeds contibute to "bottle" caries (Fig. 1.25). As with breast feeding the frequency of feeds can in the first few days be left to the demands of the infant. Some may start with six or eight feeds at 2–3-hourly intervals and proceed to four feeds at 4-hourly intervals as their capacity for taking an individual feed increases. The volume of feed offered should be related to the average taken by babies of that particular age and weight. Average volumes must only be considered as a guideline and the appetite and activity of the individual infant must always be considered. The normally breast fed infant does not take the same volume at each feed and there is no reason to expect bottle fed babies to be any more regular in their habits. By the 10th day of life term babies will generally be taking 150 ml/kg per 24 hours in five feeds. The 3.5 kg infant will therefore be having 100 ml per feed.

Every help must be given to mothers who require to bottle feed their infants for it is equally important that they establish a loving and happy relationship with their infant. Enormous stresses can be set up between family members where feeding, whether by breast or bottle, develops into an unhappy struggle between the mother and her infant. Any method of feeding which provides the basis for normal growth and development and which keeps the infant and mother happy is acceptable. It is important to maintain a balanced view about the methods of feeding required by human infants. The change in fashion from a situation where every infant was breast fed or did not survive to a situation where 90% were artificially fed led to mothers being thought to be "less sophisticated" if they breast fed their infants. This was manifestly nonsensical. On the other hand where a mother cannot breast feed through no fault of her own it is most important that she realises that reasonably satisfactory nutrition can be derived from the use of artifical formulae and that she has not "failed" her infant. The professionals involved in advising mothers about feeding matters must be aware of the social pressures and anxieties experienced by all mothers in their desire to do their best for their infant. Overanxiety by parents or attendants, frequent handling of the baby at every whimper, attempts to give feeds when they are not wanted, all create an atmosphere of tension which distresses the infant as much as the father and mother and which may persist into later life as a factor affecting normal emotional development. Feeding is a social occasion in which mother and infant establish a very close contact which should be enjoyed by both. The infant not only enjoys the satisfaction of hunger relief but welcomes the feeling of warmth and security of the nursing process and being handled and spoken to. These stimuli are an important early requisite to the infant's emotional development as well as a critical factor in the infant's communication and language development. Mothers also experience considerable pleasure from satisfying their infant's needs.

WEANING

Weaning is a process of expanding the diet to include food and drink other than breast milk or infant formula. Weaning allows the infant to meet changing nutritional needs and to become less nutritionally dependent on milk. Most infants should not be given solid foods before the age of 4 months but a mixed diet should be offered by the age of 6 months. There are health benefits for infants who are exclusively breast fed during the first months of life. Solid food should be introduced between the ages of 4 and 6 months when the infant's physiology and development have matured and the diversity of the weaning diet can be handled. Weaning too early or too late or with inappropriate foods or in inappropriate manners may result in behavioural and health problems and in family stress. At around 4–6 months of life a more energy and nutrient dense diet is needed than can be provided by milk alone. However, weaning should not start before neuromuscular co-ordination has developed sufficiently to allow the infant to eat solids, nor before the gut and kidney have matured to handle a more diverse diet. Infants double their birthweight in the first 5 months of life and as their size increases and the growth rate remains rapid their dietary needs can no longer be met with milk fluids. The capacity of the infant's stomach limits the volume of milk that can be consumed. The quantity of calories, protein and vitamins A and D particularly are likely to become inadequate by 6 months. Adequate dietary sources of iron and zinc at this stage are also recognised to be very important. In spite of adequate iron stores normally present in healthy term infants and in spite of highly efficient absorption of iron from breast milk, additional sources of absorbable iron are required from the diet from the age of 6 months if the infant is not to become iron deficient and at risk of anaemia. By 4–5 months the infant can begin to form a bolus of semi-solid food and move it from the front to the back of the mouth and should be able to accept soft pureed foods from a spoon, form a bolus and swallow it. Infants of 5 months can sit with support, hold objects and put them to their mouths. These skills can be encouraged by providing foods for the infant to hold. Infants can chew from about 6 months of age but if not encouraged this ability may not readily develop and the teaching of older infants to chew can be difficult.

From about the age of 7 months infants learn to shut their mouths, turn their heads and indicate refusal to feed. They may use this manipulatively and may make weaning particularly difficult if the child has not yet accepted new tastes and textures. Semi-solid foods should be given from a spoon and not mixed with milk or other drinks in a bottle. From 6 months of age infants should be introduced to drinking from a cup and after the age of 1 year, bottle feeding should be discouraged. Normal growth and development of the infant should be the principal determinant of the diets of children under 5 years of age. A variety of foods should be offered at each meal and protein sources should be mixed. Most dietary fat during weaning comes from milk whether as breast milk, infant formula or cows' milk. Milk also makes important contributions to the intakes of several nutrients as well as energy. Cows' milk is not recommended as a main drink during infancy. During the second year whole cows' milk is suitable as a main drink and it contributes particularly energy, calcium and fat-soluble vitamins which may not be readily available from other sources. After the age of 2 years semi-skimmed milk may be introduced provided the diet is varied and adequate to meet fully the energy and nutrient needs.

As the contribution from fat to the total energy requirements reduces, the deficit should not be made up with large intakes of non-milk extrinsic sugars but by natural starchy foods such as bread, potatoes, pasta and rice. A recent report from the UK Department of Health Committee on Medical Aspects of Food Policy (COMA) on diet and cardiovascular disease recommends that the population aged 5 years and older should consume no more than about 35% of calories from fat and about 10% of calories from saturated fatty acids. Children under 5 years are not included in this recommendation. Growth in infancy and young childhood must be safeguarded and this cannot be achieved without adequate fat intake. Diets for the under 5s should offer a wide diversity of foods and tastes and are to be enjoyed. At a time of life when individual children show a wide but normal diversity low fat diets intended to provide "healthy eating" usually result in restricting this dietary diversity and run the risk of providing inadequate energy intakes.

Non-starch polysaccharides form a complex group of polymers derived largely from plant cell walls and are generally known as dietary fibre. The effects of high intakes of foods rich in non-starch polysaccharide which also often contain high phytate levels and in association with a low fat intake may predispose to "toddlers' diarrhoea". The proportion of energy supplied as starch should increase as the proportions supplied as fat decrease. Non-milk extrinsic sugars should be limited to no more than about 10% of total dietary energy intake and should be confined to main mealtimes in order to safeguard dental health. Non-wheat cereals and pureed fruit, vegetables and potatoes are suitable first weaning foods. Salt should not be added and additional sugar should be limited to that needed for palatability of sour fruits. Between 6 and 9 months of age the amount and variety of foods including meat, fish, eggs, cereals and pulses should be increased and the number of milk feeds reduced. Food consistency should proceed from pureed through minced/mashed to finely chopped. By the age of 1 year infants should be feeding on a mixed and varied diet.

Where there is a family history of atopy or gluten enteropathy, mothers should be encouraged to breast feed for 6 months or longer. Weaning before 4 months should be discouraged and the introduction of foods traditionally regarded as allergenic should be delayed until 6 months at the earliest. For infants who are allergic to cows' milk protein, soya infant formula provides a reasonably adequate source of nutrition in the early months of life and should be continued as part of a mixed diet. Infants weaning on to diets restricted in animal protein should be introduced to weaning foods no later than 6 months and should be advised to continue on infant formula beyond the first year of life. Additional vitamin C should be ensured and an energy supplement from a fat source may be required if there is an inadequate intake of energy.

Infants and young children who are failing to thrive should be identified as early as possible and a nutritional cause investigated. Advice to prevent obesity should be given to children who are becoming excessively fat at the age of 1 year or when the parents are obese.

Weaning is a process which should be enjoyable for the weanling and the weaner. It is, however, a time when antagonisms can arise and clashes of will may develop. There are many ways in which to wean a child and the process should not be looked upon as a challenge. There is still a great deal to learn about the range of weaning practices adopted in many different societies dependent upon a multitude of different food sources. There is now a bewildering supply of manufactured foods for infants which offer a degree of convenience but which should not be allowed to exclude introducing infants to the range of normal family foods. There is still much to be learned about the process of weaning and the optimal weaning diet. The report of the Department of Health Working Group on the Weaning Diet is an additional source of information and advice.

NORMAL GROWTH AND DEVELOPMENT

Growth progresses from conception through to maturity though not at a steady state throughout. Many factors determine the size of normal children and a measurement close to the population mean does not necessariliy mean normality. Centile charts are available for many body measurements and show the population distribution and change with growth from birth until maturity. The 50th centile is the mean, with half of the population having measurements greater and half less. The 50th centile is not necessarily the average of the measurements in the population; for many dimensions such as weight and skinfold thickness the distributions are asymmetrical. Population measurement on the 3rd centile and 97th centile are indicators of the population distribution for any specific growth measurement. Most of the data, however, for centile charts have been derived from cross-sectional observations augmented over the years of puberty by repeated measurements on the same children. Centile charts are relevant only to the population from which they were derived and at that time. Racial differences and differences between social categories in individual countries may not have the same centile distribution. It must also be remembered that centile charts show a population as it is and not necessarily the ideal for that population. For example, most of the infant growth data currently available is from a population of largely artificially fed infants. Racial and population differences may be due to true genetic variations but may equally well result from suboptimal growth in underprivileged or under- or overnourished children. As it is impracticable to obtain data appropriate for every population group, reference is usually made to a standard national chart. Preterm birth and differing times of onset of puberty can alter the individual infant and child growth patterns. Growth data are usually presented as distance centiles of body measurements at particular ages which represent the total accumulated over the past, or as velocities which show the change in a dimension over a limited period of time. Perinatal growth charts from 22 or 24 weeks gestation allow the plotting of birth measurements and subsequent ages are plotted appropriately for the length of gestation. After 2 years of age the significance of the effect of being born preterm can be ignored. Velocities of many body measurements are greatest at or before birth and rapidly decline over the first 2–3 years of life, then remain relatively constant over the subsequent prepubertal years. By tradition length is measured up to the age of 2 years and height thereafter. Height velocity continues to slow down after the age of 2–3 years and is at its slowest immediately before the acceleration of puberty. Growth of the head reflects growth of the brain and is fastest in the first few years of life. At puberty, growth of the limbs is at its most rapid and is completed before that of the trunk. Weight gain velocity increases steadily between the ages of 4 years and puberty but skinfold measurements show a much more undulating pattern. Lean body mass is the main component of weight gain at some ages and weight changes should not be considered as solely due to changes in body fat. Skinfold measurements are useful indicators of body fat and its changes. Growth velocity increases dramatically at puberty and this precedes the cessation of bone growth. Bone development in girls is considerably advanced compared with boys throughout childhood but does not become apparent clinically until puberty. Signs of puberty in girls appears about a year before those in boys and the ages of maximal growth and cessation of growth occur 2 years earlier. In early puberty the average girl is taller than the average boy of the same chronological age but finally measures about 12 cm less. The timings of the various changes of puberty relative to each other vary greatly from one individual to another and may follow family predispositions. The first observational change in boys is growth of the testes and peak growth rate in boys is late in the sequence of changes. A boy well advanced in sexual development may still have considerable growth potential. In girls the age of most rapid growth is relatively early in puberty and invariably precedes the menarche after which growth velocity slows down and little residual growth will occur thereafter. In two-thirds of girls breast development is the first observed change of puberty and precedes the appearance of pubic hair. Weight gain is proportionately greater in puberty than height. In delayed puberty the slow prepubertal velocities of height and weight persist and the relative decrement in weight from the average centile line is much greater than that of height. This can give a false impression of being underweight. A useful method of describing the position of a child's height, weight, etc. in relation to the normal population is the standard deviation score (SDS):

$$SDS = \frac{X - M}{SD}$$

where X is the child's measurement. M is the mean measurement in the normal population at the child's age and SD is the standard deviation in the normal population at the child's age.

Skeletal age (radiological bone age) is that age to which the bony development of the child corresponds when compared with standards derived from the normal population. The stage of physical maturity of the child may not correspond with the chronological age but may correlate with bone age. By convention the bones of the left wrist and hand are used for estimating bone age. There is considerable variation in skeletal age within the normal population and centile distributions are wide. Again there are variations between populations of different racial, geographical and cultural backgrounds. At puberty as with height growth the bone age of an individual does not adhere to the composite pattern of change in the normal population but will frequently cross skeletal age centiles. Usually when the phase of rapid physical growth at puberty occurs there will be an accompanying acceleration in bone age compared with the standards.

Factors affecting physical growth

Some of the influences responsible for physiological differences in growth such as racial, familial and environmental factors can be assessed and adjustments made to the expected growth centiles for the individual child. Other influences cause pathological deviations in growth (Table 1.18).

Knowledge of the centile positions of height and weights of siblings as well as both parents can be valuable in identifying one child who is conspicuously different from the other family members. In extremely tall or short individuals the fact that a parent is similarly tall or small must not always be taken as a reason to assume that there is no underlying pathology. For example, there may occasionally be a dominantly inherited abnormal growth pattern, e.g. in certain bone dysplasias, growth hormone deficiency and Marfan syndrome. Many other characteristics may be inherited such as fatness and thinness. The family pattern in age of puberty may influence the age of menarche or rapid growth in children and late onset of adolescence in one or both parents may

TABLE 1.18 Factors resulting in abnormal growth

Abnormalities of nutrition (quantitive and qualitive)
  Undernutrition
    inadequate intake
    abnormal digestive, absorptive and/or metabolic processes.
    excessive alimentary loss (vomiting, regurgitation, malabsorption, diarrhoea)

  Overnutrition – obesity
    Adverse antenatal factors (small for dates infant)
    Inherited metabolic and other disorders
    Chronic ill health and disease processes
    Adverse psychosocial and emotional influences
    Abnormal endocrine function

be reassuring in a short statured child with delayed puberty.

A genetic abnormality may affect growth prenatally so that the infant is born small for gestational age. Bone dysplasias (e.g. chondrodysplasias) and chromosomal anomalies such as Turner syndrome may be clinically obvious.

A child's state of physical development in contrast to intellectual development may not correspond well with chronological age. Skeletal age estimations help to establish whether a child's physical development is advanced, retarded or commensurate with actual age. A component of short stature may be delayed onset of puberty in which case the child may continue to grow for a longer period of time until skeletal maturity and ultimately achieve a taller stature. Some late developing boys may still be growing after the age of 20 years. The mean difference in adult height between the sexes is 12.5 cm and this is mainly due to the fact that girls enter puberty before boys and on average complete their growth 2 years earlier. Undernutrition can be a potent factor in delaying puberty whereas exogenous obesity is associated with early onset puberty. Weight loss for any cause delays pubertal development and is a common cause of primary or secondary amenorrhoea. Adverse psychosocial circumstances and chronic ill health sometimes suppress endocrine function and delay puberty. Endocrine disorders such as deficiencies of thyroxine or growth hormone are associated with delayed puberty. There has been a secular trend of advancement in pubertal age throughout most developing countries but different geographical areas have different patterns of pubertal onset which may not necessarily be entirely nutritionally related. Climatic influences such as altitude, temperature and daylight hours affect growth. Children grow faster during the spring and summer than in autumn and winter. Emotional deprivation or psychological trauma not only delays puberty but can also produce growth retardation not always as a result of an inadequate nutritional intake. It may be that there is either supression of hormonal release or reduced receptor response of end organs.

Diagnosis of significant growth abnormalities

Table 1.19 shows some of the aspects to be considered in the recognition of growth disorders at an early stage. The earlier a diagnosis is made the greater time there is for treatment and growth correction. Routine measurements of children at clinics, schools and in hospital outpatient departments with appropriate interpretation of the measurements could prevent many unnecessary delays in therapy. Once the child

TABLE 1.19 Indicators of abnormal growth

Body measurements above the 97th or below the 3rd centile for the population
  Deviation with time from a centile line (except at puberty)
  Gross disparity in height and weight centile
  Gross deviation from parental and sibling pattern
  Abnormal body proportions
  Inappropriate size at birth
  Inappropriate or delayed sexual development
  Gross abnormality in skeletal age
  Other abnormal clinical features

has entered puberty and the skeletal age is well advanced the remaining growth potential is small. Bony epiphyses fusion will prevent further increase in height. Even when growth disorders are diagnosed and no treatment available an early diagnosis is none the less important in the recognition of possible hereditary implications and also to predict likely subsequent growth. This will allow the child, parents, teachers and others to adjust and cope with the problem.

Obesity

A diagnosis of obesity is sometimes defined as 10% or more overweight for height at a given age. Skinfold measurements interpreted on centile charts are of value in confirming that excessive weight is due to fat and will give a measurement of the severity of the obesity. Impedence measurements can also give an indirect estimate of the body fat content. In short stature associated with short limbs the weight/height relationship may be high without the child being obese because of the greater contribution of the trunk to total height. Very few obese children have an underlying recognisable pathology (endogenous obesity). Most of these children have retarded bone age. The majority of overweight children are exogenously obese and are frequently taller than expected with advanced bone age. Children with Turner or Down syndrome or with Prader–Willi syndrome may be obese due to lack of exercise and overeating. If one parent is obese, half of the children will be obese and if both parents are obese then over three-quarters of the children will be similarly affected. Fifty per cent of children who become obese acquire their obesity before the age of 5 years. Early recognition of a tendency to obesity is critical if family diet is to be influenced sufficiently to reduce the child's obesity. Simple exogenous obesity is now the most important form of malnutrition in the western world. Fat children are physically less active and agile than other children. They are subject to derisive name calling at school and this often results in a degree of unhappiness. Obese infants are unduly susceptible to respiratory infections, skeletal development tends to be advanced and on average bone age is one year ahead of the chronological age. The body mass index is obtained by applying the formula wt/ht^2 (g/cm^3) and ponderal index is obtained by applying the formula wt/ht^3 (g/cm^3) and high indices will indicate obesity. In both sexes the onset of puberty also occurs about one year earlier. Pickwickian obesity can lead to cardiorespiratory failure or the hypoventilation syndrome. The typical features are long-standing obesity with dyspnoea on exertion, cyanosis, tachycardia, raised central venous pressure, cardiac dilation, hepatomegaly and peripheral oedema.

Treatment

The principle of treatment is to ensure that intake of energy is less than output. It is a difficult and disappointing condition to treat. The only way that a fat child can safely be made to lose weight is by limitation of the food intake. An 800–1000 kcal diet, if strictly enforced, will prove an effective, although often remarkably slow, method of treatment. Such a diet should contain approximately 60 g protein and 40 g fat; the main restriction should fall on the carbohydrate intake which will be reduced to 100 g. A major difficulty is to ensure strict adherence to this diet for so often the parents remain overindulgent in spite of the dietary advice given. In severe cases it will be necessary to admit the child to hospital for a period to become accustomed and trained to the diet although relapse may occur on return home. Drugs which curb appetite are best avoided altogether in children. In less severe cases the child can at least be prevented from becoming more obese by a qualitative dietary limitation of carbohydrates such as bread, cakes, steamed puddings and sweets. Again the major problem is to obtain the parents' full cooperation. In older children who are themselves anxious to lose weight the outlook is more optimistic. Because treatment of obesity is difficult and the long-term results disappointing, prevention should be the aim. Preventive measures may be instituted in the prenatal period, in infancy and in later childhood.

Development

There are tables available which describe the normal range of attainment for a wide range of developmental progress. Such measures as gross motor, fine motor and the acquisition of language can be applied to population groups and developmental quotients and intelligence quotients derived. Measures of emotional development, social development and the development of self-esteem are at present the subject of much debate. It will be interesting to have such measures and to begin to delineate the pathogenesis and detect the early onset of deviations from normal development in these aspects of human behaviour. Until these aspects of infant and child development can be measured it is difficult to relate deviant patterns to genetic and environmental factors such as nutrition. A longer-term aim will be to relate the physical, intellectual, emotional and social growth of the infant to the home, educational and nutritional background of the individual child, the family, and the community.

2

Assessment of the Child and the Family

THE HISTORY

Introduction

At all times the doctor must show genuine concern and interest when speaking with parents. The parents and the child must feel that the doctor has the time, interest and competence to help them. A physician who greets the child by name irrespective of age will convey an attitude of concern and interest. Parents tell us about the child's signs and symptoms although children contribute more as they grow older.

The doctor–patient relationship gradually develops during history-taking and physical examination. Considerable tact and discretion are required when taking the history, especially in the presence of the child: questioning on sensitive subjects should best be reserved for a time when the parents can be interviewed alone. It may therefore be necessary to separate the parent and the child–patient when taking the history especially when the problems are related to behaviour, school difficulties and socio-economic disturbances in the home environment.

The medical student having been instructed in the history-taking and physical examination of adults needs to appreciate the modifications necessary when dealing with the child–patient. A basic template for history-taking is useful and serves as a reminder of the ground to be covered (Table 2.l). Initially the medical student may be confused because of the need to obtain information from someone other than the patient, usually the mother. Useful information may be obtained by observing the infant and young child during the history-taking. The older child should be given an opportunity to talk, to present their symptoms and to tell how they interfere with school and play activities.

TABLE 2.1 History-taking – the paediatric patient

Presenting problem
History of the presenting problem
Previous history:
   Pregnancy and delivery
   Neonatal period and infancy
   Subsequent development
   Other disorders or diseases
   Dietary
   Immunisation
Family history
   Parents
   Siblings
   Others

The simple act of offering a toy, picture book or pen-torch is often an effective step toward establishing rapport. Rigid adherence to routine is both unnecessary and counterproductive. A lot may be learned of the family constellation and the parent–child relationship by simply observing the parent(s) and child during the history-taking and physical examination. Therefore watching, listening and talking are of paramount importance in paediatric practice and are invaluable in arriving at a working diagnosis.

History of present complaint

Even before language develops in the infant (Latin – without speech) parents can detect altered behaviour and observe abnormal physical signs. It is sensible to commence with the history of the presenting observations because that is what the parents have come to talk about. In the newborn infant the history from the attending nurse and medical staff is important.

Every endeavour should be made to ask appropriate questions and discuss relevant points in the history in order to identify the nature of the child's problems and come to a tentative diagnosis. The doctor should ask what the child is called at home and address the child with this name since otherwise he/she may be less forthcoming. The parents should be allowed to give the history in their own way and the doctor should then ask specific questions, such as: how severe are the symptoms; have the symptoms changed during the past days, weeks or months; has there been any change recently in the child's appetite, energy or activities; has the child been absent from school; has anyone who cares for the child been ill; has the child been thriving or losing weight; what change in behaviour has there been; has there been a change in appetite, sleep, micturition or bowel habits. An articulate older child can describe feelings and symptoms more accurately, as the child's memory for the time and sequence of events may be more precise, than the parents.

Past medical history

The past history is the documentation of significant events which have happened in the child's life and which may be of relevance in coming to a diagnosis. Therefore the doctor should try to obtain relevant information concerning the past from the family and any other sources that are available. It is useful if the events are recorded in the sequence of their occurrence. A careful history should contain details of pregnancy, delivery, neonatal period, early feeding, the child's achievement of developmental milestones and details of admissions to hospital, with date, place and reason for admission. A complete list of current medication including vitamins and other supplements should be obtained. An enquiry should be made of any drug or other sensitivity which should always be prominently recorded. Details of immunisation and all previous infectious diseases should be elicited.

Mother's pregnancy, labour, delivery and the neonatal period

The younger the child, the more important is the information about the period of intrauterine life. The history of pregnancy includes obstetric complications during the pregnancy; history of illness, infection or injury and social habits, e.g. smoking by the mother are important. Drug or alcohol ingestion and poor diet during pregnancy may have an adverse effect on the fetus and lead to problems. The estimated length of gestation and the birthweight of the baby should be recorded. Details of any intrapartum or perinatal problems should be recorded.

Dietary history

The duration of breast feeding should be recorded or the type of artificial feed and any weaning problems. The dietary history can be of major importance in paediatric history-taking. If the patient is not thriving or has vomiting, diarrhoea, constipation or anaemia then the physician must obtain a detailed dietary history. The dietary history should not only include solid foods but also the consumption of liquid foods and any other supplements such as vitamins. In this way the quality of the diet and the quantity of nutrients can be assessed and compared to the recommended intake. Any discrepancy between the actual and recommended intake may have a possible bearing on the diagnosis.

Developmental history

Inquiries about the age at which major developmental milestones in infancy and early childhood were achieved are necessary when faced with an infant or child who is suspected of developmental delay. On the other hand, with the child who is doing well at school and whose physical and social activities are normal, less emphasis on the minutiae of development is needed. Some parents are vague about the time of developmental achievements unless very recently acquired, but many have clear recall of the important events such as smiling, sitting and walking independently. It can be helpful to enquire whether this child's development paralleled that of other children.

Family and social history

The health and educational progress of a child is directly related to the home and the environment. Medical, financial and social stresses within the family sometimes have a direct or indirect bearing on the child's presenting problem. It is therefore essential to know about the housing conditions and some information of parental income and working hours, as well as the child's performance in school and adjustment to playmates.

The family history should be thoroughly evaluated. The age and health of the close relatives are important to record. Heights and weights of parents and siblings may be of help, especially when dealing with children of short stature, obesity, failure to thrive, or the infant with an enlarged head. Consanguinity is common in some cultures and offspring of consanguinous marriages have an increased chance of receiving the same recessive gene from each parent and thus developing a genetically determined disease.

Finally, a history of recent travel abroad, particularly in tropical areas, is important as the child may have a disorder uncommon in the UK but having been contracted in another country where disease may be endemic.

PHYSICAL EXAMINATION

The physical examination of the paediatric patient requires a careful and gentle approach. It should be carried out in an appropriate environment with a selection of books or toys around which can be used to allay the apprehension and anxiety of the child. No special tools are required to perform an examination of a neonate and the best equipment a doctor has are his eyes. More can be learned by careful inspection than by any other single examination method. The baby should be examined in a warm environment in good light. Nappies must be removed to examine the baby fully. We look first at the baby as a whole, noting especially the colour, posture and movements, followed by a more detailed examination, starting at the head and working down to the feet: "top to toe".

It is important to realise that the child may be apprehensive with a stranger, especially when faced with the unfamiliar surroundings of a surgery or hospital outpatient department. It is essential that the doctor be truthful with the child regarding what is going to be done. The child should never by made to face sudden unexpected manoeuvres and should be allowed to play with objects such as the stethoscope. It may be useful to let him or her examine a toy animal or doll to facilitate gaining confidence. Infants and young children are often best examined on the mother's lap where they feel more secure. The doctor should ensure that his hands and the instruments used to examine the child are suitably warmed. It is not always mandatory to remove all the child's clothes, although it is often essential in the examination of the acutely ill child. Procedures which may produce discomfort such as examination of the throat, ears or rectal examination should be left until towards the end of the examination. The order of the examination may be varied to suit the particular child's needs. Awareness of the normal variations at different ages is important.

A thorough physical examination is a powerful therapeutic tool especially if the problem is one primarily of inappropriate parental anxiety. Understandably parents do not usually accept reassurance if the doctor has not examined the child properly. Examination of the infant or child is often preceded by recording the patient's height, weight and head circumference on the growth chart. This may have been done by a nurse before the doctor sees the family. These measurements are plotted on graphs or charts which indicate the percentiles or standard deviations at the various ages throughout childhood. If these measurements are outwith the 3rd to 97th centile for children of that sex and age further study is indicated. If previous records of height, weight or head circumference are available for comparison with the current measurements this may provide considerable help towards diagnosis and management. Inquiry of parental height, weight or head size may also be important.

General inspection

The general appearance of the child may suggest a particular syndrome. Does the child look like the rest of the family? The facies may be characteristic in Down syndrome and other chromosomal disorders or in mucopolysaccharidoses and hypercalcaemia. Peculiar odours from an infant may provide a clue to diagnosis of aminoacidurias, such as maple syrup disease (maple syrup-like odour), phenylketonuria (mousy odour), or trimethylaminuria (fishy odour). A more detailed examination should then be performed. The most valuable of the doctor's senses are his eyes as more can be learned by careful inspection and also on watching the patient's reactions than any other single procedure.

General inspection should include the following.

Colour

Colour should be pink with the exception of the periphery which may be slightly blue. Peripheral cyanosis is a feature of the relatively polycythaemic newborn who has enough reduced haemoglobin to give the appearance of cyanosis. Congenital heart disease is only suggested if the baby has central cyanosis. A pale baby may be anaemic or ill and requires careful investigation to find the cause. A blue baby may have either a cardiac anomaly or respiratory problems. If jaundice is present in an infant the serum bilirubin level should be checked.

Posture and movements

A term baby lies supine for the first day or two and has vigorous, often asymmetric movements of all limbs. In contrast, a sick baby adopts the frog position with legs abducted, externally rotated and is inactive. Older infants and children should be observed for abnormal movements, posture and gait.

Skin

The skin is a major body organ which, because of the larger surface area in relationship to weight, of the young means that the skin is relatively more important in the immature. It forms a barrier against environmental attack and its structure and function reflect the general health of the child, i.e. in states of malnutrition and dehydration. The presence of any skin rash, its colour and whether there are present macules, papules, vesicles, bullae, tumours or pustules should be recorded. The skin texture, elasticity, tone and subcutaneous thickness should be assessed by picking up the skin between the fingers. A newborn infant may have a dry scaly skin which is the result of placental insufficiency. The skinfolds in the groin, axilla and neck should be examined as they are sometimes the sites of infection. Pigmented naevi, strawberry naevi, haemangiomata or lymphangiomata may be present and may vary in size and number. They may be absent or small at birth and grow in subsequent days or weeks. A number of babies may have transient erythematous rashes on the trunk which are of little significance although perinatal viral infections may be identified in some.

Head

The head should be inspected for size, shape and symmetry. Measurement of the head circumference (occipital frontal circumference – OFC) with a non-elastic tape by placing it to encircle the head just above the eyebrows around the maximum protuberance of the occipital bone should be performed and charted. In the infant the skull should be palpated to determine the size and tension in the fontanelles and to assess the skull sutures (Fig. 2.1). In the neonate the posterior fontanelle may be very small and subsequently closes by 3 months of age but the anterior fontanelle is larger, only closing at around 18 months. It varies considerably in size from baby to baby. A normal baby will have a concave anterior fontanelle when quiet and held in the upright position and pulsation synchronising with the heart may be seen. A tense fontanelle suggests raised intracranial pressure and a deeply sunken one suggests dehydration. Many normal babies have separated sutures and

there may be some overlapping as a result of the moulding which occurs during delivery. By 24 hours the caput succedaneum should be gone and a cephalhaematoma may not become obvious until later. A depressed fracture which is usually frontal or parietal is obvious but linear fractures of the vault bones are even more rare. The risk of any skull fracture is in its associated cerebral damage with haemorrhage resulting in brain damage or hydrocephalus as a secondary complication. Fractures heal very rapidly. The amount of hair on the scalp of a baby varies from almost nothing to "a mop".

Large fontanelles, separation of sutures, delayed closure of the fontanelles may be associated with raised intracranial pressure or other systemic disorders such as hypothyroidism.

Ears

Position and configuration of the ears should be observed. Whilst abnormalities such as low setting of the ears is frequently associated with renal tract anomalies, absence of an ear or non-development of the auricle will require early referral to an otolaryngologist It often requires the parent to hold the child on his or her lap and provide reassurance during the examination. A method of doing this is illustrated in Fig. 2.2. Parents are usually very competent in detecting hearing impairment. The exception to this is where the child is mentally retarded. All infants should be given a screening test for hearing at 6 months of age. Simple testing materials are required,

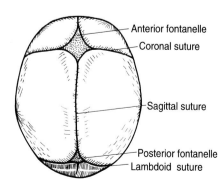

FIGURE 2.1 Top of head – anterior fontanelle and sutures.

Anterior fontanelle
Coronal suture
Sagittal suture
Posterior fontanelle
Lambdoid suture

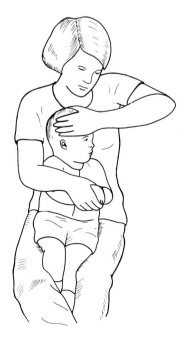

FIGURE 2.2 Method of restraining a child for examination of the ear.

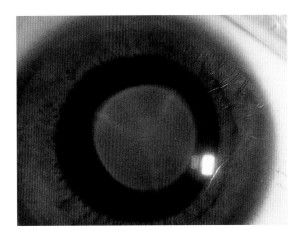

FIGURE 2.3 Congenital cataract.

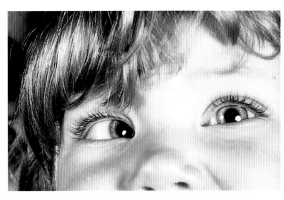

FIGURE 2.4 Squint – corneal light reflections

e.g. a cup and spoon, high and low pitched rattles, devices to imitate bird or animal sounds, or even snapping of finger tips are usually effective if hearing is normal. The sounds should be made quietly at a distance of 2–3 feet out of view of the child. By 6 months of age a child should be able to localise sound. To pass the screening test the child should turn and look directly at the source of the sound.

Eyes

These should be inspected for subconjuctival haemorrhages which are usually of little importance, for cataracts (Fig. 2.3), or other congenital abnormalities such as colobomata. "Rocking" the baby from the supine to vertical position often results in the eyes opening so they can be inspected. Squint is a condition in which early diagnosis and treatment is important. There are two simple tests which can be carried out to determine whether or not a squint is present:

1 The position of the "corneal light reflection" should normally be in the centre of each pupil if the eyes are both aligned on a bright source of light, usually a pen-torch. Should one eye be squinting then the reflection of the light from the cornea will not be centred in the pupil of that eye (Fig. 2.4). It will be displaced outwards if the eye is convergent and inwards towards the nose if the eye is divergent. It may be displaced by such a large amount that it is seen over the iris or even over the sclera, where of course it may be rather more difficult to identify, but with such obvious squints the diagnosis is usually not in doubt.
2 In the "cover test" one chooses an object of interest for the child, e.g. a brightly coloured toy with moving components. When the child is looking at the object of interest the eye thought to be straight is covered with an opaque card and the uncovered

eye is observed to see whether it moves to take up fixation on the object of interest. If the child has a convergent squint then the eye will move laterally to take up fixation, and this is the usual situation since convergent squints are four times more common than divergent squints. If the eye were divergent it would move medially.

The commonest cause for apparent blindness in young children is developmental delay. Assessment of whether a young baby can see is notoriously difficult. *Fixation* should develop in the first week of life but an early negative response is of no value as the absence of convincing evidence of fixation is not synonymous with blindness. The failure to develop a fixation reflex results in ocular nystagmus, but these roving eye movements do not appear until the age of 3 months.

A misleading response may be obtained when a bright light stimulus is applied to a child, preferrably in a dimly lit room. The normal response is a blinking or "screwing up" the eyes and occasionally by withdrawing the head. This is a subcortical reflex response and may be present in babies despite them having cortical blindness. The absence of this response increases the probability of blindness.

Face

Abnormalities of facial development are usually obvious and an example is the infant with cleft lip. Associated with this there may be a cleft palate but full visual examination of the palate including the uvula is necessary to ensure that the palate is intact and there is not a submucous cleft of the soft palate or a posterior cleft. Submucous and soft palate clefts cannot be felt on palpation.

Small areas of dilated capillaries are common between the upper eye lids, on the forehead and in the nape of the neck. These "stork marks" or salmon patches become less obvious as the infant grows.

Mouth

Inspection of the mouth should include visualisation of the palate, fauces and the dentition. A cleft lip is obvious but the palate must be visualised to exclude a cleft. The mouth is best opened by pressing down in the middle of the lower jaw. A baby is rarely born with teeth but if present these are almost always the lower central incisors. The soft palate should be inspected to exclude the possibility of a submucous cleft which could be suggested by a bifid uvula. Small fibromata are sometimes seen in the gums. They are white and seldom require treatment. These are normal. The lower jaw should be seen in profile as a receding chin (micrognathia) may be the cause of tongue swallowing or glossoptosis (Pierre Robin syndrome) and it may be associated with a cleft palate. These babies very often have feeding difficulties as well as respiratory problems. Average times of eruption of primary and secondary dentitions are shown in Table 2.2. The mean age for shedding deciduous teeth is 75 months for central incisors, 86 months for lateral incisors, 122 months for canines, 100 months for the first molars and 109 months for second molars.

Neck

Examination of the neck may reveal congenital goitre and midline cysts which may be thyroglossal or dermoid in origin. Lateral cysts may be of branchial origin or sometimes there may be extensive swellings which may be cystic hygroma or lymphangiomata. In early infancy a sternomastoid tumour may be palpable in the mid region of the sternomastoid muscle. Associated with this there may be significant limitation of rotation and lateral flexion of the neck. Palpation along the clavicle will define any tenderness or swelling suggestive of recent or older fracture or absence.

Chest

The shape, chest wall movement and the nature and rate of the breathing (30–40 per minute) as well as the presence of any indrawing of the sternum and rib cage should be noted. In a normal baby without respiratory or abdominal problems the abdomen moves freely during breathing and there is very little chest movement. Most of the movements of the breathing cycle are carried out by the movement of the diaphragm. The nipples and axillary folds should be assessed to exclude conditions such as absent pectoral muscles.

Cardiovascular

Examination of the cardiovascular system of infants and children is carried out in a similar manner to that

TABLE 2.2 Average times of eruption of primary and secondary dentitions

Deciduous teeth	Average time of eruption
Central incisors	
lower ⎱	
upper ⎰	7th month
Lateral incisors	
lower ⎱	
upper ⎰	9th month
First molars	12th month
Canines	18th month
Second molars	24th month
Permanent dentition	
First molars	
lower ⎱	
upper ⎰	6th year
Central incisors	
lower	6th year
upper	6th to 7th year
Lateral incisors	
lower	7th year
upper	8th year
Canines	
lower	10th year
upper	10th to 11th year
First premolars	
upper	10th year
lower	10th to 11th year
Second premolars	
upper	11th year
lower	11th to 12th year
Second molars	
lower	11th to 12th year
upper	12th year
Third molars	20th year

of adults. The examiner should always feel for femoral pulses and ascertain whether there is any radiofemoral or brachiofemoral delay as this would suggest the possibility of coarctation of the aorta. The most important factor in recording the blood pressure of children is to use a cuff of the correct size. The cuff should cover at least two-thirds of the upper arm. If the cuff size is less than this a falsely high blood pressure reading may be obtained. In small infants relatively accurate systolic and diastolic pressures as well as mean arterial pressures can be obtained by use of the doppler method. The apex should be visible and palpable and the position noted. The precordial areas should be palpated for the presence of thrills. Right ventricular preponderance in the first few days makes the apex beat easier to see and palpate. If the apex beat is not obvious it should be sought on the right side of the chest as there could be dextrocardia or a left-sided congenital diaphragmatic hernia with the heart pushed to the right or collapse of the right lung. All areas should be auscultated while the baby is quiet. The rate is approximately 120 per minute and the sounds are much more evenly spaced than in older children with a "tic-tac" rhythm. Systolic murmurs may be very harsh and can be confused with breath sounds.

Lungs

Small children frequently cry when the chest is percussed and when a cold stethoscope is applied. If the mother holds the child over her shoulder and soothes him it is often easier to perform a thorough chest examination. Light percussion can be more valuable than auscultation in some situations but the basic signs are similar to those found in an adult. Breath sounds are usually harsh, high pitched and rapid. Any adventitious sounds present are pathological. Percussion of the chest in a newborn baby may be helpful to pick up the presence of a pleural effusion (stony dull), collapse, consolidation of a lung (dull) or a pneumothorax (hyper-resonant). These pathological states are usually associated with an increase in the respiratory rate, as well as clinical signs of respiratory distress.

Abdomen

In the infant the abdomen and umbilicus are inspected and attention should be paid to the presence of either a scaphoid abdomen, which in a neonate may be one of the signs of diaphragmatic hernia or duodenal atresia, or a distended abdomen which suggests intestinal obstruction especially if visible peristalsis can be seen. Peristalsis from left to right suggests a high intestinal obstruction whereas one from the right to the left would be more in keeping with low intestinal obstruction. Any asymmetry of the abdomen may indicate the presence of an underlying mass. Abdominal movement should be assessed and abdominal palpation should be performed with warm hands.

Palpation of the abdomen should include palpation for the liver, the edge of which is normally felt in the newborn baby, the spleen which can only be felt if it is pathological and the kidneys which can be felt in the first 24 hours with the fingers and thumb palpating in the renal angle and abdomen on each side. The lower abdomen should be palpated for the bladder and an enlargement can be confirmed by percussion from a resonant zone, progressing to a dull zone. In the baby with abdominal distension where there is suspicion of perforation and free gas in the abdomen, the loss of superficial liver dullness on percussion may be the only physical sign present early on. Areas of tenderness can be elicited by watching the baby's reaction to gentle palpation of the abdomen. There may be areas of erythema, cellulitis, oedema of the abdominal wall and on deeper palpation crepitus can occasionally be felt from pneumatosis intestinalis (intramural gas in the wall of the bowel).

Auscultation of the abdomen in the younger patients gives rather different signs than in the adult. The infant even in the presence of peritonitis may have some bowel sounds present. However, in the presence of ileus or peritonitis breath sounds become conducted down over the abdomen to the suprapubic area and in even more severe disorders the heart sounds similarly can be heard extending down over the abdomen to the suprapubic area. As gut tone is gradually re-established the heart sounds recede up towards the chest and are followed by the breath sounds. As this is occurring the patient will be able to start tolerating oral feeds.

Perineal examination is important in both sexes. Examination of the anus should never be omitted. If it is visible and the child has passed meconium then nothing more need be done. Occasionally the anus is ectopic, e.g. placed more anteriorly than it should be, stenotic or even absent. The rectal examination is an invasive procedure and should be carried out in a comfortable warm environment, preferably with the child in the left lateral position and the mother holding the hand of the child at the top end of the bed. It is desirable to have a nurse to keep the lower limbs in the flexed position. The examiner should be talking to the child and to the mother and explaining what is about to happen. There is nothing more intimidating to the child or to the mother than to carry out this procedure without any explanation. It is advisable to place one hand on the pelvis, while with the gloved hand one should retract the buttocks to inspect the anus. The position of the anus should be noted because at times it may be in an ectopic position, i.e. more anterior than in the normal situation. The presence of soiling will also be obvious and inspection of the perineum and the anus, especially with breathing movements and asking the child to strain during this inspection procedure, can provide some useful information with regard to the tone of the anus whether there are varicosities, fissures or anal skin tags. The lubricated index finger is then placed at the anal verge and gradually levered into the anal canal whilst all the time talking to the patient and mother, explaining what is being done. The finger is then gradually inserted up to its hilt and then palpation of the four areas of the anal and rectal canal should be carried out anteriorly, laterally and posteriorly. During this examination it is also important to be able to feel the sacrum and the coccyx to make sure there is no abnormality or absence of these segments. In very small babies the little finger should be used rather than the index finger to avoid damage to the anal sphincter. In some situations it is possible to do a bimanual examination with the index finger in the rectum and the other hand over the abdominal region. It is possible to locate a pelvic mass or confirm an inguinal hernia in a small baby. Excessive discomfort during this procedure might indicate the presence of an anal fissure or even an inflamed pelvic appendix. When the finger is withdrawn from the anal canal it should be carefully inspected for faeces, blood, mucus or threadworms. Following this procedure it is important to wipe the bottom of the child and make the child comfortable.

In the absence of any hypoxic episode during delivery or birth trauma 95% of term babies pass meconium within the first 24 hours. The baby who has failed to pass meconium in the first 48 hours could be considered abnormal and the possibility of Hirschsprung disease considered. The baby with an ectopic or stenotic anus should be treated in order to avoid a ballooned rectum, resulting in rectal inertia which is very difficult to treat when it is picked up later in infancy. The baby with an absent anus may have a high or low anorectal anomaly (supralevator or intralevator anomaly). The presence of a fistula in a boy with passage of meconium per urethrum is very suggestive of a high anomaly. Careful inspection of the perineal region after 24 hours, looking for a small bead of meconium, suggests the presence of a low anomaly. In females the presence of a single opening suggests a cloacal anomaly, the presence of two openings, an intermediate or high anomaly and the presence of three openings an intermediate or low anomaly. It is important to palpate the sacrococcygeal region carefully in these babies because bony segments may be missing and could also be associated with severe renal anomalies. The testes in boys born at term should be in the scrotum. The prepuce cannot be and should not be retracted. It is several months or years before the prepuce can be retracted and stretching is both harmful and unnecessary. In girls the labia should be separated and the genitalia examined. Vernix is almost always present and there may be oedema of the genitalia, especially after a breech delivery.

The presence of a swelling in the scrotum or high in the groin may suggest torsion of a testis and requires urgent attention. Unfortunately many of these are necrotic and the testis is permanently damaged by the time they are diagnosed. The testis which cannot be palpated in the scrotum and cannot be manipulated into the sac, indicates the presence of an undescended testis which will need to be explored and corrected before the age of 2 years. A swelling in the scrotum which has a blueish hue to it suggests the presence of a hydrocele due to a patent processus vaginalis and one can get above such a swelling in most children. Palpation of the scrotum is initially for testes but if gonads are not present then palpation in the inguinal, femoral and perineal regions to determine the presence of undescended or ectopic testes should be carried out.

Conditions such as hypospadias, epispadias, labial adhesions or imperforate hymen should be diagnosed on this initial inspection. Phimosis which is always an acquired disease may be noted at later examination.

Limbs

Upper and lower limbs are examined in detail. The hands should be examined for gross abnormalities, e.g. lobster-claw deformity, and for more subtle disorders such as abnormal palmar creases and dermatoglyphics. Hands and feet should be examined for signs and those experienced in dermatoglyphics may define a finger print pattern which is consistent in various syndromes. The presence of a simian palmar crease may suggest trisomy 21 (Down syndrome) and thumb clenching with neurological disease. The feet, ankles and knees should be examined for the range of movement in the joints and tone of the muscles. Orthopaedic help should be sought if there is fixed deformity or limitation of the normal range of movement.

The femoral head may be outside the acetabulum at birth in true dislocation of the hip or it may be dislocated over the posterior lip of the acetabulum by manipulation, in which case the hip is described as unstable, dislocatable or lax. There are conditions in which the acetabulum is hypoplastic and shallow and the femoral head itself is distorted. Congenital dislocation of the hip is more common after breech deliveries in girls and in certain parts of the world. All newborn infants should be screened shortly after birth. The infant is placed supine with the legs towards the examiner and each hip is examined separately. The knee and hip of the baby are flexed to 90% and the hip fully abducted by placing the middle finger over the greater trochanter and the thumb on the inner side of the thigh opposite the position of the lesser trochanter. When the thigh is in the mid-abducted position, forward pressure is exerted behind the greater trochanter by the middle finger. The other hand holds the opposite femur and pelvis steady. A dislocated femoral head is felt to slip over the acetabular ridge and back into the acetabulum as a definite movement. This part of the test is called the Ortolani manoeuvre (Fig. 4.29). The second part of the test is the Barlow procedure. With the infant still on his back and the legs and hands in the same position, the hip is brought into the position of mid-abduction with the thumb exerting gentle pressure laterally and posteriorly; at the same time the palm exerts posterior and medial pressure. If a hip is dislocatable the femur can be felt to dislocate over the posterior lip of the acetabulum. There is need for caution in performing this test and no force should be employed. Caution is particularly required in infants born with neural tube defects and paralysis of the lower limbs. Similar care in examining the shoulder girdle and upper limbs is necessary.

The knees, ankles and feet should be examined. Dorsiflexion of the feet should allow the lateral

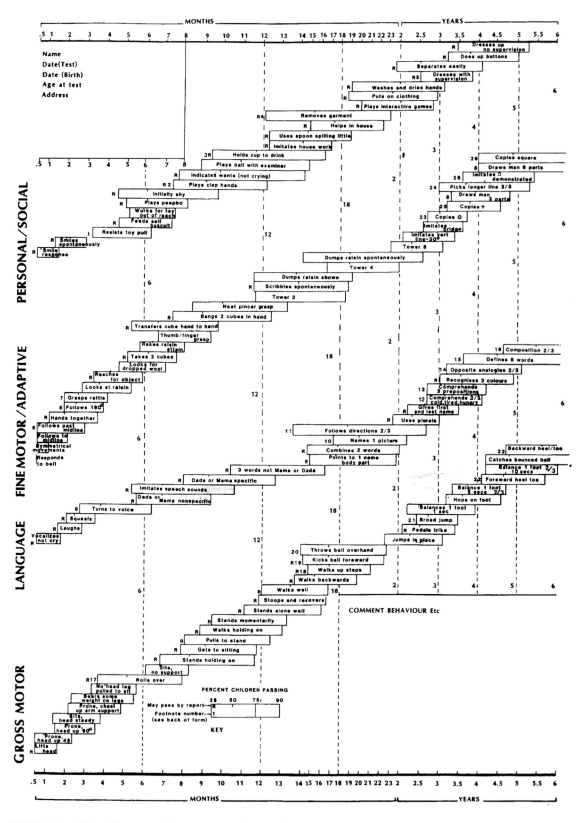

FIGURE 2.5 Cardiff modification of the Denver Developmental Screening tests.

border to come in contact with the peroneal compartment of the leg. Failure indicates a degree of talipes equino-varus (TEV) which is of concern to the parents although with simple physiotherapy there are seldom long-term problems in the absence of underlying neurological abnormality.

Spine

With the baby held face downwards fingers should be run along the spine excluding spinal defects such as spina bifida and noting the presence of the common post-anal dimple, if present. A Mongolian blue spot is commonly seen over the sacrum in Asian babies. The presence of a posterior coccygeal dimple or a sacral pit is common in babies and is due to tethering of the skin to the coccyx. When one stretches the skin and the base of the pit can be seen then nothing needs to be done about it. Very rarely there is communication with the spinal canal which could be the source of infection and cause meningitis.

Stool and urine examination

Examination of a stool which is preferably fresh is often informative. The colour, consistency and smell are noted as well as the presence of blood or mucus. Urine examination is also important in children since symptoms related to the urinary tract may be non-specific. Pyuria is of greater significance than bacteriuria alone in the diagnosis of a urinary tract infection.

Neurological examination

The neurological examination of the young infant and child is different from that routinely carried out in the adult. Muscle tone and strength are important parts of the examination. In infants muscle tone may be influenced by the child's state of relaxation. An agitated hungry infant may appear to be hypertonic but when examined in a cheerful post-prandial state the tone reverts to being normal. The examination of the neurological system cannot be complete without the evaluation of the child's development level relating to gross motor, fine motor, language and social skills (Fig. 2.5; Cardiff modification of the Denver Developmental Screening Test). All older children should be observed for gait to detect abnormal co-ordination and balance

Older children may be tested for sense of touch and proprioception as in adults. Tests of sensation as well as motor power must be performed in the paediatric patient but are difficult to assess in the very young child. The normal newborn has a large number of primitive reflexes (Moro, asymmetric tonic neck, glabellar tap, sucking and rooting process). The *Moro reflex* is a mass reflex which is present in the early weeks after birth. Its absence suggest cerebral damage. It consists of throwing out of the arms followed by bringing them together in an embracing movement. It can be demonstrated by making a loud noise near the child. The *sucking reflex* is present at birth in the normal baby as is the *swallowing reflex*. If the angle of the baby's mouth is touched by the finger or teat the baby will turn his head towards it and search for it. It is looking for its mother's nipple and is known as the *rooting* or *searching reflex*. Excessive salivating may suggest the presence of oesophageal atresia.

The *grasp reflex* is illustrated by gently stroking the back of the hand so that the fingers extend and on placing a finger on the palm of the baby it takes a firm grip. Similar reflexes are present in the toes. If the baby is held up under the arms so that his feet are touching a firm surface, he will raise one leg and hesitatingly put it down in front of the other leg, taking giant strides forwards. This is the *primitive walking reflex*.

Tendon reflexes such as the biceps and knee jerks are easily obtainable but the ankle and triceps jerks are not readily elicited. Important as an indication of nervous system malfunction are muscle tone, posture, movement and the primitive reflexes of the newborn that have been described. Plantar reflex is usually extensor and is of little diagnostic importance in the first year. Delay in disappearance of the primitive reflexes suggests cerebral damage.

3

Head and Neck

Extensive birth marks of the face and facial anomalies distress parents more than any other overt developmental malformations.

EYES

Complete absence of the eyes is very rare and usually associated with other anomalies which are often lethal. Micro-ophthalmia is an uncommon congenital abnormality where impaired growth and development of one or both eyes may cause defective vision. Micro-ophthalmia may also be part of a more generalised syndrome, the other components of which are often of a more serious nature. The sclera of the eye is usually white in colour but in newborn babies it may be blue. The presence of blue sclera in the older infant may suggest the presence of osteogenesis imperfecta (brittle-bone disease) (Fig. 4.13). Jaundice of sclera should be fully investigated but other pigmented spots of the sclera may be due to a congenital deficiency in the wall of the sclera with pigmentation showing through. Colobomata are not infrequent in children and usually present with a slit iris. This usually extends to the anterior chamber of the eye but may involve the retina and cause visual defects. Retinal colobomata may cause no visual problems but occasionally they may be part of a syndrome including other more major visceral

defects. Glaucoma (buphthalmos) (Fig. 3.1) in a child may be heralded by severe headaches and irritability. Examination reveals increased tension in the eyeball and also alterations in the pupillary reflexes of the iris. Retinoblastoma may be inherited in a dominant fashion and can affect one or both eyes. There is loss of the normal pink reflex from a light shone into the eyes (Fig. 3.2). The eyelid is a common site for haemangiomas and lymphangiomas. If a haemangioma protrudes over the eye, preventing vision, then it should be removed as soon as possible because of

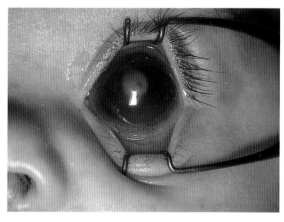

FIGURE 3.1 Buphthalmos.

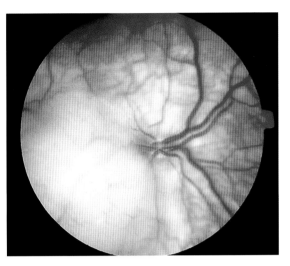

FIGURE 3.2 Retinoblastoma.

the danger of amblyopia and loss of vision in the obstructed eye. Treatment with systemic steroids or interferon may be effective and worth a try before resorting to surgical excision. Where vision is not affected, the haemangioma can be left to resolve spontaneously over the next 5 years at which time a less major procedure can be used for any remaining excess tissue. Dermoid cysts around the eye are quite common in childhood. The external angular dermoid found at the lateral angle of the eyebrow is a firm swelling which grows with the child and often appears to be attached to the underlying bone (Fig. 3.3). These can be treated by surgical excision. There is very rarely intracranial extension of these angular dermoids. Internal angular dermoids, sited at the medial end of the eyebrow are less common. Squints in childhood may be due to neurological or structural problems (see Chapter 2).

EARS

Accessory or supernumerary auricles are common and should be excised with their central core of carti-lage (Fig 3.4). Sometimes they can be bilateral and may appear along the line between the ear and the angle of the mouth. Pre-auricular sinuses are less common. The opening is found at the root of the helix and a blind ending track runs downwards and slightly forwards. These sinuses are prone to infection and excoriation of the skin. If the opening to the surface of the skin is occluded a cyst may form. Treatment is by complete excision.

Complete absence of the pinna or external ear is rare and does not necessarily mean that the middle and inner ear are also absent. Under-development of

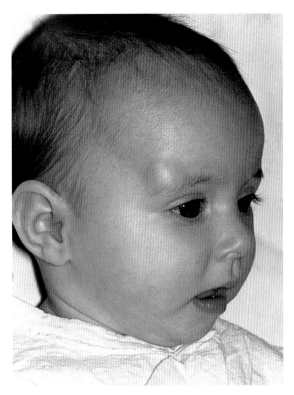

FIGURE 3.3 External angular dermoid.

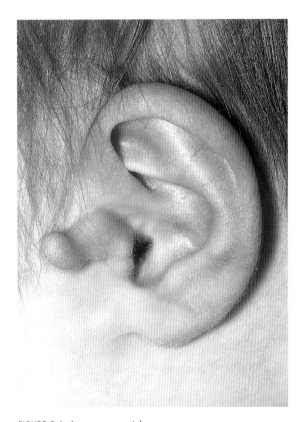

FIGURE 3.4 Accessory auricle.

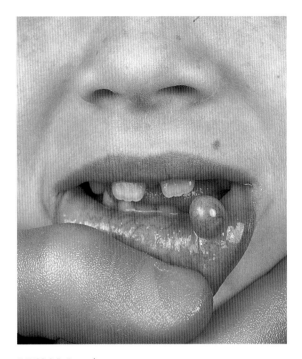

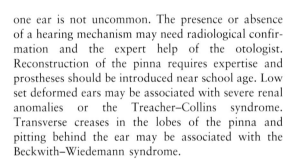

FIGURE 3.5 Buccal cyst.

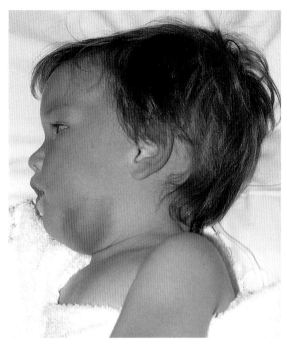

FIGURE 3.6 Submandibular lymphadenitis.

one ear is not uncommon. The presence or absence of a hearing mechanism may need radiological confirmation and the expert help of the otologist. Reconstruction of the pinna requires expertise and prostheses should be introduced near school age. Low set deformed ears may be associated with severe renal anomalies or the Treacher–Collins syndrome. Transverse creases in the lobes of the pinna and pitting behind the ear may be associated with the Beckwith–Wiedemann syndrome.

Bat ears

Marked protrusions of the ears, particularly in boys, may be the focus of cruel criticism as well as jibes at school and consequently may lead to a life of misery at school. Correction by surgery (pinnaplasty) is completed usually before school age.

MOUTH

Tongue-tie (ankyloglossia) is due to a short frenulum that tethers the tongue to the base of the mouth and prevents it from being extruded. The tongue curls on itself. Parents are concerned that it will cause problems with feeding but this is never the case and reassurance is all that is needed in most cases. Another fear is that it delays speech and causes lisps. This may

occur but should not be blamed entirely on a tongue-tie. If the tongue cannot be protruded beyond the teeth, the frenulum can be divided transversely under a general anaesthetic. A short frenulum of the upper lip is invisible and rarely causes a disability. In later life it may be associated with a wide gap between the central incisor teeth. If the frenulum extends between the incisor teeth and if the deformity persists in the second dentition, the frenulum should be excised completely under a general anaesthetic.

RANULA

This is a soft translucent bluish swelling under the tongue, usually confined to one side of the frenulum. It can vary in size from a small pea to a large swelling deforming the tongue. A ranula may be subject to recurrent infections and become painful. Rarely it may be the cause of dysphagia. Deroofing of the cyst and suturing of its edges (marsupialisation) will cure this condition. Mucous glands are present in abundance in the oral cavity and may become blocked, in which case the mucus is retained as a mucous retention buccal cyst or a mucocele (Fig. 3.5). These appear on the mucosal aspect of the lips and may disappear spontaneously. Treatment of persistent mucoceles is simple excision. Congenital pits in the lower lip rarely cause any clinical problems but can be associated with a cleft lip. If they cause an

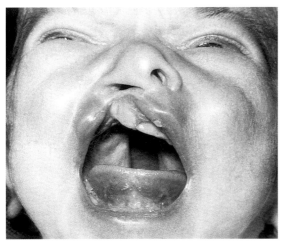

(a)

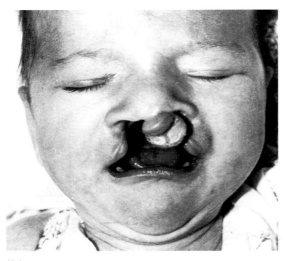

(b)

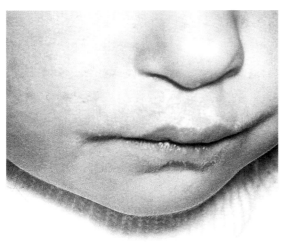

(c)

FIGURE 3.7 (a) Cleft lip and palate (before repair).
(b) Bilateral cleft lip and palate.
(c) After repair (unilateral).

unsightly appearance they may be excised before school age.

TONSILS AND ADENOIDS

Tonsils and adenoids are lymphoid aggregates which form the ring of Waldeyer. This is a protective mechanism which traps and destroys pathogenic organisms entering the body through the oral/nasal cavity. As a consequence, they are very often the seat of infection and inflammation and may enlarge and cause problems with breathing. Persistent infection in these tissues may require removal of the tonsils and adenoids. A very common problem for the paediatric surgeon is the presence of cervical lymph nodes that are secondarily infected. The jugulodigastric lymph node is very commonly enlarged and the seat of reactive hyperplasia secondary to tonsillar infections (Fig. 3.6).

CLEFT LIP AND PALATE

These anomalies occur in approximately 1:600 births and there is a family history in 10% of patients. If a child is born with a cleft lip or palate the risk of a similar anomaly in a sibling is approximately 1:25. The degree of involvement of the alveolus in cleft lip and palate is the factor of greatest importance with regards to treatment and outcome. It is usual to describe the deformities as;

1 Pre-alveolar clefts:
   (a) incomplete – lip only involved,
   (b) complete – lip and nostril involved.
2 Alveolar clefts where the cleft involves the lip, alveolar ridge and the palate.
3 Post-alveolar clefts in which the cleft is confined to the palate.

They may be unilateral or bilateral (Fig. 3.7).

Treatment is aimed first at correcting function by restoring the parts to their proper anatomical position in order to allow normal growth and the establishment of proper swallowing and speech. Second, treatment should correct the disfigurement. This last may not be fully achieved until adequate nasal growth has been established. Where the cleft involves the alveolus this is closed at the same operation as the cleft of the lip. Palatal clefts are usually treated separately and at a later date.

CLEFT LIP

This malformation may occur alone or in association with cleft palate. It may be present as a cleft to the right or left of the midline which may vary from a slight notching to a complete cleft running right up to the nostril. When the cleft is bilateral and complete the premaxilla is displaced forward and the columella is shortened. The premaxilla in these situations looks like a proboscis. In unilateral cases the nostril on the affected side is flattened and the nasal septum displaced toward the sound side.

Treatment

Treatment is initially aimed at correction of alignment by the orthodontist through prostheses and strappings which need to be reapplied regularly to bring the edges of the tissues into line. The repair of the lip and alveolus is usually carried out at around 3 months of age where closure of the defect in its component layers, i.e. mucosa, muscle and skin, is undertaken. There is rarely functional disability but feeding may be difficult and it may be necessary to use a special teat or spoon for feeding purposes.

CLEFT PALATE

The two halves of the hard palate fuse followed by the soft palate. Incomplete fusion may produce a variety of defects:

1 A bifid uvula.
2 Cleft of soft palate.
3 Cleft of soft palate and hard palate.
4 Cleft of soft palate and hard palate with unilateral cleft of the alveolus usually associated with a unilateral cleft lip.
5 Cleft of soft and hard palate with bilateral cleft alveolus usually associated with bilateral complete cleft lip.

Clinical features

Feeding and speech require an efficient nasopharyngeal mechanism. Regurgitation of feeds from the mouth into the nose interferes with feeding and may lead to malnutrition, nasopharyngeal and middle ear infection and aspiration pneumonia. Later, the defect may cause difficulty in phonation and be responsible for nasal speech.

Treatment

Operation is essential to close the gap and to provide a soft palate sufficiently long and mobile to meet the posterior pharyngeal wall, thus permitting closure of the sphincter between the nasopharynx and oropharynx. It is important that a specialist team including a paediatric surgeon with a special interest in plastic surgery, or a plastic surgeon with a paediatric interest, orthodontist, speech therapist, ear nose and throat surgeon, dentist experienced in oral orthopaedics and prosthetics as well as an audiologist and a nurse experienced in feeding problems of infants should deal with these problems. Repair is performed in the latter part of the first year of life. Subsequent pharyngoplasty may be necessary if the child has persistent "nasal escape" when speech has developed.

SUB-MUCOUS CLEFT

This is a condition in which the palatal muscle layer is incomplete and has not met in midline. On inspection the palate may appear normal but full visualisation of the soft palate will show a bidid uvula and poor palatal movement. This requires surgical correction.

SWELLINGS IN THE NECK

The differential diagnosis of midline swellings in the neck includes:

1 Lymph node, submental node, resulting from a dental root abscess.
2 Dermoid.
3 Thyroglossal cyst/abscess.
4 Median cleft.
5 Solitary thyroid nodule.

Lateral swellings in the neck are usually lymph nodes (submandibular and jugulodigastric lymph nodes) enlarged because of a reactive hyperplasia from an infection. More recently atypical mycobacteria have superseded tuberculosis in the UK. Other rare causes of lateral swellings in the neck include lymphoma (Hodgkin's and non-Hodgkin's) and metastases from tumours elsewhere. Other lesions in the differential diagnosis are:

1 Developmental remnants such as branchial cysts, sinuses and fistula.
2 Cystic hygroma/lymphangioma.
3 Neonatal goitre.
4 Salivary glands (submandibular and parotid).
5 Sternomastoid tumour or/and torticollis.

SALIVARY GLANDS

Recurrent painful enlargement of the parotid gland is not uncommon in childhood (Fig. 3.8). The condition

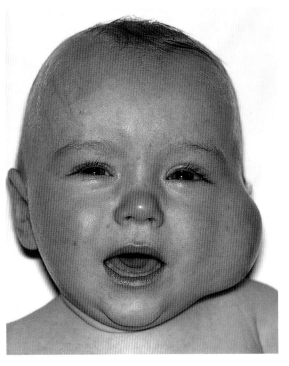

FIGURE 3.8 Parotid swelling.

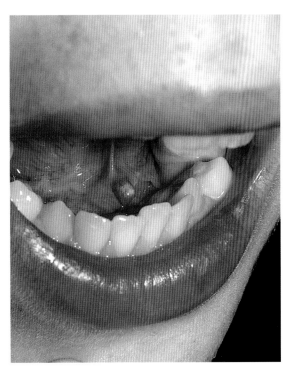

FIGURE 3.9 Submandibular calculus.

is usually unilateral and is seldom due to a calculus. The swelling may subside spontaneously in a day or so but can persist for several weeks. The child has a very tender inflamed parotid gland and the orifice of Stenson's duct in the mouth will appear red and gentle parotid pressure may express a little fluid. Treatment is with appropriate antibiotics and sialogogues. A sialogram may show obstruction of the duct or more often a congenital sialectasis. Very rarely is surgery needed and, when it is, it is difficult and demands great skill and expertise to avoid damage to the branches of the facial nerve which are sandwiched between the superficial and deep lobes of the parotid gland. Recurrent enlargement of the submandibular gland is rare in childhood and may be due to a calculus which can be felt or even seen at the tip of the duct on the undersurface of the tongue (Fig. 3.9). At other times this stone may be where the duct is acutely angled at the posterior part and is seen on X-ray.

OSTEITIS OF THE JAWS

The maxilla used to be the most common site for haematogenous osteitis in infancy. There are clinical signs of swelling, redness under the eye, and the lids may become swollen to simulate an orbital cellulitis. The organism is usually *Staphylococcus aureus*. It usually responds to flucloxacillin treatment. The abscess may point to the hard palate at the alveolus or at the lower orbital ridge. A root abscess in an older child may simulate an osteitis.

NECK

Pharyngeal arch defects

Epithelial remnants derived from the branchial arches are common and can give rise to cysts, sinuses and fistulae. Infection of these can result in a localised cellulitis and may progress to an abscess. Portions of the branchial arches and clefts may persist and give rise to several anomalies. These developmental anomalies may arise from segments of the first and second branchial clefts.

In persistence of the first cleft, the lower end opens below the border of the mandible and the upper end in the external auditory canal.

Persistence of the second cleft is commoner and opens in the tonsillar fossa and the skin over the anterior border of the lower half of the sternocleidomastoid muscle. The track passes between the internal and external carotid arteries over the glossopharyngeal nerve. Branchial cysts are not commonly seen in infancy but may become apparent

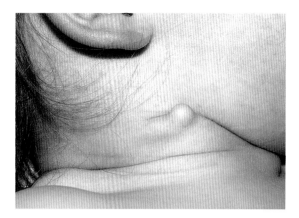

FIGURE 3.10 Branchial remnants.

during childhood. They usually present as a painless cystic swelling over the lower sternocleidomastoid muscle. These cystic swellings may be difficult to differentiate from cervical lymphadenopathy but when identified the cyst is often removed *in toto* (Fig. 3.10). A branchial fistula is usually unilateral although bilateral fistulae do occur. As the opening on the less obvious side may be microscopic it is important to massage the area of the fistulous tract to identify a bead of clear or opulescent fluid at the small orifice which can be found anywhere along the anterior border of the lower half of the sternomastoid. The whole fistulous track should be excised when it is diagnosed as it may be subject to recurrent infection.

Thyroglossal cysts are midline swellings (Fig. 3.11) arising from remnants of the thyroid anlage which can be found along a track from the foramen caecum at the base of the tongue to the thyroid isthmus. Cysts may have squamous, mucous, or respiratory epithelium and can have multiple tracks in the midline. They vary from the size of a few millimetres to 3 cm. The cyst moves up and down on deglutition and especially on protruding the tongue. They are subject to recurrent infection and can present as a thyroglossal abscess. These may rupture to form a fistula. A thyroglossal cyst in the suprahyoid portion occasionally may cause respiratory problems and require early surgical intervention. Total surgical removal (Sistrunk's operation) includes excision of the middle portion of the hyoid bone. Inclusion dermoid cysts may be difficult to differentiate from thyroglossal cysts but excision is the treatment and the pathologist establishes the diagnosis.

MIDLINE CERVICAL CLEFT

This uncommon anomaly may be mistaken for a thyroid fistula. It arises as a dimple or pit of the skin in the midline of the neck. The cleft is excised and the skin repaired by a Z-plasty.

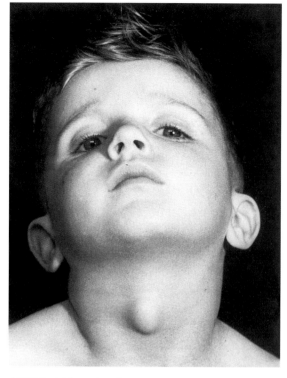

FIGURE 3.11 Thyroglossal cyst.

TORTICOLLIS

Torticollis is a restriction of the lateral movements of the neck, usually due to a shortening of the sternomastoid muscle. Historically it was first mentioned by Plutarch in describing Alexander the Great. The first operation was done by Isaac Minius in Amsterdam in 1641. The differential diagnosis includes fibrosis of the sternocleidomastoid muscle which usually follows trauma to the muscles as a result of traumatic breech delivery or the use of forceps. Other causes of torticollis include cervical hemivertebrae, cervical adenitis, imbalance of ocular muscle squint and neuromuscular inco-ordination.

Secondary effects of torticollis include rotation of the head to the opposite side, plagiocephaly and hemihypoplasia of the face on the affected side.

STERNOCLEIDOMASTOID TUMOUR

The pathology involves the deposition of collagen fibrobasts around individual muscle fibres which undergo atrophy (endomesiofibrosis) *in utero* and may cause obstetric difficulty (Fig. 3.12). The natural history of the sternomastoid tumour is that 50% disappear by the age of 6 months with no residual

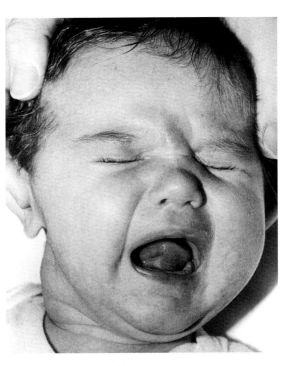

FIGURE 3.12 Sternomastoid tumour.

fibrosis. Thirty per cent disappear with residual fibrosis and no torticollis by the age 12 months. The remaining 20% have persistent torticollis and require physiotherapy.

CYSTIC HYGROMA OF THE NECK

The Greek word hygroma means "moist or watery tumour". The cyst, sac or bursa is usually distended with fluid. It is a tumour of the lymphatic system occurring predominantly in the neck of infants and children. It was first described by Redenbeker in 1828, and Koester in 1872 suggested for the first time the possibility of derivation from lymphatic cysts.

Embryology

It arises from sequestration of portions of lymphatic tissue from primitive lymphatic sacs surviving embryonic life. The incidence of cystic hygroma is 0.4% of all neck masses, 50–60% appear before the age of 1 year, there is an equal male to female incidence with no racial predisposition. The natural history is variable growth and regression. Growth occasionally is arrested by infection or spontaneous regression may occur. The pathology is that of a typical hamartoma. It is composed of multilocular cysts which may or may not communicate. Very often there is

infiltration of the surrounding tissues including the neck muscles and the base of the tongue.

The clinical picture is that of a soft fluctuant, lobulated mass in the neck which transilluminates (Fig. 11.16). Compression effects are rare but often there are secondary complications such as infection and haemorrhage into the hygroma. Treatment is complete excision which may prove difficult.

KLIPPEL–FEIL SYNDROME

This syndrome is characterised by fusion and partial absence of the upper cervical vertebrae, giving an abnormally short neck and low hairline posteriorly. Other developmental anomalies may be associated with the Klippel–Feil deformity such as webbing of the neck and can be improved by plastic surgery. Also associated may be congenital elevation of the scapula (Sprengel deformity). Webbing of the neck also occurs in Turner syndrome.

CERVICAL LYMPHADENITIS

Inflammation of the lymph nodes of the neck may be secondary to infection in the scalp, face, oro-nasal cavities or the external ear. In spite of systematic search, the primary focus may never be found. The glands affected most commonly are in the anterior triangle or in the submandibular region and they may become matted together to form a firm tender mass. Discoloration of the skin and fluctuation are not early features as the glands lie deep to the deep cervical fascia. Abscess formation is not infrequent when the causal organism is a penicillin resistant *Staphylococcus aureus*. Evacuation of the pus is mandatory with insertion of a wick to allow complete drainage.

MAIS INFECTION

Mycobacterium avium, *M. intracellulare* and *M. scrofulaceum* (MAIS) are atypical mycobacteria which invade the reticulo-endothelial cells of lymph nodes. Children with these infections present with enlarged lymph nodes which may suppurate and produce persistent chronic sinuses. There may be a moderate reaction to the Mantoux test or no reaction. Differential testing with antigens prepared from specific atypical mycobacteria is more likely to produce a larger reaction than that with PPD. Anti-tuberculous treatment is of little value and surgical removal of affected lymph nodes is the treatment of choice.

4

Trunk and Limbs

TRUNK

BREAST AND NIPPLE

The breasts of many newborn babies of both sexes enlarge during the first week and may produce secretions of white fluid (witches' milk). This is a response to the withdrawal of maternal oestrogens. No treatment is needed. Rarely, cellulitis or a breast abscess may develop (Fig. 4.1). Since the organism is usually a staphylococcus, the appropriate initial treatment is flucloxacillin. If an abscess is present a radial incision is made to evacuate pus and to avoid damage to the ducts. A wick is left *in situ* to allow the cavity to heal from below.

In older children breast lumps are a common feature and rarely cause concern since reassurance that this is *not a cancer* is very often all that is needed. The commonest causes are breast tissue responding to hormonal stimuli, underlying lymphangioma and haemangioma or even a lipoma. Pain and swelling of the breast may occur in both sexes between the ages of 7 and 14 years. The condition may be unilateral or bilateral and a button-like swelling may develop beneath the areola. These lesions usually subside after 6–18 months and no adequate explanation is available. Early onset of puberty in the female may present with unilateral breast enlargement. Persistent hypertrophy of the male breast (gynaecomastia) may be unilateral or bilateral and a mastectomy may be indicated for cosmetic reasons. Rarely, an underlying hormonal secreting tumour arising from the adrenal gland may be responsible for breast hypertrophy in the male. Atelia (absence of the nipple) is usually associated with amastia (absence of the breast) and absence of the sternal portion of the pectoralis major (Poland syndrome) and this is a rare anomaly. Developmental absence of the pectoralis major is more common but causes little disability. There may be an underlying associated deficiency of ribs but the resulting paradoxical respiration is seldom sufficient to warrant attempts to stabilise the thoracic cage. This is a rare phenomenom in boys. Supernumerary nipples (polythelia) are common. They are symmetrically situated in the primitive mammary line below

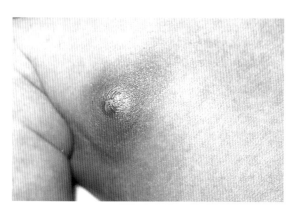

FIGURE 4.1 Breast abscess in a neonate.

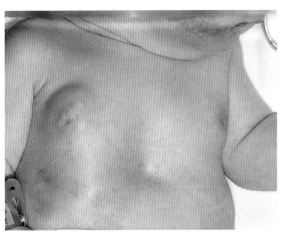

FIGURE 4.2 Pectus excavatum with right-sided gynaecomastia.

the normal nipples. These may be pigmented and may be excised for cosmetic reasons.

PECTUS EXCAVATUM (funnel chest)

Minor depression of the lower sternum requires no treatment whereas severe deformity may be associated with kyphosis and may impair heart and lung function. Cosmetic correction is delayed until after the age of 4. The intercostal cartilages are divided or resected and the sternum is partially transected and elevated. The cause is not known, although some people have attributed the pectus excavatum to abnormal attachments of the diaphragm to the sternal ridge (Fig. 4.2).

PECTUS CARINATUM (pigeon chest)

Pectus carinatum (pigeon chest) is a condition in which there is a marked sternal prominence which rarely causes a clinical upset but may rarely require surgery for cosmetic reasons.

HARRISON'S SULCUS

Harrison's sulcus is a depression of the bony component of the chest wall which runs in a transverse fashion beneath both pectoral muscles. This is seen predominantly in children who have asthma or rickets but at times may be idiopathic. No treatment is necessary. This sulcus is most prominent in the under 10-year-olds but as they grow older and

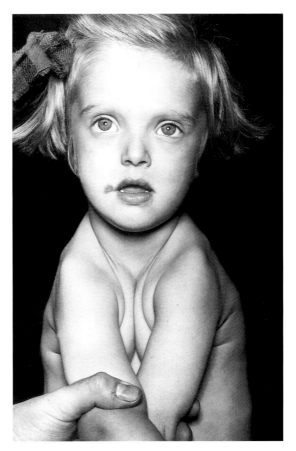

FIGURE 4.3 Craniocleidodysostosis.

develop more musculature and subcutaneous fat, it becomes less of a cosmetic problem.

Absence of the clavicle occurs in the condition craniocleidodysostosis (Fig. 4.3).

OTHER CHEST WALL DEFORMITIES

The 11th and 12th ribs are often designated as floating ribs. This is a variation of normal anatomy and may be confused with an abnormal abdominal wall mass. Reassurance is all that is necessary. The xiphoid process may assume a variety of shapes, some of which involve eversion of the process and produce a prominent lump beneath the skin in the midline. At times, this may be deviated to one side or another. This variation of normal causes no problems and very rarely is surgery indicated. Reassurance of the parents is all that is necessary. In association with tracheo-oesophageal fistula and oesophageal atresia in the VACTERL group of anomalies, an extra set of ribs may be present (Fig. 4.4). This is an interesting radiological finding but of little clinical significance.

V	Vertebral/rib anomaly
A	Ano-rectal anomaly
C	Cardiac anomaly
T **E**	Tracheo-oesophageal fistula
R	Renal anomaly
L	Limb deformity

FIGURE 4.4 VACTERL anomalies.

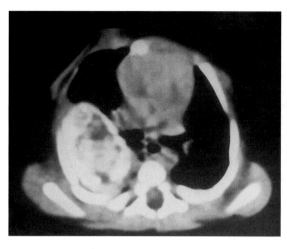

FIGURE 4.5 Mesenchymoma.

Chest wall deformities such as fused ribs or enchondromata may be due to previous thoracotomies. Very rarely is cosmetic surgery necessary to correct this. Another complication of thoracotomy is a "winged" scapula due to damage to the long thoracic nerve of Bell. Some children have a flattening of the lower portion of the chest wall after repair of a congenital diaphragmatic hernia. This is partly due to the congenital abnormality caused by the deficiency of the diaphragm on that side, and partly due to the repair which creates considerable tension on the edges of the diaphragm, pulling the chest wall inwards. This deformity becomes less of a problem as the child grows older.

TUMOURS OF THE CHEST WALL

Haemangiomas and lymphangiomas may occur on the chest wall. Haemangiomas tend to resolve spontaneously even when they are of the giant variety. Neoplasia may arise from the rib, cartilage, muscle, fascia or fat. These are often sarcomas and are highly malignant. Treatment is by chemotherapy and surgical excision. Two types of tumour need special mention here. The first is a mesenchymoma of the rib which presents as an expansile tumour of the ribs which may encroach on the thoracic viscera, especially the lung and mediastinum (Fig. 4.5). It is a benign tumour which is locally invasive and complete excision provides a cure. There is no tendency for malignancy to supervene in this tumour. The other is the Askin tumour which is a primitive neurectodermal tumour, the histology of which resembles that of a neuroblastoma, and it arises from the chest wall. It is very malignant, highly anaplastic and treatment with chemotherapy, surgery and radiotherapy is very often disappointing. Congenital malformations of the osteochondral junctions which present as a chest wall lump which grows with the patient may be confused with malignant conditions. Chest X-ray should be performed to make sure there is no underlying

condition. They do not require surgical intervention. Another lump which may be confused with a malignant condition is a swelling at the costochondral junction caused by local injury. This may result in a swelling with some bruising and usually subsides within 2–3 weeks. Attempts at biopsying any of these lesions should be strongly resisted. Simple chondromas may arise in the centre of a rib; a prominence at the costochondral junction is usually due to a developmental angulation.

LUNG ABSCESS

Lung abscesses may complicate inhalation of a foreign body, a pneumonia or a developmental sequestration of lung tissue in which there is an isolated segment of lung with an atretic bronchus. An acute lung abscess results in a very sick child with severe toxaemia and with pyrexia and a cough. There is localised dullness to percussion and impaired air entry. The diagnosis is confirmed by radiography. In most instances drainage of the abscess is necessary either percutaneously or through an open thoracotomy. The underlying diseased lung should be excised as a segmental resection, otherwise recurrence of the lung abscess is possible.

Intrathoracic cysts and primary tumours

These rare lesions can provoke acute respiratory distress and may present incidentally without symptoms. They are usually revealed by X-ray examination. In young patients the mostly common anterior mediastinal lesions are infantile enlargement of the thymus, a thymoma or a dermoid cyst.

Posterior mediastinal lesions are more common. They include ganglioneuroma, neuroblastoma, cystic hygroma, embryonic prevertebral posterior enteric remnants such as enterogenous, bronchogenic or teratomatous cysts and oesophageal duplications. The enteric remnants may be associated with abnormalities in the vertebral bodies, including anterior spina bifida. Thoracic neuroblastoma may produce catecholamines leading to an increased urinary excretion of catecholamine breakdown products such as vanillylmandelic acid (VMA). Rarely these neuroblastomas may extend into the spinal theca in a dumbbell fashion resulting in paraplegia. Another intrathoracic tumour which may be present and cause acute respiratory problems is lymphoma which grows rapidly and sometimes necessitates urgent chemotherapy. In general, most of these lesions justify thoracotomy with a view to total excision but lymphoma usually responds to chemotherapy.

THE ABDOMINAL WALL

In the newborn the abdomen is relatively larger than the chest. Most of the breathing is diaphragmatic and very little chest movement is observed. Abdominal distension may cause splinting of the diaphragm and respiratory difficulties. Between the 6th and 8th week of fetal life, the midgut grows rapidly and herniates into the base of the umbilical cord. At about the 10th week the abdominal cavity enlarges at an accelerated pace and midgut is then withdrawn into the abdomen. If the development of the anterior abdominal wall is delayed, then abnormalities of the umbilicus and the abdominal wall may result.

The embryological structures transmitted by the umbilical cord include the umbilical vein, which is a large structure that goes to join the portal vein and thence to the right side of the heart, the vitello-intestinal duct, which communicates with the ileum and two umbilical arteries that descend into the pelvis to join with the iliac arteries. There is also a communication with the bladder which is called the urachus. When the ring of fibrous tissue which surrounds these structures at the level of the umbilicus is larger than normal an umbilical hernia may result. After clamping of the umbilical cord at birth, the vessels rapidly fibrose and inflammatory changes in them result in atrophy of these vessels, resulting in cord-like structures with no lumen. The vitello-intestinal duct usually disappears completely; if a remnant remains then a vitello-intestinal cyst tethered to the umbilicus or even a Meckel diverticulum which communicates with the lumen of the ileum may be found. The urachus is rarely the seat of any problem since it disappears very quickly and forms the median ligament of the bladder. If it does persist it may cause

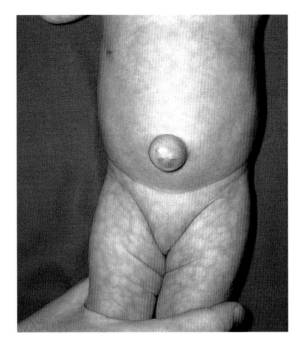

FIGURE 4.6 Umbilical hernia.

a cyst or an abscess on the dome of the bladder and present as an abdominal mass. Persistence of the urachus may be suspected at birth when there is a very thick umbilical cord with a lot of Wharton jelly. This is due to the presence of urine absorbed into the Wharton jelly. Very rarely after birth a patent urachus may result in intermittent discharge of urine from the umbilicus. This condition has to be differentiated from a granulating umbilicus and a vitello-intestinal fistula. Instillation of radio-opaque dye will show a connection with the bladder or intestine.

Umbilical discharge

Serious inflammation around the umbilicus (omphalitis) is rare, but when it does happen it may have serious consequences since a spreading cellulitis of the abdominal wall may cause septicaemia. Umbilical vessels may remain patent in the first few weeks of life and infection may spread to the portal vein resulting in portal vein thrombosis and abscesses in the liver. Portal hypertension may ensue at a later date.

Granulation tissue around the umbilicus with persistent infection may result after the cord has sloughed. These granulations usually disappear if treated with a silver nitrate pencil. A persistent discharge from the umbilicus is most likely to be due to a vitello-intestinal fistula which may communicate with the lumen of the bowel. Surgical exploration is necessary to remove the vitello-intestinal remnant.

Umbilical hernia

Umbilical herniation is common in infants and children. The hernial ring has a firm edge and is usually confined to the peri-umbilical region. Umbilical herniae are more common in girls than boys and can vary in size from a tiny protruberance to a bulge which may be up to 3 cm in diameter (Fig. 4.6). A hernia is rarely the cause of underlying problems. Complications such as incarceration or spontaneous rupture are virtually unknown.

Treatment

Most umbilical herniae are spontaneously cured before the child goes to school. Even very large ones at birth usually resolve spontaneously and up to 80% of them have disappeared by the age of 2 years. Persistence beyond this age is usually an indication for surgery. No strapping of the hernia is necessary since it is more likely to cause complications by trapping the bowel. It is much better to allow the contents of the hernial sac to pop in and out of the abdominal cavity without any obstruction. It is important that during operative repair of the umbilical hernia, an omphaloplasty is performed to remove the excess redundant skin present so that a normal umbilical appearance is maintained. If a child is constantly crying and screaming and has an umbilical hernia it is important to look for the source of discomfort elsewhere since the umbilical hernia is not likely to be the cause. The presence of an umbilical hernia may signify an associated condition such as the Beckwith–Wiedemann syndrome or hypothyroidism. Rarely it may be associated with raised intra-abdominal pressure from a space-occupying lesion.

Supraumbilical hernia

In this relatively rare hernia, the defect in the abdominal wall is just above the umbilical cicatrix and the bulge is directed obliquely downwards. Spontaneous cure is less likely and surgery is more commonly required.

Epigastric hernia and divarication of the recti muscles

These conditions are very common in children and present with a bulge in the midline usually above the umbilicus midway between the xiphoid process and the umbilicus. When the child attempts to sit up from a supine position the bulge is most obvious. This is a feature of great worry to some parents and examination usually reveals that the recti muscles have failed to join in the midline to the linea alba. At times it is possible to insert the hand through the absent linea alba and touch the vertebral bodies. A simple epigastric hernia may be present due to a deficiency of the linea alba at various points, and there may be multiple herniae present. These are rarely the source of any symptoms and give rise to more concern because of parental worry. Occasionally a bit of epigastric fat may be trapped and cause some discomfort, in which case surgical intervention is necessary. Operations for divarication of the recti are not required and most of these deformities correct themselves. Advice usually given to the parents is that as the child grows older the abdominal wall musculature strengthens and the defect gets smaller as the muscles enlarge.

Polyps of the umbilicus

Epithelial polyps of the umbilicus are not uncommon. They usually result from growth of skin over a granuloma which has been present since birth. Excision of these polyps can be performed on a day-case basis.

Absence of the abdominal wall musculature – the prune belly syndrome

This is a condition where there is absence of the mesoderm or part of the mesoderm of the abdominal wall. The skin looks wrinkled and very much like a prune, hence the condition known as prune belly syndrome. The underlying viscera can usually be seen and visible peristalsis is normal in this situation. These children usually have associated renal abnormalities and in boys undescended testes. Although they have no obstructive uropathy their urinary tract is usually tortuous and dilated.

Abdominal wall defects

Upper abdominal wall defects are rare and may involve congenital heart disease, absence of the diaphragm, sternal defect, and even ectopia cordis (Cantrell's pentalogy). Much more common are abdominal wall defects around the umbilicus which fall into two main groups – exomphalos and gastroschisis. Abdominal wall defects affecting the lower abdomen usually involve the bladder and may present as extrophy of the bladder or vesico-intestinal fissures. These are usually associated with deficiencies of the pelvic bone and the pubic symphysis and abnormal genitalia. In the female there is usually wide separation of the labia and in the male there is epispadias.

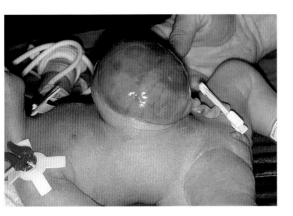

FIGURE 4.7 Exomphalos.

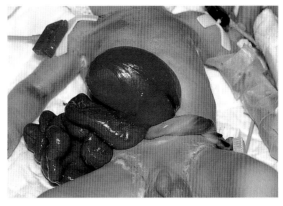

FIGURE 4.8 Gastroschisis.

Hernia into the cord

This is a condition in which the umbilical cord enters into the abdominal wall through a defect which allows bowel, very often small intestine, to prolapse into the umbilical cord. This is clinically obvious at birth where the cord appears to be thickened and contains small bowel. This condition is not associated with any underlying major congenital abnormalities and its treatment involves elective surgical exploration of the defect, replacement of the prolapsed bowel into the abdominal cavity and closure of the umbilical defect, leaving an umbilicus. Attempts at twisting the cord to reduce the bowel into the abdominal cavity and application of clamps should be strongly resisted since at times the tearing of adhesions between the bowel, appendix, or a Meckel diverticulum can damage the bowel and cause peritonitis.

Exomphalos

This defect involves the umbilical cord (Fig. 4.7). There may be a thin-walled sac covering the intestines, liver or other abdominal organs which are visible. The defect varies from a few centimetres in diameter (exomphalos minor) to a swelling the size of a large grapefruit and may involve the whole of the anterior wall (exomphalos major). The latter usually contains liver. The umbilical cord arises from the apex of the caudal base of the sac. In most cases the sac is intact, but in some it is damaged during delivery and may not be so obvious. During the first day of life the sac is usually moist and pliable. After this it becomes dry, friable, more opaque and may rupture and allow evisceration. Introduction of maternal plasma α-fetoprotein screening and fetal ultrasound examinations has increased the numbers of prenatally diagnosed infants. A detailed ultrasound examination can usually differentiate exomphalos from gastroschisis. Infants with exomphalos major are large at birth

and 50% may have other underlying abnormalities. These may be congenital defects of the heart, kidneys or gastrointestinal tract. The mortality in this group is high because of the associated malformations. The treatment of exomphalos major is fraught with many problems. A primary closure of the defect, if possible, gives the best results. In many instances, however, the small size of the peritoneal cavity and the large viscera which are in the exomphalos prevent this from happening. Raised intra-abdominal pressure will inhibit diaphragmatic movements and interfere with effective respiration. Raised intraperitoneal pressure can also affect renal perfusion and cause acute renal shutdown post-operatively. Because of these effects the creation of too much tension in a primary closure should be avoided. Alternative methods of treatment involve the application of a "plastic" pouch to contain the organs and gradually reduce the size of the pouch over a period of a week, whereby delayed primary closure can be obtained. Another alternative is to create a ventral hernia to allow skin closure over the abdominal organs. This ventral hernia will require surgical repair at a later date. In the past, intact membranes were painted with mercurochrome which allowed escharisation of the defect and eventual epithelialisation. Toxic levels of mercury were produced in some of these infants and this method is no longer appropriate.

In exomophalos minor primary closure with good healing is easily obtained. Post-operative management of babies with exomphalos includes ventilation and paralysis until adequate spontaneous respiration is possible. Parenteral feeding and antibiotics have improved the outcome.

Gastroschisis

This condition, which in the past was confused with exomphalos, has a very different clinical picture and should be regarded as a separate entity (Figs 4.8 and

Exomphalos   Gastroschisis

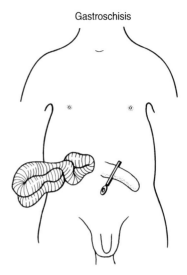

FIGURE 4.9 Comparison of abdominal wall defects: exomphalos and gastroschisis.

4.9). The gastroschisis typically arises as a punched out lesion in the anterior abdominal wall lateral to the umbilicus. There is usually a bridge of epithelium between the defect and the umbilical cord which is usually intact, and predominantly occurs on the right-hand side of the abdominal wall. Through this defect, which is usually small, protrudes intestinal contents, small bowel, large bowel and at times even an ectopic testis or an ovary. After delivery there is a risk that the vascular pedicle of the prolapsed bowel will twist and compromise the intestinal blood supply. The application of a layer of clear plastic (cling film) to the abdominal wall immediately after delivery will allow a clear view of the bowel colour and, should any torsion be observed, allow the position of the bowel to be readjusted. It also prevents excessive loss of heat and fluid. Affected infants can be observed continuously during transport from the maternity to the surgical unit where corrective procedures can be performed. Babies with gastroschisis usually tend to be light for their gestational age and smaller than babies with exomphalos major. They very rarely have associated abnormalities which are life threatening. Malrotation of the intestines is a common association when the bowel has not been properly positioned when it re-enters the abdominal cavity. After the bowel has been exposed to air for some time it becomes thickened and covered with fibrin. Hence, it is important to try to replace the bowel within the peritoneal cavity as soon as possible. Primary closure should always be attempted after adequate stretching of the peritoneal cavity and evacuation per anus of as much of the meconium from the bowel as possible. A nasogastric tube should also be inserted to aspirate any excessive fluid that may be present in the upper gastrointestinal tract. If primary closure is not possible then a silo made of a silastic pouch should be created and the bowel contents reduced gradually into the peritoneal cavity over a period of a week. This can be done in the incubator in the ward without any anaesthetic. At the end of the week, under cover of antibiotics, delayed primary closure of the abdominal wall with skin cover should be possible. Post-operatively there is usually a delay of several weeks before proper gastrointestinal tract peristaltic function is regained and during this time total parenteral nutrition will be required.

Ectopia vesicae and epispadias

Both deformities arise from midline deficiency of the infra-umbilical abdominal wall (Fig. 4.10). The lower abdominal wall is usually reinforced by fusion of the

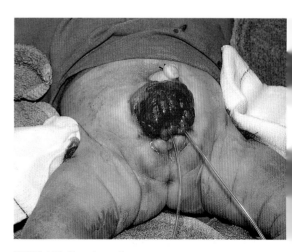

FIGURE 4.10 Ectopia vesicae.

genital tubercules. If these tubercules develop a little caudal to their normal position and then fuse in the midline, the lower abdominal wall will not be reinforced by mesoderm. The thin covering consisting of one layer of ectoderm and one layer of entoderm will break down, causing the deformity of ectopia vesicae (extroversion or extrophy of the bladder) with a dorsal urethral groove on the penis. If the genital tubercles develop even further caudally, the hypogastric area and the cloacal membrane break down to cause the rare deformity of *vesico-intestinal fissure*.

Ectopic vesicae

The lower abdominal wall and the anterior bladder wall are absent and the vesical mucosa prolapses through the defect. The umbilicus is usually lower than normal and represented by a scar at the apex of the bladder. There may be an associated exomphalos. The trigone and ureteric orifices lie exposed and often urine can be seen spurting from the ureteric orifices. Pubic bones are widely separated and the pubic symphysis is absent. In the male, the penis is short, thick set and uptilted. The urethra forms a groove on the dorsal surface of the penis and the prepuce is split dorsally (epispadias). The scrotum is normally fused but may be separated (bifid scrotum) and it may be empty. In the female, a vaginal orifice lies below the bladder and the clitoris is divided and lies below and posterior to the urethra. The exposed vesical mucosa is tender and the urinary incontinence soon causes severe excoriation of the skin. Treatment of this condition has varied over the years and primary neonatal closure is now attempted in most cases. This may be with or without sacroiliac osteotomies prior to the procedure. If a functional bladder cannot be fashioned in the neonatal period a free ileocolonic loop into which the ureters drain can form a urinary conduit. Many of these children have severe psychological problems in later life with suicidal tendencies because of the severe deformity of the penis. All children with ectopia vesicae have wide separation of the pubic symphysis and have a waddling gait resembling that of a child with bilateral congenital dislocation of the hip.

Epispadias

This is discussed in Chapter 8.

DAY BED SURGERY

There are many surgical procedures which may be carried out in children on a day basis. They are usually admitted to the day bed area in the morning, having been fasted from a specific time before their procedure. They are then interviewed and examined by the house doctor in order to make sure they are fit for surgery and at the same time to confirm that they do have their original complaint. The anaesthetist then visits the child to make sure that he/she does not have any upper respiratory tract problem or rashes or a hyperpyrexia that may have been missed or developed since the first examination. During this interview, he explains to the parents what is going to happen to the child and at the same time anaesthetic cream (Emla) is applied to the dorsum of both hands to anaesthetise the area prior to injecting anaesthetic agents. The child is taken to the anaesthetic room with the parents in attendance and then is anaesthetised either by an intravenous injection or mask inhalation. Once the child is asleep the parents leave the anaesthetic room and the procedure is performed in the operating theatre.

Procedures that may be performed as day cases include:

1 Lumps, bumps and pigmented lesions for biopsy.
2 Inguinal hernia.
3 Hydrocele.
4 Umbilical hernia.
5 External angular dermoids and pre-auricular sinuses.
6 Tongue tie, excision of ranulae and mucous retention cysts in the mouth.
7 Removal of foreign body.
8 Ingrowing toenails which require surgical treatment.
9 Undescended testes.
10 Upper gastrointestinal tract endoscopies.
11 Lower gastrointestinal tract endoscopies including sigmoidoscopy and colonoscopy.
12 Genitourinary procedures such as circumcision, urethroscopy, cystoscopy and retrograde procedures.

These procedures form a large part of paediatric surgical practice and there are advantages of doing them as day cases. The child and parents are separated for a minimum amount of time and do not require expensive hospital overnight admission. There is a rapid turnover of patients and therefore hospital beds can be made available for emergencies and more major surgical procedures.

HERNIA AND HYDROCELES

Inguinal hernia

Inguinal hernia in childhood is almost invariably of the indirect type (Fig. 4.11). They are ten times more common in males than in females and the incidence in both sexes under 12 years of age is 10 per thousand live births. The right testis descends at a

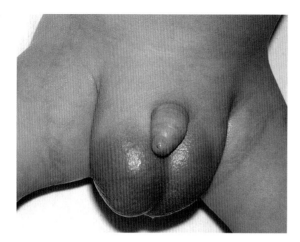

FIGURE 4.11 Bilateral inguinal hernia.

later date than does the left, and accordingly the processus vaginalis is closed off later on the right side. This probably accounts for the greater frequence of right-sided inguinal hernia (60%) than left-sided (20%).

An indirect inguinal hernia passes down the tract of the processus vaginalis through the inguinal canal to appear near the skin surface at the external inguinal ring. The hernia usually contains the pampiniform plexus of veins, the vas deferens and its artery and the cremasteric coverings.

Clinical features

A hernia may be discovered at or shortly after birth and very large scrotal herniae may appear during the first few weeks of life. Most commonly herniae are first noticed during the second or third month and recognition may follow a period of coughing, crying or straining. The hernia may be empty or it may contain intra-abdominal contents, especially bowel. The contents usually reduce spontaneously when the child ceases to cry or strain. If that does not occur, then they usually can be reduced with ease by simple taxis. The hernia may be small and appear at the external ring or may be elongated and extend beyond the inguinal canal into the scrotum. Examination of an older infant or child with an inguinal hernia is carried out by a bimanual procedure. First of all, it is important to gain the confidence and cooperation of the child and the inguinal area and scrotum should be inspected before touching it. If the child wishes to stand he may be allowed to do so and coughing in the erect position may induce the hernia to bulge. If a bulge is visible, then attempts should be made to try to reduce this and if it does reduce easily then it can only be an inguinal hernia. The testes should also

be palpated to ensure that they are present and properly descended. An undescended testis may be mistaken for a hernia and is not uncommonly complicated by the presence of a hernia. The swelling of a simple hernia is elastic and painless on palpation while that of an undescended testis is firm and tender.

Sometimes there may be a good history of recurrent swelling but no inguinal swelling can be found during the examination. Thickening of the spermatic cord on the side of the hernia will help confirm the diagnosis. The middle finger is placed on the spermatic cord as it crosses the pubic bone and by rolling the cord from side to side with the thumb, one can with practice estimate the thickness of the structures within. If the hernia is unilateral the cord will be found to be slightly thicker on the affected side even though the hernial sac is empty. When there is a left inguinal hernia the parents should be warned that a hernia is likely to appear on the right ride at a later date and therefore bilateral exploration is desirable in these cases.

Incarcerated hernia

An incarcerated hernia is one which defies reduction by simple taxis. Although strangulation of the contents of an inguinal hernia is rare in childhood, incarceration is not uncommon and occurs in approximately 5%. The local swelling is usually painful and the child or infant may show signs of great discomfort. Even if the intestine is present in the sac there may be no signs of intestinal obstruction, but reflex vomiting is not uncommon. Incarceration is most common in the first 6 months of life and rarer in older children. The differential diagnosis is made difficult in this age group, and torsion of the spermatic cord or the appendix testis may also resemble incarceration of a hernia. A very tense hydrocele may also be confused. If there is any doubt about the diagnosis of an incarcerated hernia, then a digital rectal examination should be performed. If there is an incarcerated hernia then bowel can be felt entering into the deep inguinal ring and it may be possible to manipulate it and withdraw it bimanually.

Intestinal obstruction is a serious complication and may proceed to gangrene of the bowel when strangulation occurs. When this has happened there is evidence of cellulitis of the scrotal and groin region and any attempts to try to reduce the hernia should be strongly resisted. These children need emergency surgery to define the problem and relieve a vascular obstruction. Another complication from an incarcerated or strangulated hernia is that extrinsic pressure on the pampiniform plexus of veins can induce a venous infarction of the ipsilateral testes. If a hydrocele is present its relationship to the testes and cord is defined. In infancy, both herniae and hydroceles are *translucent*.

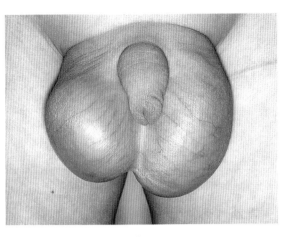

FIGURE 4.12 Bilateral hydroceles.

Hydrocele of the tunica vaginalis

There is usually a bluish hue to this swelling which appears at the inguinal scrotal region (Fig. 4.12). It is often possible to get above a hydrocele and impossible to reduce it since it contains fluid and the neck of the hydrocele which is part of the persistent tunica vaginalis has valve-like flaps which prevent the fluid from returning into the peritoneal cavity. Most hydroceles disappear spontaneously by the age of 2 years (80%). The remainder require ligation and division of the patent processus vaginalis together with drainage of the hydrocele. The aetiology of a hydrocele of a child is very different from that in an adult. In a tense hydrocele it is important to define the testis and make sure it is not the seat of any underlying pathology. Transillumination of a hydrocele, although helpful, is not absolutely diagnostic since children's tissues contain a lot of fluid and transilluminate easily. A testicular tumour in a child has been mistakenly diagnosed as a hydrocele because it transilluminated.

An encysted hydrocele of the cord is a localised collection of fluid incorporated within the spermatic cord and is irreducible. It may extend into the scrotum and simulate a hydrocele of the tunica vaginalis but it does not envelop the testis which is easily palpated. The swelling is frequently mistaken for an incarcerated hernia although there are none of the other features. It is usually possible to palpate a normal cord above the upper limit of the swelling.

In a female, an inguinal hernia is a rare event although sometimes it does occur and presents as a lump in the groin. The child is usually well with no complaint. This hernia may contain a prolapsed ovary and pain may be caused by attempts to reduce it into the peritoneal cavity. During surgical exploration it is important to ensure that the hernia does contain an ovary and not a testis because in a number of cases these children have an underlying testicular feminisation (androgen insensitivity) syndrome. If uncertain, a biopsy to confirm the nature of the gonad should be carried out since testes would have to be removed because of the high incidence of malignancy in later life.

Operative treatment for inguinal hernia

The operative treatment in infants and children is safe and can be performed at any time with highly satisfactory results. The procedure performed in infants and children, where there is no weakness in the musculature of the inguinal canal, is different from that performed in adults. The length of the canal is short and it is possible to bring the neck of the sac into view at the external ring and thus perform a radical cure without opening the inguinal canal in children under the age of 5. The operation is a herniotomy and not a herniorrhaphy as in the adult and can be carried out as a day procedure. The exceptions are preterm infants who need to be monitored post-operatively because of the risk of apnoea and aspiration.

Femoral hernia

This is a rare condition in childhood and often is diagnosed at the time of exploration of a femoral lump.

Haematocele

Haematocele may result from crushing injury to the testes or may follow operation for hernia or hydrocele when haemostasis has been less than perfect. Absorption of blood from the tunica vaginalis usually occurs more rapidly in childhood than in adult life.

MUSCULO-SKELETAL DISORDERS

There are some general conditions which affect the skeleton and produce characteristic clinical pictures which, although rare, should be considered briefly as they may enter into the differential diagnosis of more common conditions encountered in infancy and childhood. These disorders may affect predominantly one component of the neuromusculo-skeletal system as in achondroplasia or they may have secondary effects as in limbs paralysed as a result of a neural tube defect. The effect of the paralysis on the limb may affect the structure as well as the function. There is usually

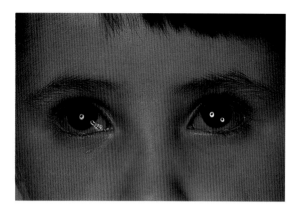

FIGURE 4.13 Osteogenesis imperfecta.

1 The thick boned variety, where newborn babies have numerous fractures and stunted limbs, and may be mistaken clinically for other causes of dwarfism.
2 The slender fragile bone type, in which fractures occur postnatally.
3 Osteogenesis imperfecta cystica where the bones are honeycombed and the deformity progresses with advancing years. No treatment is available for this condition apart from protection from injuries and effective, prompt management of the fractures.

severe wasting of the muscles in the limb and weakness of the skeletal matrix, resulting in oesteoporosis which increases the possibility of fractures. The blood supply to the affected limb has poor vasomotor tone and is unaided by the muscular pump so that the skin is more likely to suffer from trophic ulcers.

The osteochondrodysplasias

This group of disorders have in common abnormalities of collagen which affect cartilage and bone growth and structure. In some the condition may be evident at birth and lethal, e.g. thanatophoric dwarfism, osteogenesis imperfecta lethalis, asphyxiating thoracic dystrophy and achondrogenesis; achondroplasia and Ellis–van Creveld syndrome are non-lethal but obvious at birth and dysplasias which present in later childhood include metaphyseal chondrodysplasia, hyperchondroplasia and mesomelic dwarfism. It is important to reach a diagnosis if possible by careful clinical and radiological examination and to exclude metabolic bone disease secondary to renal, parathyroid or vitamin D disorder. Confusion with mucopolysaccharide and peroxisomal bone disorders can sometimes occur. The underlying molecular defects in collagen are beginning to be identified in some of the osteochondrodysplasias.

Osteogenesis imperfecta (fragilitas ossium)

This condition is dominantly inherited and is characterised by excessive fragility of skeletal bone. The sclera are usually deep blue in colour and the infant may have prenatal fractures (Fig. 4.13). This condition may progress to osteosclerosis if the individual lives beyond a third decade. Three main types of osteogenesis are described:

Osteopetrosis (marble bones; Albers–Schönberg disease)

In this condition there is excessive radiographic density of the bones with or without fragility due to absence or dysfunction of osteoclasts. There is a severe recessive form of the disease which presents at birth or in early infancy with failure to thrive, anaemia, generalised lymphadenopathy and splenomegaly. Failure of bone medulla caused by ineffective osteoclast activity results in bones of greatly increased radiological density and poor trabecular pattern. Optic atrophy, deafness, facial palsy and hydrocephalus may develop as a result of failure of skull foraminae to enlarge normally. Extramedullary haemopoiesis in the reticulo-endothelial system will fail to compensate for the obliteration of the bone medullary cavities and bone marrow transplant to allow colonisation with effective osteoclasts before severe anaemia and neurological deficit develop offers the best chance of survival. There is an autosomal dominant form of the disorder (osteopetrosis tarda) which presents in later childhood with pathological fractures and anaemia but is compatible with a normal life span.

Pyknodysostosis

Pyknodysostosis is an autosomal recessive condition with generalised osteosclerosis but without the anaemia and cranial nerve disorders of osteopetrosis. There is increased risk of bone fractures in a child of short stature, delayed closure of cranial sutures and dentition, mid facial hypoplasia with narrow palate and failed mandibular angulation and in some instances developmental delay.

Dyschondroplasia (Ollier disease; multiple enchondromata)

In this condition there are rounded masses of unossified cartilage in the metaphysis and diaphysis of the long bones of the limbs, as well as in the metacarpals and phalanges. The lesions are essentially endosteal

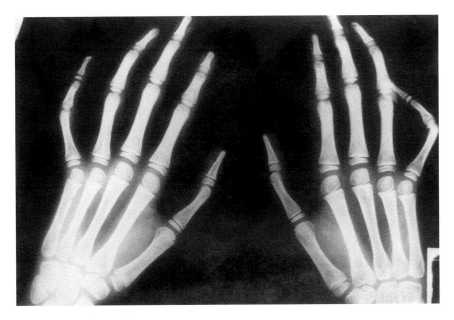

FIGURE 4.14 Marfan syndrome.

and not projections from the bone surface. Enchondromata in the hands may lead to gross deformity. Treatment is symptomatic.

Chondro-osteodystrophy (Morquio–Brailsford disease – mucopolysaccharidosis IVA and IVB)

The outstanding features of this autosomal recessive condition are dwarfism, kyphosis, knock knee, flat foot and progressive changes in the femoral head and acetabulum. Unlike the other forms of mucopolysaccharidosis, the dysplastic joint changes affect predominantly the lower limbs. Intelligence is usually unaffected, there is little or no coarsening of facial features but cardiac valvular lesions, dental enamel dysplasia and corneal opacities develop during childhood.

Achondroplasia

In this autosomal dominant (90% are new mutations) condition there is interference with endochondral ossification and the condition is characterised by short limb dwarfism, a large head, and trident hands. Bones at the base of the skull, which are cartilagenous, grow poorly, whereas skull vault, which is formed from membranous bones, grows normally. Hydrocephalus is a not uncommon complication of the poor basal skull growth which causes obstruction to CSF outflow.

Fibrodysplasia ossificans (myositis ossificans)

Swellings arise in association with connective tissue, fascia and tendons and progress to ossification. The muscles are only affected secondarily. There is characteristic shortening of the thumbs and great toes. The joints are stiffened and the neck becomes immobile. The patient becomes bed-ridden and susceptible to recurrent chest infections.

Craniocleidodysostosis

In this condition there is deficient formation of ossification of the membranous bones in the body which include the clavicles and the vault of the skull. The patient can usually approximate the tips of the shoulders to each other below the chin (see Fig. 4.3). There is no disability or discomfort and no treatment is called for.

Neurofibromatosis (von Recklinghausen disease)

This is an hereditary disease transmitted as a dominant trait. There are pigmented (café-au-lait) patches on the skin. Cutaneous fibromata, multiple neurofibromata and in some cases skeletal changes may be found. Skeletal disorders include scoliosis, diminution in the growth of affected bones and bowing of the tibia which may have pathological fractures which proceed to non-union. Sarcomatous changes are known to have occurred in fibromata in later life.

Arachnodactyly (spider fingers; Marfan syndrome)

The essential features are extreme length of the digits, slender build with poorly developed muscles and

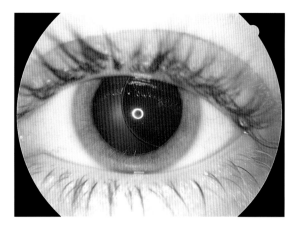

FIGURE 4.15 Marfan dislocation of the lens.

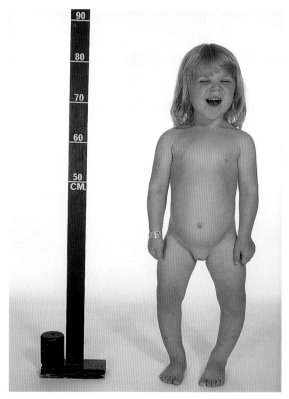

FIGURE 4.16 Deformities of rickets: genu varum.

hyperextensibility of the wrists, ankles and digits (Fig. 4.14). There is a congenital dislocation of the lens (Fig. 4.15) in half of the patients and congenital heart disease is found in one-third. There is also a tendency to weakness of the wall of the aorta and lax cardiac valves resulting in valvular incompetence and dissecting aneurysms in later life.

Fibrocystic disease of bone

Osteitis fibrosis cystica due to hyperparathyroidism is a rare phenomenon but can be found in the newborn and in childhood. Fibrocystic disease may appear in two forms: bone cysts and polyostotic fibrous dysplasia.

Solitary bone cyst

This may appear in any long bone, may present with pain and swelling and pathological fractures may occur. The cyst is cured by simple curettage of the thin-walled cavity and the defect then filled with bone chips.

Polyostotic fibrous dysplasia

There are multiple lesions in the skeleton without general decalcification or disturbance of calcium metabolism. In 30% of cases there are areas of pigmentation in the skin with precocious puberty in females (Albright syndrome). The major long bones are principally affected and the skull may be involved as in leontiasis ossea. Fractures are common but unite readily. The bone changes are arrested when growth ceases.

Infantile scurvy

This disease, now rare, is characterised by haemorrhages and disturbances in ossification due to lack of vitamin C. Scurvy may still be seen in some children with spina bifida who have low ascorbic acid levels present due to deficient intake or an abnormality in the metabolism of vitamin C. There is often visible and palpable swelling of a limb with pain, pseudoparalysis and tenderness accompanied by fever, and the condition can be mistaken for osteitis. Most cases present between 6 and 12 months of age and the infant may lie in a frog-like position with thighs abducted and knees flexed. Haemorrhage may occur at any site but in the gums is most typical. The radiographic appearances are diagnostic and are due to subperiosteal haemorrhages with secondary calcification. The response to vitamin C is dramatic with marked improvements within 24 hours. The pain settles completely within 1 week.

Rickets

Deformities such as genu varum and genu valgum may occur in neglected cases of infantile rickets, resistant rickets or renal rickets (Figs 4.16 and 4.17). Most bones show a remarkable return to normality with vitamin D supplementation. To prevent severe deformities occurring, splintage may be necessary. In renal rickets as in Fanconi syndrome (renal glycosuria with hypophosphataemic rickets), orthopaedic management is supportive.

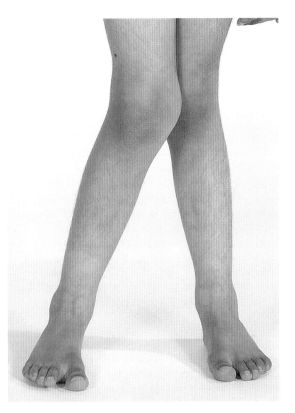

FIGURE 4.17 Deformities of rickets: valgum.

Infantile cortical hyperostosis

This condition is characterised by periostitis affecting the clavicles, mandible, scapula, ribs and long bones. The mandibular swelling gives the infant a charac-teristic appearance. The disease appears in the early months of life and in its early phase may closely resemble neonatal osteitis. The aetiology is unknown. Complete recovery takes place spontaneously usually within a year.

Neoplastic conditions

Certain neoplastic conditions may present with bone or muscular pain, in particular; these may be very misleading and result in delay of diagnosis. Bone lesions are common in leukaemia in children and may take the form of decalcification, osteoporosis, or subperiosteal shadows. Usually the presenting complaint is that of pain in the limbs, and bone changes may be mistaken for a low grade osteitis or even at times growing pains. Another malignancy which presents with bony involvement is neuroblastoma which can be mistaken for an inflammatory condition of the bones or the joints.

Langerhans cell histiocytosis used to be known as "histiocytosis X". Stage I, single lytic bone lesion, and stage II, multiple lytic bone lesions (both formerly known as eosinophilic granuloma of bone), can present with isolated bone pain.

Osteochondritis (osteochondrosis)

This is a non-inflammatory derangement of the normal process of growth which occurs at various centres of ossification during the period of their greatest activity. Before puberty, the common sites are the femoral head (Perthes disease; Fig. 4.18) and the tarsal scaphoid (Köhler disease). Osteochondritis can

FIGURE 4.18 Perthes disease.

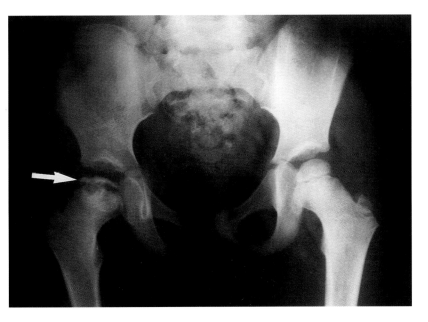

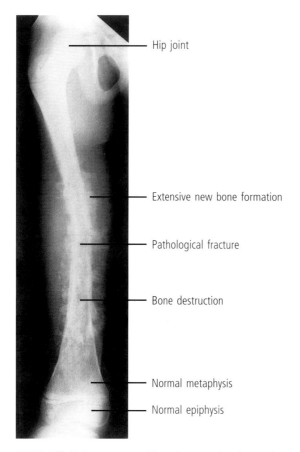

Hip joint

Extensive new bone formation

Pathological fracture

Bone destruction

Normal metaphysis

Normal epiphysis

FIGURE 4.19 Ewing sarcoma. There is extensive destruction of the femoral shaft with marked new bone formation. There is a pathological fracture through the mid-shaft.

also affect the tibial tubercle (Osgood–Schlatter disease) and calcaneum (Sever disease) the second metatarsal (Freiberg disease) and the vertebral epiphyses (Scheuermann disease) but tend to occur at puberty. They are self-limiting diseases that may require immobilisation of the affected limb for periods of 6–8 weeks with physiotherapy to maintain muscle tone and power.

Osteosarcoma

Sarcoma of bone is more common in the young adult while Ewing sarcoma is more common in early childhood. In osteosarcoma the long bones are primarily affected and there is early spread of the disease to the lung. Children usually present with bone pains and diagnosis is made on X-ray. Improvement in survival has been dramatic since the introduction of chemotherapy plus surgery as compared with previous poor results with surgery alone. In Ewing sarcoma the malignancy may be of primitive neural cells and presents with bone pain and tissue swelling. It is radiosensitive as well as responsive to chemotherapy (Fig. 4.19).

Kyphosis

Increased posterior curvature is seen in adolescent kyphosis or Scheuermann disease. This osteochondritis of the epiphyseal plates of the vertebrae causes pain in the back and is treated by physiotherapy. Angular kyphosis may be congenital and due to hemivertebrae or due to infection such as tuberculosis. Kyphosis may occur in other situations such as achondroplasia or Von Recklinghausen disease of bone as part of the general deformity of the skeleton.

Scoliosis

Scoliosis is lateral curvature of the spine and may be congenital or acquired. In a few infants congenital scoliosis is consequent on intrauterine position and in this group the condition corrects spontaneously. In others malformation of the vertebrae, often malsegmentation with rib anomalies also present, may be the cause of scoliosis (Fig. 4.20). It becomes obvious as the child grows and adopts the upright posture.

Acquired scoliosis particularly affects females in the second decade of life. This may progress and referral to a physiotherapist to encourage good posture may help. Infection, particularly tuberculosis, was a frequent cause of interference with vertebral growth, and consequent scoliosis, although more often it resulted in kyphosis or a mixed deformity (kyphoscoliosis). Some children with neurological disorders may have muscle imbalance so that scoliosis develops.

Patients with scoliosis should be seen when the curvature becomes apparent by an orthopaedic surgeon who is experienced in the management of this problem. Initially the infant, child or adolescent will be assessed and the position documented. Subsequent reviews will show if the scoliosis is static, increasing or decreasing. Treatment by bracing, e.g. using the Milwaukee brace, is used less frequently now and has been replaced in some patients by spinal fusion to stabilise the affected segment.

Lordosis

An exaggerated lumbar curvature is seen in bilateral congenital dislocation of the hips and rarely in older children with spondylolysthesis as well as children and adults with neural tube defects.

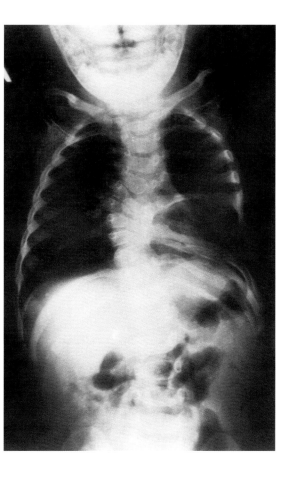

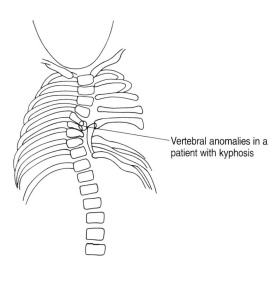

Vertebral anomalies in a patient with kyphosis

FIGURE 4.20 Kyphosis.

Osteitis

The term osteitis is preferred to osteomyelitis as the bone marrow plays only a small part in this infection. The most common infecting organism is *Staphylococcus pyogenes*. Streptococcal osteitis is more common in infancy. The route of infection is blood borne and may come from septic lesions such as boils, abrasions, infected teeth and tonsils. In the neonatal period infection probably enters through the respiratory or alimentary tract or umbilical cord and may be a consequence of a septicaemic episode.

In childhood, infection can lie latent for long periods and the initial lesion is often healed and forgotten for 2–3 weeks before the onset of the disease. Acute osteitis is essentially a disease of childhood. Apart from the neonatal osteitis which is usually secondary to a septicaemia, the disease is relatively uncommon in the first 2 years of life. It is commoner in boys and trauma is a predisposing factor. The bones of the lower extremity are most liable to infection and the tibia and femur are by far the most common sites. The septicaemic phase may be of short duration or last several days. Circulating organisms settle in the vascular metaphases of a long bone and lead to acute suppurative inflammation.

This may progress to abscess formation where periosteal vessels are obliterated and superficial portions of bone may undergo necrosis resulting in sequestrae at a later stage. Usually the diagnosis is made before this stage is reached and antibiotic treatment arrests the progression of the disease. This condition is still prevalent in underdeveloped countries where there is a delay in the diagnosis and unavailability of drugs to treat it adequately.

Clinical features

The disease begins with acute pain affecting the limb which may be preceded by a variable period of malaise. There may be a history of a recent injury or a primary focus of infection. The child is usually ill, flushed, restless and the affected limb is kept still. There is resentment to any examination of the limb. There is usually a pyrexia and a rapid pulse. In the early stages there is no swelling of the limb but by gentle palpation an area of maximum tenderness is found over the affected metaphasis. Swelling of the limb is associated with a subperiosteal effusion but cellulitis does not appear until the periosteum ruptures. There is a very high polymorphonuclear leucocytosis and an ESR which is markedly raised.

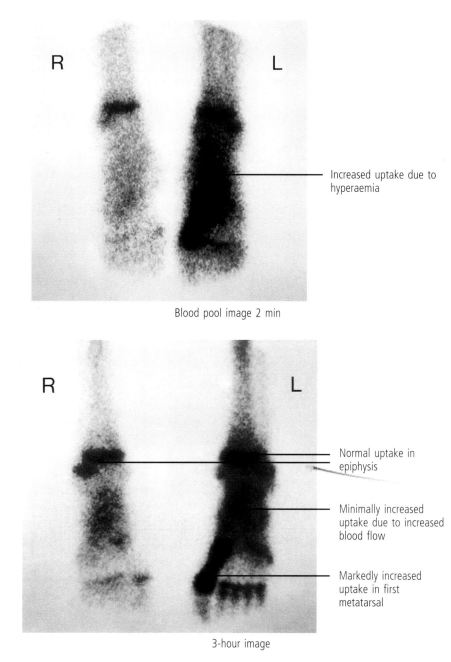

FIGURE 4.21 Osteitis. Typical bone scan of left foot showing hyperaemia of the left foot with increased activity in the first metatarsal. The X-rays were normal and the appearances are those of osteitis of the first metatarsal.

No radiographic changes are seen in the first week of the illness. Thus radiography has nothing to offer in the early diagnosis of acute osteitis. Bone scans may prove helpful (Fig. 4.21). Subsequently there is evidence of elevation of the periosteum and a translucent area of decalcification in the affected metaphasis. In more advanced cases sequestrae, areas of devascularised bone, may be seen.

After cultures have been taken, treatment should be started promptly. The affected limb is immobilised and an intravenous infusion of flucloxacillin started. If an abscess has formed then operative intervention is necessary to allow the pus to discharge. Sequestrae may have to be resected if prompt effective treatment is not instituted rapidly enough to prevent devascularisation and necrosis of substantial areas of bone.

SHOULDER AND UPPER LIMB

SHOULDER GIRDLE – THE CLAVICLE

The clavicle forms the only bony connection between the shoulder girdle and the trunk. It is one of the most commonly fractured bones in the body. The clavicle is liable to break when force is applied to the outstretched hand, elbow or shoulder. Injuries to the clavicle may present with a pseudoparalysis and pain when the arm is moved. It must be differentiated from Erb palsy (Fig. 4.22), osteitis of the clavicle, scapula or upper humerus. At times, children present with a swelling due to massive callus over the clavicle after the initial injury has been missed. In children, reduction of a fractured clavicle is rarely necessary under the age of 6 years. Attempts at mobilisation encourage healing of this bone.

Persistent non-union of the clavicle after a fracture may result in a pseudoarthrosis. The radiographic appearance is of bone sclerosis and expansion at the site of non-union. Improvement in appearance can be obtained by excision of the defect and the excessive bone with bone grafting and internal fixation.

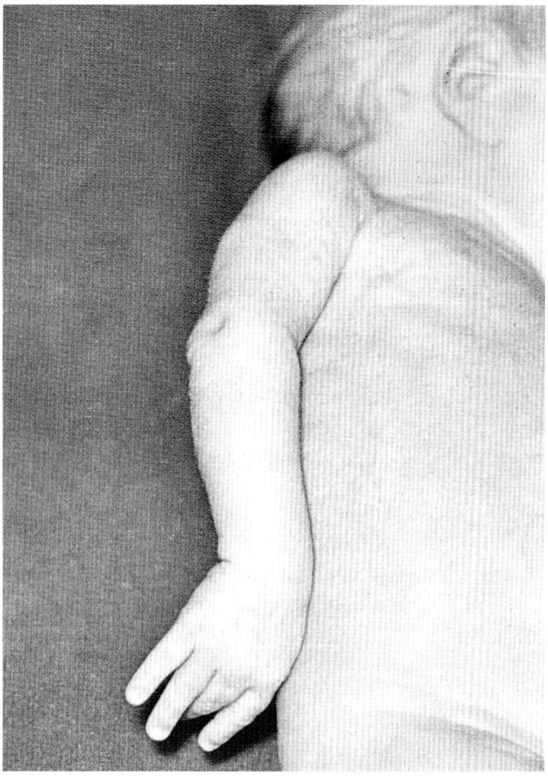

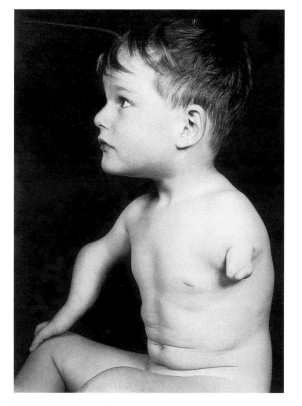

FIGURE 4.22 Erb palsy.

THE SCAPULA

In normal, especially in thin subjects, vigorous movement of the scapula girdle may cause loud crepitus as the scapula and its surrounding muscles move over the ribcage.

Congenital high scapula (Sprengel shoulder)

Congenital absence of the pectoralis major muscle occurs as an isolated entity or associated with abnormalities of the hand (Poland syndrome). There is little dysfunction except from some weakness of shoulder adduction. A thin web of skin over the site of the absent muscle may be unsightly and Z-plasty may help to conceal this. Breast development in girls with this condition is deficient and breast tissue and the nipple may be hypoplastic or absent. In girls cosmetic surgery to the breast area may be performed.

UPPER ARM

Congenital anomalies in the arm vary from almost complete absence (ectromelia), as occurred in 1959/1962 following the use of thalidomide in

FIGURE 4.23 Phocomelia.

pregnancy, to relative minor failure of differentiation of parts of the limb as in syndactyly. Gross failure of limb bud growth may leave the child with a small flipper-like limb (phocomelia) or a more substantial part to which an arm prosthesis may be attached (Fig. 4.23).

Increased sophistication of upper limb prostheses continues with steady improvement in the prognosis for those with arm reduction deformities. More subtle embryonic failure may leave the child with abnormalities such as congenital dislocation of the radial head with partial loss of elbow and forearm movement or with synostosis of radius and ulna with loss of forearm rotation. With these anomalies the forearm tends to be shorter. There is no effective treatment for these conditions although forearm osteotomy may be considered to put the hand in a more favourable position. In the distal part of the limb bud, developmental disorders may give rise to congenital absence of the radius in variable degree. The forearm is shorter, the thumb may be absent or hypoplastic, and the hand deviates to the radial side due to lack of support by the radius. This can occur as part of the VACTERL association in oesophageal atresia (see Fig. 4.4). Some correction of hand position is possible to improve appearance and to a lesser extent function by surgical release of soft tissue deformity and repositioning of the carpus over the end of the ulna.

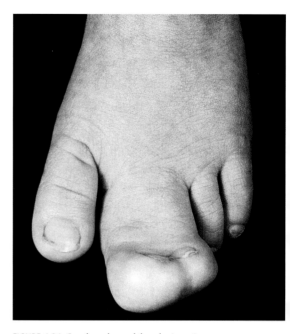

FIGURE 4.24 Syndactyly and local gigantism.

Radioulnar synostosis

The upper ends of the radius and ulna are fused in this condition and the forearm is fixed in pronation and the palm cannot be turned upwards. The results of surgery are disappointing.

Syndactyly (webbed fingers)

Differentiation of the complete upper limb bud is usually complete by the seventh or eighth week of intrauterine life and during the remainder of this period the emphasis is on development. Differentiation proceeds in a centrifugal direction, i.e. the upper arm appears before the forearm and the hand. The earlier the interference the greater will be the abnormality. At 6 weeks of intrauterine life there is a flipper-like broadening of the distal end of the upper limb bud before four grooves appear. These deepen until the flipper becomes separated into five parts. The thumb is first to separate and the fingers separate first at their distal ends. Two or more adjacent fingers may not separate and this failure may be partial or complete. Webbing of the fingers, syndactyly, is a common anomaly and may be associated with microdactyly or ring stricture. Minor

degrees of webbing (zygodactyly) is a normal and sometimes familial feature. Lower limbs may be affected by the same failure of separation of toes (Fig. 4.24). In syndactyly surgical separation of the webbed digits with skin grafting of denuded areas, where there is insufficient local skin to allow primary suture, is usually carried out at the age of 4 years. The quality of result will depend upon how much separate development has occurred in bones, joints, tendons and nerves. Multiple syndactyly occurs in hands and feet associated with cranial deformity in Apert syndrome.

Polydactyly

This is where there are supernumery digits which may be attached either to the radial or ulnar side of the hand (Fig. 4.25). Less commonly the digit may be fully formed with a separate metacarpal. A bifid thumb may arise from the thumb metacarpal. Congenital absence of the thumb constitutes a serious disability. It is usually associated with absence of all or part of the radius as in the VACTERL association.

Growth defects such as lobster claw hand (ectro-dactyly) are difficult to explain embryologically. Despite the ugliness of these hands, function is surprisingly good as a pinch grip between the digits is maintained. Attempts should not be made to improve appearance at the possible expense of loss of function.

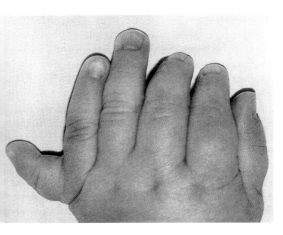

FIGURE 4.25 Polydactyly.

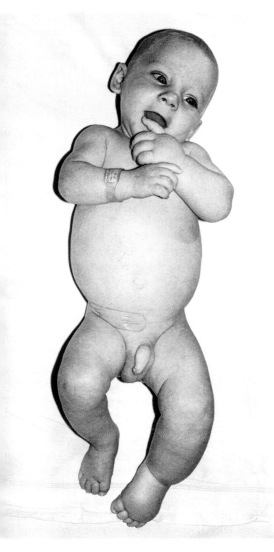

FIGURE 4.26 Hemihypertrophy.

Local gigantism (macrodactyly)

One or more digits may be almost adult size at birth (Fig. 4.24). The disproportion may become greater or less marked with increasing age. The results of plastic procedures in this condition are disappointing.

Hemihypertrophy

Hemihypertrophy may affect the whole of one side of the body (Fig. 4.26). Occasionally an arm may show hypertrophy associated with extensive haemangioma/lymphangioma formation. This may be associated with malignancies such as nephroblastoma and hepatoblastoma in later life.

Contracture

Congenital contracture of the fifth finger is common, often bilateral and causes little trouble. The proximal interphalangeal joint lacks about 30% of extension but is associated with compensatory hyperextension of the metacarpophalangeal joint. No treatment is needed and attempts to improve the interphalangeal joint extension commonly fail. Minor adduction deformity of the little finger commonly occurs due to a small deformed middle phalanx of the digit. If sufficiently severe cosmetic improvement can be obtained by osteotomy in the middle phalanx but the finger remains rather short.

Trigger thumb (stenosing teno-vaginitis)

This is a common disorder in children and attention is drawn to it following some minor injury. The condition results because the fibrous flexor sheath of the flexor policis tendon is stenosed at the level of the thumb metacarpophalangeal joint. The tendon develops a thickening which cannot slide into the sheath although passive extension can force the thickened tendon to pass into the sheath when the thumb jerks into extension. When actively flexed, the thumb jerks, triggering into its flexed position. The lump of the thickened tendon at the mouth of the fibrous sheath can be palpated in front of the metacarpophalangeal joint. The condition readily responds to the simple procedure of slitting the proximal part of the sheath in its long axis. This deformity may be bilateral and can be identified at birth.

Adductor thumbs

Many babies are born with their thumbs adducted. Quite soon, the thumbs assume their normal ability to abduct. Occasionally thumb adduction is associated with X-linked hydrocephalus. Another abnormality found in the digits of children is a benign recurrent digital fibroma of childhood. This is a soft tissue tumour made up of fibrous bundles which is diagnosed histologically. The condition is benign and has no malignant connotation but may recur locally or indeed in other digits both in the upper and lower limbs.

Ganglion

This simple lesion commonly found around the wrist, dorsum of the hand, and about the ankle and foot, causes little upset except for the presence of the lump itself and the parental worry (Fig. 4.27). The ganglion consists of a fibrous sac containing gelatinous material. The sac is usually closely adherent to but not communicating with underlying synovial sheaths or joints. Many ganglia will disappear spontaneously in the course of months. The only effective cure for the persisting ganglion is complete excision. Bursting by direct blow, aspiration, injection of steroids, and the use of drainage and suture are all unreliable methods of treatment.

Spasticity in the upper limb

Cerebral palsy of infancy producing spastic paralysis is not usually apparent in the early months of life, but as the normal arm and hand develops skills the affected hand is seen to be clumsy and less used. Any child reported to show dominance in one hand early in life is indicating there is something wrong with the other. In half the children the perinatal history indicates some harmful insult or hypoxic episode.

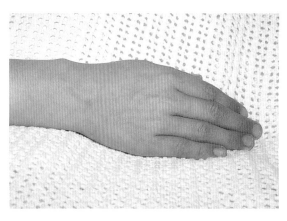

FIGURE 4.27 Ganglion.

Increased muscle tone and tendon jerks and abnormal posture of the arm confirm the diagnosis. Spasticity may be present in other limbs. The affected arm nearly always shows spastic pronation of the forearm and in diminishing degrees, elbow flexion, wrist and finger flexion, a thumb clasped in the palm and limitation of shoulder abduction. If distracted into running, the arm is held out from the body in an odd posture – the bat wing arm. Every attempt is made to prevent fixed deformity by instructing the parents to maintain mobility, stressing passive manipulation into supination, elbow, wrist and finger extension and shoulder abduction. Skilled physiotherapy to instruct the parents and maintain their enthusiasm is most important in maintaining as full a range of movement as possible.

In the lower limb the spasticity results in a characteristic gait with equinus position of the foot and scissoring of the lower limbs. Release of muscles, tendon lengthening or altering the position of muscle insertion improves the mobility of some children, but surgical intervention in the upper limb is rarely of any benefit.

Pseudoparalysis

The unwillingness of a young child to actively move a limb arm or leg is a most important physical sign. In a child too young to be able to indicate the nature of the complaint, a limb found to be left unmoved is a limb in which there is pathology of some sort, particularly trauma or infection.

Gross fracture should be obvious but careful examination will be needed to find a mild injury. Two common causes of the child being presented with a parental statement that "he won't use his arm" are fracture of the clavicle and a pulled elbow seen in children up to the age of 4. With the latter there is usually a history of the young child being pulled or lifted by the hand. The subluxed head of the radius can be manipulated back into position by pronation and supination of the flexed elbow.

THE LOWER LIMBS

Examination of the musculo-skeletal system should start with observation of the infant or child. The position of the limbs and the gait often give a clue to a problem which is subsequently confirmed on more detailed examination. Having inspected the lower limbs of an infant for signs of dissimilarity in the skin creases, girth, gross abnormalities such as bowing of the leg due to congenital absence of the tibia, size and length of the limbs, a systematic examination is

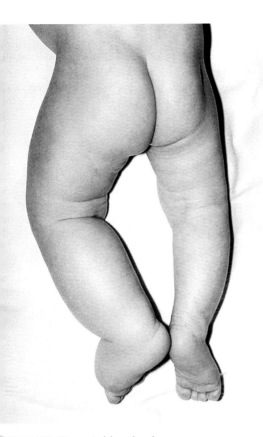

FIGURE 4.28 Congenital lymphoedema.

undertaken. An assessment of muscle tone, power, sensation and reflexes is followed by measurement of limb length and girth. The true length of the legs is measured from anterior superior iliac spine to the medial malleolus or from umbilicus to the malleolus. Discrepancy between the thighs or calf girths is measured at comparable levels above the patella or below the tibial tuberosity and recorded. Discrepancy is usually due to muscle wasting or poor development which may be due to a neurological problem, but on occasion it is the larger limb which is abnormal due to hypertrophy, lymphoedema, or a malformation (Fig. 4.28). Symptoms arising from the musculo-skeletal system are most often due to inflammatory conditions which may be infective or non-infective. The infections of osteitis and myositis are considered elsewhere and the inflammatory disorders are discussed under the connective tissue disorders, e.g. juvenile chronic arthritis.

THE HIP

In assessing movement, assuming that the other hip is normal, the ranges of flexion, extension, rotation, abduction and adduction are simply compared but one must beware that a loss of full extension (i.e. a flexion contracture) may be concealed by the mobile lumbar spine assuming a lordotic posture. To demonstrate this flexion contracture, the other hip is flexed fully to flatten the lumbar spine and in so doing the suspect leg assumes its true position of flexion. This is known as the Thomas test.

Congenital dislocation of the hip

This condition occurs more commonly in the female (five in every six will be girls) and in one to two babies in every thousand births. In 10% there will be a family history of a close relative with this condition. The causation probably depends on a number of factors such as high birth weight, full maturity, the presence of joint laxity and breech delivery – 17% of babies with congenital hip dislocation are breech presentations compared with 4% of all deliveries being breech. It is thought that extreme flexion of the hip in the conduct of breech delivery levers the head of the femur out of the acetabulum. The joint capsule is stretched and the head of the femur comes to lie above the acetabulum with the hip extended and behind the acetabulum when flexed. The condition is commoner in north Italy and Brittany and rare in India and Africa. Excluding those with a neurological basis, e.g. myelomeningocele, in less than 5% the dislocation is prenatal and associated with other pathology such as arthrogryposis. In the vast majority the condition occurs during or shortly after birth and is detectable by the appropriate clinical tests. If undetected at birth, congenital dislocation of the hip may pass unnoticed. It is painless and there is no striking abnormality, apart from limitation of abduction of the hip which may be noted during routine infant examination or the "clicking" hip when the child is specifically tested or when the child stands about 1 year to 18 months later when she may be

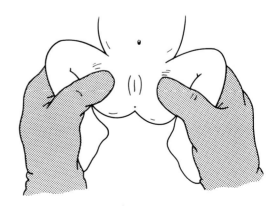

FIGURE 4.29 Ortolani test.

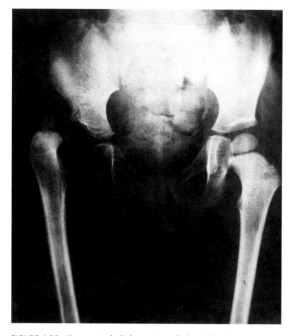

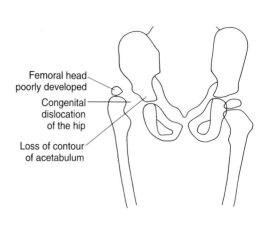

Femoral head poorly developed

Congenital dislocation of the hip

Loss of contour of acetabulum

FIGURE 4.30 Congenital dislocation of the right hip.

noted to have a short leg and a limp. Attention is drawn to the diagnosis.

Diagnosis

In the newborn infant the diagnosis is clinical and depends upon the signs found when doing the Ortolani test (Fig. 4.29). The technique is to examine the baby by grasping the flexed thigh and gently abducting the hip. In the normal hip full abduction occurs smoothly but if the hip is dislocated abduction is limited until, with a jerk, the upper thigh moves forward as the head reduces into the acetabulum. On allowing adduction, the femoral head and proximal thigh can be felt and seen to slip backwards. The Ortolani test usually ceases to be useful after the first 2–3 months. X-rays are unhelpful in finding congenital dislocation of the hip (CDH) and a trial of the efficacy of ultrasound in the routine screening for CDH is currently being undertaken in the newborn. When performing the Ortolani test, sensitive hands may detect a faint clicking sensation but provided no displacement of the upper femur occurs these hips should be regarded as normal.

In the older child, before walking, upward migration of the femur has not occurred and the only clinical sign is limited abduction – few children are detected at this age. Later the child has a short leg and extra skin creases due to bunching of the soft tissues. On walking, there is a characteristic dip when weight-bearing on the affected side – Trendelenburg sign. With the femoral head no longer in joint to

provide an eminence, there is a hollow in the groin at the mid-inguinal point. As seen in Fig. 4.30 the affected hip socket is shallow and saucer-like and the femoral head lies above and outside this socket. The ossific nucleus is often smaller than the other side although the cartilaginous head is generally normal in size. There may even be a notch of a false acetabulum on the ilium above the true acetabulum due to pressure from the femoral head.

Treatment

Treatment of congenital hip dislocation consists essentially of replacing the head in the acetabulum and maintaining it there until stable with acetabular development.

In the newborn the act of carrying out the Ortolani test has produced reduction and this is maintained with the hips held flexed and fully abducted in a suitable divaricator splint. This is worn continuously, being adjusted at intervals of 1 or 2 weeks and allows outpatient management. After about 6 weeks it is customary to change to a simpler removable divaricator worn most of the time but allowing freedom to bath the baby. This is worn until about 3 months when treatment ceases. Follow-up should show normal hip development in almost all.

In the older child, reduction requires release of the tight adductor muscles by tenotomy at their pelvic origin while manipulative reduction is attempted under general anaesthesia. In 75% of children in the early part of the second year, a stable reduction will be obtained and a plaster cast from waist to ankles is applied in the "frog" position. In the remaining 25%, closed reduction will fail and an open reduction is required to undo whatever soft tissue obstruction prevents reduction – notably the tight psoas tendon across the lower part of the acetabulum, or a down-turned lip of the acetabulum (the limbus) obstructing the entrance to the acetabulum.

After a period in wide abduction, in which the other leg also has to be held to stabilise the pelvis, a less flexed position, allowing more hip movement, is chosen – with "Batchelor" plasters applied. In this type of plaster, it will be found that inward rotation of the femur corrects for the anteverted (forward turned) femoral neck usually present at this age. To allow the upper end of the femur to remain so corrected a rotation osteotomy, with internal fixation, is needed at upper femoral shaft level to leave the lower leg facing forwards. After 10–12 months the acetabulum will be found to be developing and treatment can cease.

The longer the child walks undetected on the dislocated hip, the poorer the results will be.

The results of treatment will be a normal or nearly normal hip in about 90% but at the expense of a number of hospital admissions, anaesthetics, and one or two operations. The less satisfactory minority may need further salvage procedures beyond the scope of this book. Provided the hip is nearly normal in its radiographic appearance there is little risk of osteoarthritis in later life. A general restoration of load-bearing anatomy permits development of a fairly normal pelvic shape and it would be relatively straightforward to carry out a hip replacement arthroplasty if osteoarthritis developed later. Such replacement arthroplasty has not proved a solution in the totally untreated hip dislocation.

Osteochondritis of the femoral head (Perthes disease)

This occurs largely in boys (five out of six will be boys exactly the reverse of the sex ratio in congenital dislocation of the hip). Although it may occur between the ages of 2 and 10 years, the peak incidence is between 4 and 7 years. The condition occurs about once in every 2000 children. A small number have a family history of the condition and 10% will have both hips affected but not necessarily at the same time.

Perthes disease is due to loss of blood supply, in part or in whole, to the femoral capital epiphysis which then undergoes avascular (aseptic) necrosis. The cause of the loss of blood supply is uncertain but children have a relatively tenuous blood supply to the femoral head under normal conditions. The articular cartilage is not primarily involved. The death of the capital epiphysis usually causes synovitis of the joint, giving rise to mild symptoms.

The pathology and natural process of repair are paralleled by X-ray changes (see Fig. 4.18). In the very earliest stages, not often seen, the joint space may be enlarged by synovial effusion and thickening of the articular cartilage. The affected femoral head may seem relatively dense due to rarefaction in healthy, vascular bone of the pelvis and femur but this is followed by compression of the dead head, its reduction in height and the absolute increase in its density. At this time the natural process of repair involves an ingrowth of blood vessels with gradual revascularisation, the accompanying removal of dead bone and its replacement with living bone (creeping substitution). The dense bone mass appears to fragment radiologically and the portions of dead bone gradually become absorbed, being replaced with less dense living bone. This process takes 1–2 years and during this time the femoral head is softened and may also be partly subluxed from the acetabulum and is at risk of deformation due to weight-bearing forces so that the new live bone may be produced in a deformed shape leading to restriction of movement and possibly to osteoarthritic changes in later years.

Symptoms and diagnosis

The child usually presents with relatively mild complaints. Nearly all have a history of weeks or months of intermittent or continuous limp but only 50% admit to moderate pain at hip, thigh or knee. The child will be generally well. Examination will confirm the limp and some slight wasting of the thigh is usually seen. Hip movements are usually free except for limitation of internal rotation and abduction. The hip X-ray is usually diagnostic although occasionally the X-ray changes may lag some months behind the physical signs. It is usual to admit the child for a few weeks to allow bedrest with traction during which time the irritability of the hip settles and full movements return.

Orthodox treatment has been the relief from weight-bearing by bedrest, the use of a weight relieving caliper, or most commonly by the use of crutches with a sling to suspend the affected leg. In the latter device a return to home and school is possible and the regimen would continue for about 1 year.

In recent years carefully controlled studies have cast doubt on the value of this treatment and with grading of the degree of involvement of the femoral head, with the age of the child it may be possible to achieve a good result without such treatment. Hips showing lateral subluxation are best managed by containment of the femoral head in an abduction plaster – like a Batchelor plaster for congenital hip dislocation.

Slipped upper femoral epiphysis (adolescent coxa vara)

Although much less common than congenital hip dislocation or Perthes disease, this condition is important and early diagnosis will avoid possible crippling deformity and complications. The condition occurs in the pre-pubertal child usually within the age groups of 10–14 years in girls and 12–16 years in boys. Three-quarters of these children are frankly obese or taller than average – often strikingly so.

The pathology is one of weakness at the upper femoral epiphyseal plate so that relative to the neck and shaft of the femur the femoral head epiphysis slips *backwards*. Although the alternative name of coxa vara would suggest a medial and downward slip the main direction of movement is backwards. The slip of the femoral head is insidious and initially the symptoms are slight, with limp and pain at the hip but such pain is often referred to thigh and knee. Depending on the severity of symptoms the adolescent may be detected early with a minimal slip or may proceed over months to a severe deformity and superimposed upon the gradual slip may be a sudden detachment of the femoral head so that symptoms are severe and the child resembles one with a femoral neck fracture. The child thus tends to present in one of three different ways – with minimal slip, massive chronic slip, or with an acute severe displacement.

The diagnosis should be suspected in any adolescent particularly if heavily built or tall, who presents with a limp and pain. In the early minimal slip there may be little clinical abnormality except for slight restriction of flexion, abduction and internal rotation. As the degree of slip increases a frank external rotation deformity will develop. In advanced slips the condition will be obvious in antero-posterior X-rays but in minor degrees the A-P view may appear normal and it is essential to have lateral view X-rays which are needed to demonstrate the backward slip.

Treatment

In minimal slips, internal fixation to prevent further slip is carried out using an appropriate nail or multiple pins inserted under X-ray control. When the epiphyseal plate fuses (usually early) no further risk of slip exists and the nail can be removed.

In chronic massive slip, with or without prior internal fixation, an osteotomy either at femoral neck or intertrochanteric level is carried out to return the femoral head to a normal attitude for weight-bearing.

When an acute displacement is the mode of presentation, an attempt to reduce the deformity may be made or an open reduction carried out, followed by internal fixation.

As the condition ultimately proves to be bilateral in 30%, the other hip must be kept under periodic review with lateral X-rays to detect early any tendency to slip so that this can be internally fixed.

The following complications may arise:

1 Avascular necrosis may develop especially after acute slips as the blood supply to the femoral capital epiphysis is mainly by vessels on the posterior surface of the neck of the femur. Vigorous attempts at closed reduction of such slips may also produce vascular damage.

2 With any mode of slip, but especially with larger degrees of displacement, acute cartilage necrosis at the hip may occur when the articular cartilage of both the femoral head and acetabulum undergoes severe degeneration leading to a painful stiff hip or possibly ankylosis.

3 Following upper femoral epiphyseal slip and its treatment, the epiphyseal plate tends to fuse early, abolishing growth at this point. A small amount of leg length shortening, usually 1 cm, may develop.

Synovitis of the hip

Young children commonly develop a benign, transient inflammation or effusion in the hip, probably as the result of minor injury. Pain in hip, thigh or knee develops with a limp or inability to stand on the leg and these symptoms frequently are found first on rising in the morning after a previous day's normal activity.

Clinically the hip is found to have limitation of internal rotation and of abduction but other movements are usually free. There may be some muscle spasm on passively moving the hip but there is no wasting. X-rays are normal except for soft tissue shadows which may indicate some hip joint distension. These findings exclude most other pathology but it is important to rule out the possibility of acute septic arthritis in its early stages, although in that condition all hip movements are affected.

Treatment

In the straightforward mild condition it is reasonable to explain the affliction as a minor sprain of a hip to be treated by bedrest for a few days and restricted activity for a further week. If any doubt exists, hospital admission for bedrest with traction, and observation and investigation are indicated. If the hip gives rise to serious doubt regarding possible infection, the joint should be aspirated and antibiotics administered as for septic arthritis. Even in the more severe cases of synovitis most will settle in a few days following which it is usual to apply the adjective "transient" to the synovitis. As Perthes disease occasionally appears with a history of past attack of synovitis of the hip some months earlier, it is wise to advise that the child

TABLE 4.1 Comparison of important hip disorders – an aid to differential diagnosis

DIAGNOSIS	USUAL AGE (YEARS)	SEX	SYMPTOMS	DURATION OF HISTORY	SIGNS	X-RAY APPEARANCES
Congenital dislocation of the hip	0–3	F/M 5/1	Limp, difference in appearance of legs	Since birth – obvious since walking	In neonate – Ortolani sign. Later – limp, short leg, skin creases, limited abduction	Diagnostic in older child. Ultrasound in infancy
Perthes disease	4–7	M/F 5/1	Limp, ± pain in hip/thigh or knee	Weeks or months	Wasted thigh. Limited abduction and internal rotation	Dense flattened femoral head
Slipped upper femoral epiphysis	F 10–14 M 12–16	M = F	Limp + pain in hip, thigh or knee. May be sudden/severe	Weeks or months or sudden	Tall/obese. Limited flexion, abduction and internal rotation	Lateral X-ray (check contralateral)
(Transient) Synovitis of hip	1–6	M > F	Pain in hip, thigh, or knee. Limp or refuses to stand/walk	1–3 days, often on rising from bed	Child well. No wasting. Limited abduction and internal rotation. Muscle spasm	Normal
Septic arthritis	0–10	M = F	Acute pain. Unable to stand/walk. Pseudo-paralysis in infants	Hours or days	Child is ill. All movement is painful. Joint tenderness and fullness	At early stage – normal. Later bone erosion, joint distension/dislocation
Tuberculosis of the hip	2–10	M = F	Pain in hip/thigh or knee. Stiffness/limp – worsening	Weeks or months	Wasting. Restriction of all movements	Diffuse bone porosis/outlines "fuzzy"

returns if there is any unexplained limp or pain in hip, thigh or knee.

Adductor origin strain

An uncommon cause of hip pain and limp, usually in athletic boys of 10 years or older, is a strain of the origin of adductor longus at the pubic tubercle. There is pain on active use of the leg and passive abduction produces pain at the adductor origin where tenderness will also be found. There are no X-ray changes. The symptoms tend to disappear spontaneously and reassurance and advice to restrict physical activity are all that is needed.

A summary of the conditions affecting the hip joint is tabulated in Table 4.1.

THE KNEE

Congenital deformity of the knee is rare, the most common being congenital hyperextension which may be the result of an *in utero* position in its simpler form, treated by gentle manipulation into flexion or fixation in progressively flexed plaster casts until a full range of movement is restored. Severe grades of this deformity are usually associated with fibrous contracture of the quadriceps muscle requiring surgical release.

Derangement within the knee joint

The lateral meniscus is occasionally congenitally deformed as a discoid lateral cartilage. This may give rise to no symptoms but can cause a loud clicking on flexion/extension movements possibly with mechanical disturbances of locking and instability. If the symptoms are persistently troublesome lateral menisectomy is needed.

Tears of normal menisci, so common in the adult male, are rare in children but if symptoms of mechanical disturbance are troublesome menisectomy is indicated.

The most common derangement within the knee is osteochondritis dissecans, usually found in boys over 10 years. An islet of bone, perhaps 1–2 cm in diameter, usually on the intercondylar aspect of the medial femoral condyle surface, separates from the underlying bone. This may be the result of trauma or disturbance of the local blood supply. The button-like fragment of bone is avascular and, covered by the articular cartilage which holds it in place, lies in a bed of sclerosed bone. The articular cartilage may break down to allow the bone fragment to separate from its bed and become a loose body in the knee joint.

The symptoms are usually of discomfort felt in the region, worse after activity, and often accompanied by a small joint effusion. There may be local tenderness but physical examination is usually unhelpful. X-rays will demonstrate the lesion especially if an intercondylar view is requested.

In the younger child, with restriction of weight-bearing and rotational strains as occur in football etc., the condition can be expected to heal over a period of 1–3 years. In the adolescent, the bone fragment may separate to become a loose body which should be removed. Although a defect in the articular surface is left, this tends to smooth off with cartilage growth.

Derangement outwith the knee joint

This concerns dislocation of the patella, bursal conditions, osteochondritis of the bones about the knee and stress fracture of the tibia.

Dislocation of the patella

Although involving the knee joint, the tibio-femoral articular is not concerned in this condition. The patella always dislocates laterally and this may proceed to become a recurrent condition as the soft tissues about the medial side of the patella become slack with stretching. There are three distinct types of pathology to be found:

1 Fibrosis in the lateral part of the quadriceps muscle may develop – usually the result of injection of antibiotics in infancy. The resulting fibrous tether from the origin or belly of the muscle to the lateral part of the patella becomes tense as the knee flexes and pulls the patella laterally so that eventually it dislocates. Should the patella be held in place passively, knee flexion will be found to be limited. This type of patellar dislocation is treated by division or excision of the fibrous tether, with plication of the stretched soft tissue attachments medial to the patella.
2 Dislocation of the patella may occur in the absence of the above fibrous tether where there is generalised laxity of the soft tissue capsules of the joints and a relatively long patellar tendon or an increase in the valgus angulation of the knee or in various combinations of the above. These are best treated by soft tissue plication on the medial side of the knee together with realignment medially of the lateral part of the patellar tendon insertion to the tibia.
3 Rarely the patella may be found dislocated congenitally – lying permanently on the lateral side of the knee – for this no treatment is advised.

Prepatellar bursitis

The bursa directly overlying the superficial aspect of the patella may be acutely swollen with blood or serous fluid following a local injury. This usually subsides with protection of the part and chronic bursitis (housemaid's knee) is rare in children. Acute infection as a result of a penetrating injury or secondary to local soft tissue infection should be treated with antibiotics and possibly with surgical incision and drainage. Until positive bacteriological information is obtained, an antistaphylococcal antibiotic should be used on a "best guess" basis.

Semi-membranosus bursa (Baker's cyst)

This bursal swelling is relatively common – usually presenting as a painless, non-tender swelling in the medial part of the popliteal aspect of the knee just lateral to the tendon of semi-membranosus. The swelling is tense and most apparent with the knee extended, disappearing into the relaxed soft tissues as the knee bends. This bursa is deeply attached to but not in communication with the back of the knee joint. If large or persistently present the bursa can be excised but as it may disappear spontaneously this treatment should be postponed for a year or more.

Osteochondritis

Osgood–Schlatter disease, although commonly referred to as an osteochondritis of the tibial tubercle, is really a chronic traction injury due to the pull of the patellar tendon inserted at that site. Commonly found in athletic boys in the 10–14 years age group, the complaint is often of many months of pain at the tibial tubercle, worse after exertion and accompanied by enlargement of the tibial tubercle which is tender to touch or on kneeling. These features are easily confirmed on examination and active extension of the knee against resistance will cause pain at the site. An X-ray usually shows some avulsion and fragmentation of the tibial tubercle.

Less common, but basically similar, is the strain of attachment of the patellar tendon to the lower pole of the patella, usually called Johansson–Larsen disease. Here there will be localised tenderness at the site and an X-ray may show a small flake of patellar bone detached.

In these conditions, about half the children will sooner or later have bilateral disease. The conditions are self-healing and all that is required is to reduce the child's activities to a level at which symptoms can be tolerated, i.e. less football, but allowing cycling and swimming which demand less of the extensor apparatus of the knee. After 1–2 years the symptoms will disappear.

Stress fracture of the tibia

Due to the physical demands of athletics a stress (or fatigue) fracture may occur in the upper third of the shaft of the tibia. This is usually in active boys of 10 years or older and the complaint, usually of a few weeks' duration, is of pain at the site on weight-bearing eased by rest. Later a distinct local thickening and local heat may be noted. An X-ray at a very early stage may show no abnormality but after a few weeks layers of periosteal new bone will appear, usually on the posterior cortex, together with a zone of sclerosis across the bone. Occasionally the local heat and swelling may give rise to suspicion of osteitis, or the X-ray appearances of periosteal new bone may suggest an osteosarcoma, but both these diseases are usually initially confined to the metaphysis rather than the shaft of the bone. The only treatment needed is reduction of physical activity for some weeks as the fracture is self-healing and will leave the bone a little thicker to withstand stress in the future.

Bow leg and knock knee

Uncommonly, leg deformity may occur due to nutritional or renal rickets, or more rarely, to a general skeletal malformation or due to some local abnormality in the bone. When suspicious of these possibilities an X-ray of the leg bones and other appropriate investigations are indicated. The vast majority of leg deformity in young children is to be regarded as physiological.

Bow leg usually appears late in the first year and up to about 2 years. In some it may be a genuine varus angulation between femur and tibia such that there is a gap between the knees when the ankles touch. More often the legs are straight but the soft tissue contour of the calf in a fat child gives the appearance of bowing of the lower leg.

If in doubt an X-ray (A-P) of knees and tibiae will show the lower femoral and upper tibial and lower tibial epiphyses to exclude rickets etc., and will demonstrate, particularly for the parents, the straightness of the tibia and fibula. No treatment is needed beyond reassurance for the parents.

Knock knee is equally common but appears later than bow leg – usually in the age group 2–5 years. This is a genuine deformity with a gap between the medial malleoli best measured with the leg straight and the knees touching while the child lies on a flat surface. The valgus deformity is usually more obvious and persists longer in children of heavier or taller build than average. Only in cases of extreme deformity proving persistent is corrective osteotomy of the tibia needed. The parents should be reassured but if they are still worried, the child can be reviewed from time to time.

Splay footed and in-turned gait

The vast majority of external or internal rotation gait abnormalities are due to the posture of the whole leg at the hip joint, although evidence of foot deformity or tibial torsion should be looked for.

Splay footed stance or walking is common in children about 1 year of age due to persistent fetal posture. It can be demonstrated that the hip joint possesses a far greater range of external than of internal rotation. No action is called for as the vast majority become normal after 6–12 months of weight-bearing.

In-turning is common in children in the 2–5 years age group and can be shown to be due to a greater range of inward than outward rotation at the hips. Habits of kneeling with the legs inwardly turned or sleeping on the face make the posture more persistent. An appropriate demonstration of these features should be made to the parents who are asked to carry out walking re-education and to stop abnormal rotation postures being adopted.

ANKLE AND FOOT

Congenital foot deformities

Talipes means "ankle and foot", i.e. the part of the body being described. Equinus means to be in a toe-down, plantar-flexed position whilst calcaneus, "the prominent heel", is the opposite. Varus deformity involves medial deviation of the distal part of the limb while a valgus deformity is the opposite.

Talipes equinovarus: club foot

This common deformity occurs two to four times in every 1000 births, i.e. about twice as common as congenital dislocation of the hip. The male is twice as often affected as the female, and in half the affected children both feet are deformed. The diagnosis is obvious on inspection, the deformity being in three parts: the heel is drawn up, the foot inverted and the forefoot adducted, i.e. an equinovarus position (Fig. 4.31). In a small minority the deformity is postural and can be corrected easily by manipulation to neutral and beyond. Repeated manipulation is sufficient treatment. The majority have rigidly deformed feet. In most this is the only problem but club foot deformities are also found in such conditions as arthrogryposis, trisomy 18 and in spina bifida cystica.

Initially the treatment is carried out as inpatient with daily manipulation of each element of the deformity. The correction obtained each day is maintained

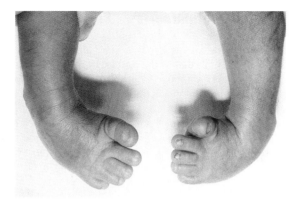

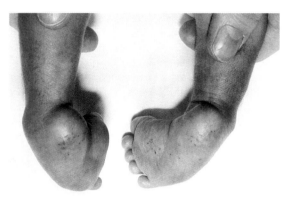

FIGURE 4.31 Talipes equinovarus: club foot.

with the careful application of a Denis Browne splint to the foot (or feet); as the deformity is overcome progressively the splint may be bent to hold a greater degree of correction and then connected to the other foot (normal or affected) by a connecting bar to hold the correction more effectively. Over a period of 7–14 days the foot will reach the over-corrected position and the baby can be sent home in the splints. It is necessary to continue to maintain an over-correction by remanipulation and reapplication of the splints as an outpatient every 2 weeks until the child starts to stand late in the first year. Alternative regimens to hold the correction obtained by manipulation involve the use of elastoplast strapping or plaster of Paris.

For walking the splints are discarded and boots with an outer raise to the sole are supplied, with night boots and connective bar for night wear. The parents are instructed to manipulate the foot into the over-corrected position. Over the next few years these treatments can be abandoned gradually with a view to the child going to school at 5 years with normal footwear and a foot which is slightly small and stiffer than usual. If the foot is found to be inadequately corrected during the first year, or to be relapsing during the later years, a soft tissue release operation on the medial and posterior aspects of the foot and ankle is needed. About half the affected feet will need

this procedure and in a few with severe deformity, bony correction will be necessary.

Talipes calcaneovalgus

As the name implies, this is exactly the opposite deformity from that of club foot. This is usually the result of *in utero* posture in that the foot has been caught in an upturned position with the sole against the uterine wall. The deformity is ugly but the prognosis is excellent as natural improvement occurs with active movement on release from the uterus. All that is needed is for the mother to manipulate the foot into equinovarus frequently and the deformity resolves permanently within a few weeks.

Metatarsus varus

In this less common deformity the forefoot is deviated inwardly in relation to the hind foot, as in club foot, but without equinus or inversion. This is best treated as early as possible with serial well padded moulded plasters until the forefoot remains straight. In a small proportion surgical exploration is needed to release a tight medial tether.

Arthrogryposis multiplex congenita

This name is used for a congenital condition affecting joints which may be localised or generalised. Differentiation of primitive mesoderm is impaired and the joints and soft tissues are deformed and almost completely rigid. The muscles are atrophic and fibrous and the skin is tight so that the limbs resemble hosepipes. Arthroplasty has always failed to provide useful movement and the only treatment is to stabilise the affected joints in good position.

Minor toe abnormality

Overlapping fifth toe

From birth the smallest toe lies on the dorsum of the base of the fourth toe in a medially deviated position. This is the only common toe abnormality in childhood to need surgical correction on most occasions in order to avoid trouble with shoe fitting. From about 3 years of age a minor plasty surgical correction allows the toe to return to its normal position.

Curly toes

It is normal for the fifth and fourth toes to be a little flexed and curled medially, but if the third toe, instead of being straight, shares this flexed and medial deformity, the second toe is usually deformed such that it lies on a higher plane than the others and curls laterally, overlying the third toe. This curious pattern of deformity is very common but it is seldom the cause of trouble, although tight shoes and socks should be avoided.

Occasionally a single toe, usually the fourth, is more flexed and adducted than usual and if it comes to cause pressure on the group with the side of the nail discomfort is felt. The toe can be straightened without damaging the growth potential by transferring the insertion of the long flexor tendons to the extensor tendons on the dorsum of the toe.

Hallux valgus

Although usually regarded as an adult affliction, girls from about 10 years may present with increasing valgus of the great toe. Osteotomy of the distal shaft of the first metatarsal is the recommended procedure and long-term satisfactory correction is achieved.

Painful lesions about the foot

Sever calcaneal apophysitis

In may ways similar to Osgood–Schlatter disease of the tibial tubercle this condition troubles children in the 10–14 years age group with pain at the point of the heel, usually worse during or after athletics. The calcaneal apophysis is tender as the heel strikes the ground and even on tiptoes is painful due to the pull of the insertion of the tendo Achilles. In half the children the condition may be bilateral. The diagnosis depends upon the history and finding tenderness about the point of the heel. X-rays are normal. The treatment is simply to restrict activity to a level at which the symptoms are tolerable. Cycling and swimming are useful alternatives to football or netball. An absorbent rubber heel to the shoe may cushion heel strike and in 1–2 years the symptoms will disappear.

Köhler disease of the navicular

An osteochondritis, similar to Perthes disease of the hip, affects the navicular bone causing vague pain about the mid-foot and locally the part may be tender. An X-ray shows changes of increased density and collapse of the navicular. With minimal treatment by temporary supportive bandaging the symptoms will disappear and the X-ray appearances will become normal in 1–2 years.

Stress fracture of a metatarsal (march or fatigue fracture)

As occurs in the upper tibia, an increase in physical activity may so stress a metatarsal (usually the second) to produce an undisplaced self-healing fracture. Local pain, tenderness and swelling will be found with X-ray changes similar to those in the tibia. Modest rest for a few weeks will result in a cure.

Freiberg disease

In the capital epiphysis of the second (occasionally the third) metatarsal, osteochondritic change similar to Perthes disease may occur, with the head of the bone becoming enlarged and tender. X-rays show an irregular increase in density with flattening of the front of the head. This may end up with a large square-shaped metatarsal head which later in life may need excision, but in childhood no specific treatment is needed as symptoms disappear with rest.

Peroneal spastic flat foot

In the age group beyond 5 years, due to the presence of a tarsal anomaly giving rise to pain, the foot is held in eversion with the peroneal muscles in spasm – this is protective spasm as the foot is more comfortable in this position.

If it is possible to demonstrate the tarsal anomaly, commonly a calcaneo-navicular bar or joint, then surgical removal of the anomaly will restore normal anatomy and permanently relieve the symptoms. If this anomaly (possibly cartilaginous) cannot be seen, then forced manipulation under general anaesthetic into inversion, with a short leg plaster to maintain the position for 4–6 weeks will produce improvement in the foot.

Occasionally juvenile rheumatoid arthritis affecting the tarsus presents in a similar way but local warmth, a raised ESR and the presence of another joint involvement usually indicates the correct diagnosis.

Pes cavus

There is a wide variation in the height of the arch of the foot but when this is seen to be marked and unilateral, it must be regarded as pathological. The affected leg is often a little thinner and short and with the raised arch, the foot is often smaller. This condition develops in the early years and it is probable that all have a neurological cause, mostly due to minor anomalies of the cord in the lumbo-sacral region. As occasion may justify, investigation by myelography, MRI or direct surgical exploration will demonstrate a lesion such as intraspinal lipoma, angioma, etc. Attempts to deal with the fundamental neurological defect are generally unrewarding and are associated with hazard to continence. Accordingly attention should be directed to the foot deformity, tackling whichever feature is most troublesome.

As the foot becomes more arched, shoe fitting is made difficult, weight-bearing is confined to smaller areas of the sole and the toes become clawed. Correction of heel shape by calcaneal osteotomy may be useful, or division of tight plantar soft tissues may release some of the cavus. Tendon transfers help toe-clawing and in the worst cases wedge tarsectomy produces an improved foot shape.

Flat foot

Many young children when first standing have such *fat* feet that as the adipose tissue is pressed to the ground the hollow beneath the arch is obliterated and the foot looks flat. This is not pathological and the parents should be reassured.

Older children very frequently have flattening of the longitudinal arch on standing but the arch reasserts itself on standing on tiptoe – this is the usual mobile flat foot and no specific treatment is needed beyond getting the child to practise toe walking and walking on the inverted feet. As the limb matures a normal arch will appear. In severe cases a longitudinal arch support (a Whitman brace) may be worn for a few years.

Toenails

An isolated deformity of nail pushed up by a sub-ungual exostosis or fibroma arising from a terminal phalanx may occur, accompanied by tenderness at the part. This can be dealt with by avulsion of the nail and removal by curettage of the exostosis or fibroma. When the nail regrows it will be normal. Ingrowing toenails are not common in children but when they occur they give the same trouble as in adults due to pressure of the over-wide nail on the soft tissues of the nail fold. The usual management is to keep the nail fold clean and let the corner of the nail grow free of the soft tissues (cutting the nail square across is helpful). If this fails and recurrent sepsis occurs then wedge resection of the nail bed is indicated.

Onychogrypotic nails which have an appearance like a piece of sheep's horn are normally thought of as a complaint of the elderly but do occur in children (Fig. 4.32). If the shape of the nail causes trouble which cannot be made tolerable by cutting or filing, the radical removal of the nail and the nail bed is needed.

GENERAL AFFLICTIONS OF THE LEG

Leg length discrepancy may develop due to a variety of causes and in all but rare events, such as an arterio-venous malformation in which the leg overgrows, or occasionally following acute osteitis, the short leg is the pathological one. Shortening may be due to malunion of a fracture, but this is not a

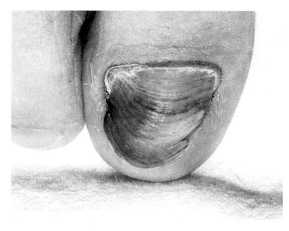

FIGURE 4.32 Onychogryposis.

progressive shortening as occurs when epiphyseal growth plates are damaged by trauma or infection. A flaccid (as opposed to spastic) paralysis deprives the limb of the growth stimulus of muscle contraction and poliomyelitis has in the past given rise to severe leg length discrepancy. Less than 3 cm can be dealt with simply by an appropriate shoe or heel raise, but greater deficiencies may be dealt with by:

1 shortening of the longer leg; or
2 by retarding growth in the longer leg by destroying or stapling the epiphyseal plates above and below the knee; or
3 by lengthening the short leg, usually in the tibial segment, although this latter method requires great attention to avoid complications.

Poliomyelitis

Although rare since the introduction of oral vaccination, poliomyelitis may occur and leave the child with a variable degree of flaccid paralysis, quite unpredictable in its pattern. Sensation remains normal. The problems are due to loss of function, the acquisition of deformity due to the unbalanced pull of muscles no longer opposed by paralysed muscles, and loss of growth potential due to lack of muscle pull and weight-bearing. Each patient is an individual problem. Unstable legs may be supported by calipers, etc. and stiffening of joints or possible tendon transfers may control deformity and improve function. Leg length problems will have to be dealt with as outlined above.

Spina bifida cystica

Spina bifida cystica in its neurological effect in the legs must be considered in the light of the patient as a

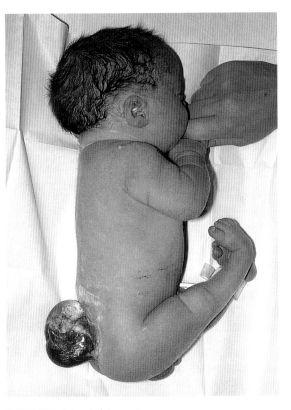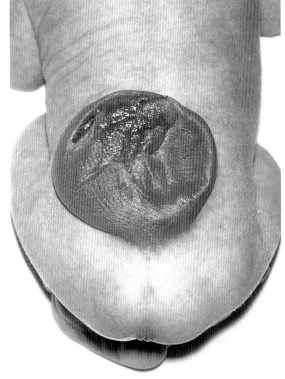

FIGURE 4.33 Spina bifida cystica.

whole – a child in whom there is a 98% chance of urinary and faecal incontinence, whose hydrocephalus has required drainage and in whom cerebral palsy and congenital anomalies may be present (Fig. 4.33).

In the legs the sensory loss may be extensive depending on the degree of nerve root or spinal cord damage. The motor dysfunction is largely due to root damage giving flaccid paralysis but areas of spasticity may be present due to higher cord damage with intact lower cord segments and lower motor neurone function, together with a potential to develop severe deformity. Some problems are reasonably predictable; for example, a common level of lesion about L4 will leave the roots of femoral and obturator nerves largely intact while the sciatic nerve will be paralysed. As a result the hip, subject to the pull of flexors and adductors but with no extensor or abductor muscle function, will dislocate. At a lower level active quadriceps, unopposed by paralysed hamstrings, will produce recurvatum of the knee. The foot may be deformed in any direction and loss of the normal weight distribution on the sole of the foot will readily lead to trophic ulceration in the anaesthetic foot.

By a variety of procedures leg deformity may be controlled and function improved by caliper bracing. Any success in getting the child to stand or walk in some way with various aids will depend upon the child's intelligence, the degree of neurological damage, and the possible presence of spinal deformity, all of which are not under our control. One factor which may be controlled is obesity which makes standing and walking more difficult. A wheelchair existence is the likely result in many children and indeed later many may choose this as an easier way of life. The sensory loss gives rise to the problems of trophic ulceration. Any ill-fitting appliance or footwear may initiate this and the ulcer can be very deep as well as slow and difficult to heal. Trophic ulceration is a much more common problem in the second decade of life than in the first.

5

Cardiovascular Disorders

CONGENITAL HEART DISEASE

Incidence, aetiology and classification

Developmental abnormalities of the cardiovascular system come a close second in terms of frequency to those of the nervous system. Remarkable though surgical advances in the correction of cardiac anomalies have been in recent years, it must be realised that some cases are still inoperable. The main efforts of the paediatric cardiologist and surgeon are now directed towards the malformations which so often cause death during early infancy. The marked fall in the incidence of rheumatic fever in the more prosperous countries has now resulted in congenital heart disease causing more morbidity than rheumatic heart disease.

The aetiological factors in congenital heart disease are only vaguely perceived at the present time. However, they may be divided into four categories: environmental, chromosomal, genetic and multifactorial causes. It is known that certain environmental factors operating in early pregnancy can result in malformations, e.g. rubella embryopathy, heavy consumption of alcohol, maternal diabetes, phenylketonuria and systemic lupus erythematosus. In most cases, however, no specific cause can be detected. Genetic influences seem not to be of great importance, although the relatives of affected children are more often similarly abnormal than would be expected to occur by chance. The risk of a sibling of an index patient also having congenital heart disease is of the order of 1 in 50 against a frequency of about 1 in 100 in the community at large. There are, however, individual families in which the risk is much greater. In addition, cardiac malformations are well recognised to be the frequent accompaniment of several syndromes, e.g. trisomy 21 (atrioventricular septal defect, ventricular septal defect, atrial septal defect, tetralogy of Fallot), trisomy 18 (ventricular septal defect, patent ductus arteriosus, double outlet right ventricle, single umbilical artery), trisomy 13 (ventricular septal defect, atrial septal defect, dextrocardia, single umbilical artery), 45 XO Turner syndrome (coarctation of the aorta, aortic stenosis), Noonan syndrome (pulmonary stenosis, hypertrophic cardiomyopathy), Marfan syndrome (defects of the aorta), polydactyly (ventricular septal defects), triphalangeal thumbs (atrial septal defects in the Holt–Oram syndrome).

No classification of congenital heart disease is entirely satisfactory. It is convenient to subdivide malformations into those which cause central cyanosis due to shunting of blood from the right to the left side of the heart, and those in which cyanosis is absent. The separation is not absolute. Less severe forms of anomalies such as tetralogy of Fallot may not cause cyanosis during the early months of life. Children with anomalies such as patent ductus arteriosus or ventricular septal defect, where there is a left to right shunt, may later develop cyanosis if pulmonary hypertension causes a reversal of the shunt through the defect. In every child with central cyanosis care must be taken to avoid making a diagnosis of congenital heart disease in the rare case of congenital methaemoglobinaemia. The possible combinations and variations of cardiac malformations are so numerous that precise diagnosis frequently demands an extremely high standard of clinical expertise, plus skilled investigations.

Improvements in ultrasound techniques over the last decade have led to a steady increase in the use of these risk-free non-invasive methods and a decrease

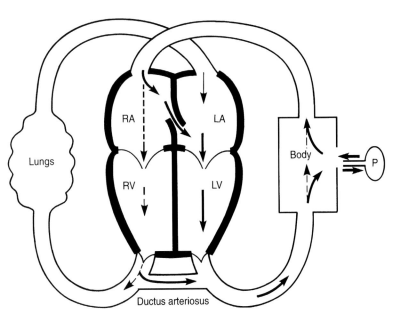

FIGURE 5.1 Fetal circulation. A, atrium; L, left; R, right; V, ventricle; P, placenta.

in the need for diagnostic cardiac catheterisation and angiocardiography which, being invasive, do carry some risk. With two-dimensional echocardiography providing detailed anatomical data and M-mode adding functional information, together with the addition of doppler ultrasound to assess valvular function and colour-flow doppler giving detail of flow direction and velocity, the cardiologist is in most cases able to make an accurate assessment of the nature and severity of complex lesions and plan management. The value of risk-free echocardiography in the sick newborn need not be emphasised.

Ultrasound techniques have not rendered cardiac catheterisation and angiocardiography obsolete and they are sometimes essential. Interestingly, as their need in diagnosis has lessened they are acquiring an increasing role in the interventional manoeuvres which allow some lesions to be treated without recourse to conventional surgery. Balloon atrioseptostomy is long established in the palliation of certain cyanotic lesions, particularly transposition of the great arteries. Balloon dilatation of pulmonary valve stenosis is now the preferred treatment for that lesion and the technique may be applied to aortic valve stenosis and coarctation of the aorta. Devices to occlude the ductus arteriosus at catheterisation are increasingly employed and similar devices to close atrial and ventricular septal defects are being developed. Stenting of stenosed pulmonary and other vessels is now possible by catheter techniques. The full potential for these interventional methods has not yet been achieved in most paediatric cardiac units. However, conventional surgery remains the accepted management for common lesions as well as for complex defects.

CYANOTIC CONGENITAL HEART DISEASE

Transposition of the great arteries

This is the most common type of cyanotic congenital heart disease presenting in the neonatal period. Boys are affected two to three times as frequently as girls. No definite aetiological factors have been identified. Emergency palliative treatment is frequently required to save the infant's life.

Anatomy

The aorta arises from the right ventricle and the pulmonary artery from the left ventricle. The venae cavae and the pulmonary veins drain normally to the right and left atria respectively. Thus the fundamental physiological derangement in complete transposition is that the systemic and pulmonary circulations are separate. This causes few if any problems in the fetus because the entire venous return is normally distributed through the right atrium and ductus venosus (Fig. 5.1). After birth there is a major problem with functional closure of the ductus venosus and arteriosus so that oxygenated pulmonary venous blood is unable to reach the systemic circuit and the systemic venous return cannot reach the lungs for oxygenation (Fig. 5.2). This results in severe systemic arterial desaturation. In transposition of the great arteries, unless there is a coexisting shunt at atrial or ventricular level or through the ductus arteriosus, life cannot be sustained.

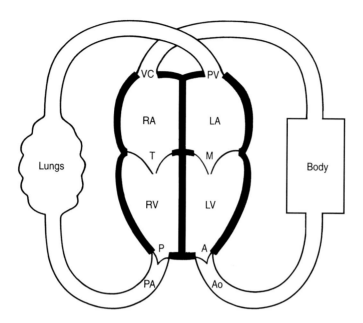

FIGURE 5.2 Postnatal circulation. A, aortic valve; Ao, aorta; LA, left atrium; LV, left ventricle; M, mitral valve; P, pulmonary valve; PA, pulmonary artery; PV, pulmonary vein; RA, right atrium; RV, right ventricle; T, tricuspid valve; VC, vena cava.

Clinical features

Affected infants fail to thrive and are usually markedly cyanosed from birth. Dyspnoea may be present at rest with subcostal recession and it is more obvious during feeds. Finger clubbing may develop early in life. The precordium is seen to be prominent and palpation reveals the notable left parasternal impulse of right ventricular hypertrophy. Thrills are absent. There may be no murmurs but a loud systolic murmur may be heard best at the left lower sternal border. The pulmonary second sound is not remarkable. Cardiac enlargement of gross degree develops rapidly and infants develop congestive cardiac failure. The characteristic cardiac silhouette in postero-anterior radiographs shows an enlarged heart with a narrow supracardiac shadow, rather like an egg lying on its side (Fig. 5.3). Lung vascularity may be increased. The crucial initial investigation in infants with cyanosis is the demonstration by arterial blood gas analysis of systemic arterial hypoxaemia. In those infants without major intercirculatory mixing the arterial P_{O_2} is in the range of 12–25 mmHg (1.6–3.3 kPa) and even with associated ameliorating shunts the P_{O_2} rarely exceeds 40–50 mmHg (5.3–6.6 kPa). Administration of 100% O_2 results in a rise of arterial P_{O_2} but rarely above 180 mmHg (23.9 kPa).

The electrocardiogram shows right axis deviation with right ventricular or biventricular hypertrophy, and there may be a P pulmonale. Real-time echocardiography will reveal the aorta arising from the right ventricle and the pulmonary artery from the left. Cardiac catheterisation will reveal that the catheter leaves the right ventricle by the aorta. The pulmonary artery blood has an oxygen concentration above that in the aorta. Various other shunts can be demonstrated according to their site.

Prognosis

Most infants go into cardiac failure in the early months of life with increasing dyspnoea, cyanosis, cardiomegaly and hepatomegaly. This is frequently precipitated by intercurrent respiratory infection. If untreated, 90% of children with complete transposition die by 1 year of age and 95% by 5 years of age.

Treatment

Balloon atrial septostomy

The introduction of the Rashkind balloon catheter has considerably lowered the early mortality rate in this condition. A catheter is passed through the foramen ovale into the left atrium and its balloon distended with fluid to 2–4 ml capacity. It is then withdrawn against the atrial septum until resistance is felt whenever it is tugged back sharply towards the IVC, thus tearing the septum and creating an atrial septal defect. This technique usually results in a considerable improvement of the hypoxia and mixed respiratory metabolic acidosis from which these infants suffer and most survive long enough to undergo more radical surgery. It is, however, essential to perform the procedure as early in life as possible so that diagnostic echocardiography has become an emergency procedure in deeply cyanosed newborn infants.

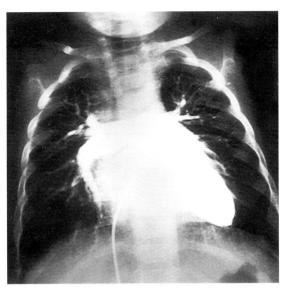
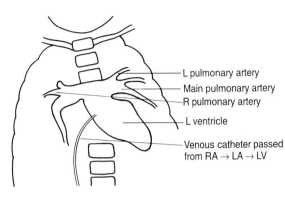

L pulmonary artery
Main pulmonary artery
R pulmonary artery
L ventricle
Venous catheter passed from RA → LA → LV

FIGURE 5.3 Transposition of great arteries. LV angiogram. LA, left atrium; LV, left ventricle; RA, right atrium.

Definitive surgical treatment

When possible, radical surgery is carried out promptly and the favoured operation is anatomical correction by switching the aorta with the coronary artery's origins to the left ventricle and the main pulmonary artery to the right ventricle. For this to succeed it has to be done before pulmonary pressure falls so that the left ventricle continues to sustain the systemic circulation at the necessary pressure. The operation is generally done in the neonatal period.

When arterial switch is not possible the physiological correction would be performed using the Mustard or Senning techniques both of which involve creating a baffle between the atria which redirects the venous returns appropriately: the venae caval flow across to the mitral valve and hence from the left ventricle to the pulmonary artery, the pulmonary venous return across the tricuspid valve and hence from the right ventricle to the aorta.

Total anomalous pulmonary venous drainage

Anatomy

All the pulmonary veins, as well as the venae cavae, enter the right atrium. There must, of course, be an atrial septal defect for life to continue at all. There are several possible anatomical variations. Most commonly the pulmonary veins form a common vessel which empties into a persisting left superior vena cava, less often into the right superior vena cava. The pulmonary veins may also unite to form a common trunk which drains directly into the right atrium or into the coronary sinus. Rarely, the pulmonary veins drain beneath the diaphragm into the inferior vena cava or even into the portal vein.

Clinical features

These infants fail to thrive, are cyanotic, and become dyspnoeic on slight exertion. They are extremely prone to respiratory infections. Cardiac pulsation is forceful over the left parasternal area, that is, over the right ventricle and its outflow tract. The precordium may bulge. Auscultation often reveals triple or quadruple rhythm and there is usually a blowing systolic murmur. The electrocardiograph shows right axis deviation, severe right ventricular hypertrophy and a P pulmonale. Radiographs show right atrial and right ventricular enlargement with pleionaemic lungs. In the common type of anomaly with a persisting left superior vena cava the supracardiac shadow is very broad, giving rise to the so-called "cottage-loaf", "figure-of-eight" or "snowman" heart (Fig. 5.4). Echocardiography will usually confirm the diagnosis. Cardiac catheterisation reveals the same oxygen concentration in the right atrium, right ventricle, pulmonary artery and femoral artery; the pressures in the right ventricle and pulmonary artery are above normal. The diagnosis can also be confirmed by selective angiocardiography when opaque medium is injected into the pulmonary artery and pulmonary venous return to the right atrium is demonstrated (Fig. 5.5)

Prognosis

Most affected infants develop right heart failure early with progressive dyspnoea, cardiomegaly and hepatomegaly.

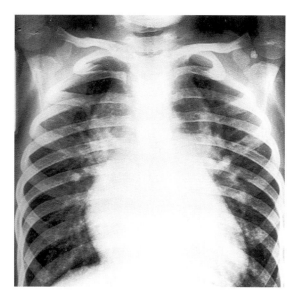

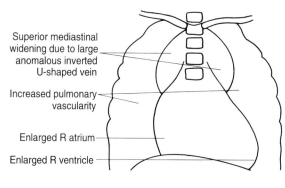

Superior mediastinal widening due to large anomalous inverted U-shaped vein

Increased pulmonary vascularity

Enlarged R atrium

Enlarged R ventricle

FIGURE 5.4 Chest X-ray, total anomalous pulmonary venous drainage.

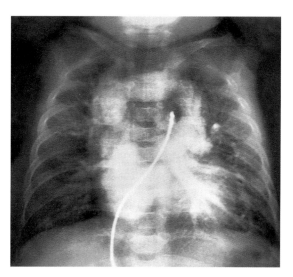

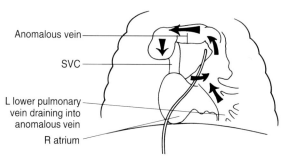

Anomalous vein

SVC

L lower pulmonary vein draining into anomalous vein

R atrium

FIGURE 5.5 Total anomalous pulmonary venous drainage, angiogram into the main pulmonary artery. SVC, superior vena cava.

Treatment

The most common type of operation is based upon anastomosis of the common pulmonary venous trunk to the back of the left atrium. The atrial septal defect is closed and the connection with the right atrium, vena cava or coronary sinus is obliterated. After the age of 1 year this type of correction carries a low mortality and gives good results, but when surgery has to be undertaken as an emergency in the newborn a higher mortality must be expected.

Tetralogy of Fallot

This is the most common type of cyanotic congenital heart disease in children over the age of 1 year. Males and females are equally affected. As with many congenital cardiac anomalies, the precise aetiology is unknown.

Anatomy

The classical tetrad consists of pulmonary stenosis (rarely atresia), ventricular septal defect with right to

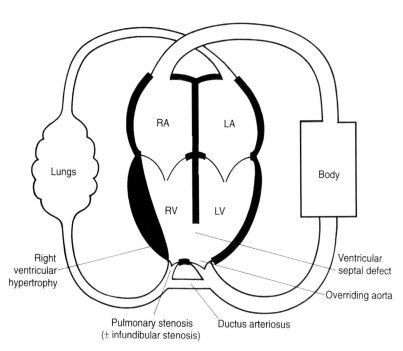

FIGURE 5.6 Tetralogy of Fallot. LA, left atrium; LV, left ventricle; RA, right atrium; RV, right ventricle.

Lungs

RA

LA

Body

RV

LV

Right ventricular hypertrophy

Ventricular septal defect

Overriding aorta

Pulmonary stenosis (± infundibular stenosis)

Ductus arteriosus

left shunt, dextroposition (or rightward deviation) of the aorta which receives blood from both ventricles, and right ventricular hypertrophy (Fig. 5.6). There are many variations depending upon the degree and type of pulmonary stenosis, the size of the ventricular septal defect and the degree of overriding of the aorta. In most instances the pulmonary stenosis is infundibular, there being a long, narrow separate infundibular chamber; in others it is a valvular stenosis. In some cases there is a right-sided aortic arch, a matter of importance to the thoracic surgeon.

Clinical features

Clinical presentation is dominated by the degree of right ventricular outflow tract obstruction. Cyanosis may be marked from early childhood, although it is often absent in the first few months of life. It may be quite slight in less severely disabled children. Cyanosis is associated with stunting of growth, clubbing of the fingers and polycythaemia. Affected children usually show marked breathlessness on exertion and take frequent rests in a very characteristic squatting position. The most severely affected infants with severe pulmonary stenosis have episodes of deep cyanosis, dyspnoea, unconsciousness and convulsions. These hypercyanotic attacks occur typically on waking in the morning but may be precipitated by crying, defaecation, eating, exercise and hot weather. These are accompanied by marked metabolic and respiratory acidosis due to the severe degree of hypoxia. It has been postulated that these spells are due to infundibular spasm or shutdown. Also it has been demonstrated that some of the

haemodynamic consequences of an increase in infundibular stenosis can be alleviated by a beta-adrenergic blocking agent. The heart is not enlarged and the apex beat may be difficult to locate. Right ventricular pulsation, however, can be readily felt over the left parasternal area where there is often a systolic thrill. In most cases a loud systolic murmur is heard down the left sternal border but this may be slight or absent when pulmonary stenosis is severe. The second pulmonary sound is often quiet and may be single. The characteristic radiographic appearances (Fig. 5.7) show a small heart with concavity in the region of the pulmonary artery and with the apex raised above the left diaphragm (*coeur en sabot*). The lungs are oligaemic due to diminished pulmonary blood flow. The electrocardiogram shows marked right axis deviation and right ventricular hypertrophy.

Echocardiography will confirm the diagnosis (Fig. 5.8). Cardiac catheterisation reveals a high right ventricular pressure and the presence of an infundibular chamber or a valvar stenosis can be demonstrated. The catheter may leave the right ventricle through the overriding aorta. Angiocardiography shows simultaneous filling of the pulmonary artery and the aorta. It is also associated with other anomalies such as the VACTERL anomalies.

Prognosis

Tetralogy of Fallot is not compatible with long life and the child's exercise capacity becomes progressively more limited. Indeed, only half the children with this anomaly survive their third birthday

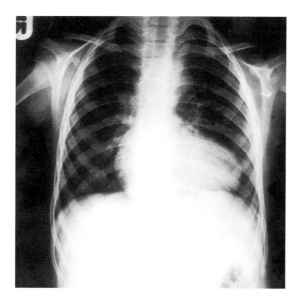

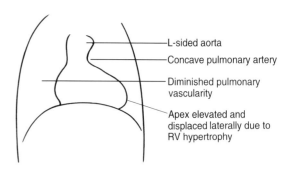

L-sided aorta

Concave pulmonary artery

Diminished pulmonary vascularity

Apex elevated and displaced laterally due to RV hypertrophy

FIGURE 5.7 Chest X-ray, tetralogy of Fallot. RV, right ventricle.

without surgical intervention. Severely affected infants who have hypoxic episodes require early operation to ensure survival. There is a tendency to the development of brain abscess in this disease especially after a Blalock–Taussig shunt. It often follows a respiratory infection but the mechanism of its production is not understood. It should be suspected whenever an affected child develops neurological manifestations. These may also be due to severe anoxia or thrombosis, e.g. sudden hemiplegia. Their investigation necessitates lumbar puncture, computed axial tomography (CAT scan) or investigation by nuclear magnetic resonance (NMR) in addition to electroencephalography.

Treatment

The asymptomatic child with tetralogy of Fallot requires surgical correction any time towards the end of the first year of life. As regards the treatment of hypercyanotic spells, the drug of choice during an attack is a beta-adrenergic blocking agent such as propranolol. Severely cyanotic infants and children can be dramatically improved by means of some type of anastomosis between the systemic and pulmonary arteries which will greatly augment blood flow through the lungs. A major decision in the symptomatic patient is whether to palliate or whether to attempt total correction. The issue is still unresolved, since many surgeons obtain excellent results when performing primary correction in infancy in all but those with severely hypoplastic pulmonary arteries. The palliative operation which has been most frequently employed is the Blalock–Taussig shunt between the end of the ipsilat-

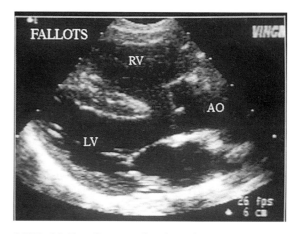

FIGURE 5.8 Two-dimensional echocardiogram (long axis view) from a child with tetralogy of Fallot. The right ventricle (RV) and left ventricle (LV) are separated by the ventricular septum. The aorta (AO) and aortic cusps can be seen to override the ventricular septum.

eral subclavian artery and the side of the pulmonary artery. This operation relieves the cyanosis and encourages growth of the pulmonary artery as the child reaches the stage when radical corrective surgery may be considered.

Complete correction of all the defects by open heart surgery using heart–lung bypass may be performed during the second year of life or even earlier as the initial procedure, or it may follow a previous shunt operation. The mortality rate is now under 10% in those cases of tetralogy of Fallot where the pulmonary arteries are well developed. In

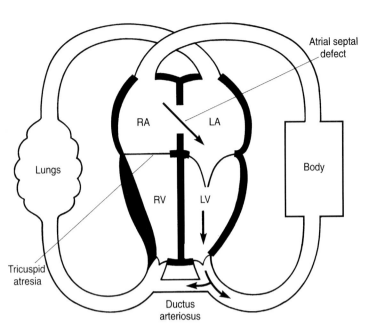

FIGURE 5.9 Tricuspid atresia. LA, left atrium; LV, left ventricle; RA, right atrium; RV, right ventricle.

cases where the pulmonary trunk is hypoplastic and requires widening by means of a pericardial patch, the mortality is considerably greater and some surgeons are content to leave the patient with a palliative shunt. In major centres nowadays 90–95% of patients can be expected to survive corrective surgery and the same percentages reach adult life.

Tricuspid atresia

This is a relatively rare condition but it must be considered in the differential diagnosis of every child with cyanotic congenital heart disease. There is little sex difference in the incidence.

Anatomy

The basic defect is the absence of communication between the right atrium and the right ventricle, so that all blood entering the right atrium from the venae cavae must cross an atrial septal defect to mix in the left atrium with blood from the pulmonary veins (Fig. 5.9). There are several variations. Most often there is a patent ductus arteriosus which diverts some of the blood entering the aorta from the left ventricle into the lungs. In some cases there is a ventricular septal defect allowing some blood from the left ventricle to enter the undeveloped right ventricle; in these cases the great vessels are transposed and there is then always a large ventricular septal defect. The pulmonary valve which, in such cases, forms the exit from the left ventricle may or may not be narrowed. Thus in all cases of tricuspid atresia there is complete systemic and pulmonary

venous admixture. If there is substantial pulmonary blood flow cyanosis may be slight.

Clinical features

As a rule cyanosis is marked from birth with dyspnoea on feeding, failure to thrive and early clubbing of the digits. Anoxic attacks of unconsciousness may occur. The heart is frequently but little enlarged and the pulsation often felt in the left parasternal region arises from the left ventricle. There is a loud systolic murmur at the left sternal border. The second pulmonary sound may be quiet and single. The cardiac contour on radiographs may simulate that seen in tetralogy of Fallot, but oblique films will reveal underdevelopment of the right ventricle. An important diagnostic clue is to be found in the electrocardiogram which shows left axis deviation and left ventricular hypertrophy. This may be associated with a P pulmonale due to high pressure in the right atrium. Echocardiography will confirm the diagnosis.

Prognosis

The overall prognosis without treatment for patients with tricuspid atresia is poor. Few affected infants survive for more than 1 year. Cardiac failure occurs with progressive dyspnoea, hepatomegaly and oedema.

Treatment

Surgical operations devised for tricuspid atresia have all had the objective of improving pulmonary blood

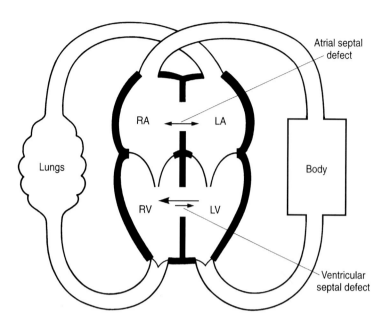

FIGURE 5.10 Septal defects. LA, left atrium; LV, left ventricle; RA, right atrium; RV, right ventricle.

flow. None is very successful. Arterial shunts such as the Blalock–Taussig procedure are sometimes combined with enlargement of the atrial septal defect. In the Glenn operation the superior vena cava is anastomosed to the right pulmonary artery.

A more definitive surgical approach is the Fontan procedure in which the right atrium acts as a pumping chamber (unidirectional) by means of closure of the atrial septal defect and the insertion of a conduit leading from the atrium to the pulmonary arteries.

Other types of cyanotic congenital heart disease

These are numerous although each occurs infrequently. In *single ventricle* the child is underdeveloped and unduly dyspnoeic. Cyanosis is variable in degree. Cardiomegaly is gross. A systolic thrill and murmur are found, sometimes also a mid-diastolic murmur. The electrocardiogram may show a left ventricular hypertrophy pattern. This difficult diagnosis has been rendered easier by echocardiography which reveals only one A-V valve, one large ventricular chamber and one diminutive one. In *persistent truncus arteriosus* a common arterial trunk drains both ventricles thus giving origin to the systemic, pulmonary and coronary circulations. Pulmonary arteries may arise from the common truncus or the blood flow to the lungs may depend entirely on the bronchial arteries, so that the degree of oxygen unsaturation is very variable. There may also be pulmonary hypertension in some patients. Therefore, the presenting clinical features are largely dependent on the volume of pulmonary blood flow and the presence or absence of associated significant truncal valve insufficiency. Thus, cyanosis may be severe or slight. Cardiomegaly is marked. A systolic or continuous murmur may be found. The second pulmonary sound is single. The chest X-ray may show absence of a pulmonary conus but a large aortic shadow which can be seen by echocardiography to override the ventricular septum. The electrocardiogram shows left ventricular or biventricular hypertrophy. Precise diagnosis of these anomalies is often impossible without cardiac catheterisation or angiocardiography although the use of cross-sectional sector echocardiography and colour doppler has greatly increased the ability to make the diagnosis of truncus noninvasively.

In the *Ebstein malformation* the posterior and septal cusps of the tricuspid valve arise from the wall of the right ventricle near the apex so that part of the right ventricle is, in fact, incorporated within the right atrium. There is, in addition, tricuspid incompetence. It is exceedingly rare. In severe cases symptoms occur in the first months of life. The child is dyspnoeic on exertion, cyanosed to a variable degree and poorly developed. Death ultimately takes place from right heart failure. On examination of the child the neck veins are distended. Auscultation reveals triple or quadruple rhythm and there may be both presystolic and soft systolic murmurs. The radiograph shows a huge atrium and the lung fields are often oligaemic. The electrocardiogram shows a large notched P wave and some degree of right bundle branch block. These patients are subject to atrial extrasystoles and to attacks of paroxysmal tachycardia. Cardiac catheterisation is dangerous but echocardiography will

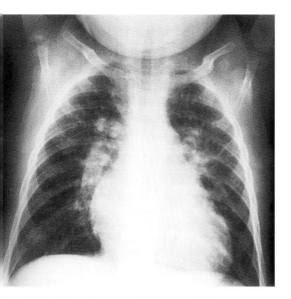

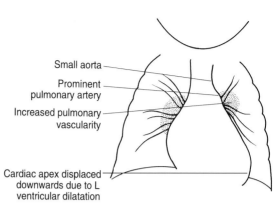

Small aorta
Prominent pulmonary artery
Increased pulmonary vascularity
Cardiac apex displaced downwards due to L ventricular dilatation

FIGURE 5.11 Chest X-ray, ventricular septal defect.

establish the diagnosis. There is no effective medical treatment for the malformation, although patients suffering symptomatic arrhythmias should benefit from appropriate drug therapy. Surgery provides the only possibility of radically ameliorating the haemodynamic problems. As with other cyanotic malformations the spectrum of severity varies and surgical intervention may not be required for many years.

ACYANOTIC CONGENITAL HEART DISEASE WITH LEFT TO RIGHT SHUNTS

Ventricular septal defect

Defects in the interventricular septum can occur as isolated anomalies or in association with many other defects. Undoubtedly isolated ventricular septal defect is the commonest form of congenital heart disease (Fig. 5.10). The pathophysiology of ventricular septal defect is determined by the size of the defect and the state of the pulmonary vascular resistance. These two features govern the direction and magnitude of flow through the defect, and thus the clinical features and symptomatology. The site of the defect within the septum has little influence; the size of the defect is dominant. The defect may be small in size and relatively benign or large and associated with a reduction in life expectancy. When the ventricular defect is large, pressures in the systemic and pulmonary circuits remain equal (as in the normal fetus) or nearly equal. This results in a very high pulmonary blood flow (pleionaemic lungs) and in some cases in the develop-

ment of pulmonary vascular obstruction. In babies with large ventricular septal defects the sudden drop in pulmonary vascular resistance which follows the first few breaths of life in the normal newborn is less marked. Subsequently, in some infants, the normal involution of the muscular media of the fetal-type pulmonary arterioles fails to occur to any extent. As life goes on the medial and intimal changes in these arterioles may increase progressively with increasing pulmonary vascular obstruction until the left to right shunt is reversed due to severe pulmonary hypertension (Eisenmenger syndrome). The other serious complication of large ventricular septal defects is congestive cardiac failure which usually occurs within the first 6 months of life, but almost never in the early neonatal period. Infective endocarditis may affect small as well as large ventricular septal defects but this is not a very common complication during childhood. Surgical closure of defects does not eliminate the chance of contracting the infection. The risk can be minimised by the use of antibiotic prophylaxis before dental extractions or tonsillectomy.

Clinical features

Ventricular septal defects are rarely clinically detectable at birth, since it takes a few weeks for the pulmonary vascular resistance to fall from the high intrauterine levels. Thus it is rare for a ventricular septal defect to be diagnosed at routine postnatal examination on the first day of life.

Small ventricular septal defects

This child is symptomless and normally developed. The heart is normal in size and minimally enlarged.

A palpable systolic thrill in the left parasternal area is associated with a harsh systolic murmur maximal at the fourth left interspace. The electrocardiogram is normal or shows slight left ventricular preponderance. Most patients seem to remain trouble-free for many years.

Large ventricular septal defects without pulmonary hypertension

The child is often underdeveloped and sooner or later develops undue dyspnoea on exertion. There is often marked susceptibility to respiratory infections. The heart is enlarged with a forceful apex beat. A systolic thrill and loud pansystolic murmur are maximal at the left sternal border at the level of the fourth interspace. Radiographs show left or biventricular enlargement and pleionaemic lungs (Fig. 5.11). The electrocardiogram shows left ventricular hypertrophy. Cardiac catheterisation reveals a higher concentration of oxygen in the blood in the right ventricle than in the right atrium, and the catheter may be induced to traverse the septal defect to enter the left ventricle. In some cases the pressures in the right ventricle and pulmonary artery may be elevated due to the large volume of blood being shunted across the defect from the powerful left ventricle. However, in this "dynamic" type of pulmonary hypertension there is no true pulmonary vascular obstruction. Until recently the definitive diagnosis of isolated ventricular septal defect depended upon cardiac catheterisation and angiocardiography. Now the diagnosis can be made with certainty in the majority of cases using cross-sectional echocardiography and colour doppler. Therefore, echocardiography is invaluable in differentiating isolated defects from more complex anomalies and should be performed in all symptomatic infants suspected to have ventricular septal defect.

Large ventricular septal defects with peripheral pulmonary hypertension (Eisenmenger syndrome)

In this type of case symptoms are usually present from early infancy with failure to thrive, dyspnoea on exertion such as feeding, and repeated respiratory infections. When the pulmonary hypertension is severe, and especially if there is some overriding of the aorta, the right to left shunt so occasioned may cause constant or intermittent cyanosis to be present. Cardiomegaly may not be marked but palpation reveals not only a powerful apical thrust but excessive pulsation over the right ventricle and its outflow tract in the left parasternal area. There is no thrill and any systolic murmur is short. The second heart sound at the pulmonary area is loud and booming and usually single. Radiographs confirm the presence of enlargement of the main pulmonary artery and hilar branches with translucent peripheral lung fields. The electrocardiogram indicates biventricular hypertrophy

or right ventricular hypertrophy and there may be tall P waves due to enlargement of both atria. Cardiac catheter studies will show high pressures in the right ventricle and in the pulmonary arteries.

Prognosis

The natural history of ventricular septal defects has been considerably clarified in recent years and it is now clear how variable may be the outcome of such lesions. The majority of children with isolated ventricular septal defects live normal lives both in terms of duration and quality. Approximately 50–60% close spontaneously. This usually happens during the first 5 years of life but spontaneous closure can occur at any age. Infants with large defects and dynamic pulmonary hypertension may die during the first 6 months of life in congestive cardiac failure with hepatomegaly, pulmonary oedema and crepitations or from intercurrent bronchopneumonia. In other cases, the infant who was in congestive cardiac failure due to a large septal defect with torrential pulmonary blood flow survives only to develop later progressive pulmonary vascular obstruction. He may then become an adult with severe cyanosis, polycythaemia and dyspnoea. Another outcome in some cases of large ventricular septal defects is the development in time of acquired infundibular stenosis due to narrowing of the right ventricular outflow tract by muscular hypertrophy. By the second or third decade the left to right shunt is replaced by a right to left shunt due to severe subvalvular pulmonary stenosis and the clinical picture becomes indistinguishable from that of tetralogy of Fallot. Rarely, the development of infundibular obstruction is associated with spontaneous closure of the ventricular septal defect and the picture alters radically to that of an isolated pulmonary stenosis. Yet another unfavourable development in some cases of ventricular septal defect is prolapse of the right coronary aortic cusp into the left ventricle with consequent aortic regurgitation. This most commonly occurs towards the end of the first decade. At first a faint, high-frequency diastolic murmur appears in addition to the systolic murmur of the ventricular septal defect. In the course of time the classical signs of aortic regurgitation replace those of the septal defect. This complication greatly worsens the prognosis and death may ensue either from congestive cardiac failure or infective endocarditis. It is recommended that surgical treatment be offered as soon as significant aortic regurgitation is recognised.

Treatment

When a child presents in early infancy the outcome is always in doubt. Small ventricular defects should be left alone and those patients should be encouraged

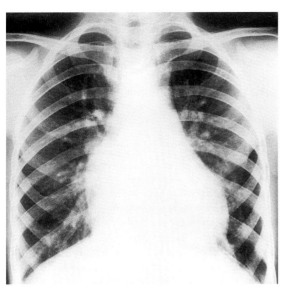

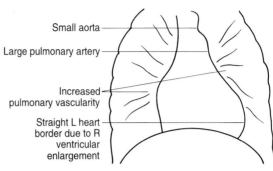

Small aorta
Large pulmonary artery
Increased pulmonary vascularity
Straight L heart border due to R ventricular enlargement

FIGURE 5.12 Chest X-ray, atrial septal defect.

to undertake full physical activities in all respects. These are children with normal pulmonary arterial pressures. Asymptomatic infants should be closely followed with echocardiographic assessment of the anatomy and doppler assessment of intracardiac pressures. Those remaining asymptomatic with no signs suggesting pulmonary hypertension require no treatment. They should take no precautions other than prophylactic measures against infective endocarditis. When the defect is large with high pulmonary blood flow and pressure it should be closed, although the indications for operation vary in different centres. In young infants with severe pulmonary hypertension closure of the defect is imperative to prevent irreversible pulmonary vascular disease. The final decisions in these difficult cases should be taken by a cardiac team containing both physicians and surgeons who have specialised in this field of paediatric medicine and surgery. It is rare for surgery to be required for an isolated defect after the age of 1 year. Occasional patients who have escaped detection with a large left to right shunt and cardiomegaly may need surgical closure in childhood.

Atrial septal defect

Traditionally atrial septal defects are divided into "primum" and "secundum" types. The more common is a failure of closure of the ostium secundum, which is in the upper part of the interatrial septum. This defect is not uncommonly associated with partial anomalous pulmonary venous drainage so that one or both veins from the right lung enter the right atrium. Much less common, but more

serious and arising at an earlier stage of embryogenesis, is failure of closure of the ostium primum in the lower part of the septum. The base of this defect commonly involves the mitral and tricuspid valves so that one or both may be rendered incompetent. Furthermore, there is a high ventricular septal defect in many of these cases (atrioventricular septal defect)

Clinical features

Ostium secundum defect

These children are usually symptomless save for undue susceptibility to respiratory infection. Girls are more often affected than boys and they frequently have a somewhat characteristic slender asthenic body build. The sternum may be unduly prominent with accompanying Harrison grooves. The heart varies in size from normal to very large but right ventricular pulsation is excessive over the left parasternal area. A soft systolic murmur is best heard at the second or third left interspace and the second pulmonary heart sound is wide and persistently split. A mid-diastolic murmur may be heard at the tricuspid area when the atrial septal defect is large with a greatly excessive pulmonary blood flow. The X-ray shows a large pulmonary conus and pleionaemic lungs (Fig. 5.12). Echocardiography is usually diagnostic (Fig. 5.13).

The electrocardiogram shows partial right bundle branch block (RsR pattern). There may be prolongation of the P-R interval or right ventricular hypertrophy. An increased oxygen concentration is demonstrable in the right atrium during cardiac catheterisation; a level about 95% suggests the presence of an anomalous pulmonary vein which has,

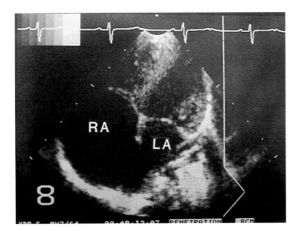

FIGURE 5.13 Two-dimensional echocardiogram from a child with an ostium secundum ASD. The plane is adjusted to give an optimal image of the atrial septum separating the right atrium (RA) and the left atrium (LA). The ASD appears as a gap in the atrial septum.

in fact, been entered by the catheter from the right atrium. The catheter frequently crosses the atrial septal defect into the left atrium, but this can happen in a normal heart through the foramen ovale and is not by itself a significant occurrence. The precise site of the atrial septal defect can be determined by angiocardiography although this information is not essential before operation.

Ostium primum defect (atrioventricular septal defect)

The child in this situation usually fails to grow normally from infancy. There may be episodes of cardiac failure and respiratory infections are often severe. Cardiomegaly is associated not only with a powerful right ventricular thrust in the left parasternal area, but also with a displaced heaving apex beat due to left ventricular hypertrophy. When there is mitral regurgitation a pansystolic murmur is heard at the apex and propagated into the axilla. A palpable systolic thrill is usually detected. There may be an apical mid-diastolic murmur. The pulmonary second sound is loud and widely split. The most characteristic electrocardiographic changes are left axis deviation, partial right bundle branch block and right ventricular hypertrophy. When mitral regurgitation is marked there may be evidence of hypertrophy of the left or both ventricles. Heart block may be present when there is a complete atrioventricular septal defect. The diagnosis can be confirmed by echocardiography.

Prognosis

In ostium secundum defects of large size, increasing cardiomegaly is associated with increasing limitation of exercise tolerance. This can be aggravated by the late development of peripheral pulmonary vascular obstruction. An increased susceptibility to rheumatic fever may lead to superimposed mitral stenosis (Lutembacher syndrome). Patients with smaller defects may, however, live to a good age. In ostium primum defects the expectation of life is considerably curtailed.

Treatment

The timing of elective surgery does not seem to be crucial, but surgical repair between 4 and 6 years of age is recommended. Earlier surgical closure of ostium secundum defects is indicated in every case in which there is cardiac enlargement, growth failure or congestive heart failure. The mortality rate is now very low. The repair of ostium primum defects always necessitaties the use of heart–lung bypass. On the whole, an atrial septal defect is an important congenital heart disorder because it is relatively common and because its surgical treatment is so successful. Children born with this cardiac malformation when suitably treated should be able to enjoy a normal life expectancy free from cardiovascular morbidity.

Patent ductus arteriosus

Isolated patent ductus arteriosus results in shunting of blood from one side of the circulation to the other (Fig. 5.14). The shunt volume depends on the length and internal diameter of the duct and on the systemic and pulmonary vascular resistances. As pulmonary resistance is usually much lower than systemic, the blood flow is from the aorta through the ductus to the pulmonary artery, and the lungs are pleionaemic. In a minority of cases where the ductus is very wide, the pulmonary and right ventricular systolic pressures may be so elevated as to approach systemic levels with the development of pulmonary vascular obstruction. This entirely alters the picture, and, indeed, in severe cases the blood flow may be right to left through the ductus with consequent cyanosis (Eisenmenger syndrome). This type of peripheral pulmonary vascular obstruction must be distinguished from the "dynamic" pulmonary hypertension commonly found in the larger pulmonary arteries in cases of patent ductus arteriosus and due only to the torrential flow of blood reaching them from the aorta. The former situation is irreversible whereas "dynamic" pulmonary hypertension can be completely relieved by simple closure of the ductus.

Clinical features

In the vast majority of cases patent ductus arteriosus produces no cardiac symptoms during childhood. The

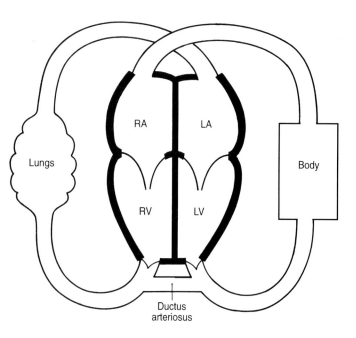

FIGURE 5.14 Patent ductus arteriosus. LA, left atrium; LV, left ventricle; RA, right atrium; RV, right ventricle.

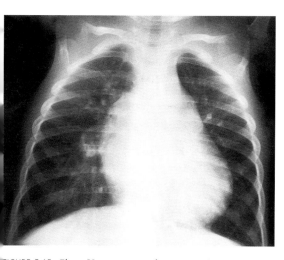

FIGURE 5.15 Chest X ray, patent ductus arteriosus.

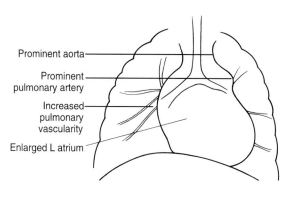

special problems associated with patent ductus arteriosus in the preterm infant with the respiratory distress syndrome have already been considered in Chapter 1. However, even the child without symptoms is frequently rather underdeveloped for his age, and the dramatic growth spurt and increase in physical activity which is sometimes seen after successful closure of the ductus reveal in retrospect a degree of previous incapacity. The diagnostic physical sign is a continuous (machinery) murmur, loudest during systole but extending into diastole, maximal at the pulmonary area and well conducted under the left clavicle. It may be associated with a systolic thrill at the second left interspace. The murmur is caused by turbulent flow through the ductus itself. The pulses are collapsing in type due to a large pulse pressure. The heart may or may not be enlarged. X-ray will reveal prominence of the main pulmonary artery with increased lung vascularity. There may also be enlargement of the left ventricle (Fig. 5.15). The electrocardiogram is often normal but may show some left ventricular preponderance. In young infants the diastolic component of the murmur is not always audible.

When the patent ductus is complicated by peripheral pulmonary hypertension a vastly different clinical picture presents itself. The child is markedly underdeveloped, highly susceptible to respiratory infections and unduly breathless on exertion. Cardiomegaly is marked with a very large pulmonary artery and the presence of combined ventricular hypertrophy can be demonstrated on radiographs, echocardiograms and electrocardiograms. The lung roots show severe engorgement but the periphery of the lung fields on radiographs are characteristically clear and translucent. The typical continuous murmur is no longer audible, being replaced by foreshortened systolic murmur. The second pulmonary sound, which tends to be obscured in a typical case of patent ductus, is now loud and booming. A systolic thrill is not always palpable. A large pulse pressure with collapsing pulses are still the rule. When the shunt is reversed from right to left the presence of cyanosis makes differentiation from transposition of the great vessels with patent ductus a difficult matter without echocardiography.

Most cardiologists would not consider cardiac catheterisation a necessary investigation for patients with typical clinical findings of a patent ductus arteriosus. However, cross-sectional echocardiography will help rule out other structural malformations.

Differential diagnosis

Other causes of continuous murmur may create confusion. A congenital aortopulmonary fenestration will be differentiated from patent ductus by ultrasound examination. More typical, the communication is large and does not cause a continuous murmur. A venous hum is usually best heard in the supraclavicular fossae. When it is loud it may be transmitted below the clavicle. Hence it may be misdiagnosed as being from a patent ductus arteriosus. The murmur of a venous hum varies with position whereas that of the patent ductus is constant.

Prognosis

Even with a simple patent ductus arteriosus cardiac enlargement sooner or later develops. Death takes place from cardiac failure or infective endocarditis before middle age. When pulmonary hypertension complicates the picture, death is likely to occur in infancy or early childhood from cardiac failure or pneumonia.

Treatment

Every case of uncomplicated patent ductus arteriosus should be treated. Most centres still perform surgical ligation but the technique of occlusion by interventional cardiac catheterisation will be increasingly used. Recanalisation of the duct is rare with modern surgical techniques. Closure is best performed before schooling begins. It may have to be carried out in infancy if cardiac failure, failure to thrive or signifi-

cant cardiac enlargement form part of the picture. The presence of "dynamic" hypertension in the larger pulmonary arteries is a clear indication for operation. On the other hand, the presence of pulmonary vascular obstruction makes closure hazardous and it may fail to help the patient. Against this must be set the fact that without closure the patient's expectation of life is very short and it has been our practice in such cases to advise this in spite of the risks involved unless cyanosis due to a right to left shunt is already established.

ACYANOTIC CONGENITAL HEART DISEASE WITHOUT SHUNTS

Pulmonary stenosis

This defect occurring alone is usually due to fusion or malformation of the semilunar cusps. Infundibular stenosis in which there is a narrow infundibular chamber between the valve and the right ventricular cavity may also occur alone, but is more often associated with other anomalies (see tetralogy of Fallot). Fixed stenosis of the infundibulum coexisting with valvar stenosis is rare. Uncomplicated pulmonary stenosis is a common condition.

Clinical features

Most affected children are symptomless and they are often well developed with somewhat highly coloured cheeks and lips. Slight cyanosis is seen only in a few very severe cases. Palpation reveals a powerful right ventricular thrust over the left parasternal area and a systolic thrill at the second left interspace. At this area there is a harsh systolic murmur of ejection type which is conducted into the neck, under the left clavicle and through to the back. The second pulmonary sound is quiet and usually single because the low pressure in the pulmonary artery makes the valve closure inaudible. Radiographs reveal post-stenotic dilatation of the pulmonary artery and translucent oligaemic lung fields. The electrocardiogram shows right ventricular hypertrophy; there may be P pulmonale and partial right bundle-branch block. Cardiac catheterisation demonstrates a high right ventricular pressure, with a steep pressure gradient between the ventricle and the pulmonary artery. Withdrawal tracings differentiate clearly between valvular and infundibular stenosis. Both cross-sectional and M-mode echocardiography techniques may appear normal in the presence of mild stenosis. If the valve is thickened it should be detected on cross-sectional examination. Doppler studies will provide a satisfactory assessment of the gradient across the stenosed valve.

Prognosis

Mild degrees of pulmonary stenosis are compatible with long life, but the more severe cases end in cardiac failure before middle age. Apart from the risk of infective endocarditis, they do not die prematurely. Routine prophylaxis is therefore indicated throughout life in all patients, irrespective of the site or severity of stenosis.

Treatment

The accepted treatment for isolated pulmonary valve stenosis nowadays is balloon valvoplasty performed at catheterisation and this technique has a substantial success rate.

Surgical correction under direct vision should be advised in those cases where the pressure gradient across the pulmonary valve is more than 40 mmHg, when balloon valvoplasty fails. The mortality rate is now extremely low.

Aortic stenosis

In most cases there is fusion of the cusps of the aortic valve. Less commonly there is a fibrous ring round the left ventricular outflow tract (subaortic stenosis). In rare instances the stenosis is supravalvar with a discrete ring of narrowing of the aorta. This defect has sometimes been associated with single or multiple constrictions along the major branches of the pulmonary artery. In some of the cases with supra-aortic stenosis there has also been present a characteristic facies, mental retardation, an association with the severe form of idiopathic hypercalcaemia of infancy and this syndrome is called the William syndrome. Isolated aortic valve stenosis is always congenital. When seen in association with a mitral lesion it may be either congenital or rheumatic. A chromosomal abnormality (deletion chromosome 7 for the elastin gene) has recently been identified in some instances of this syndrome.

Clinical features

This defect is more common in boys. Most are symptomless but in a few anginal pain develops on effort. The danger of sudden death during exertion is well known although it is, in fact, an uncommon event. Affected children are usually well grown. The maximal cardiac impulse is at the apex although the heart is not commonly enlarged. A systolic thrill is palpable at the second right interspace and also along the carotid arteries and in the suprasternal notch. A harsh systolic murmur is best heard in the aortic area and there may be a short soft diastolic murmur. The pulse is anacrotic and of small volume. The pulse

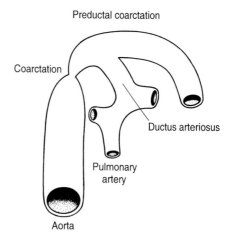

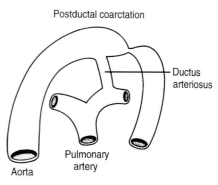

FIGURE 5.16 Pre- and postductal coarctation of the aorta.

pressure is low. The heart may appear quite normal in radiographs. The electrocardiogram often shows left ventricular hypertrophy in these cases. The pressure gradient across the aortic valve can be assessed by doppler ultrasound and confirmed by left heart catheterisation when operation is considered to be a possibility. The non-invasive technique is free of risk and may be repeated at intervals.

Treatment

Most children with aortic stenosis are likely to live well into middle age. This makes an operation which may leave the patient with the more severe disability of aortic regurgitation hazardous. Surgery is probably only to be advised in the more severe cases with anginal symptoms. It is wise, however, in this congenital lesion to depart from the usual practice in other acyanotic congenital defects and to forbid arduous competitive games. Some centres perform balloon valvoplasty by catheterisiation to manage aortic valve stenosis but others feel this technique by lacking the precision of surgical valvotomy, is unduly risky.

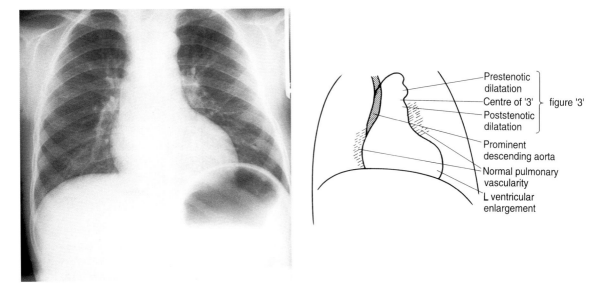

FIGURE 5.17 Chest X-ray, coarctation of the aorta "figure 3 sign".

Coarctation of the aorta

This is a relatively common anomaly and one so amenable to surgical correction that palpation of the femoral arteries should form part of the physical examination of every patient of any age. The common site of narrowing of the aorta is just beyond the origin of the left subclavian artery and of the ligamentum arteriosum. The earlier classification into "adult" and "infantile" types should be abandoned. As most lesions are found in preductal position and a small minority in postductal location, it has become fashionable to describe coarctation as preductal and postductal respectively (Fig. 5.16); those opposite the ductal mouth are described as "paraductal" coarctation. About 2% of coarctations are associated with Turner (XO) syndrome while around 15% of patients with Turner syndrome have coarctation.

Clinical features

Isolated severe coarctation of the aorta may occasionally cause heart failure with pulmonary oedema in the young infant. The onset of cardiac failure is almost always within the first 3 months of life, but many infants present in the first week of life. Coarctation of the aorta is the commonest structural anomaly causing heart failure in the first week of life in an acyanotic infant. In the vast majority of cases, however, the child is well developed and symptomless. The murmur, which may be discovered during routine medical examination or during an intercurrent illness, is systolic in time. It is well heard at the aortic area, in the suprasternal notch, and in both interscapular areas. The apex beat is forceful due to

left ventricular hypertrophy but it may not be displaced for many years. The femoral pulses are absent or only weakly felt in comparison with the radial or brachial pulses. A marked blood pressure difference can be shown between the arms and legs and in time hypertension is established in the upper extremities, head and neck. In adolescence dilated and tortuous collateral vessels may be visible around the scapulae. Thus the combination of weak or absent femoral pulses and an arm/leg blood pressure gradient is virtually diagnostic of aortic coarctation.

Radiographs may show no abnormality during childhood but ultimately left ventricular enlargement develops. An overpenetrated film may reveal a notch in the aortic shadow at the site of the coarctation and the narrow aortic arch above with some dilatation of the aorta below this notch produces an outline somewhat like the figure three (3) (Fig. 5.17). Notching of the inferior borders of the ribs by the enlarged intercostal arteries is seen in later childhood. The electrocardiogram may reveal left ventricular hypertrophy but in the young infant with a severe degree of aortic obstruction the ECG will show right ventricular hypertrophy as blood supply to the abdomen and lower limbs may be via the ductus arteriosus from the pulmonary artery. Cross-sectional echocardiography will usually demonstrate a coarctation and is invaluable in demonstrating any associated abnormality.

Prognosis

Coarctation presenting with heart failure in infancy is a lethal condition. Those who survive infancy may live into late middle age. Some die suddenly from a cerebrovascular accident. Most die in cardiac failure before the age of 40 years. A few develop rheumatic fever or infective endocarditis.

Treatment

Surgical resection of the narrowed segment of the aorta with direct anastomosis or the insertion of a graft is now so safe and satisfactory that operation should be advised in all cases. This is best performed before the age of 4 years. In young infants with cardiac failure operation is essential and performed as an emergency procedure. Interventional relief of coarctation of the aorta by balloon angioplasty is practised in some centres but its long-term benefits and risks have yet to be assessed.

Hypoplastic left heart syndrome

This syndrome comprises a wide variety of related anomalies associated with hypoplasia of the left ventricle and of the ascending aorta and aortic arch. Other constant findings include a large pulmonary artery, dilatation and hypertrophy of the right ventricle and a patent ductus arteriosus. The hypoplastic aortic arch may show a preductal coarctation, or that part of the arch between the left subclavian artery and entrance of the ductus arteriosus may be atretic and represented only by a solid core of tissue. Other common anomalies include atresia (or hypoplasia) of the mitral and/or aortic valves. Severe endocardial fibroelastosis may affect the left ventricle (only when the mitral valve is patent) or the left atrium. In cases where there is atresia of the aortic or mitral valve it is obvious that the right side of the heart has to maintain both the systemic and pulmonary circulations, and the pulmonary return to the left atrium has to be shunted across to the right side of the heart so that the right atrium becomes a mixing chamber for both oxygenated and venous blood. If the mitral valve is atretic and the aortic valve atretic or hypoplastic, and if there is no ventricular septal defect, the right ventricle alone is the propelling force for both pulmonary and systemic circuits. This explains the dilated pulmonary artery, while the patent ductus arteriosus which appears to continue into the large descending aorta permits a retrograde flow of blood into the arch of the aorta, so supplying the brachiocephalic and coronary arteries. It will be readily understood that this syndrome is incompatible with life. Furthermore, there are frequently associated non-cardiac abnormalities.

Clinical features

The hypoplastic left heart syndrome is the commonest cardiac cause of death in the neonatal period, and it ranks next only to transposition of the great arteries as a cause of death in all infants with congenital heart disease. The actual life span of affected infants depends on the severity of the obstructive valvar lesions. When the aortic or mitral valves are atretic life is usually sustained for only a few days, whereas when the valves are hypoplastic survival is longer and may extend for a few weeks. The clinical presentation is with the rapid development of severe dyspnoea, hepatomegaly, gross cardiomegaly and oedema. Cyanosis is common and in cases with a right to left flow through a patent ductus the lower half of the body may show a more severe degree than the head and arms. Some of those babies may initially be seen in severe cardiovascular collapse. Hypotension is common, as is the inability to maintain normothermia. Hypoglycaemia and a disseminated intravascular coagulopathy may occur in severely ill infants. Cardiac murmurs are inconstant as are the electrocardiographic changes. Precise diagnosis is now established by echocardiography which shows a very small left ventricle, a small or absent aortic root and the mitral valve echo is absent or greatly reduced. In most cases cardiac catheterisation, which carries great risk, can be avoided.

Prognosis and treatment

Most die in the first week of life and by 1 month of age more than 90% will have succumbed. The response to medical measures is usually poor and transient. Successful surgical treatment for the hypoplastic left heart syndrome is now being achieved in some centres. Perhaps cardiac transplantation will offer more prospect in due course.

Duct-dependent anomalies

There are a number of congenital cardiac malformations in which continued patency of the ductus arteriosus is essential for survival. In such life-threatening situations the continuous infusion of prostaglandins PGE_1 and PGE_2 can prevent closure of the ductus until appropriate investigations followed by surgical management have been achieved.

In pulmonary atresia with intact ventricular septum, pulmonary atresia with ventricular septal defect, severe pulmonary stenosis, tetralogy of Fallot and tricuspid atresia where deepening cyanosis from birth is a common clinical feature, the continuous intravenous or intra-arterial infusion of prostaglandin can be life saving. The initial dosage should be low to avoid the unwanted side effects of bradycardia and apnoea and we suggest 0.01–0.02 µg/kg/min increasing by increments of 0.01 µg/kg/min as necessary to 0.1 µg/kg/min. In most cases the infusion needs to be maintained for 12–24 hours while metabolic acidosis

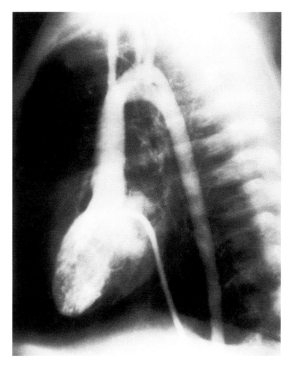
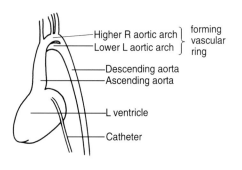

FIGURE 5.18 Left ventricular angiogram showing double aortic arch: lateral view.

is corrected and, when indicated by investigations, surgery is arranged.

Infants with hypoplastic left heart syndrome and coarctation of the aorta, where systemic rather than pulmonary blood flow is dependent upon patency of the ductus arteriosus, may also be helped by infusions of prostaglandin. In infants with complete transposition of the great arteries, where balloon atrial septostomy has failed to achieve adequate increase in arterial P_{O_2}, infusion of prostaglandin can, by dilating the ductus and reducing pulmonary vascular resistence, improve tissue oxygenation until surgical excision of the interatrial septum (Blalock–Hanlon operation) or other corrective procedure can be performed. Infusion may also be helpful in cases where balloon septostomy has been unduly delayed.

Prolonged administration of prostaglandin appears to be safe although reported side effects include fever, bradycardia, apnoea, hypotension and jitteriness. Assisted ventilation should be immediately available and the infusion should be reduced or discontinued until the unwanted effects have abated.

Vascular ring

Several aberrations can occur in the formation of the large arteries in the superior mediastinum. Amongst the most common are double aortic arch, right aortic arch with left ligamentum arteriosum, anomalous right subclavian artery and anomalous innominate artery (Fig. 5.18). In all these situations the trachea and oesophagus may be compressed by vessels which run normally in front of them and abnormally behind them. The term "vascular ring" has been used to decribe a variety of such vascular abnormalities.

Clinical features

Clinical manifestations of aortic arch anomalies vary with the severity of encroachment of the abnormal vessel on the trachea, bronchus or oesophagus. The features vary considerably in severity. The typical picture is of an underdeveloped infant with feeding difficulties and with constant laryngeal or tracheal stridor, wheezing and cough. The child may find relief with extreme extension of the neck. When symptoms are delayed until later infancy dysphagia may be obvious. There may be repeated severe respiratory infections. Patients with a double aortic arch tend to have signs at an earlier age than patients with other types of vascular rings. The diagnosis is confirmed by fluoroscopy visualising the tracheal compression and during a barium swallow, when indentations of the oesophagus by the aberrant vessels can be visualised (Fig. 5.19). It is frequently possible to identify the precise anomaly by this technique. Tracheobronchoscopy and further investigations by digital subtraction angiograph will better define the pathology.

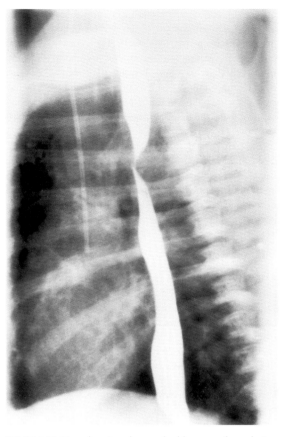
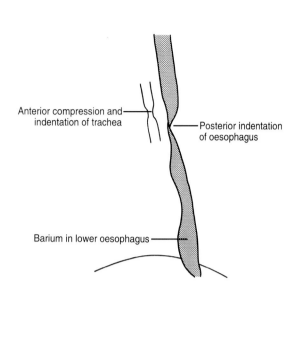

FIGURE 5.19 Vascular ring due to double aorta (lateral view of barium swallow).

Treatment

The simple existence of a vascular ring is not an indication for surgical intervention. However, it is generally accepted that surgical intervention should be undertaken whenever there is significant airway compromise. Thoracotomy and division of the aberrant vessel provides complete relief in the great majority of cases.

ENDOCARDIAL FIBROELASTOSIS

The incidence of this disorder of infancy seems to have diminished in recent years. The aetiology is obscure although it is probably an acquired disease process which nearly always, if not always, has its onset during intrauterine life. This seems a more likely explanation than a developmental anomaly. The pathological changes consist of a fibroelastic thickening which involves the endocardium and subendocardial tissues. They are most marked in the left atrium and left ventricle where the endocardium has a thickened and milky appearance. The disease may occur alone and is also seen in combination with those anatomical abnormalities which involve the aortic valve and arch. The condition behaves functionally like constrictive pericarditis, causing impairment of left ventricular filling, diminished systolic ejection and narrowing of the pulse pressure.

Clinical features

The first signs which may appear at any time during infancy are due to left heart failure and, therefore, are dominated by respiratory problems. Right heart failure is usually a late phenomenon. Feeding problems, vomiting, and failure to thrive are common. Murmurs are frequently faint or absent. X-ray reveals a markedly enlarged hert. The electrocardiogram usually shows severe left ventricular hypertrophy and T-wave inversion and echocardiography reveals poor left ventricular function with a dilated and poorly contracting left ventricle but normal overall anatomy.

Treatment

Apart from the treatment of cardiac failure nothing can be done. Recovery is extremely uncommon although in some cases life is prolonged for several years.

ACQUIRED DISEASES OF THE HEART

The most common cause of acquired heart disease in childhood is acute rheumatic fever. Apart from causing death during childhood from extensive myocardial involvement leading to congestive cardiac failure, the rheumatic process may result in severe valvular deformities which for mechanical reasons give rise to trouble in adult life, e.g. mitral stenosis and incompetence and/or aortic stenosis and incompetence. It is common to find mitral and aortic regurgitation singly or together in children who have active rheumatic endocarditis in addition to myocarditis. On the other hand, acquired stenosis of the mitral or aortic valves is rare in childhood because several years must elapse before constriction of the valve rings can develop. Rheumatic fever has shown a greatly reduced incidence in the more prosperous countries of the world in recent years.

Other acquired diseases of the heart are rare in childhood but sufficiently important as causes of death or severe illness to justify adequate description.

Myocarditis

Aetiology

There are several widely different causes of myocardial disease in childhood. In the paediatric age group two main causes of non-rheumatic inflammatory heart disease can be recognised, namely infectious myocarditis and generalised autoimmune myocarditis. Infectious myocarditis can occur as a complication of almost any infectious disease. Diphtheritic myocarditis was once a common cause of death, signs appearing usually in the third week of illness, but in Britain today it is virtually unknown. Almost any viral disease can be complicated by myocarditis. The most important viruses are Coxsackie, influenza, ECHO, mumps and rubella. Viral infections are by far the most important in the Western world, but in other parts of the world parasitic infections such as schistosomiasis, malaria and trypanosomiasis may rank highest.

Clinical features

The clinical onset of myocarditis usually occurs after a latent period following the onset of a systemic viral infection. Abdominal pain, fever, anorexia, dyspnoea and cough develop suddenly in a young child who has previously been perfectly well. He quickly becomes seriously ill with pallor, cyanosis of peripheral type, and frequently diarrhoea and vomiting. The signs of congestive cardiac failure which predominate are cardiac enlargement, gallop rhythm without a murmur, crepitations over the lungs, and increasing hepatomegaly. Oedema is often slight or absent. The chest X-ray shows generalised cardiac enlargement (Fig. 5.20) and often bilateral pleural effusions. The electrocardiograph (ECG) shows abnormalities of a non-specific character in the S-T segments and T waves and arrhythmias of different types may occur. Echocardiography will show poor left ventricular action.

Differential diagnosis

At the onset of illness the severe abdominal pain may simulate acute appendicitis. There is usually less muscular rigidity in myocarditis, and enlargement of the liver should direct attention to the heart. It is often difficult during life to exclude other causes of cardiac failure in early childhood such as endocardial firbroelastosis, anomalous left coronary artery, glycogen storage disease of the heart and mitochondrial cardiomyopathies. Acute myocarditis is more likely when the child has been in good health prior to the onset of the illness and when his nutritional state is obviously good. "Acute benign pericarditis" also enters the differential diagnosis; indeed the two diseases are often caused by the same virus and may coexist. All available diagnostic procedures should be used in an attempt to identify the micro-organism. IgM antibodies may indicate a recent virus infection.

Treatment

The prognosis is grave and many cases end fatally. Some, however, show a marked response to treatment. Cardiac failure should be treated with digitalis and diuretics as mentioned in the section on cardiac failure in infancy. The course of the disease should be controlled by regular radiographic and electrocardiographic observations, especially as some patients show undue susceptibility to digoxin. None the less, digitalisation should be maintained for many weeks after recovery from the acute attack. Also patients with an infectious myocarditis should be closely monitored for the occurrence of arrhythmias and should be treated according to the currently accepted regimens.

Autoimmune myocarditis

Myocarditis can occur in connective tissue disorders and is described in the chapter on connective tissue disorders (Chapter 15).

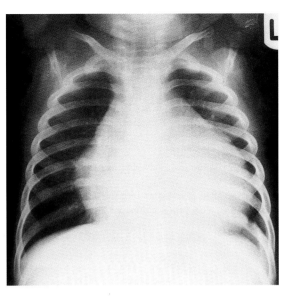
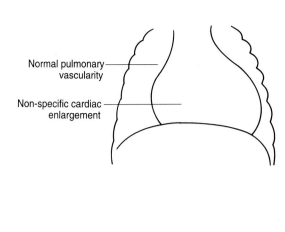

Normal pulmonary vascularity

Non-specific cardiac enlargement

FIGURE 5.20 Chest X-ray showing marked cardiomegaly due to viral myocarditis.

Pericarditis

Aetiology

The aetiology of pericarditis differs considerably from one part of the world to the other. Infectious causes (such as tuberculosis) and pericarditis due to a generalised autoimmune disease (such as rheumatic fever) are rare in developed countries. Within the past 20 years both these varieties of pericarditis have become quite uncommon. Indeed, in recent years we have seen pericarditis associated with rheumatoid arthritis as frequently as with rheumatic fever. In the former, of course, endocarditis and myocarditis are usually absent. Septic pericarditis was once a common complication of pneumonia and left-sided empyema and of pyaemia due to a variety of pyogenic organisms. The micro-organisms most commonly involved are *Staphylococcus*, *Pneumococcus*, *Meningococcus*, *Haemophilus influenzae* and *Streptococcus*. It has been almost abolished by modern antibacterial drugs. Pericarditis may develop in the child dying from uraemia. This is thought to be due to chemical irritation of the pericardial endothelium. Pericardial effusion may result as an uncommon complication of central lines where the catheter has eroded into the pericardial sac, or in patients with hydrocephalus treated by ventriculo-atrial drainage. Cardiac tamponade can develop.

Clinical features

While these vary to some extent according to the aetiology, certain features are common to all types of pericarditis. One of the most characteristic is pain. This may be severe in rheumatic or viral cases and is often slight in tuberculous cases. The pain is most often retrosternal, but it may be in the upper abdomen or in the left shoulder. Other general features are dypsnoea, fever and a tendency on the part of the child to lean forwards. The most valuable diagnostic sign is, of course, pericardial friction which may have a double or triple rhythm and which, in any event, is not synchronised to the heard sounds as are murmurs. It is best heard with the patient leaning forwards and with the stethoscope placed firmly against the chest wall. It is not heard in every case, nor is its presence indicative of the amount of fluid in the pericardial sac. The area of cardiac dullness is usually demonstrably increased upwards as well as to the left and right. A common finding is dullness and bronchial breath sounds at the inferior angle of the left scapula (the Ewart or Bamberger sign). Its cause has been variously attributed to pleural effusion, pulmonary compression by the pericardial sac and "rheumatic" pneumonia. When there is a lot of fluid in the pericardial sac with cardiac tamponade, the heart sounds are distant and muffled, the neck veins are visibly distended, hepatomegaly develops and the pulse pressure is reduced due to inadequate cardiac output. There may be pulsus paradoxus in which the systolic blood pressure is reduced during inspiration. The most reliable diagnostic confirmation of a pericardial effusion is by echocardiography. The heart shadow on radiography is usually much enlarged with a short, wide supracardiac shadow – "water bottle" shape. Fluoroscopy reveals much diminished cardiac pulsation. The heart shadow in pericarditis frequently fluctuates rapidly in size, a useful distinguishing feature from gross cardiac enlargement due to rheumatic pancarditis, in which cardiomegaly recedes only very slowly, if ever. The characteristic electrocardiographic changes are low voltage, and elevation and convexity of the S-T segment in all the left ventricular leads. Indeed the electrocardiogram may occasionally remain completely normal.

Diagnosis

In rheumatic pericarditis there is almost invariably a loud apical systolic murmur in addition to pericardial friction. The child is pale, toxic in appearance, and may have other manifestations such as arthritis or nodules. The antistreptolysin 'O' (ASO) titre is usually raised. It is unusual to find a large volume of fluid in pericarditis of rheumatic origin and paracentesis is rarely indicated. On the other hand, in tuberculous cases large collections of straw-coloured lymphocytic exudate with cardiac tamponade are the rule in the early stages of the disease. The Mantoux test will be positive and there may be other signs of intrathoracic or disseminated tuberculosis. Septic pericarditis is associated with gross suppuration elsewhere. Cardiac tamponade is common and a large volume of pus may be found in the pericardial sac. In viral pericarditis there are usually no signs of disease in other systems of the body. The heart sounds may be muffled, and if there is a systolic murmur it is soft and unimpressive. There is frequently a history obtainable of a recent preceding upper respiratory infection.

Treatment

General measures include bed rest. Cyanosis demands the use of oxygen therapy. Anti-rheumatic treatment with a combination of salicylates, corticosteroids and penicillin should be given in rheumatic pericarditis, although the child is likely to be left with a severe permanent cardiac disability from the associated myocarditis and endocarditis. Tuberculosis cases require the energetic use of antituberculous drugs. Whenever there is cardiac tamponade the fluid should be removed from the pericardial sac by paracentesis. Patients with septic pericarditis must have intensive antibiotic treatment according to the sensitivities of the causal bacteria. It is essential also to empty the pericardial sac either by paracentesis or thoracotomy. There are no specific drugs available for Coxsackie virus infections. It should be stressed that in large pericardial effusions from any cause, paracentesis can be life saving, whereas digitalisation is ineffective.

Infective endocarditis

The term "infective" is more appropriate to bacterial endocarditis since fungal, rickettsial and probably viral agents can also initiate endocarditis. This is not a common disease in childhood. The customary subdivision into "acute" and "subacute" forms is not really satisfactory and cases are better classified according to their infecting organism. The majority are due to *Streptococcus viridans* but many organisms can cause the disease, e.g. staphylococci, β-haemolytic streptococci, pneumococci, enterococci and coliforms. Staphylococcal cases are more common in children than in adults. The vast majority of infections are superimposed upon pre-existing rheumatic or congenital heart disease, the latter forming a much higher proportion than is the case in bacterial endocarditis in adults. It is well known that the bacteraemia which must precede bacterial endocarditis is sometimes related to the extraction of teeth or the removal of tonsils, but in most cases there is no such defined preceding event. In recent years cases have been seen following cardiac surgery or cardiac catheterisation in which the causal organism has been *Staphylococcus albus* and in which diagnosis and treatment can be particularly difficult. In the young infant a rather different category of bacterial endocarditis is occasionally encountered. This forms but part of a generalised pyaemic process with other septic foci such as osteitis, empyema and pyoderma. There is no underlying cardiac malformation in these infants and the endocarditis is only one factor in causing death. With the increasing use of central venous lines for intravenous nutrition endothelial trauma is the likely predisposing factor to the establishment of endocarditis by bacteria or fungi such as *Candida*.

Pathology

The typical finding is of large, crumbling vegetations on the valve cusps along the lines of apposition. These are composed of fibrin, leucocytes and bacteria. In some cases the process is not found on the valves. For example, in cases complicating patent ductus arteriosus the vegetations are commonly found on the wall of the pulmonary artery opposite to the site of entry of the duct – bacterial endarteritis. In cases complicating ventricular septal defect the vegetations may be on the right-hand surface of the ventricular septum or on the wall of the right ventricle – mural endocarditis. When rheumatic heart disease is present, the aortic and mitral valves are commonly involved. The blood stream carries off small portions of these vegetations to result in embolism in many organs, e.g. lungs, kidneys, brain and spleen.

Clinical features

The diagnosis should be suspected whenever a child with rheumatic or congenital heart disease develops fever, leucocytosis, an alteration in the character of

TABLE 5.1 Antibacterial prophylactic therapy in relation to congenital or acquired heart disease

1   Uncomplicated defects – dental surgical treatment, local anaesthesia
    Amoxycillin (by mouth) 1 hour before and 6 hours after procedure
    Dosage: under 10 years, 1.5 g; over 10 years, 3 g
2   Uncomplicated defects – dental surgical treatment, general anaesthesia
    Ampicillin (IM) 1 hour before procedure
    Dosage: under 10 years, 500 mg; over 10 years 1 g
    AND
    Amoxycillin (by mouth) 6 hours after procedure
    Dosage: under 10 years, 1.5 mg; over 10 years, 3 g
3   Patients in categories 1 and 2 but allergic to penicillin or already on penicillin prophylaxis
    Erythromycin (by mouth) 1 hour before and 6 hours after procedure
    Dosage: under 10 years, 1 g; over 10 years, 2 g
4   Defects repaired with a fabric patch or prosthetic valve (should be referred to hospital)
    Ampicillin and *Flucloxacillin* (IV) 1 hour before and 8 and 16 hours after procedure
    Dosage: under 10 years, 500 mg of each; over 10 years, 1 g of each
5   Patients having GI or GU surgery
    Gentamicin (IM or IV) 1 hour before and 12 hours after procedure
    Dosage: 2 mg/kg (dose not to exceed 80 mg)
    AND
    Ampicillin (IM)
    Dosage: under 10 years, 500 mg; over 10 years, 1 g
6   Patients in categories 4 and 5 above but allergic to penicillin or already on penicillin prophylaxis
    Gentamicin (IM or IV) 1 hour before and 12 hours after procedure
    Dosage: as in 5 above
    AND
    Vancomycin (IV infusion)
    Dosage: 20 mg/kg (dose not to exceed 1 g)

the cardiac murmurs, and embolic phenomena such as splenomegaly, haematuria, petechiae and subungual flame-shaped haemorrhages. Osler's nodes, raised, tender red spots on the fingertips, are uncommon in children. Clubbing of the fingers is of diagnostic significance in the absence of preceding cyanotic congenital heart disease. In cases due to *Streptoccocus viridans* fever is not usually above 39°C (102°F) and progressive muddy pallor is common. In staphylococcal cases high fever, 39–40°C (102–104°F) is the rule and the disease runs a rapid course. In mural endocarditis of the right ventricle, pulmonary embolism may cause pain in the chest, dyspnoea, haemoptysis and clinical and radiographic signs of infarction. The diagnosis can be confirmed by isolation of the organism in blood cultures, which should be taken at least three times daily as soon as the diagnosis is suspected. When blood cultures are repeatedly negative the clinician is faced with a diffi-

cult problem, but in the child acutely ill with cardiac and embolic signs treatment should rarely be delayed for longer than 72 hours. Both M-mode and cross-sectional echocardiography can be used to demonstrate vegetations attached to valvar structures in children with infective endocarditis. However, it should be emphasised that lack of demonstration of vegetations does not rule out the diagnosis. More than 90% of patients will have at least microscopic haematuria. Its absence makes diagnosis unlikely.

Treatment

An antibiotic, bactericidal rather than bacteriostatic, chosen according to the bacterial sensitivities, should be given by the intravenous route in large doses for at least 6 weeks. If blind therapy is required it would be advisable to start in children with a high dose combination of penicillin and gentamicin or possibly streptomycin. Effective treatment of endocarditis should result in subsidence of fever along with the return to normal of the sedimentation rate and the white blood cell count. Also, the major indication for surgical intervention in children with infective endocarditis is when foreign material has been previously inserted, e.g. for closure of a septal defect.

Prophylaxis

Minor surgical procedures such as dental extraction or tonsillectomy should always be "covered" with antibiotic prophylaxis in children known to have organic disease of the heart. A suitable antibacterial prophylactic therapy programme is shown (Table 5.1).

ARRHYTHMIAS

Cardiac arrhythmias are less common and usually of less serious import in children than in adults.

Sinus arrhythmia

In this phenomenon the heart rate increases during inspiration and slows during expiration. The condition has been related to increased vagal activity. It is commonly found in perfectly healthy children, although it is considerably overstating the case to suggest that sinus arrhythmia in itself indicates a normal heart.

Extrasystoles

Ectopic cardiac beats arise from impulses which have their origin outwith the sino-atrial node, e.g. the atria, the atrioventricular node or the ventricles. They are not, in themselves, of serious significance. Indeed they may occur in apparently healthy children. In present-day Britain, enquiry as to cigarette smoking is not superfluous in the case of the older child. Extrasystoles may also complicate organic disease of the heart or the action of digitalis. They may cause the child to become aware of his heart action but are more often symptomless. In the case of ventricular extrasystoles the premature beat is followed by a compensatory pause which fully compensates for the preceding short diastole. In atrial or nodal ectopic beats the following compensating pause is not marked. The diagnosis should be confirmed by electrocardiography. Extrasystoles which occur in a healthy heart are usually abolished by exercise, whereas they may be rendered more frequent in underlying cardiac disease. Ectopic beats in healthy children do not require treatment unless they are producing excessive anxiety, when nitrazepam 2.5 mg twice daily may provide some relief.

Paroxysmal tachycardia

This is most often seen in supraventricular form in infants or children. While it may be associated with cardiac anomalies, in the great majority of cases the heart is structurally normal. Most cases are re-entry tachycardias with an ectopic focus in atrial muscle or the junctional tissue. In a significant proportion of cases the resting electrocardiogram shows typical characteristics of the Wolff–Parkinson–White syndrome, namely, a very short P-R interval, delta wave and prolonged duration of the QRS complex. In this "pre-excitation" syndrome there are two conduction pathways between atria and ventricles: the A-V nodal–His pathway and an accessory pathway. The latter may go from left atrium to left ventricles (type A) or from right atrium to right ventricle (type B). The type A syndrome is particularly related to supraventricular paroxysmal tachycardia in young infants with a good prognosis as the accessory pathway seems to cease being used as the infant gets older. Type B, however, is commoner in older children, sometimes associated with complex cardiac anomalies (e.g., Ebstein anomaly) and it may be resistant to drug therapy. Other much less common abnormal conduction pathways with characteristic electrocardiographic changes have also been described.

Fortunately, ventricular tachycardias are rare in children, as they carry a serious prognosis and may cause sudden death. They are generally related to uncommon cardiac disorders, e.g. coronary artery abnormalities, cardiomyopathy and tumour.

Clinical features

The young infant with paroxysmal tachycardia quickly develops congestive cardiac failure. He looks anxious and ill with dyspnoea, restlessness, subcostal recession, greyish cyanosis, and reluctance to feed. Cardiomegaly and hepatomegaly are marked. There may be facial or generalised oedema. Crepitations over the lungs may be due solely to cardiac failure or in part to the respiratory infection which sometimes seems to precipitate the tachycardia. The heart rate is over 280 per minute. There may be a systolic murmur which disappears after the attack has been brought under control. Radiographs show an enlarged heart and passive congestion of the lungs.

In older children cardiac failure ultimately develops if the paroxysm lasts for over 24 hours. Accurate diagnosis of the nature of the tachycardia can only be reached by electrocardiography and it is particularly helpful to have 24 hour ECG monitoring available.

Treatment

Supraventricular tachycardia in the infant

The infant will often have signs of congestive cardiac failure. Vagal manoeuvres are ineffective. Pharmacological measures are too slow and may not be successful. DC cardioversion is the treatment of choice using a single shock of 1 joule/kg, repeated if necessary, under general anaesthesia or sedation. The tachycardia may recur and digitalistion should be carried out immediately after DC conversion as described in the section on cardiac failure in infancy. It is essential that initial drug treatment is controlled by electrocardiography and preferably by continuous ECG monitor.

If the infant is seen before congestive cardiac failure develops, rapid treatment is still indicated. Vagal manoeuvres (e.g. diving reflex – face covered with an ice-filled plastic bag) are unlikely to work but are worth trying. Electrocardioversion on digitalisation is usually effective in controlling the tachycardia. An alternative therapy is intravenous propranolol 0.1 mg/kg followed by oral propranolol 2 mg/kg/day. Drug therapy may usually be withdrawn at 1 year of age without further problem.

Supraventricular tachycardia in the child

While the prognosis in the young infant is good, the outcome in older children is less predictable. Vagal stimulation should be tried first (e.g. by pressure over one carotid sinus in the neck or by the Valsalva manoeuvre) before using one of the drugs mentioned above. However, when the tachycardia proves resistant to such measures recourse must be had to DC electric shock. Verapamil is the treatment of choice for supraventricular tachycardia in paediatric patients beyond the infant age group who do not respond to vagal manoeuvres and who are not in congestive cardiac failure. It may be given intravenously at a dose of 0.1 mg/kg over a 60–120 second period. Once the tachycardia has been controlled careful electrophysiological investigation is important to detect accessory pathways, and to control the effect of drugs given to prevent recurrences. Adenosine (3 mg/ml in physiological saline) by rapid IV injection has recently been introduced for the treatment of paroxysmal supraventricular tachycardias in specialist centres. In the rare case of ventricular paroxysmal tachycardia the child will be critically ill with pallor, restlessness and hypotension. The diagnosis must be confirmed by electrocardiography. Reversal to sinus rhythm is best achieved by DC electric shock. Alternatively lignocaine may be given intravenously in an initial dose of 1 mg/kg followed by continuous infusion of 0.2% solution under ECG control. Subsequent investigations may require echocardiography and angiocardiography.

Atrial flutter and atrial fibrillation

These serious arrhythmias are rarely seen in children and they are almost invariable associated with grave rheumatic or congenital lesions. In flutter there is a regular tachycardia, and in fibrillation an irregular irregularity. The diagnosis should be confirmed by electrocardiography. Congestive failure is the rule because the heart is already seriously damaged. The drug of choice in each case is digoxin in the dosage recommended for cardiac failure in infancy. Electrical cardioversion may also be used to restore sinus rhythm in cases of atrial flutter and fibrillation.

Bradyarrhythmias

Sinus bradycardia

Sinus bradycardia is a relatively uncommon cause of a slow heart rate in infants and children. It is a transient finding in severe systemic disease, hypoxic episodes, head injuries and increased intracranial pressure in young infants.

Heart block

In childhood, heart block is often congenital and it is then usually complete. In some cases there are cyanotic or acyanotic congenital anomalies; in others no cardiac abnormality can be detected. Incomplete heart block may also be unassociated with detectable cardiac disease, but in most cases there is a discoverable cause, e.g. rheumatic, diphtheritic or viral myocarditis; congenital anomalies such as atrial septal defect or the Ebstein anomaly; and digitalis overdosage. There appears also to be a peculiar association between congenital heart block and

mothers who have, or later develop, systemic lupus erythematosus. The autoantibody associated with the "neonatal lupus syndrome" is anti-SSS/Ro antibody. These antibodies are of the IgG classes and are passed across the placenta even from some mothers who are asymptomatic.

Incomplete heart block

In first-degree block the PR interval on the electrocardiogram is longer than is normal for the age of the patient. In second-degree block some P waves fail altogether to be followed by ventricular QRS complexes. In the Wenckebach phenomenon there is progressive lengthening of the P-R intervals until finally a QRS complex is missed. In other cases, the block may involve every third, fourth or fifth complex in a regular manner.

Complete heart block

In third-degree block there is complete dissociation of the contractions of the ventricles and the atria. In children the ventricular rhythm is usually set at about 40 per minute, rising rarely more than 20 after exercise. The electrocardiograph shows, of course, the P waves have a rhythm which is totally unrelated to that of the QRS complexes. Stokes–Adams attacks are rare in children and the prognosis of heart block is that of the primary cardiac condition. Most children with congenital heart block are asymptomatic, but a few develop congestive cardiac failure or Stokes–Adams attacks during the neonatal period. Nevertheless, as children reach adult life a number develop severe bradycardia with attacks of dizziness or syncope and require the insertion of pacemakers. Life-long follow-up is recommended in all cases.

Treatment

Specific treatment will be required for the underlying cardiac disease when this has been acquired. In congenital heart block treatment is unnecessary in the absence of the symptoms. If Stokes–Adams attacks or episodes of extreme dizziness occur the implantation of a permanent pacemaker is indicated.

For reflex anoxic seizures see Chapter 9.

CARDIAC FAILURE IN INFANCY

Aetiology

Congestive cardiac failure in infancy is not uncommon. It may be due to paroxysmal tachycardia when the long-term prognosis is excellent. Various congenital anomalies can result in heart failure in the early

TABLE 5.2 Digoxin dose regimen

AGE/WEIGHT	DIGITALISING DOSE (µg/kg over 24 hours)		MAINTENANCE DOSE (µg/kg twice daily)	
	IV	Oral	IV	Oral
Preterm under 1.5 kg	20	30	2	3
Preterm 1.5–2.5 kg	30	40	3	4
Term neonate to 2 years	35	50	3	5
Over 2 years	40	40	4	4

days or weeks of life, especially coarctation of the aorta, hypoplastic left heart syndrome, transposition of the great vessels and patent ductus arteriosus with or without pulmonary hypertension. Other causes include endocardial fibroelastosis, viral myocarditis and glycogen storage disease of the heart.

Clinical features

Breathlessness on exertion takes the form of slowness and difficulty with feeds during infancy. The infant becomes dyspnoeic with subcostal recession and may become unduly cyanosed. Venous congestion may be manifest as dilated scalp veins and hepatomegaly is marked and easily found. The heart is usually grossly enlarged, tachycardia is present, and there is often a loud murmur. Oedema is a late sign. It appears first in the face of the young infant, then in the genitalia and lumbosacral area before the feet. Crepitations over the lungs may be misinterpreted as due to respiratory infection; indeed such an infection may be the precipitating cause of the cardiac failure and it is important to recognise the true significance of the other signs of heart disease.

Treatment

The infant should be nursed with the head well raised above the feet. Cyanosis and restlessness are indica-

tions for oxygen therapy controlled and monitored by T_{CO_2} saturation. Digoxin should be administered as recommended in Table 5.2. Diuretics are the mainstay of treatment for cardiac failure. Their effect is to remove excessive extracellular fluid. If oedema is marked, frusemide is given in a dose of 0.5–l mg/kg intravenously two or three times daily or 0.5–3 mg/kg orally two or three times daily. When diuretics are being given the serum potassium level should be measured frequently and an electrocardiograph record made at regular intervals. Hypokalaemia should be treated with oral potassium chloride 2 mmol/kg/day.

CARDIAC FAILURE IN OLDER CHILDREN

The clinical picture of cardiac failure in older children is very much the same as that with which we are familiar in adults and a detailed description is unnecessary. Pure left heart failure is uncommon in childhood but may occur in renal hypertension, aortic stenosis, coarctation of the aorta, mitral stenosis and patent ductus arteriosus. It is characterised by pulmonary oedema and crepitations, left-sided hydrothorax, gallop rhythm, cardiac asthma and pulsus alternans. Pure right heart failure is more common in the form of increased venous pressure, hepatomegaly, peripheral oedema and right hydrothorax. It may be caused by pulmonary stenosis, atrial septal defect, transposition of the great vessels and anomalous pulmonary venous drainage. However, in children the most common form of congestive cardiac failure involves both ventricles. It may be due to most of the causes mentioned above, to myocarditis, most often rheumatic, to paroxysmal tachycardia, or to pericarditis. In most children with congestive heart failure initial therapy will be with diuretics and digoxin. A lower total dose of digoxin should be used in the presence of myocarditis or cardiomyopathy because of the increased risk of inducing arrhythmias.

6

Respiratory System

INTRODUCTION

Successful treatment of severe bacterial infections of the respiratory tract has contributed to the rapid fall in mortality rates during infancy and childhood in the past three decades. Deaths due to respiratory infection have not been eliminated and continue to be a common cause of morbidity, particularly in the children of large families of low socio-economic status. The majority are now associated with viral infections and only a minority are due to bacterial or other infection. This chapter will discuss first of all the congenital anomalies of the respiratory system which are all uncommon, followed by acquired disorders which are common.

CONGENITAL ANOMALIES

The respiratory system develops in early intrauterine life with bronchial tree, bronchi, and bronchioles forming by the 16th week after conception. Subsequently the alveoli develop and this development continues postnatally, particularly in the first year of life (Fig. 6.1). The number of alveoli continue to increase to approximately 300×10^6 by 8 years of age. Further growth is simply one of size rather than number. Growth ceases when the chest wall ceases to increase in size. The periacinar blood vessels follow the development of the bronchial tree, and the intra-acinar the alveoli. Abnormalities such as diaphragmatic hernia when established early in intrauterine life can inhibit bronchial branching and alveolar development. Postnatal problems primarily affect the alveoli and the pulmonary vasculature.

CONGENITAL ABNORMALITIES

The respiratory tract, in contrast to the nervous, cardiovascular or urinary systems, is infrequently the site of anatomical malformations.

Choanal atresia

Choanal atresia may be complete or partial, bilateral or unilateral, bony or membranous. A newborn baby breathes through the nose and the technique of mouth breathing is acquired slowly during the first three months of life in most infants. Thus bilateral choanal atresia results in severe dyspnoea, or apnoea during feeds, and thick gelatinous mucus in the nasal cavities. In partial cases the symptoms are similar but less severe. When the condition is unilateral the risk to life is much less. The most important feature is constant unilateral nasal obstruction and thick secretion which may cause excoriation of the skin of the nostril. Feeding difficulties are experienced because of the inability to suck and breathe at the same time. Diagnosis can be confirmed by finding that the

16 weeks   24 weeks   32 weeks

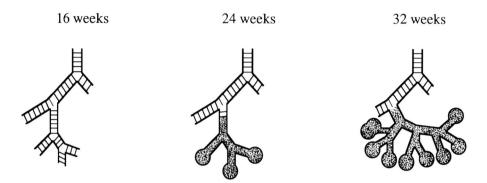

FIGURE 6.1 Diagram of lung developments at 16 weeks showing branchial branching; 24 weeks, initial alveolar development; 32 weeks, with secondary alveolar development. The increase in alveoli continues to approximately 8 years of age, thereafter growth is due to increase in size of alveoli.

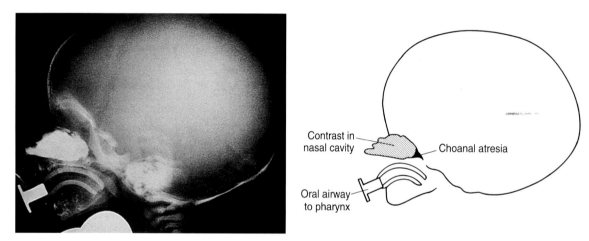

FIGURE 6.2 X-ray of choanal atresia showing dye in the obstructed choanal region.

passage of a catheter is arrested at the level of the choana about 30 mm from the nostril. Furthermore, a dye such as methylene blue, when instilled into the nostril, will fail to appear in the pharynx. Radiographs should also be taken after the nasal cavities have been cleared of secretions and contrast medium inserted (Fig. 6.2). Treatment is surgical. This may have to be performed during the neonatal period but it is sometimes possible, even in bilateral cases, to avoid operation until an older age by orogastric tube feeding for some weeks when the infant learns how to breathe through the mouth and feed from a spoon.

Congenital laryngeal stridor

Congenital laryngeal stridor (laryngomalacia) is common and soon after birth produces inspiratory stridor with suprasternal indrawing. The noise of stridor varies with respiration and increases during crying or with mild airway obstruction secondary to upper respiratory tract infection. Respiratory difficulty is rarely severe enough to interfere with the infant's general well-being or nutrition. The common cause is an unusually long and curved epiglottis, which can be seen on direct laryngoscopy to become drawn down against the arytenoids during inspiration. In children in whom the symptoms are typical and if the child is thriving and feeding normally, no further tests are indicated. However, when there is a doubt about the diagnosis, further investigations such as lateral neck X-ray, chest X-ray, barium swallow to exclude extrinsic tracheal and oesophageal compression and laryngoscopy should be considered. Spontaneous recovery takes place within the first 2–3 years of life. They very seldom require any other treatment. Other anomalies of the larynx such as laryngeal or subglottic stenosis or compression by hamartomas such as cystic hygroma or haemangioma may require emergency tracheostomy and later repair.

Tracheomalacia

Tracheomalacia is the condition where the normal struts of cartilage which maintain the trachea patent are either malformed, as is the case in a number of infants with tracheo-oesophageal fistula, or are compressed by vessels. This allows collapse of the trachea. The infant may suffer attacks where apnoea occurs and resuscitation is necessary. Intubation of the baby relieves the apnoeic attack. Aortopexy in the infants who had tracheo-oesophageal fistula and compression of the trachea by the aortic arch, or division of the vascular ring if present, relieves the symptoms.

Agenesis of the lung

Agenesis of the lung is rare. Bilateral pulmonary agenesis is extremely rare and incompatible with life. When one lung or one lobe is absent the patient is usually symptomless, although the heart is displaced into one hemithorax. In these cases there may or may not be a bronchial bud present. The diagnosis is frequently made during a routine medical examination and can be confirmed radiologically. There is no specific treatment and the prognosis is good since the other lung is normal.

Pulmonary hypoplasia

Bilateral pulmonary hypoplasia is often associated with oligohydramnios which during prenatal life commonly is secondary to fetal urological abnormalities. Severe bilateral pulmonary hypoplasia is typically found in Potter syndrome where it is associated with renal agenesis. It is frequent in babies with congenital diaphragmatic hernia. The degree of pulmonary hypoplasia varies in this latter group from being severe with arrest of development estimated at 10–12 weeks in some infants with large left-sided diaphragmatic hernia to minor degrees which do not interfere with function.

Pulmonary sequestration of the lung

Pulmonary sequestration of the lung may be intralobar, extralobar or complete, depending upon whether the segment of lung tissue which has no communication with the main bronchial tree is within a lobe of the lung, is outside the lung although still attached to it, or is completely separated from the lung. In the case of the extralobar and complete types the arterial blood supply is from the aorta and the venous return to the hemiazygous vein, whereas in the intralobar variety there may be a pulmonary artery supply with

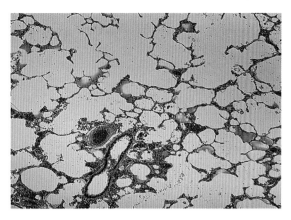

FIGURE 6.3 Histology of congenital lobar emphysema showing overdistension of "normal" lung alveoli.

venous return by a pulmonary vein. The extralobar and complete sequestrations are most often on the left side, sometimes in association with a diaphragmatic hernia. Radiographic interpretation may be difficult without bronchography to demonstrate the absence of communication with the bronchial tree. Barium studies may demonstrate communication to the oesophagus or stomach. Symptoms occur only if infection is superimposed.

Cystic disease of the lungs

Cystic disease of the lungs may be congenital or associated with acute infection. Congenital lung cysts may be either duplication cysts or congenital cystic adenomatoid malformation. The latter usually affects the lower lobes and these may also become infected. Duplication cysts may be found on chest X-ray in infants or children presenting with respiratory distress. These lesions require surgical removal and the results of surgery are usually excellent.

Congenital lobar emphysema

This postnatal overdistension of one or more lobes of a histologically normal lung are thought to result from cartilagenous deficiency in the bronchial tree (Fig. 6.3). The lobe usually affected is the left upper lobe which expands across the superior mediastinum and compresses the left lower lobe, causing the infant increasing respiratory distress (Fig. 6.4). Treatment of the disorder when the baby is severely compromised is lobectomy. Less severely affected infants may be helped by maintained positive airway pressure until the bronchi stabilise and gas exchange can occur freely.

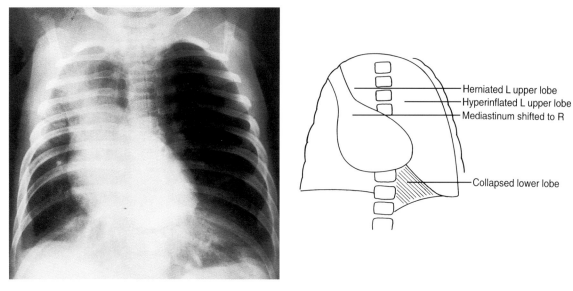

FIGURE 6.4 X-ray of congenital lobar emphysema of left upper lobe.

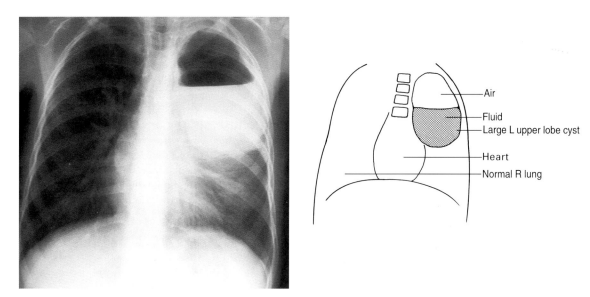

FIGURE 6.5 X-ray of chest showing lung cyst with air/fluid level.

Cystic adenomatoid malformation

This may be a single or multicystic mass in pulmonary tissue in which there is a proliferation of bronchial structures at the expense of alveoli. The cysts are lined by cuboidal or columnar epithelium which may appear to be of alimentary tract origin. The disease is considered a focal pulmonary dysplasia or some prefer to designate it a hamartoma. In some cases there is skeletal muscle in the cyst walls. The abnormality more often affects the lower lobes and is detected on X-ray of an infant with respira-

tory distress. Treatment is excision which must be complete to avoid the later possibility of malignancy arising in the cyst wall.

Bronchogenic cyst

Bronchogenic cyst is a discrete cyst of non-functioning pulmonary tissue, the cysts being lined by ciliated columnar epithelium and often including smooth muscle, glands and cartilage. There is no communication with the tracheo-bronchial tree and symptoms

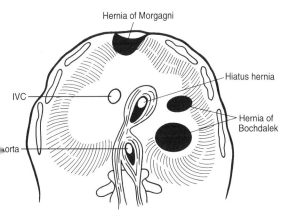

FIGURE 6.6 Various anatomical openings of the diaphragm.

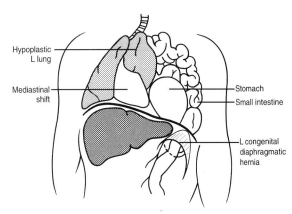

FIGURE 6.7 Diagram showing congenital diaphragmatic hernia.

may be caused by pressure on the trachea or bronchi. X-ray shows a soft tissue swelling with an air fluid level (Fig. 6.5). Treatment is excision and is usually a simple procedure.

Congenital diaphragmatic hernia

The primitive, pleural and peritoneal spaces communicate freely through the pleuro-peritoneal canal (Fig. 6.6). Between the 8th and the 10th weeks these canals are obliterated by fusion of the dorsal pleuro-peritoneal membrane with the ventral septum transversum. Failure of closure of the pleuro-peritoneal can results in the congenital diaphragmatic hernia of Bochdalek, commonly left sided (Fig. 6.7). During this process the bowel, returning to the abdomen, finds its way, together with the liver, into the chest and is partly responsible for the poor development of the lung with consequent pulmonary hypoplasia (Fig. 6.8).

In pulmonary hypoplasia there is a low ratio of lung weight to body weight. The severity of pulmonary hypoplasia is a major factor in the survival of neonates with congenital diaphragmatic hernia. In a series of 13 babies with congenital diaphragmatic hernia who died the ipselateral lung weighed 3.7 g whereas the contralateral lung weighed 13.3 g. A normal lung of the newborn should weigh 35 g. Histologically the developmental arrest appears to

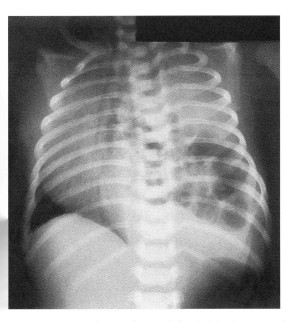

FIGURE 6.8 X-ray of chest showing left-sided diaphragmatic hernia.

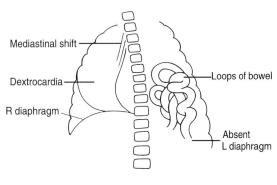

occur between 10 and 12 weeks in a left-sided congenital hernia, whereas it is a little later, 12–14 weeks, in right-sided congenital diaphragmatic hernia.

Clinical features

Within the first hours of birth the infant develops respiratory distress which worsens as air enters the bowel lying in the chest. If left alone this progresses to death from mediastinal compression and cardiac tamponade. Physical examination reveals a tachypnoeic, tachycardiac, cyanotic mottled baby with a bow shaped chest and a scaphoid abdomen.

The trachea will be deviated to the side opposite the hernia and the apex beat will be displaced. The clinical findings may be confused with those of dextrocardia in a left sided hernia.

Investigations

These include an X-ray showing all the chest and abdomen. Gas filled loops of bowel are seen in the chest. Measurements of blood gases and acid–base status are necessary to assess the level of hypoxaemia and acidosis.

Preoperative treatment

This should include early insertion of a large bore nasogastric tube with continuous suction to prevent further inflation of the bowel in the chest. The position of the tube must be confirmed by an X-ray. Oxygen should be administered via a head box if the baby is breathing adequately and, if distressed, via an endotracheal tube. Face mask oxygen must be avoided as it only encourages more air into the stomach and the chest. There is a great risk at this stage of a contralateral tension pneumothorax if the pressure needed to ventilate the baby is high. Sudden deterioration of such a baby should suggest the possibility of a contralateral tension pneumothorax and the need for a chest drain to be inserted. The urgency to operate on these babies has now been replaced by delayed surgery in order to resuscitate, stabilise the baby and assess the state of the pulmonary circulation. Operative correction is done through the abdomen and the hernia contents are replaced into the abdomen. The lung is inspected and the degree of hypoplasia is assessed. Large defects and agenesis of the diaphragm, causing a worse prognosis, are usually repaired by prosthesis. The post-operative course of these babies depends on the degree of pulmonary hypoplasia and pulmonary hypertension that may develop. Shunting can occur at three levels, at the level of foramen ovale, patent ductus arteriosus and ventilation/perfusion shunting in the lung tissue. All this results in hypoxaemia, acidosis and hypercapnia which causes worsening of the state of pulmonary hypertension. Introduction of vasodilators, such as

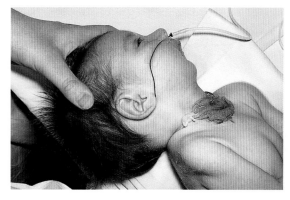

FIGURE 6.9 Pierre Robin syndrome.

tolazoline, prostacyclines and enoximone may be of value in these dire situations. More recently the introduction of ECMO (extracorporeal membrane oxygenation) and HFO (high-frequency oscillation ventilation) has allowed some of these babies to survive who would otherwise have died. Currently the value of fetal procedures is being assessed.

ACQUIRED DISORDERS

Acquired disorders of the respiratory system are common in infancy and throughout childhood. Respiratory distress in the neonatal period where the infant has tachypnoea, tachycardia, laboured breathing often with jerky movements and the accessory muscles of respiration being utilised are the end result of a variety of different causes. The infant may have peripheral or central cyanosis. The aetiology of the respiratory distress must be determined and clinical examination with chest X-ray elucidate most causes although, as always, the preceding history is of importance. The cause may be upper airway obstruction, e.g. choanal atresia; micrognathia with the tongue obstructing the airway in Pierre Robin syndrome (Fig. 6.9); secondary to space-occupying lesions e.g. cystic hygroma, congenital laryngeal anomalies; laryngeal oedema; meconium aspiration; hyaline membrane disease; tracheo-oesophageal fistula; congenital diaphragmatic hernia; or infective causes resulting in laryngotracheobronchitis, bronchiolitis or pneumonia (Table 6.1).

INFECTIONS OF THE RESPIRATORY TRACT

Every year between October and March there is a high incidence of respiratory infection in children and

TABLE 6.1 Respiratory emergencies in the newborn

CONDITION	TREATMENT
Bilateral choanal atresia	Oral airway followed by perforation of bony or cartilaginous obstruction occluding posterior nares
Pierre Robin syndrome	Nasopharyngeal suction, postural treatment, and skilled nursing
Oesophageal atresia (often with tracheo-oesophageal fistula)	Aspiration of proximal pouch. Division and closure of tracheo-oesophageal fistula and reconstruction of oesophagus
Subglottic stenosis	If severe, tracheostomy – later, correction
Pneumothorax	Needle aspiration, if severe, intercostal water-seal drain
Congenital lobar emphysema	Lobectomy
Congenital diaphragmatic hernia	Laparotomy and repair of hernia
Congestive cardiac failure	Emergency medical investigation and treatment: early operation when appropriate

adults in the countries of the northern hemisphere. Indeed, respiratory illnesses account for more disability than any other infections. Every 2 or 3 years there is a virtual epidemic of bronchiolitis among infants. The peak incidence of the respiratory infections in general is during the months December to February. These infections tend to run through individual households and there is a higher attack rate among families of four or more persons. The attack rate is higher among children than adults and is especially severe in those under 3 years.

The causal agents are a wide variety of viruses and bacteria, the former only infrequently being followed by secondary invasion of the respiratory tract by the latter. A wide range of clinical patterns, from the trivial to the fatal, can be produced by many viruses, each of which may produce an essentially similar clinical illness.

Classification of the acute respiratory disease is difficult because the isolation of viruses requires laboratory facilities which are not universally available and probably some viruses which cause respiratory disease have still to be identified. An anatomical classification is not entirely satisfactory because a single virus can affect the respiratory mucous membrane, which is continuous from the nose to the alveoli, throughout the whole or any part of its extent. In clinical practice an anatomical diagnosis, such as nasopharyngitis, tracheitis or bronchitis, indicates merely the point of maximum impact by the infective agent. It gives no indication as to its identity or total distribution. Furthermore, some of the viruses (e.g. ECHO and Coxsackie) do not confine their ravages to the respiratory tract but may also invade the gastrointestinal tract, mesenteric lymph nodes, nervous system and meninges.

Several groups of viruses are known to cause respiratory disease and each group contains a bewildering variety of serologically identifiable types. There are three main groups. The myxoviruses include the parainfluenza group, respiratory syncytial virus and influenza viruses A, B and C. The adenoviruses contain a large number of different types, some being regarded as "endemic", others as "epidemic". The picornaviruses are of two types: enteroviruses such as

Coxsackie, ECHO and Coe virus; and rhinoviruses of many serological types. There is no doubt that the respiratory syncytial virus (RSV) is now the major pathogen encountered in the severe respiratory infections of infants and young children, and that it is capable of causing death in the absence of any secondary bacterial invaders. The parainfluenza and adenoviruses, and the enteroviruses, are more likely to cause upper respiratory tract infections, which are generally less dangerous than the severe lower respiratory involvements with RSV. There is some evidence that a small percentage of children with acute respiratory disease have been infected with herpesvirus despite the fact that the conventional herpetic rash is absent. The rhinoviruses are an important cause of "colds" in adults but they do not seem to be an important cause of acute respiratory disease in very young children.

Pneumonia due to the Eaton agent of *Mycoplasma pneumoniae* is described later in this chapter, but there is evidence that this agent is also responsible for some of the upper respiratory tract infections of childhood.

Whilst a few viral infections will respond to antiviral therapy, only life-threatening infections are at present treated with these antiviral agents. None is vulnerable to the presently available antibiotics, and the vast majority of children with respiratory infections will recover safely without their use. On the other hand, antibiotics have enormously reduced the mortality from respiratory illnesses in children when they are bacterial in origin. A major problem in young children is to isolate the causal bacteria at an early stage of the illness and thus to determine the antibiotic sensitivities. The existence of a good local laboratory service, however, will allow the clinician to be kept informed of the most frequent bacterial causes of respiratory illness and of the prevalent antibiotic sensitivities.

Sudden infant death syndrome

The sudden infant death syndrome (SIDS) became a registerable cause of death in 1971 in England and

Wales. There was an apparent increase in incidence but this was largely attributable to a change in diagnostic categorisation from respiratory causes to SIDS. The cause of SIDS is still unknown but accounts for 30–50% of post neonatal infant deaths throughout the world. In Scotland in 1981–82 the SIDS rate was 2.3/1000 live births. Throughout the 1980s the rate remained stable with fluctuations between 1.9 and 2.3/1000 live births. Since 1989 the rate has dropped precipitously to 1.3/1000 live births and this may be related to improvement in four modifiable risk factors. These are prone sleeping, maternal smoking, lack of breast feeding and bed sharing. The most likely associated factor in Scotland for the reduced mortality is a reduction in prone sleeping and correction of the other important factors should result in a further decrease.

Although no clear association has yet been established between SIDS and the presence of bacterial or viral pathogens there is a suggestion that infections may act as thermal stressors which, together with other aggravating factors, such as heavy wrapping of the infant, prone position and bed sharing might result in unexplained death. In the UK there is scope for further public health action to reduce the numbers of infants sleeping in the prone position, to change parental smoking habits and to avoid excessive wrapping, particularly in infants who are unwell with upper respiratory infections.

Upper respiratory infections

Aetiology

The vast majority of cases, including those in which tonsillitis is present, are due to the viruses already mentioned. A few cases of tonsillitis and pharyngitis are due to β-haemolytic streptococci, but this is not true of the majority in whom throat swabs fail to yield pathogenic bacteria.

Clinical features

Upper respiratory infections vary widely in their clinical presentation depending upon the area of maximum involvement, the age of the patient and the causal agent. Rhinitis with nasal obstruction and a mucopurulent discharge may seriously interfere with feeding in the infant, whereas a similar "common cold" in the toddler may result only in mild malaise, low-grade fever, and nasal discomfort. In most cases, however, the pharynx shows acute hyperaemia and some oedema. There may be cervical adenitis. The presenting features are often brisk fever, irritability and anorexia. When the cause is adenovirus type 3, conjunctivitis and posterior triangle cervical lymphadenitis are often present. A generalised

convulsion may usher in the illness. Indeed, the existence of an upper respiratory infection is frequently discovered only by direct inspection of the throat because the young child rarely complains of sore throat. The importance of careful inspection of the throat and tympanic membranes in every ill, fevered child cannot be overemphasised. In other cases there is a tendency for inspiratory stridor to develop suddenly, usually during the night, so that the child awakens distressed and struggling for breath, and with a noisy, barking cough. In this type of laryngitis stridulosa the morning usually sees the child relieved, but careful medical supervision is required as in a few cases a severe and dangerous degree of laryngeal obstruction develops. When the trachea predominantly is inflamed the outstanding sign is a harsh cough, sometimes causing retrosternal pain, often worse during the night and of a character which tends to alarm parents unduly. In other cases, the prominent complaints are abdominal pain and vomiting, presumed to be due to involvement of the mesenteric lymph nodes. The differential diagnosis from appendicitis may be difficult, but the viral infections are associated with higher fever and a flushed, hot skin whereas consistent tenderness and muscle rigidity are often absent. In a few cases headache and neck stiffness may arouse the suspicion of meningitis. It is always wiser to perform a lumbar puncture than to risk leaving a pyogenic meningitis inadequately treated.

When the tonsils bear the brunt of the attack they are grossly hyperaemic and swollen. Small patches of yellow to white exudate may appear in the crypts – acute follicular tonsillitis. The lymph nodes at the angles of the jaw are usually enlarged and tender and the child is fevered, ill and miserable. While some of these cases are caused by β-haemolytic streptococci, they cannot be distinguished on clinical grounds alone from those of viral aetiology.

Scarlet fever is to be regarded as no more than streptococcal tonsillitis accompanied by a rash. It is, nowadays, a relatively mild disease.

Treatment

In the great majority of cases, simple measures will suffice. The room should be reasonably ventilated and with an ambient temperature of around 18°C (65°F). A good intake of fluids and glucose in the form of sweetened drinks must be encouraged and paracetamol may be given to reduce fever. The diet should be light and palatable and the intake of calories is unimportant in a short illness. The common practice of prescribing antibacterial drugs for every child with fever and respiratory signs is to be deplored. In most cases they can do no good, and their hurried use may mask an early meningitis, leading to inadequate or misdirected treatment. A throat swab should always be taken for culture when the pharynx is inflamed although most pharyngeal infections are viral in origin.

Complications of upper respiratory infection

The most common is spread to the lower respiratory tract in various forms – bronchitis, bronchiolitis, pneumonia – which are separately discussed. When chest radiographs are taken of children with upper respiratory infections, it is quite common to find areas of atelectatic pneumonitis or aspiration pneumonia which are segmental or lobar in distribution. While this condition may produce physical signs such as diminished resonance but good air entry, or a few crepitations, it is often only recognised radiologically. Indeed, this type of aspiration pneumonia is much more common than purely clinical diagnosis might suggest. Resolution is usual and may be assisted by physiotherapy and forced coughing. Complications of upper respiratory infections are less common and much less dangerous since the availability of antibiotics. It is sensible to observe each child carefully until recovery takes place, or until a definite bacterial complication justifies the use of an antibacterial drug.

Acute otitis media

This is a relatively common complication, especially in young infants who lie supine for much of the day and in whom the Eustachian tube is short and straight. It can only be diagnosed by making inspection of the tympanic membranes through an auriscope part of the routine examination of every infant. Older children will usually, although not invariably, complain of earache. Fever and malaise are usual and meningism may be present. In catarrhal otitis media the drum is red and injected. In suppurative cases it is seen to be bulging and it may pulsate. In neglected cases perforation of the drum occurs and it is then obscured by a profuse purulent discharge. Spread to involve the mastoid air cells has become uncommon. The commonest organisms in otitis media are *Pneumococcus* and *H. influenzae* and a number of other less common bacteria and viruses such as influenza, parainfluenza and RSV.

Treatment

Treatment of the acute infection involves symptomatic measures to relieve pain and reduce the fever with paracetamol. Antibiotics are commonly used, the most frequent being penicillin, amoxycillin, erythromycin or trimethoprim. Treatment is usually given for 5–7 days but may be longer if inspection of the tympanic membrane does not reveal a satisfactory

response. Drainage of the middle ear may be necessary on occasion when the infection is not responding to conservative treatment. Acute mastoiditis is much less common and similarly failure to respond to antibiotic therapy is the indication for surgical drainage. It is also valuable in identifying the causative organism by culture of the pus.

Acute sinusitis

Some degree of sinusitis occurs in most upper respiratory infections and most often recovers spontaneously. In older children acute empyema of a sinus may occasionally develop and cause severe pain. This is usually over the maxillary antrum or the frontal sinus. However, when the sphenoidal sinus is involved the pain is suboccipital in distribution, and it may be over the temple and mastoid when the ethmoid cells are involved. Radiographs will reveal opacity of the affected paranasal sinus. Pathogenic organisms causing this problem include pneumococci, group A streptococci, *Haemophilus influenzae* and occasionally staphylococci.

Treatment

Treatment consists of symptomatic measures to reduce pain and fever and the administration of antibiotics including amoxycillin, erythromycin or trimethoprim.

Acute retropharyngeal abscess

This once common emergency has become rare. The child has severe difficulty in swallowing. He often assumes a characteristic position with his elbows on a table, head supported on his hands and neck hyperextended so as to widen the airway and relieve his respiratory difficulty. Lateral radiographs of the neck will reveal the mass in the pharyngeal region. This method of examination also serves to exclude the rare case in which the abscess is secondary to tuberculosis of the cervical spine. Life can be in serious danger if a retropharyngeal abscess is allowed to rupture spontaneously because the pus may flood into the larynx, burst into a blood vessel with severe haemorrhage, or even reach the mediastinum.

Treatment

Flucloxacillin should be started without awaiting the results of the preliminary throat swab. Drainage of the abscess should be performed but the pharyngeal oedema is potentially a serious problem to the child's airway and an experienced anaesthetist is necessary.

Peritonsillar abscess (quinsy)

This is common in childhood. It usually follows an acute streptococcal tonsillitis and is exceedingly painful. It interferes with swallowing, speech becomes "thick" and a characteristic sign is difficulty in opening the mouth. The tonsillar area is swollen, red and the oedematous uvula is often displaced to the opposite side.

Treatment

If fluctutation is present it is better to incise the abscess than to let it rupture spontaneously and this should be followed by an interval tonsillectomy.

ACUTE INFLAMMATORY OBSTRUCTION OF THE UPPER AIRWAYS

The two commonest causes of acute inflammatory obstruction in children are croup and epiglottitis (Table 6.2).

Acute laryngotracheobronchitis (croup)

Croup is a disorder in which the child develops stridor, a barking cough and respiratory difficulties, usually worse at night time. A variety of names for the disorder collectively known as croup have been used in the past and include laryngotracheobronchitis, laryngitis and laryngotracheitis. Viral croup usually occurs in children between the ages of 18 months and 3 years. There is a bacterial or pseudomembranous croup which is a severe form of tracheitis affecting children usually over the age of 5 years. In this less common disorder an inflammatory, membranous exudate lines the tracheal and subglottic areas.

Aetiology

The most common infectious agent is the parainfluenza virus but RSV and rhinoviruses can be implicated. In bacterial croup *Staphylococcus aureus*, streptococci and *H. influenzae* are the commonest pathogens. These may be secondary to a preceding viral infection.

Clinical features

A coryzal illness develops over 1–2 days and is complicated by a harsh barking cough with marked inspiratory stridor when the child is disturbed. He may be restless with cyanosis and subcostal and inter-

TABLE 6.2 Features of croup and epiglottitis

	CROUP	EPIGLOTTITIS
Age	<3 years	2–7 years
Aetiology	Parainfluenza virus	*H. influenzae* type b
Prodromal	Coryza	Sore throat, dysphagia and unable to talk
Temperature	<38°C	>38°C
Breathing	Barking cough	Drooling
	Loud stridor	Muffled stridor
	Rarely need intubation (3%)	Almost all will require intubation

costal indrawing, suggesting impending obstruction. Although respiratory obstruction rarely occurs in viral croup it is important that these signs are treated seriously. On occasion the bacterial form of croup, like epiglottitis, is a more severe illness. Other causes of croup should also be considered, mainly foreign body inhalation, an acute allergic reaction, retropharyngeal abscess and diphtheria in a child who has not been immunised. The main differential diagnosis is from acute epiglottitis. A small number of children have recurrent episodes of croup. These may be viral or allergic in origin and an underlying abnormality, such as subglottic stenosis, could be a predisposing factor. If epiglottitis is suspected no attempt should be made to visualise the throat unless facilities for endotracheal intubation are immediately available because of the risk of acute airway obstruction.

Treatment

The decision of when to admit a child to hospital because of croup is a difficult one. Severe continuous stridor with marked chest recession, restlessness, tachycardia and irritability also suggest significant upper airway obstruction and immediate admission to an intensive care facility is essential. The child should not be separated from the parents as crying may exacerbate the severity of the inflammation in the throat. When children are admitted to hospital many will not require oxygen but with the use of transcutaneous oxygen saturation monitors it is possible to decide readily when to administer additional oxygen. A number of treatments have been recommended including increased humidity both cold and hot, corticosteroids and sedatives but none has been proven in standard clinical trial conditions. Humidified oxygen therapy will be given on the basis of oxygen saturation measurements and a broad spectrum antibiotic, such as a third generation cephalosporin, should be given intravenously for bacterial croup. Antibiotics are not required for the treatment of viral croup. If the child deteriorates with exhaustion, tachycardia and hypoxaemia, a skilled paediatric anaesthetist will be required to induce anaesthesia and carry out orotracheal inspection and an endotracheal tube inserted. Fortunately only 3% of all cases of croup require such therapy.

Epiglottitis

This is a disease of sudden onset and rapid progression occurring in children slightly older than those who develop croup (2–7 years). There has usually been a preceding sore throat and pyrexia with difficulty in swallowing which precedes the stridor and breathing difficulties. Unlike croup, the breathing may be muffled and quiet and is usually accompanied by the signs of upper airway obstruction. Often the child will be sitting up supported by his hands (tripod sign) and over a period of 2–3 hours can become very ill with drooling, hoarseness and loss of voice and the development of a greyish cyanosis. As the hypoxia increases both the respiratory and heart rates increase and the child may develop respiratory arrest.

Aetiology

The most common pathogenic organism involved in acute epiglottitis in childhood is *Haemophilus influenzae* and it can often be isolated in blood cultures. In some cases the haemophilus may have been preceded by infections with the respiratory syncytial virus or occasionally the parainfluenza viruses, types l, 2 and 3, more commonly associated with croup.

Treatment

On admission to hospital the first essentials are oxygen, high humidity and a cool environment. Intravenous antibiotics should be given after a blood culture has been taken. It is essential that before distressing procedures, such as blood sampling, are undertaken, intensive care facilities are immediately available. If a clinical diagnosis of severe epiglottitis has been made then the withdrawal of blood should be delayed until after intubation. Also no attempt should be made to visualise the throat because of the risk of acute airway obstruction. After induction of anaesthesia, on laryngoscopy typically a large swollen ocdcmatous cherry-red epiglottis is seen. Chloramphenicol or a third generation cephalosporin should be used since an increasing number of *Haemophilus influenzae* are resistant to ampicillin. If not already intubated, arrangements for laryngeal intubation or tracheotomy should be kept in constant readiness and if such a life-saving procedure is considered it should be undertaken earlier rather than later. It should be performed in any patient in whom the respiratory difficulty worsens in spite of treatment and when there is diminishing air entry over the lungs. An adequate fluid intake is important, by mouth if possible. The usefulness of steroid therapy is very doubtful. The prognosis for children who recover from acute epiglottitis is excellent and the recurrence of this condition is uncommon. With the introduction of *Haemophilus influenzae* b (Hib) immunisation there should be a reduction in the prevalence of acute epiglottis.

ACUTE BRONCHITIS

Aetiology

Most cases of acute bronchitis are due to an extension downwards of an upper respiratory viral infection, or they form part of the clinical spectrum of diseases such as measles, influenza, whooping cough or typhoid fever. Secondary bacterial infection by pneumococci, *H. influenzae* or staphylococci infrequently aggravates the damage to the bronchial tree.

Clinical features

The usual history is of a preceding upper respiratory illness with sudden worsening of fever, cough, malaise and anorexia. Most children are not very ill, although infants may become dyspnoeic and toxic.

The cough is initially unproductive but later sputum may be coughed up by the older child or vomited during spasms of coughing by the infant. Physical signs over the lungs consist of rhonchi and crepitations which vary considerably in severity and do not have a close correlation with the severity of the illness. Recovery usually begins after a week and serious sequelae such as bronchiectasis are rare.

Treatment

In the vast majority of cases the simple palliative measures described under "upper respiratory infections" will be sufficient treatment and spontaneous recovery can be expected. There is no evidence that the so-called expectorant mixtures have any useful effects and the use of cough suppressants is illogical. Antibiotics are rarely required but they should be used when the child is toxic or dyspnoeic. Oxygen is only rarely required for children with simple bronchitis.

ACUTE BRONCHIOLITIS OF INFANCY

Aetiology

This is a disease which is only seen in infancy. It occurs in epidemic form every 2 or 3 years during the

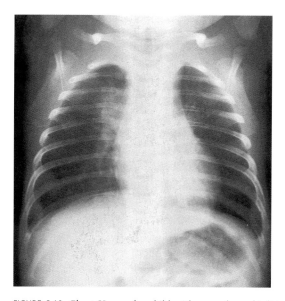

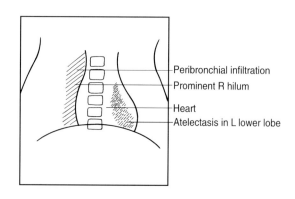

Peribronchial infiltration
Prominent R hilum
Heart
Atelectasis in L lower lobe

FIGURE 6.10 Chest X-ray of a child with acute bronchiolitis.

winter months. The great majority of cases are due to respiratory syncytial virus (RSV) which is, indeed, the most common cause of lower respiratory tract infections in infants and young children, although other viruses including parainfluenza and adenovirus can cause similar symptoms.

Clinical features

There is normally a preceding history of upper respiratory catarrh and slight cough. The infant then becomes acutely ill with inspiratory difficulty, resulting in visible subcostal and intercostal recession, but there is also marked expiratory difficulty and wheezing or grunting. Severe spasms of coughing may so interfere with feeding as to lead to dehydration. This is further aggravated by tachypnoea and increased insensible loss of water from the lungs. Hypoxia is reflected in agitation and restlessness and there may be cyanosis. Tachycardia is marked but the temperature rarely rises above 38°C (101°F) and may, in fact, be normal. Bilateral obstructive emphysema causes the chest to be held in the inspiratory position and the percussion note is hyper-resonant. The breath sounds are diminished and there may be rhonchi or numerous crepitations. Radiographs of the chest show increased lung markings due to interstitial infiltrations and often overinflation with increased translucency of the lungs (Fig. 6.10). In the most distressed infants the P_{O_2} of arterial or arterialised capillary blood may be found to be dangerously low, and in these circumstances the P_{CO_2} is likely to be raised with a low blood pH. This respiratory acidosis and hypoxaemia may further be associated with a metabolic acidosis.

It is now possible for the virologist to confirm rapidly the presence of respiratory syncytial and other viruses in the nasopharyngeal secretions by means of immunofluorescent antibody techniques.

Treatment

Treatment is mainly supportive. The infant should be nursed propped up in a humid atmosphere enriched with oxygen. The absence of cyanosis is an unreliable indication of a normal arterial oxygen tension, and our practice is to monitor transcutaneous oxygen saturation in very dyspnoeic infants. The arterialised capillary blood P_{O_2} should whenever possible be maintained above 70 mmHg (9.3 kPa) and oxygen saturation above 97%. In a very few cases it is impossible to achieve satisfactory P_{O_2} levels even in high oxygen concentrations, and when the P_{CO_2} level in these circumstances rises to 70 mmHg (9.3 kPa) or higher, tracheal intubation and intermittent positive-pressure ventilation may save the infant's life.

An adequate fluid intake is important and if the infant refuses feeds a dextrose-electrolyte fluid such as BPC, BNF sodium chloride, dextrose oral powder small size, or Dioralyte may be substituted. Maintenance of hydration may also require feeds or fluids to be given by nasogastric tube and it is occasionally necessary to give intravenous fluids.

Antibiotics are not given unless there is evidence of secondary bacterial infection. Infants with severe disease should be screened for cystic fibrosis and immune deficiency as both can present in this way. The most useful agent for specific treatment of this infection is ribavirin, an antiviral agent that has activity against RSV. Specific indications for treating high-risk hosts include proven RSV infection in newborns, immunocompromised patients and in those with serious underlying pulmonary or cardiovascular conditions. Ribavirin is aerosolised directly into the trachea or into the inspired air via mask, hood or tent over 16–18 hours usually for 3–7 days. Most infants with RSV bronchiolitis appear to make a complete clinical recovery. However, some infants who recover continue to have recurrent wheezing attacks.

ACUTE BACTERIAL PNEUMONIA

An aetiological classification of the bacterial pneumonias would be of more practical value to the clinician, who is now armed with effective antibacterial drugs, than the traditional subdivision into bronchopneumonia and lobar pneumonia.

Unfortunately, sputum is rarely obtainable from young children, and bacteria grown from the nose or throat are not necessarily those present in the lung. None the less, it is often possible from a knowledge of the epidemiology of the common pulmonary infections in a region, to hazard a shrewd guess as to the probable bacterial cause in the individual patient with pneumonia. This is also influenced by the age of the patient.

Bacterial pneumonia in infancy

Aetiology

In Britain today the most common bacterial causes of pneumonia during the first year of life are *Staphylococcus aureus* and *Haemophilus influenzae*. Pneumonia is frequently preceded by a viral infection of the respiratory tract which presumably damages the mucous membranes and permits its penetration by bacteria. Pneumococcal pneumonia, which was the common type in the pre-antibiotic era, has become relatively rare in the young infant. Occasional cases are due to streptococci and coliforms.

Pathology

The striking features in the staphylococcal cases are massive consolidation, destruction of tissue, abscess formation and the frequent appearances of emphysematous bullae. When these rupture into the pleural cavity the result is pyopneumothorax. In pneumococcal cases the lobular areas of consolidation rarely suppurate and empyema has become unknown.

Clinical features

There is frequently a preceding upper respiratory infection. The infant then becomes acutely ill, fevered,

irritable and restless. Feeds are taken reluctantly. Dyspnoea is associated with inspiratory dilatation of the alae nasi and expiratory grunting. There may be subcostal recession. Cough is severe and may precipitate vomiting. Diarrhoea may occur. Meningism is relatively uncommon. Early in the illness there may be only a few crepitations over the lungs. In staphylococcal cases dullness on percussion over the affected areas, with bronchial or diminished breath sounds, becomes quickly obvious. The presence of consolidation can be confirmed radiologically. As the disease progresses, radiographs frequently reveal emphysematous bullae (pneumatoceles) (Fig. 6.11) an appearance pathognomonic of staphylococcal pneumonia. Abscess formation may occasionally be demonstrable with fluid levels in the cavities.

Treatment

The mortality from bronchopneumonia in infancy is now very low, whereas in the pre-antibiotic days it was high, and staphylococcal cases were invariably fatal. Treatment is by supportive measures and with broad spectrum antibiotics until an organism has been identified. If the causal organisms can be isolated from sputum or laryngeal swab the antibiotic can be more accurately chosen according to the bacterial sensitivities. Severe dypsnoea or cyanosis is an indication for oxygen therapy. An adequate intake of fluids must be ensured. The importance of monitoring the oxygen saturation and concentration and the desirability of PCO_2 measurements in arterial or capillary blood in severely ill infants has already been discussed under the treatment of acute bronchiolitis.

Bacterial pneumonia in the older child

Aetiology

The great majority of cases are due to pneumococci which are sensitive to benzylpenicillin. Although type-specific sera are available for many of the 32 types of pneumococci, they are now rarely used.

Pathology

Post-mortem studies of pneumonia in older children are now fortunately exceedingly rare. The classical four stages of congestion, red hepatization, grey hepatization and resolution are well known. Complications such as empyema, pyopericardium, lung abscess and bacterial endocarditis are also rarely seen today.

Clinical features

The onset is sudden with high fever, malaise and cough. Pain in the chest or abdomen on the affected

Trachea

Thin-walled cysts
or pneumatoceles

Heart

Consolidation

Normal left lung

FIGURE 6.11 Staphylococcal pneumonia. Chest X-ray of 18-month-old
child with opacification of the right lung and numerous cystic areas due
to developing pneumatoceles.

side is common, but rarely as severe as in adults.
Meningism is not infrequent, especially when the
upper lobes are involved. A rigor is not common in
the child and a convulsion may herald the onset of
the illness. Tachypnoea is the rule but severe
dyspnoea or cyanosis is uncommon. Circumoral
pallor, inspiratory dilatation of the alae nasi and an
expiratory grunt frequently constitute a characteristic
clinical picture. The movement of the affected side of
the chest is diminished. Pleural friction is inconstant
and usually transient. Dullness on percussion is the
most definite sign while bronchial breath sounds and
fine crepitations are found in typical cases. In many
children the physical signs are remarkably slight in
contrast to the segmental or lobar area of consolidation revealed by radiography (Fig. 6.12). The white
cell count is raised but in childhood is of little
prognostic significance.

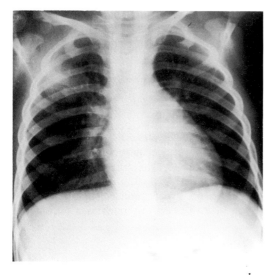

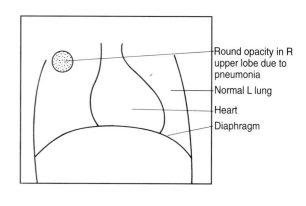

Round opacity in R
upper lobe due to
pneumonia

Normal L lung

Heart

Diaphragm

FIGURE 6.12 Chest X-ray of a child with circular pneumonia.

Treatment

The drug of choice is benzylpenicillin 500 000 units given intravenously four times daily for 3–4 days, after which oral penicillin V, 250 mg 6-hourly, may be substituted for a further few days. An adequate fluid intake is important. So-called "expectorants" or cough mixtures have no value. Oxygen is only frequently required in older children suffering from pneumonia.

Primary atypical pneumonia

This is relatively rare in children. Many cases diagnosed as "primary atypical pneumonia" are, in fact, examples of aspiration pneumonia secondary to upper respiratory catarrh but there are undoubtedly cases of primary viral pneumonia.

Aetiology

Most cases are due to a virus-like agent which is a mycoplasma – *Mycoplasma pneumoniae*. Some cases are really examples of psittacosis or ornithosis due to contact with sick parrots or budgerigars. The causal organism is in those circumstances *Chlamydia psittaci*. Another example of atypical pneumonia occurs secondary to *Coxiella burnetii* infection, the agent which causes Q fever.

Pathology

There is infiltration of the bronchiolar walls, alveolar septa and interstitial tissues by mononuclear cells. The alveoli are often free of exudate but may be filled with a mixture of fibrin and mononuclear cells.

Clinical features

The incubation period is 10–21 days. The onset is with headache, shivering, malaise and fever. Cough develops subsequently and blood staining of the sputum may be observed. There may be remarkably few physical signs over the lungs, often only a few localised crepitations, but the radiograph shows patchy consolidation confined to one or two lobes. Leucocytosis is absent. The somewhat delayed onset of cough contrasts with the situation in the much more common aspiration pneumonia, where cough has often preceded the constitutional upset. The nature of the causal organisms can be determined by sending a first specimen of blood to the virologist at the onset of the illness and a second specimen 10–14 days later. A rising antibody titre will be found for the specific agent. In the case of mycoplasma infections an early diagnosis is available from the application of immunofluorescent antibody techniques to the sputum or nasopharyngeal secretions.

Treatment

Spontaneous recovery usually takes place after an illness of 2–3 weeks' duration. Cases due to mycoplasma and *Coxiella burnetii* respond favourably to erythromycin (50 mg/kg/day).

Interstitial plasma-cell pneumonia

Aetiology

This type of lung infection is a common cause of death in early infancy in some central and northern European countries. It is, however, rarely seen in Britain or the USA, except in association with such conditions as HIV infection, hypogammaglobulinaemia, cytomegalic inclusion body disease and various malignant diseases when given immunosuppressive treatments such as radiotherapy, steroids and cytotoxic drugs. The infective agent is a protozoan, *Pneumocystis carinii*.

Pathology

The alveoli are filled with an apparently acellular exudate which shows a honeycomb appearance in sections. In the infant the alveolar septa are infiltrated by plasma cells, but these are conspicuous by their absence in cases associated with hypogammaglobulinaemia. When special staining methods are used the alveolar exudate is seen to be composed of parasites.

Clinical features

The predominant feature is progressively severe dyspnoea and cyanosis which contrast with the paucity of physical signs over the lungs. Radiographs show a characteristic symmetrical ground-glass opacity spreading outwards from the lung roots. Areas of lobular collapse may give a finely mottled appearance and emphysema is common. Interstitial emphysema or spontaneous pneumothorax may occur. The organism may be identified during life in material obtained by lung puncture or in tracheal and bronchial secretions obtained by intubation and bronchoscopy.

Treatment

Treatment of pneumocystis pneumonia consists of high-dose trimethoprim and sulphamethoxazole (20 mg/kg/day and 100 mg/kg/day respectively) for a period of 10–14 days. This should be given intravenously initially although it is also effective orally.

Good results have been reported with pentamidine isethionate 4 mg/kg/day given by intramuscular injection (but there are toxic side effects). It may be more effective and less toxic when given in nebulised form, in preventing relapse in susceptible individuals.

ASPIRATION SYNDROME – ABSORPTION COLLAPSE (ATELECTASIS) OF THE LUNGS

Resorption of air from a pulmonary segment or lobe is common in young children due to complete bronchial occlusion ("stop valve"). The thin-walled bronchi and bronchioles can be compressed by enlarged lymph nodes in tuberculosis, measles, pertussis and malignant reticulosis. The narrow lumens can be blocked by mucopus, inhaled foreign bodies or stomach contents, and by mucosal oedema due to allergy in asthmatic subjects.

Pathology

The atelectatic portion of lung occupies a smaller volume than normal. This causes compensatory emphysema of the other lobes of the lung, mediastinal shift to the affected side, a rise in the level of the diaphragm and by some falling inwards of the chest wall.

Clinical features

The features will largely depend upon the primary disease. It is important to remember that while the inhalation of a foreign body produces immediate respiratory distress with coughing, choking, gagging, stridor and cyanosis, it is possible for this short episode to pass unobserved in the case of a toddler. There may be quite a long "silent" interval before secondary bacterial infection in the obstructed bronchus produces symptoms. Foreign bodies composed of vegetable matter, e.g. peanuts, result in early severe bronchitis with fever, cough and dyspnoea, whereas metallic or plastic substances may remain *in situ* for long periods without giving rise to obvious trouble. A segment of atelectasis may be obscured clinically by compensatory emphysema and the condition becomes obvious only when postero-anterior radiographs are examined (Fig. 6.13a,b). When a lobe or whole lung is collapsed there is diminished movement of the affected side of the chest with impaired resonance, diminished breath sounds and tracheal or mediastinal shift towards the affected side. Collapse of an upper lobe can be differentiated from consolidation on the radiograph by the fact that in the former the lower border is convex, whereas in

the latter it forms a straight line. A collapsed lower lobe is visualised as a jib-shaped shadow. The airless right middle lobe is seen in the lateral view as a triangular shadow.

Treatment

This largely depends upon the aetiology and often involves the use of a suitable antibiotic. Bronchoscopy is essential wherever there is a possibility of an inhaled foreign body, or if the atelectasis fails to respond to more conservative treatment. Postural drainage with percussion over the affected lobe is valuable. Rapid re-expansion must be achieved if bronchiectasis is to be avoided.

BRONCHIECTASIS

Aetiology

Bronchiectasis is almost always an acquired disease. Two factors are commonly present:

1 bronchial occlusion with absorption atelectasis;
2 infection which is usually due to pyogenic bacteria such as pneumococcus, haemophilus and staphylococcus, but may sometimes be tuberculous.

The diseases most commonly preceding bronchiectasis are bronchopneumonia, measles, pertussis, cystic fibrosis, inhaled foreign body or primary tuberculosis. A very few cases may be related to some congenital weakness in the bronchial walls, structural abnormality of the lung such as sequestered lobe, or ciliary dyskinesia.

Social background

Bronchiectasis is nowadays much less common due to the use of antibiotics. It is mainly encountered in children from the poorer sections of the community who live in overcrowded conditions which expose them to repeated respiratory infections, who have poorer nutrition and, moreover, are less likely to receive an adequate convalescence after acute illnesses such as measles and pneumonia. A persistent cough is also less likely to receive adequate medical attention.

Clinical features

The bronchiectatic patient of a bygone era reached a pitiful state in which his putrid breath made him a burden to his fellows and himself. Sputum was abundant and malodorous. Exertion precipitated distressing outbursts of coughing and dyspnoea. Th

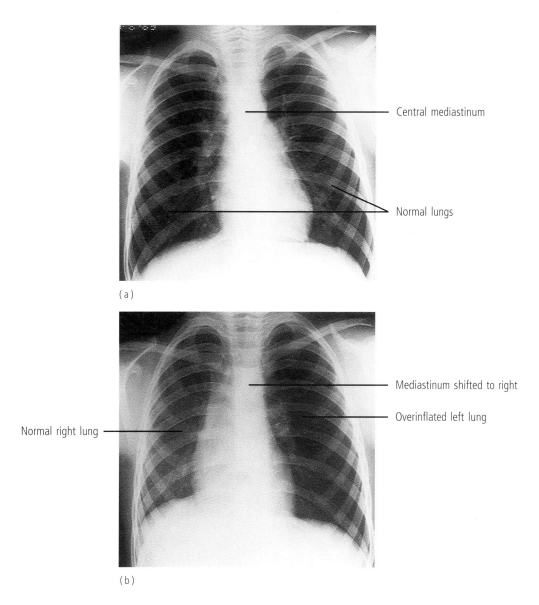

(a)

Central mediastinum

Normal lungs

(b)

Normal right lung

Mediastinum shifted to right

Overinflated left lung

FIGURE 6.13 Inhalation of foreign body. (a) The chest film is normal in inspiration. (b) In expiration the mediastinum swings to the normal right side; air is trapped in the left lung by a foreign body in the left main bronchus and the lung cannot deflate. It is overinflated and hyperlucent. The plastic top of a pen was found in the left bronchus on bronchoscopy.

fingers and toes were grossly clubbed. Cachexia was marked. Death finally resulted from empyema, brain abscess, cor pulmonale or amyloid disease.

The clinical presentation today is very different. The child is usually brought to the physician because of persistent cough, dating often from an acute respiratory illness some months or years previously. In a few male cases the bronchiectasis is a feature of congenital hypogammaglobulinaemia. In others it is part of the clinical spectrum of cystic fibrosis. Purulent sputum is obtainable but it is usually neither abundant nor malodorous. Haemoptysis, common in the adult, is a rare sign in the child. He is, however, likely to suffer from periodic episodes of fever and malaise, with aggravation of his cough, due to the retention of infected secretions within the bronchiectatic area of lung. None the less, his general condition is often remarkably good and clubbing of the fingers is usually quite slight. Physical signs over the lungs are variable. There may be an impaired percussion note, diminished breath sounds and mediastinal shift to the affected side. After the dilated bronchi have been emptied of pus by postural drainage the breath sounds may become bronchial or amphoric with whispering pectoriloquy. In some cases there are numerous crepitations over the

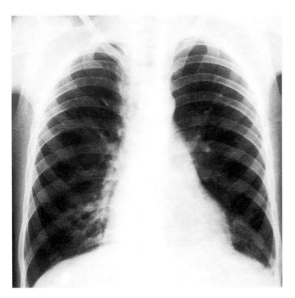
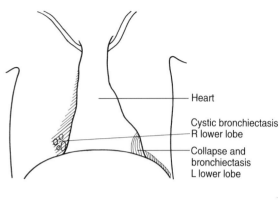

Heart

Cystic bronchiectasis
R lower lobe

Collapse and
bronchiectasis
L lower lobe

FIGURE 6.14 Bronchiectasis.

diseased lobe. Chronic sinusitis is an almost invariable accompaniment, although the causal relationship of one to the other is not clear although ciliary damage may be the common factor.

Radiographs may reveal cavities in the saccular type of bronchiectasis whereas in the more common cylindrical type there are only heavy linear markings or, sometimes, no obvious abnormality (Fig. 6.14). Confirmation of the diagnosis and estimation of the extent of the process can be obtained from well planned bronchography. Bronchoscopy is frequently informative and imperative when there is a suspicion of foreign body. Sputum should be cultured from time to time to assist in the choice of suitable antibiotics. The most common predominating organism is *H. influenzae*. When staphylococci or pseudomonas are isolated the probability of cystic fibrosis is high. In male children it is wise always to measure serum immunoglobulin values.

Treatment

Conscientiously followed medical treatment with efficient supervision usually permits the child to live a normal life, to attend school regularly and to grow into adulthood, even although established bronchiectasis is irreversible. The most important measure is postural drainage, performed at least twice daily. The child should lie prone with his head and chest over the side of the bed and supported by his hands on the floor. Vigorous coughing, assisted by gravity, produces sputum and empties the dilated bronchi. Percussion over the affected lobe helps to dislodge tenacious mucopus. Following the postural drainage the child should be encouraged to breathe slowly and deeply for

10 minutes. Febrile episodes should be treated promptly with antibiotics chosen according to the results of sputum cultures and bacterial sensitivities.

Lobectomy should only be considered after medical treatment has been tried for a prolonged period and has failed to control the recurrent infection. Operation is advisable when the bronchiectasis is confined to one, or at most two, lobes and when the remainder of the bronchial tree is reasonably free from infection. In some patients with cystic fibrosis – a generalised disease – there can still be a place for lobectomy when one lobe is acting as a reservoir from which infection spreads to the other lobes. Lung transplant may eventually be necessary.

THE CATARRHAL CHILD

The catarrhal child is one of the common and unsolved problems of paediatrics. Very little is known about the aetiological factors in this type of child and this is reflected in the widely different methods which physicians employ in management. It is important to realise that frequent "head colds" are the normal experience of children during the age period 3–8 years. Three to six such colds a year is not out of the way, but in most children recovery is complete between colds. It can be assumed that these colds are caused by a considerable variety of viruses and that in this fashion a child develops immunity. The "catarrhal child" is one who suffers from frequently recurrent respiratory infections, some of which lead to lower respiratory tract involvement with cough and wheezy rhonchi – "wheezy bronchitis".

Complete loss of symptoms rarely occurs between these episodes, these being nasal obstruction and sinusitis. Most infections are caused by respiratory viruses, bacteria being present in less than 10% of all infections. While in some children wheezy bronchitis seems to merge with asthma, most are not overtly atopic and spontaneous recovery takes place after the ages of 7–10 years.

Management

Many catarrhal children seem to possess parents who worry unduly. At least, so it has seemed to us, who have been only too familiar with the problem, but recognise from experience that at the end of the day the child will "outgrow" his susceptibility to respiratory catarrh. On the other hand, from the parents' viewpoint the physician must frequently appear comparatively impotent when called upon to bring immediate relief. Perhaps his most useful role is to take the time to explain the nature of the problem to the parents and to reassure them as to its relatively benign nature and good long-term prognosis. Some parents also need assurance that they themselves are in no way to blame for the child's repeated, but not severe, illnesses. In particular, parents frequently seek relief from their unspoken fears that the child may have tuberculosis, asthma or some other perceived grave disorder. They must be dissuaded from overprotecting the child by keeping him indoors whenever the weather in inclement, by overclothing him, and by keeping him unnecessarily away from school. In acute febrile episodes an automatic resort to antibiotics is certainly unwise. Indeed, the treatment may then prove more dangerous than the disease. They are only indicated when pathogenic bacteria are isolated from the throat swab or sputum or if the child remains highly fevered and ill after 3 days. In most cases relief can be obtained from rest in bed for a few days, and if there is nasal obstruction, from the short-term use of a nasal decongestant. The so-called expectorants are of no value.

Sooner or later the parents will raise the question of removal of tonsils and adenoids, if this has not already been discussed with them by their medical adviser. The more experienced the physician the more familiar he will have become with the disappointment of parents who have found little change in their child's catarrhal state after this operation. There is, undoubtedly, a failure by many physicians to appreciate the naturally good prognosis in sinobronchitis and a tendency too easily to succumb to the parents' pressure that "something must be done". There are, of course, certain clear indications for removal of the tonsils and adenoids:

1 recurrent attacks of acute follicular tonsillitis, especially associated with quinsy;
2 recurrent attacks of acute otitis media;
3 persistent or recurrent visible enlargement of the cervical lymph nodes.

The mere size of the tonsils is not a reliable guide to the degree of chronic infection.

EMPHYSEMA IN CHILDHOOD

During infancy and childhood obstructive emphysema is the most common type. It may involve one lobe when a primary bronchus is partially obstructed to a degree which permits the entry of air into the alveoli, but obstructs its egress during expiration (check valve). This is seen in primary tuberculosis but may also be caused by an inhaled foreign body. In lobar obstructive emphysema the lobe is overdistended with air. There is usually an "asthmatoid" wheeze at the open mouth with hyperresonance and diminished breath sounds over the affected side of the chest. The mediastinum is displaced towards the opposite side and the ribs may even be separated. The radiograph confirms this and shows increased translucency in the emphysematous lobe which may in fact herniate across the midline.

Check-valve obstruction in the bronchioles results in generalised bilateral obstructive emphysema. This can occur temporarily in acute bronchiolitis, or in a chronic form which can lead to cor pulmonale in cystic fibrosis. Generalised emphysema is uncommon in asthma during childhood. Radiographs reveal hypertranslucency in both lung fields, flattening and diminished excursions of the diaphragm and the ribs tend to be horizontally placed instead of being "tiled".

Bullous emphysema is seem most often in staphylococcal pneumonia when multiple bullae or pneumatoceles develop. If these rupture into the mediastinum a rapidly fatal *interstitial emphysema* without or with spontaneous pneumothorax results. *Subcutaneous emphysema* with palpable crackling under the skin may arise from interstitial emphysema or from perforation of the trachea, pharynx or oesophagus. It may also complicate thoracentesis. Interstitial emphysema and pneumothorax may also complicate attempts at resuscitation of the newborn by tracheal intubation and the administration of air or oxygen under pressure.

Treatment

This obviously depends upon the cause. When a tension pneumothorax develops, thoracocentesis can be life saving.

PNEUMOTHORAX

Aetiology

Establishing respiration in the neonatal period is a major change which most infants successfully achieve

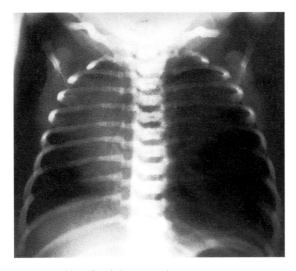

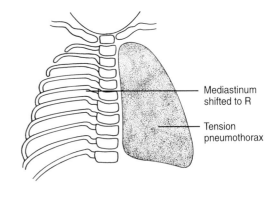

FIGURE 6.15(a) Left-sided pneumothorax.

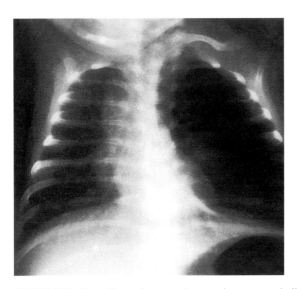

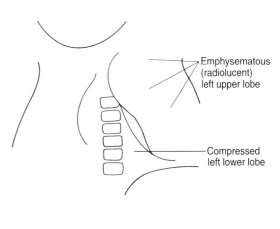

FIGURE 6.15(b) Chest X-ray showing giant emphysematous bulla.

with rapid uniform aeration of the lungs. In some infants, particularly the preterm who may have a surfactant deficiency, the lungs do not aerate evenly and the baby may generate patchy areas of high intra-alveolor pressures with resultant emphysematous ballooning of alveoli which may rupture through the visceral pleura and result in a pneumothorax. This is a more common complication in infants requiring resuscitation and intermittent positive-pressure ventilation. When air continues to leak into the pleural cavity a tension pneumothorax ensues with displacement of the mediastinum and compression of the contralateral lung.

Clinical features

When the pneumothorax is small the lung falls away from the chest wall ("relaxation collapse") but there will be no signs directly referable to the pneumothorax. A tension pneumothorax with a strongly positive intrapleural pressure ("compression collapse") causes severe pain, dyspnoea, cyanosis and circulatory collapse. There is hyper-resonance over the affected side and the breath sounds are distant or inaudible. The mediastinum and trachea may be displaced to the opposite side. When there is fluid as well as air in the pleural cavity gurgling or splashing may be heard as the child's position is moved. Transillumination or a radiograph will confirm the diagnosis, although in the infant there may be difficulty in differentiating pneumothorax from a large diaphragmatic hernia or giant emphysematous bulla (Fig. 6.15).

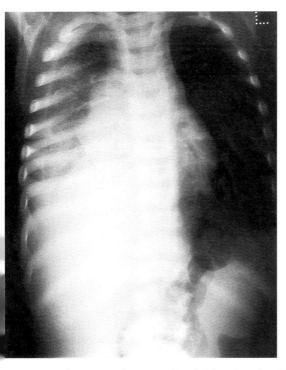
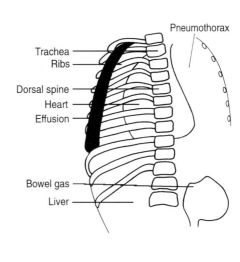

FIGURE 6.16 Chest X-ray showing right-sided lamellar pleural effusion and left-sided pneumothorax.

Treatment

Direct treatment of the pneumothorax itself is only urgently required when there is tension and acute respiratory embarrassment. Temporary relief can be obtained by aspiration with a needle or cannula inserted through an intercostal space into the pleural cavity with a three-way tap between the syringe and cannula. A suitable cannula or catheter should be inserted into the pleural cavity and plastic tubing led to below the level of the chest and an underwater seal or to a Heimlich valve. If air continues to collect and bubble out from the end of the tubing, negative-pressure drainage should be instituted. The leak usually heals spontaneously and rarely requires surgical intervention. Occasionally when a bronchopleural fistula complicates a pyopneumothorax, open thoracotomy with closure of the fistula is required.

PLEURISY WITH EFFUSION

Aetiology

In childhood serous effusions into the pleural cavity are usually tuberculous and they develop within 8–12 weeks of the primary infection. Rarely, the primary cause may be acute rheumatism, neoplasm, hydatid cyst or chylous leakage. In tuberculosis cases it is frequently possible to isolate tubercle bacilli from the fluid by culture or guinea-pig inoculation. Hydrothorax is seen in the nephrotic syndrome and cardiac failure; it is not, of course, inflammatory in origin.

Clinical features

The onset is often insidious with general loss of weight and slight fever. It may be more acute with pain in the chest, hypochrondrium or shoulder. Pleural friction may be audible but is usually transient and disappears as the effusion increases. When fluid has collected in the pleural space there is marked dullness to percussion and the affected side of the chest shows diminished movement. In large effusions the mediastinum is shifted towards the opposite side, and even the intercostal spaces may be filled in. In such cases there may be dyspnoea at rest. Above the fluid level the percussion note may have a "boxy" quality – skodaic resonance – due to compensatory emphysema of the uncollapsed portion of the lung. Auscultation over the effusion may reveal greatly diminished breath sounds and vocal resonance. In children, however, the breath sounds are sometimes well heard and bronchial in quality, so that consolidation is wrongly suspected. The postero-anterior radiograph shows a uniform opacity with a curved upper border (Fig. 6.16). When air is also present the fluid line is horizontal. Lateral and oblique films are necessary to define interlobar effusions. Thoracocentesis is necessary to confirm the

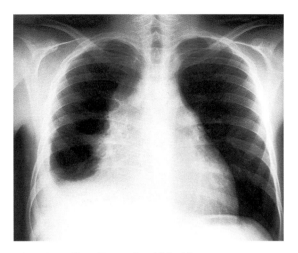
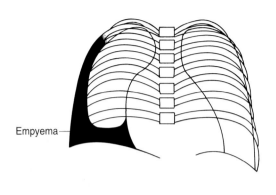

FIGURE 6.17 Chest X-ray of a child with empyema.

diagnosis and to determine the nature of the fluid. In tuberculous cases the fluid is straw-coloured and the cells are mostly lymphocytes, whereas in hydrothorax the cells are mostly of endothelial origin. The tuberculin skin test is of great diagnostic value.

Treatment

In all tuberculous cases a course of antituberculous drug treatment is necesssary. The prognosis is excellent. In other diseases the prognosis is that of the primary condition.

EMPYEMA

Aetiology

Over the past decade the aetiology of empyema – a purulent collection with the pleural cavity – has vastly altered. Whereas empyema used to be either pneumococcal or streptococcal, the great majority of cases today are staphylococcal in origin and they are mostly encountered within the first year of life. Rarely, a pneumococcal empyema is seen in an older child in whom the diagnosis of lobar pneumonia has been delayed.

Clinical features

When an empyema complicates an acute staphylococcal pneumonia in an infant, or lung sepsis in cystic fibrosis, it is only part of the continuing septic process, so that the patient's temperature may show no significant alteration from its previous pattern. The physical signs in the chest are essentially those described in pleurisy with effusion, and the frequency with which bronchial breath sounds are heard in young infants can readily mislead the physician into thinking that they indicate consolidation alone. It is not always easy to detect the shift of the mediastinum which accompanies fluid in the pleural cavity in the case of a gravely ill dyspnoeic infant. Radiography and ultrasonography (Fig. 6.17) should be used to help in diagnosis, and if not responding to conservative treatment, aspiration should be performed. A neglected empyema can lead to alarmingly rapid deterioration and death, or can become encysted.

Treatment

Treatment is by supportive measures with antibiotics, either broad spectrum until an organism has been identified or specific chemotherapy when the organism has been isolated. This regimen is often sufficient to bring about recovery. However, if the pus is very thick, or if there is pyopneumothorax, diagnosis should be followed by intercostal drainage through a catheter under negative pressure. Unpleasant manoeuvres like thoracocentesis in children should always be performed under sedation. When the pus is too thick to come through a needle operation should be performed. Repeated needle aspirations should not be continued for more than 1 week and in unresponsive cases the patient should be referred for drainage.

ASTHMA

Asthma is a common disease and affects more than 10% of children. Yet it remains commonly underdiagnosed and undertreated.

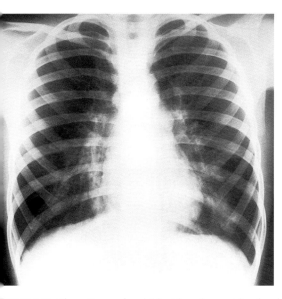
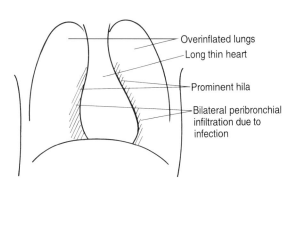

Overinflated lungs
Long thin heart
Prominent hila
Bilateral peribronchial infiltration due to infection

FIGURE 6.18 Chest X-ray of a child with asthma with related infection.

Aetiology

The existence of an allergic basis to true bronchial asthma cannot be doubted and it is due to hyper-responsiveness of the large and small airways of the trancheobronchial tree to various allergens. Rarely, attacks can be traced to exposure to one allergen, but in other cases there appears to be a plethora of possible antigens. One of the difficulties in interpretation lies in the fact that symptomless and apparently normal individuals may quite commonly react to skin tests with a variety of foreign antigens. An important observation concerns the role of house-dust mites, *Dermatophagoides pteronyssinus* and *farinae*, as causes of allergic asthma. Several workers have now expressed the view that house-dust allergy promoted by these mites is the most common cause of allergic asthma in children in the United Kingdom. House dust from floors and even more from the surfaces of mattresses may contain 500 or more *Dermatophagoides* per gram. There is overwhelming evidence that smoking and some that passive smoking produces a rapid reduction in lung function. Also a child may show evidence of allergy to the domestic pet and exposure to seasonal pollens. In children, asthma is rarely precipitated by food or drink, but if so, avoidance is indicated. The role of exercise-induced asthma is very important, especially in children who are expected to take part in regular games at school. It is also certain that emotional disturbances of a quite ordinary kind can precipitate attacks of asthma in some individuals and psychotherapeutic approaches have been shown to be of value as an adjunct to standard drug treatment. That there is a genetic influence is also clear enough in the frequency with which a family history of asthma or other allergic conditions such as eczema and hay fever, can frequently be obtained. Many children with asthma have earlier suffered from atopic eczema and they may continue to suffer from flexural eczema – the prurigo–asthma syndrome. They usually have raised total serum IgE concentrations and give positive reactions to skin tests to one or more of the common inhalant allergens. Asthmatic attacks are often precipitated by intercurrent respiratory viral infections. In some children this may be a manifestation of sensitisation to viral antigens, but the picture is confused by our not infrequent inability to distinguish true asthma from "wheezy" bronchitis where the sole aetiological role may be played by virus and bacteria. This difficulty is particularly great in the young infant in whom a diagnosis of asthma is frequently impossible until time has elapsed. Although wheeze is not synonymous with asthma, asthma is common and alternative diagnoses are rare. Gastro-oesophageal reflux with aspiration may cause episodes of wheezing (see Chapter 7).

Clinical features

The typical acute asthmatic attack is rarely seen before the second birthday. It frequently starts during the night when the child is awakened by expiratory respiratory distress. He looks frightened as well as distressed. He can be heard to wheeze with each forced expiration, and may show some cyanosis. The chest is held in the full inspiratory position and the prolonged expiratory phase can be seen to involve the use of the accessory muscles of respiration. The percussion note is hyper-resonant and there is diminution of the areas of cardiac and liver dullness. Air entry to both lungs is greatly reduced so that the breath sounds are almost inaudible in some patients. The expiratory phase is prolonged and there may be many rhonchi. Coarse crepitations are more common in very young children. The sputum is composed of sticky mucus. Microscopic examination reveals many eosinophils and mucus in the shape of spirals. The blood may also show a mild eosinophilia.

Many asthmatic children become completely free from bronchospasm between attacks. In others, expiratory difficulty and wheezing become established as a more or less permanent disability. The sternum may become unduly prominent with the development of Harrison sulci through the years. In some children chronic respiratory infection still further aggravates the situation (Fig. 6.18). Occasionally bronchial obstruction from tenacious mucus results in segmental or lobar atelectasis. This usually resolves spontaneously and bronchiectasis is a rare complication. It should also be remembered that some children with asthma present only with a persistent nocturnal cough and this may respond to the appropriate anti-asthmatic therapy. Some children with severe asthma grow slowly especially in middle childhood and most of these have a delayed bone age. The vast majority, however, will eventually attain normal height. Asthma may endanger life during childhood and it has been reported that in the UK approximately 1 in 21 000 asthmatic children die from the disease each year. Under-recognition and undertreatment of asthma contribute to these unnecessary deaths.

Treatment

Modern asthma management is based on a stepped approach with drugs tailored to the severity of the disease. A single drug, or a combination of drugs, may be used in low dose or increasing doses, as judged by symptoms and peak expiratory flow monitoring. Drugs should be prescribed in a rational sequence: beta-agonists for mild episodic wheeze; sodium cromoglycate for mild to moderate asthma; inhaled steroid for moderate to severe asthma; with xanthines, ipratropium bromide and oral steroids having their place in more persistent and severe cases. The lowest effective doses consistent with minimal or no side effects will allow the child to lead a normal life with active participation in sporting activities.

The major components of a therapeutic schedule for the child with asthma are shown in Table 6.3.

The acute attack asthma

The time-honoured use of adrenaline has now been replaced by the more selective beta 2-adrenoceptor stimulants because of the lower incidence of side effects such as tachycardia and palpitations. One of

TABLE 6.3 Therapeutic schedule for a child with asthma

Education of child and family
Recognition of precipitating factors and their avoidance, especially allergens
Drug therapy
   Beta-2-agonists – salbutamol or terbutaline
   Theophylline
   Sodium cromoglycate (Intal)
   Ipratropium bromide (Atrovent)
   Steroids – inhaled or oral
Treatment of associated disoders
   Chronic infection
   Gastro-oesophageal reflux
Psychological family support

the most important aims of asthma treatment is to deliver the "right amount of the right medicine to the right place at the right time". The beta-2-selective drugs include salbutamol and terbutaline. Various routes of administration are available, e.g. oral, intravenous or intramuscular injection, pressurised aerosol, inhalation of powder, or inhalation of nebulised solution. The last method is particularly useful in children but it requires a face mask and nebuliser. In the acutely distressed child a rapid response can be expected to intravenous salbutamol 4 μg/kg. Alternatively, salbutamol may be inhaled as a powder (400 μg capsule) by a Rotahaler for a rapid response, combined with oral administration (2–4 mg) for its more sustained effect. If the child is too young to manage a Rotahaler, the salbutamol should be given by inhalation of nebulised solution (1–1.5 ml of 0.5% salbutamol made up to 2 ml with saline). The persistence of severe bronchospasm in spite of such medication is an indication for an intravenous infusion of aminophylline, 5 mg/kg over a period of 20 minutes followed by l mg/kg/h over the next 8 hours. Care must be taken to ensure that the patient already receiving oral or rectal theophylline does not receive an overdose intravenously. Serum theophylline concentrations should be measured before instituting intravenous therapy and aminophylline should not be given intravenously if the serum theophylline values are already within the therapeutic range.

When the acute severe attack fails to yield to the treatment described the use of corticosteroids on a short term basis can be life-saving although their maximum effect will not be seen for several hours. A suitable regimen will be either oral prednisolone 1–2 mg/kg or intravenous hydrocortisone 4 mg/kg could be administered. In addition to drugs, humidified oxygen should be given in high concentrations in an oxygen tent or by face mask or nasal cannulae to maintain O_2 saturation at 90–95% if possible. The PaO_2, $PaCO_2$ and blood pH should be regularly monitored. Assisted ventilation is rarely necessary in the child with asthma, but it is indicated if the $Pa\text{CO}_2$ rises towards 70 mmHg (9.3 kPa) or the $Pa\text{O}_2$ falls towards 50 mmHg (6.7 kPa).

Milder episodes of bronchospasm can usually be aborted by the administration of a bronchodilator by mouth or inhalation. Suitable oral drugs include salbutamol, 2–4 mg 6-hourly, terbutaline 2.5–5 mg 8-hourly or orciprenaline, 10 mg 6-hourly. The same drugs may each be given by pressurised aerosol, 2 puffs three to four times daily. Salbutamol can also be given by inhalation of powder (200 or 400 µg capsules), and in the very young child both salbutamol and terbutaline are available in nebuliser solution.

Long-term management

The long-term care must aim at preventing or reducing the frequency and severity of attacks in all asthmatic children and at improving lung function in the chronic asthmatic. This involves the judicious use of drugs, avoidance of allergens possibly coupled with desensitisation, and psychological management. The most useful test of airway obstruction which can be used to monitor progress is the peak expiratory flow rate (PEFR) which can be regularly measured in the ward or the home with the inexpensive peak flow meter. Values are expressed as litres per minute or as a percentage of the predicted normal for age and height.

Drugs

While the child with recurring attacks of asthma may require bronchodilators at any time, he will also benefit from the more continuous use of a prophylactic drug. The regular use of sodium cromoglycate (Intal) frequently reduces the need for other drugs and allows considerable improvement in lung function in the child with disabling asthma. It is a remarkably safe drug having virtually no side effects. It is given by inhalation in powder form (20 mg capsule or spincap) by means of a Spinhaler two to six times daily, but the doctor or nurse must ensure that the child and his parents have been fully instructed in the use of the apparatus. The pre-school child is unlikely to manage a spinhaler, and cromoglycate is also available as a nebuliser solution (10 mg/ml ampoules) for use with a face mask and air pump. Sodium cromoglycate is also effective in the prophylaxis of exercise induced asthma. It is best given 10–15 minutes before the exercise begins. An alternative to cromoglycate is theophylline. It is being increasingly used and seems to be the equal of cromoglycate as a prophylactic. Its disadvantage lies in the considerable person-to-person variation in blood level. It is recommended that blood levels be measured after the child has been stabilised on 20–24 mg/kg/day and the dosage adjusted to ensure blood levels of 55–110 µg/ml. Slow-release preparations such as Nuelin SA and Nuelin elixir (theophylline sodium glycinate) need only be taken 12-hourly and are unlikely to cause nausea and vomiting.

Failure to respond to cromoglycate or theophylline is an indication for steroids to be given by inhalation. They are often very effective in the child with severe chronic asthma but should never be prescribed lightly. They are available as pressurised aerosols of beclomethasone dipropionate (Becotide) which delivers 50 µg per puff with each metered dose, and betamethasone valerate (Bextasol) which delivers 100 µg per puff. In either case the dose should be 1–2 puffs, two to four times daily, a dose which will not result in depression of adrenal cortical function. For the child who is unable to operate the inhaler efficiently Becotide is also available in the form of insufflation cartridges (100 µg) which allow for easier inhalation with a Rotahaler. In very young children treatment should be attempted with a metered dose inhaler (MDI) with a large volume spacer and face mask. For children unable to tolerate a face mask an MDI with a polystyrene cup may be effective for administering relief treatment only. Inhaled budesonide via a Nebuhaler and face mask has been used successfully in children aged less than 18 months. Although bronchodilator response is variable in the first year of life, it is worth trying them. It is worth remembering that the younger the child the more likely that other disorders may mimic asthma such as gastro-oesophageal relfux, cystic fibrosis, inhaled foreign body, congenital abnormalities and bronchopulmonary dysplasia. The introduction of these topical steroids has made the need for long-term treatment with oral steroids or intramuscular corticotrophin very infrequent. Nebulised beclomethasone has been successfully used in young children aged 20 months to 5–6 years although clinically it is not as effective as the capsule or aerosol preparations in older children. The response to treatment can be monitored by keeping a diary to record symptoms in addition to daily peak flow measurements.

Avoidance of allergens

This is an extremely difficult objective to achieve. None the less, to reduce contact with house dust, and house-dust mites, the child's mattress should be enclosed in a plastic bag, feather pillows should be replaced with non-allergenic synthetic materials and all surfaces should be wiped with a damp duster. Blankets and linen should be regularly aired outside when this is practicable and washed as frequently as possible. Animal contacts should be discouraged. Specific allergens such as house-dust mites, pollens, foods and animals may be identified by skin-prick tests or by the radioallergosorbent (RAST) test but a negative result does not completely exclude allergy. Desensitising solutions are commercially available, but the response of the individual child is unpredictable and usually disappointing. Recent reports of a small but significant mortality in relation to this treatment when used parenterally will remove this approach further from clinical practice in the UK.

Psychological management

The asthmatic child is likely to suffer from various stresses such as recurring illness, absences from school and disruption of social activities. He needs active support and understanding but not overprotection from his parents. He should be encouraged to take part in competitive games such as swimming, athletics and football. The more severely affected child can be greatly helped by skilled physiotherapy and postural coughing. It is the doctor's responsibility to ensure that the parents understand the nature of the disorder and that they are fully instructed in the administration of the child's drugs and of the dangers of non-compliance.

TRAUMA

Trauma to the respiratory tract is uncommon because of the protection afforded by the compliant thoracic cavity. Infants and children are at risk from inhalation of foreign bodies and children have a habit of putting objects in their mouth which inadvertently may be inhaled and cause at worst choking and death if prompt treatment is not instituted or an episode of choking with subsequent persistent respiratory signs and symptoms. A misdiagnosis of asthma may be made and the clue is the history of the acute choking episode. Inhalation of peanuts is dangerous and X-ray appearances vary from overdistension of the lung due to air trapping to collapse where the foreign body obstructs the lumen and air is absorbed from the obstructed lobe or lung. Bronchoscopy and removal of the inhaled foreign body should be performed as an emergency. Intrapulmonary trauma occasionally occurs in infants who have suffered accidental trauma in falls or road traffic accidents. Pulmonary contusion improves in most without active treatment. More severe injury to the lung is rare but a torn bronchus or haemothorax may require urgent closure or drainage. The paediatric patient's thoracic cage is so much more resilient than the more rigid adult and can withstand remarkable trauma with relatively minimal damage.

TUMOURS

Papilloma of the larynx is an uncommon cause of stridor in early childhood. In addition to hoarseness and feebleness of the voice there may be alarming attacks of dyspnoea and even fatal asphyxia. Direct laryngoscopy reveals multiple pink wart-like tumours which can be fairly easily removed by forceps. Spontaneous resolution is usual around puberty. Repeated removal is, however, often necessitated by a tendency to recurrence. In the presence of asphyxial attacks a tracheostomy may be required and it should then be maintained if the papillomata continue to recur. Haemangioma of the larynx is also rare and may be associated with haemangiomata elsewhere. Papillomata usually respond well to interferon.

Mediastinal masses

Intrathoracic tumours are rarely primary in childhood. Lymphomas arising in the thymus compress surrounding structures and result in cough, dyspnoea, stridor, venous distension, oedema of the face and arms and dysphagia. Teratomata or dermoid cysts arise in the anterior mediastinum and can be demonstrated in lateral or oblique radiographs. Calcification is uncommon in these tumours which are usually benign. The ganglioneuroma is a solid encapsulated benign tumour which may arise in the posterior mediastinum from one of the dorsal sympathetic ganglia. It may reach a large size before giving rise to symptoms or may present with symptoms or signs due to noradrenaline secretion. Neuroblastoma may also develop in this situation but, unlike abdominal neuroblastoma, is cured by surgical excision. Radiographs in all these cases will reveal the paravertebral mass to be in the posterior mediastinum. Bronchogenic carcinoma is excessively rare in childhood, but bronchial adenoma sometimes causes bronchial obstruction with obstructive emphysema or absorption collapse. The diagnosis is suggested by haemoptysis which is not otherwise common in children. It should be confirmed by CT scan. Ultrasound can differentiate cystic from solid lesions. The treatment of all intrathoracic tumours except lymphomas is surgical excision when this is possible. Lymphomas usually respond dramatically to chemotherapy.

7

Gastrointestinal System

GASTROINTESTINAL TRACT

Introduction

The alimentary tract is a complicated viscus extending from the mouth to the anus with structural differentation and adaptation according to the specific function needed. The oesophagus is a passage from the pharynx to the stomach, where digestion begins. Food then moves into the small intestine, where further digestion and absorption occurs. The large intestine reabsorbs 95% of the water and completes absorption of digested products, leaving the residue to be expelled intermittently from the rectum. Developmental anomalies of this complicated organ usually present in early infancy. The commoner ones are listed in Fig. 7.1 as are many of the later disorders affecting children.

The most common signs of alimentary tract disorders are vomiting, abdominal distension and disorders of defaecation. In the older infant and child abdominal pain becomes the most common symptom indicating dysfunction of the gut and requires investigation of its cause. An adequate history from the parents and child is most helpful in arriving at the correct diagnosis, and this may be followed by examination and investigations. Many of the causes of abdominal pain are discussed later in the differential diagnosis of acute appendicitis. Most newborn babies vomit a few times in the first weeks of life. A small quantity of milk is often regurgitated when wind is "broken" during or after feeding. Persistent vomiting and vomiting in the older child is usually a significant sign and may be associated with a wide variety of pathological conditions. Infections of the alimentary tract, such as gastroenteritis, result in the infant or child presenting with vomiting which is also a common non-specific sign in other infections, e.g. meningitis, pyelonephritis or septicaemia. Vomiting is the most consistent sign of obstruction in the newborn. It usually starts in the first day of life and becomes progressively more frequent. The vomit

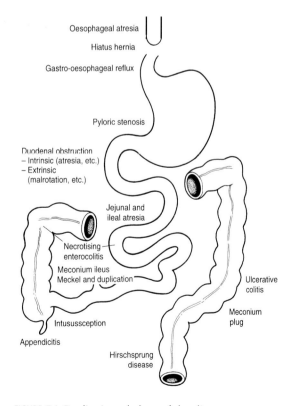

FIGURE 7.1 Paediatric pathology of the alimentary tract.

TABLE 7.1 Clinical and radiological signs of congenital gut anomalies

		COMMENT	USUAL PRESENTATION	
Duodenum	Atresia/membrane	Trisomy 21 30% Other anomalies common	Bile-stained vomiting <24 hours May pass meconium Distended stomach with peristalsis	X-ray – double bubble
	Extrinsic ± malrotation – volvulus	Isolated anomaly Male:female – 4:1	Bile-stained vomiting Passes meconium ± stool	X-ray – abnormal distribution of gas Contrast studies
Small bowel	Jejunal atresia	Isolated anomaly	Vomiting becomes bile-stained 1–2 days No meconium	X-ray – dilated loop(s) with fluid levels
	Ileal atresia	Isolated anomaly or complication of meconium ileus	Abdominal distension Vomiting becomes bile stained 2–3 days No meconium	X-ray – dilated loops with fluid levels
	Meconium ileus	Mucoviscidosis (fibrocystic disease)	Abdominal distension Palpable loops Vomiting No meconium	X-ray – very dilated bowel – few fluid levels
Large bowel	Atresia	Rare	As ileal atresia	X-ray – as ileal atresia
	Hirschsprung	Male:female – 4:1	Abdominal distension Delay in passage of meconium Vomiting Failure to thrive	X-ray – gasless rectum Contrast studies Biopsy
	Hypoplastic left colon	Prematurity Low birthweight	Abdominal distension Failure to pass meconium Vomiting	As above
Anorectal	Atresia	Rare	As colonic atresia	Rectal examination
	Anomaly			
	High	Other anomalies very common	Detected on neonatal examination	Perianal inspection (X-ray & ultrasound)
	Intermediate	Other anomalies common		
	Low	Other anomalies uncommon		

usually contains bile as it is rare for the obstruction to be above the ampulla of Vater. Bile-stained vomiting in the absence of an organic cause is rare and infants and children with bile-stained vomit should be investigated in hospital.

Normal infants should pass meconium within 24 hours of birth. Delay to do so or failure to pass meconium is an important sign which should not be overlooked. Failure to pass meconium may be due to an organic obstruction but subsequent passage may be a sign of disease such as hypothyroidism or Hirschsprung disease.

The infant normally settles into a pattern of having one, two or more bowel actions daily but diarrhoea, increased frequency of passage of stools which become more liquid, or constipation are presenting signs of a variety of disorders. In the early stages of intestinal obstruction there may be little abdominal distension, and any such distension may be difficult to distinguish from the naturally protruberant abdomen of the newborn. Visible loops of bowel and peristalsis are abnormal in the term or older infant, but in the thin-walled premature infant may not be indicative of obstruction.

The disorders affecting the alimentary tract will be considered basically in an anatomical order followed by consideration of gastrointestinal infections and infestations, chronic inflammatory bowel disease, liver and pancreatic problems. A synopsis of the congenital anomalies is given in Table 7.1.

Oesophageal atresia

Oesophageal atresia has been known for centuries. Successful treatment of the condition has only been achieved relatively recently, first by a staged procedure in 1939 and then by primary anastomosis in 1941. Since then, major improvements in management of the condition have occurred and survival is expected unless the infant has other major anomalies. Oesophageal atresia has an incidence of approximately 1:3000 deliveries. The classical case which accounts for practically 85% of infants with oesophageal atresia is that the proximal oesophagus ends blindly in the upper part of the posterior mediastinum and the distal oesophagus communicates with the posterior wall of the trachea as a

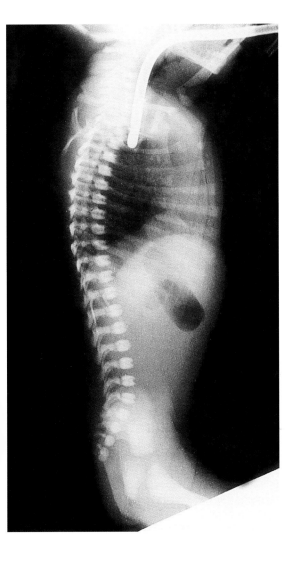

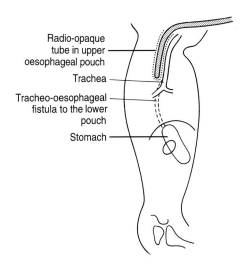

Radio-opaque tube in upper oesophageal pouch

Trachea

Tracheo-oesophageal fistula to the lower pouch

Stomach

FIGURE 7.2 X-ray showing radio-opaque tube in proximal pouch and gas in stomach indicating presence of tracheo-oesophageal fistula.

tracheo-oesophageal fistula (Fig. 7.2). In 10% of infants there is no tracheo-oesophageal fistula and in these infants the gap between the proximal and distal oesophagus is greater. The remaining infants have variations of this pattern and there may be proximal and distal tracheo-oesophageal fistulae.

Oesophageal atresia may be diagnosed ante-natally. It is looked for in ultrasound examination particularly in patients who have polyhydramnios which is an almost invariable accompaniment of the oesophageal atresia anomaly in the infant. Ultrasound examination can detect the dilated proximal blind end of the oesophagus. At birth the baby has attacks of choking, coughing and cyanosis, and "excess salivation", as saliva dribbles from the mouth because there is no passage to the stomach. The swallowed secretions or feed regurgitate and are often aspirated into the respiratory tract. These signs, particularly in an infant of low birthweight, make one suspect the diagnosis. In many neonatal units, it is routine at birth in all low birthweight infants, to try to pass an orogastric tube into the stomach and aspirate the gastric contents. The tube is held up 10 cm beyond the lips in infants with oesophageal atresia.

Diagnosis is confirmed by passage of a radio-opaque tube as far as possible into the oesophagus then taking a chest X-ray which should include the upper part of the abdomen with the field. This shows the hold-up of the radio-opaque tube at the level of the atresia. The upper abdomen shows if there is gas in the stomach, that the infant must also have a tracheo-oesophageal fistula, the air having passed down the trachea through the tracheo-oesophageal fistula and onward to the stomach and bowel.

The optimal outcome for infants with major congenital malformations requiring early surgery is when prenatal diagnosis and delivery of the infant in or adjacent to a neonatal intensive care unit with skilled neonatal surgeons in attendance can be achieved. Where this is not possible a transfer team ensuring that there is no proximal fistula, anastomosis is made between the ends of the oesophagus. Post-operatively the infant has a pleural or extrapleural drainage tube *in situ*, and the baby may be fed parenterally and ventilated for some days to assist in early healing of the anastomosis. Oral feeds are commenced 3–7 days later.

Where primary anastomosis is not possible because of an excessive gap between the ends of the oesophagus, the fistula should be divided, a temporary gastrostomy performed for feeding the infant, and the proximal pouch aspirated. Subsequently, construction of the alimentary tract is achieved by delayed primary oesophageal anastomosis, replacement of the gap between the ends of the oesophagus with a segment of large or small bowel, or mobilisation of the stomach and bringing the stomach up, which, if joined high in the mediastinum or neck to the oesophagus, does not give the major reflux problems which an oesophago-gastric anastomosis in the low mediastinum induces. The outcome of treatment of infants with oesophageal atresia is dependent on the number and severity of associated abnormalities. Infants without other anomalies have a very high survival rate but may have oesophageal dysmotility or problems with oesophageal stricture at the anastomotic level. Usually this is amenable to balloon dilatation which sometimes has to be repeated on a number of occasions. Later, the child has more chance of having dysphagia with a food bolus obstructing the oesophagus but this can be avoided by the child being encouraged to masticate food fully before swallowing it.

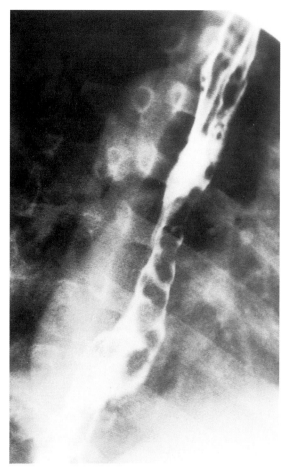

FIGURE 7.3 Barium swallow demonstrating oesophageal and gastric varices.

Oesophageal varices

Bleeding from oesophageal varices (Fig. 7.3) may be sudden and profuse and cause exanguination of the patient. Rapid and adequate transfusion is necessary. Emergency endoscopy should be undertaken in an attempt to establish this diagnosis and injection of varices with sclerosant agents may be commenced. If this is impossible, then control of the bleeding may be achieved by giving intravenous infusions of vasopressin or somatostatin. Tamponading of the oesophageal and gastric varices may be possible with a Sengstaken tube. Insertion of this tube should be done by someone experienced in proper positioning of the balloons and it should be done under imaging control. The oesophageal balloon is blown up to a pressure of 40 mmHg. This pressure will have to be released intermittently to prevent pressure necrosis. This measure should only be undertaken in an attempt to resuscitate the patient prior to more definitive treatment which may include surgical transection of the oesophagus or hemitransection of the stomach (the Tanner operation). Emergency portacaval or

from the regional fetal/neonatal unit can stabilise the infant in the referral hospital and conduct a safe transfer of the infant to the unit.

Infants with oesophageal atresia must be carefully examined. Apart from the low birthweight which has been mentioned, babies with oesophageal atresia frequently have other anomalies. These may be in the alimentary tract such as duodenal atresia or imperforate anus, or in other systems such as cardiovascular, urinary or skeletal systems. A group of infants have the so-called VACTERL association (vertebral, anal, cardiac, tracheo-oesophageal, renal and limb anomalies) (see Fig. 4.4). The disease does not usually have a hereditary or familial aspect but occasionally families have had more than one child affected.

The aim of treatment is to divide the abnormal communication with the respiratory tract and establish continuity of the alimentary tract. In the majority of infants, this can be done through a right thoracotomy. The fistula is identified, ligated, divided and after mobilisation of the proximal pouch and splenorenal shunting is rarely necessary in children. Most patients with portal hypertension and variceal bleeding can be managed by repeated injections of sclerosants into the varices, thus allowing collaterals to develop and improve the drainage from the portal venous system.

Foreign bodies

Children frequently place objects in their mouth and occasionally accidentally swallow them. Most pass down the alimentary tract and out of the anus in 24–48 hours, but occasionally the coin, pin or toy may stick in the oesophagus. This causes discomfort and inability to swallow freely. The offending foreign body may be removed by passing a catheter beyond the foreign body, inflating a balloon on the distal end of the catheter, prior to withdrawing the catheter and the object proximal to it. Removal under direct vision through an endoscope under anaesthesia is the preferred method.

Most foreign bodies which reach the stomach ultimately pass spontaneously. Two exceptions to the "wait and see" approach are the hair ball and batteries. The formation of a hair ball (trichobezoar) may be followed by poor health and vague abdominal pain as the gastric lumen becomes partially occluded by a dense mass. The history of hair eating is rarely given spontaneously by the child or the parents. A mass may be palpated in the epigastrium. Diagnosis is confirmed by endoscopy or X-ray after a barium swallow. The hair ball may be passed spontaneously but gastrostomy may be required. Small alkaline batteries (Fig. 18.4) are swallowed by children and the gastric juice may interact with them and if left may cause severe ulceration. These should not be allowed to remain in the stomach for more than 48 hours and may be removed endoscopically or by gastrotomy under anaesthesia. All other swallowed foreign bodies pass uneventfully through the gastro-intestinal tract once they have reached the stomach.

Gastro-eosophageal reflux: hiatus hernia

Vomiting in some infants becomes more troublesome than the mouthful of regurgitation which is common-place. This may be due to gastro-oesophageal reflux which occurs more frequently and more easily in the infant who has a transverse oval abdominal cavity compared to the adult vertical oval abdominal cavity and consequent altered angulation between oesopha-gus and stomach. Vomiting may be of apparently large amounts but if the infant is continuing to gain weight satisfactorily, there is no reason for major concern. When persistent, treatment with thickened feeds and the addition of Gaviscon therapy may help.

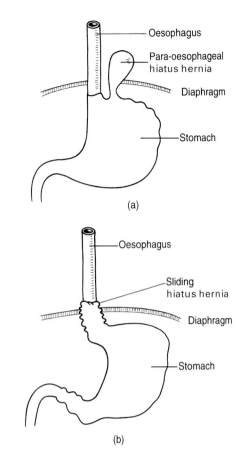

FIGURE 7.4 Diagram of (a) para-oesophageal and (b) sliding hiatus herniae.

Where barium swallow demonstrates a para-oesophageal hernia (Fig. 7.4a) operation is indicated as spontaneous cure is unlikely, whereas with the sliding hiatus hernia of infancy, 80% cure sponta-neously. A small sliding hiatus hernia is a common phenomenon in infants. The majority of these infants do not have significant symptoms, but continue to thrive satisfactorily. Treatment is by keeping the baby propped upright in a baby seat and this gives a gravi-tational effect which may help to decrease the vomit-ing. Thickening of the feeds with Carobel and the addition of medication with Gaviscon are sufficient to control the signs. In most infants the condition is a self-curing one and most children will settle to have an oesophago-gastric junction below the diaphragm with no persistent hernia. Those with a persistent hernia and with gastro-oesophageal reflux will merit surgery if they are in the group which failed to thrive or those with recurrent respiratory tract problems in consequence of the regurgitation and aspiration. Sliding oesophageal hiatus hernia occurs when the cardia and the fundus of the stomach rise into the

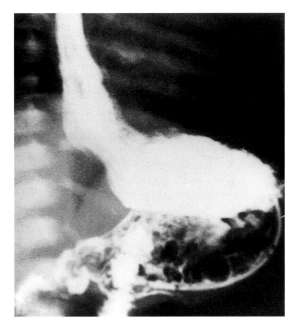 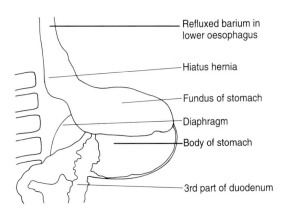

Refluxed barium in
lower oesophagus

Hiatus hernia

Fundus of stomach

Diaphragm

Body of stomach

3rd part of duodenum

FIGURE 7.5 Hiatus hernia with gastro-oesophageal reflux. Barium swallow and meal in a 2-week-old infant shows a small hiatus hernia with gross reflux of barium into the oesophagus. Gastric mucosal folds are noted within the hiatus hernia.

thorax through a loose hiatus, giving the illusion of a congenitally short oesophagus (Fig. 7.4b).

A para-oesophageal hernia is associated with an oesophagus of normal length. The cardia is still in the abdomen but part of the fundus of the stomach prolapses alongside the oesophagus. Both types produce vomiting which can predispose to "asthma" attacks, haematemesis, failure to thrive, regurgitation, rumination syndromes, dystonic neck movements (Sandifer syndrome), all of which are associated with severe gastro-oesophageal reflux (Fig. 7.5). Where symptoms and signs persist, fundoplication is performed for the sliding hiatus hernia. The para-oesophageal hernia does not have the 80% spontaneous cure rate of the sliding hiatus hernia and requires operation to reduce the hernial content to the abdominal cavity and repair the defect in the hiatus. Investigations should include a barium swallow and a meal specifically for reflux, flexible oesophagoscopy and pH monitoring.

The Barrett oesophagus, where there is presence of ectopic gastric mucosa in the oesophagus, is a particularly difficult problem to treat in childhood. The use of antacids and other drugs such as cimetidine, cisapride and Gaviscon all play a part in the symptomatic management of this condition. The long-term results of a Barrett oesophagus are difficult to assess because of reports which have described areas of dysplasia in the ectopic mucosa which could give rise to malignancy in long-term follow-up. These patients have to be kept under surveillance and have endoscopy and biopsies carried out on a regular basis to ensure that no malignancy supervenes.

Infantile hypertrophic pyloric stenosis

Hypertrophy of the smooth circular muscle of the pylorus results in a mass (tumour) that obstructs the passage of feeds from the stomach to the duodenum (Fig. 7.6). The pyloric lumen is diminished and deformed by the mucosa being compressed inwards.

Clinical features

The symptoms are those of a high obstruction with loss of fluids, electrolytes and calories. Males are more often affected and the sex ratio is 4:1. The cardinal signs are projectile vomiting, visible peristalsis (Fig. 7.7) and a palpable pyloric tumour. The infant becomes oliguric and constipated and shows evidence of dehydration with wrinkling of the skin and emaciation if not diagnosed early. Vomiting starts after the first week with regurgitation of feeds and then the vomiting becomes more forceful and frequent. The vomitus may contain blood from a secondary gastritis or oesophagitis. The common age of presentation is 3–9 weeks, but some present after the first week of life and others may not present until the infant is 3 months old. Rarely 1:100 patients with pyloric stenosis may have bile in the vomit.

The main consequences of a pyloric stenosis are:

1 Dehydration
2 Hypochloraemia
3 Metabolic alkalosis
4 Hyponatraemia

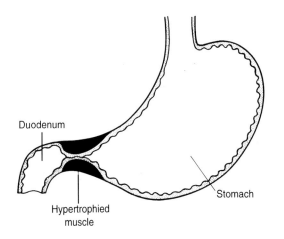

Duodenum

Hypertrophied
muscle

Stomach

FIGURE 7.6 Infantile hypertrophic pyloric stenosis: diagrammatic representation.

5 Weight loss
6 Gastritis
7 Anaemia
8 Jaundice
9 Pre renal uraemia.

The technique of examination is important if the signs are to be elicited. Seated comfortably on the left of the patient the clinician inspects the abdomen of the baby while the baby sucks either the breast or a teat. It is pointless examining the baby while restless and irritable. In a good light it is possible to see the distended stomach through the abdominal wall with visible peristalsis passing from left to right across the epigastrium (Fig. 7.7).

To palpate for the pyloric tumour, the clinician rests the fingers of the left hand gently on the abdomen and the fingertips feel slowly up under the liver edge in the central to right upper abdomen.

Palpation should be carried out while the infant is having a test feed and with patience, a rounded tumour about the size of a hazelnut can be felt. If the tumour cannot be palpated and there is doubt about the diagnosis, then an ultrasound by an experienced ultrasonographer would confirm its presence (Fig. 7.8).

Treatment of the infant is by pyloromyotomy but where there has been delay in diagnosis electrolyte imbalance has to be corrected. Adequate intravenous replacement of sodium, chloride and potassium, as well as water, is necessary prior to operation. When the infant is anaesthetised the abdomen is opened through an upper abdominal incision and a mobile pylorus is delivered and inspected. A Ramstedt pyloromyotomy is performed by making a longitudinal incision through the serosa and muscular layers. Any remaining fibres are separated with blunt forceps until the intact mucosa bulges up to the level of the serosa. Great care should be taken to avoid puncturing the mucosa of the duodenum in the distal end of the wound. If this happens, then the perforation should be closed. This can be checked by squeezing the stomach during operation to make sure there is no perforation. The procedure may be performed under local anaesthesia which may be preferred in the infant with other major problems or where a skilled paediatric anaesthetic service is not available.

Post-operatively, feeds are gradually reintroduced over 48 hours and infants usually make a quick recovery.

Peptic ulcer

Although rare in infancy and childhood, gastric and duodenal ulcers may occur. Secondary ulcers (Curling) may be associated with severe infections or extensive burns.

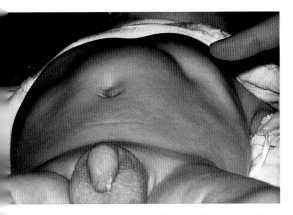
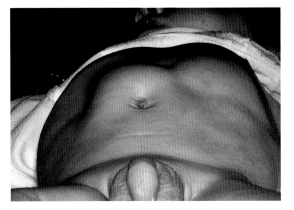

FIGURE 7.7 Infant with hypertrophic pyloric stenosis showing visible peristalsis wave passing from left to right in upper abdomen.

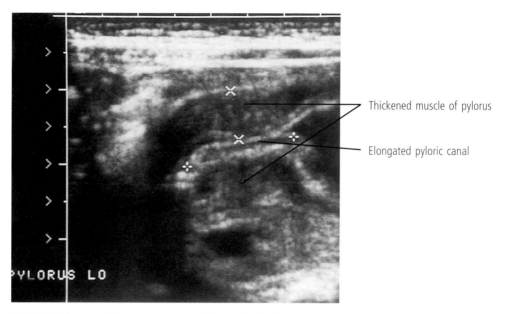

Thickened muscle of pylorus

Elongated pyloric canal

FIGURE 7.8 Hypertrophic pyloric stenosis. A longitudinal ultrasound examination showing elongation of the pylorus and thickening of the pyloric muscle.

Clinical features

Some of the vague abdominal pains which are so common in childhood may be due to undiagnosed peptic ulcer. Indeed, many of these patients may have paid several visits to the hospital and seen several consultants, and eventually been referred to the psychiatric department before an underlying peptic ulcer may be diagnosed. While the disease may run a silent course in infancy, in the older child the clinical picture is similar to that in adult life. There is epigastric pain or discomfort relieved by eating; pain at night is common. Vomiting an hour or two after food may follow pylorospasm or actual scarring of the pylorus. There may be evidence of malnutrition. The disease may present with recurrent or severe haemorrhage or with perforation into the peritoneal cavity which is very rare. Endoscopy is usually diagnostic although barium meal is less invasive and if indicated may not always reveal a peptic ulcer. During endoscopy, biopsies of the pyloric antrum and the duodenal mucosa are examined to establish the presence of *Helicobacter pylori*. The Cloe test is a spot test that can be carried out during the procedure which would elicit the presence of these organisms. If *H. pylori* are present, then the association between them and peptic ulceration is quite high and treatment should be given. The regimen for treating this infection is by a combination of bismuth (De-Nol), metronidazole and ampicillin, but eradication of the organism is not always successful and repeat treatment may be necessary. It is suggested that the initial treatment should be ampicillin for 2 weeks: 250 mg four times daily for children aged 5–10 years and 500 mg four times daily for older children together with De-Nol for 2 months 120 mg twice daily for children aged 5–10 years and 240 mg twice daily for older children. Metronidazole therapy is optional.

Duodenal obstruction

Obstruction of the duodenum in the neonatal period may be from an intrinsic lesion within the duodenum or by extrinsic pressure.

Intrinsic duodenal obstruction

Intrinsic duodenal obstruction may be complete, as in patients with duodenal atresia with a gap between the ends of the duodenum or a complete duodenum membrane, or incomplete, where in duodenal stenosis, the severity of the stenosis varies from mild to being near complete. Complete obstruction is incompatible with survival beyond 3 weeks as without treatment the infant starves. With incomplete obstruction survival for months can occur before diagnosis is established.

Intrauterine diagnosis of duodenal atresia may be made by visualising dilated stomach and duodenum in the infant. Hydramnios is not so common an accompaniment as with infants with oesophageal atresia, but occurs in 75% of infants with duodenal atresia.

The classical presentation of the infant with duodenal atresia is with bile-stained vomiting. In the great

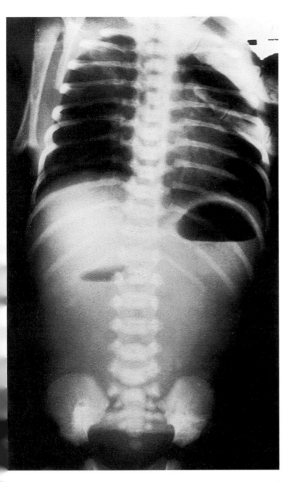

FIGURE 7.9 Double bubble sign on erect abdominal X-ray of duodenal atresia.

majority of infants, this bile stained vomiting commences within the first 24 hours of life. In 10% of infants with duodenal atresia the obstruction is proximal to the entrance of the bile ducts (ampulla of Vater) and these infants present with persistent vomiting which is non-bile stained. The diagnosis is also made on some infants presenting with another anomaly such as imperforate anus which has been obvious at birth. On screening the infant for further anomalies the duodenal obstruction is found. Approximately 30% of infants with intrinsic duodenal obstruction have trisomy 21 (Down syndrome).

The diagnosis if not made prenatally is suspected in the infant with bile-stained vomiting or persistent vomiting. Examination of the infant shows the dilated stomach with waves of peristalsis passing from left to right in the upper abdomen. X-ray of abdomen show the double bubble sign (Fig. 7.9). No contrast studies are necessary. If the diagnosis is delayed, the infant requires fluid and electrolyte correction prior to operation. Operative treatment is to perform duodeno-duodenostomy or duodeno-jejunostomy to bypass the obstruction. Gastrostomy allows insertion of a larger tube than can be passed nasogastrically into the stomach to aspirate secretions from the stomach and a transanastomotic tube passed into the proximal small bowel. This allows reintroduction of gastric aspirate and feeds into the small bowel while the anastomosis heals and tone returns to the stomach and duodenum. As the baby has had the obstruction intrauterinely for months normal propulsion of feeds from the stomach and duodenum into the small bowel may take days or occasionally weeks to return to normal. Feeding by a transanastomotic tube is safer and preferred to intravenous feeding.

The outcome of duodenal atresia, like that of oesophageal atresia, is dependent on the presence of other anomalies. If there are no other major anomalies then long-term prognosis is excellent.

Extrinsic duodenal obstruction

This form of obstruction can be caused by any extrinsic pressure on the duodenum. The usual cause is bands which are associated with incomplete rotation of the midgut loop. These peritoneal bands extend from the caecum and terminal ileum towards the right hypochondrium, undersurface of liver, gall bladder or posterior parietal wall. Obstruction usually occurs a few days after birth when the increased motility of the gut causes these bands to drag across the duodenum. Incomplete rotation, commonly referred to as malrotation, is present and this is sometimes complicated by volvulus (twisting) of the midgut loop. Extrinsic duodenal obstruction is the presenting sign but the dangerous aspect as far as the infant's health is concerned is the volvulus. The twisting of the midgut (Fig. 7.10) frequently causes venous and subsequently arterial obstruction at the root of the mesentery and so the viability of the midgut loop can become impaired. Prompt diagnosis is essential to prevent ischaemia and infarction of the bowel. The infant frequently progresses normally for the first few days and then develops bile-stained vomiting, but after the volvulus occurs there may be passage of blood per rectum. For reasons which remain unclear there is a 4:1 male to female incidence in this disorder.

On examination of the infant no clear clinical signs can be detected. If peritonism has developed, then the viability of the bowel has already become impaired. Straight X-ray of the abdomen does not give the clear cut picture obtained in intrinsic duodenal obstruction. There may be only a fluid level in the stomach. The duodenum is never dilated to the degree that it is with intrinsic obstruction. An important sign which is sometimes not appreciated is lack of normal distribution of gas throughout the bowel. This is a feature of an infant's abdominal X-ray and is different from the adult. If the straight X-rays are not diagnostic then

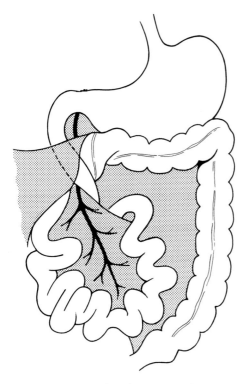

FIGURE 7.10 Diagram of malrotation with superimposed volvulus of midgut causing extrinsic duodenal obstruction.

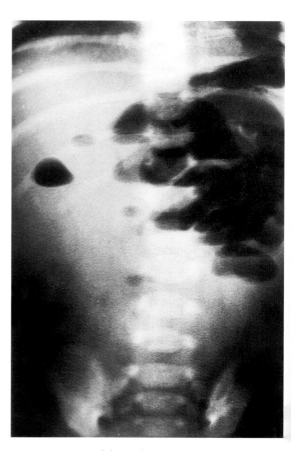

FIGURE 7.11 Erect abdominal X-ray showing dilated small bowel with fluid levels in an infant with ileal atresia.

contrast studies of the upper gastrointestinal tract will demonstrate the obstruction and treatment should be immediate laparotomy. The alternative is a barium enema which defines the "malrotation" and can also sometimes define volvulus. Treatment of extrinsic duodenal obstruction requires immediate laparotomy. Signs of peritonism indicate that bowel viability is already impaired. A Ladd procedure, i.e. dividing the peritoneal bands, broadening the root of the mesentery and returning small bowel to the left abdominal cavity and large bowel to the right, is the operation of choice.

Post-operatively there is commonly a delay of 72 hours before gut motility recovers. The long-term outlook is good but 10% of the children may in succeeding years develop an adhesion obstruction which may require laparotomy.

Jejunal and ileal atresia

If the obstruction is high in the small bowel the infant starts vomiting and the vomitus becomes bile stained within 24 hours of birth. If the obstruction is lower then much more abdominal distension occurs and the vomiting may not commence until the second or third day of life. The infant fails to pass any normal meconium. In small bowel atresia there is no sex preponderance.

Diagnosis of atresia is sometimes made prenatally when ultrasound examination shows dilated loop(s) of bowel in the fetal abdomen. Postnatally, failure to pass meconium and vomiting suggest the obstruction. X-ray of abdomen shows dilated bowel with fluid levels and a lack of gas in the distal bowel (Fig. 7.11).

Treatment is to correct any fluid and electrolyte imbalance followed by resection of the most dilated distal part of the proximal gut with end-to-end or end-to-back anastomosis. The latter is usually necessary because of the small size of the bowel distal to the obstruction. Post-operatively, feeds can start being introduced after 24 hours. The long-term prognosis for the infant is good.

Meconium ileus

Neonatal ileal obstruction occurs in one in 10 infants with cystic fibrosis. The meconium in the lower ileum is a dry green, putty-like, sticky material. Neonatal obstruction arising from impacted meconium presents a serious problem in early life. In meconium ileus, the middle or lower ileum above the obstruction is often

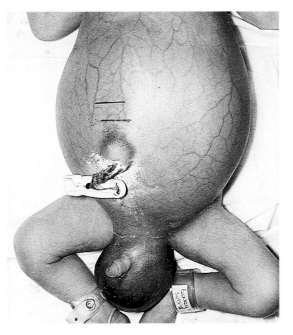

FIGURE 7.12 Abdominal and scrotal distension in infant with meconium peritonitis.

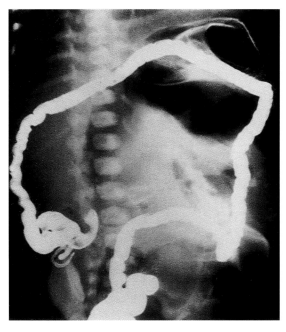

FIGURE 7.13 Gastrografin enema outlining the microcolon and passage of contrast into terminal ileum.

distended and may be complicated by volvulus of this large obstructed loop. This can result in perforation, meconium peritonitis (Fig. 7.12) and secondary atresia of the small bowel may develop. This may occur antenatally and present as a complicated meconium ileus at birth with marked abdominal distension.

Clinical features

Abdominal distension and vomiting are early features and within a day or two a ladder pattern and visible peristalsis can be seen. The putty-like mass in the ileum may be palpated in the lower abdomen. Radiography reveals distended loops of small bowel without fluid levels due to the inspissated meconium which may give a mottled or granular or ground glass appearance.

Treatment

Provided there is no associated atresia gastrografin enemata (Fig. 7.13) can often be used to treat as well as to diagnose meconium ileus. When this is not effective and/or there is a suspicion of complicated meconium ileus, then laparotomy is indicated. The dilated gut may be resected and an end-to-end anastomosis with a venting distal ileotomy performed (Bishop–Koop anastomosis). This distal ileostomy allows instillation of pancreatic enzymes and flushing

out of the terminal ileum and colon. It is important to confirm the diagnosis of cystic fibrosis.

Meconium plug

A firm plug may delay the passage of the first stools by hours or days and the infant may present with signs of intestinal obstruction. A saline rectal washout may soften the viscid meconium and promote evacuation. An underlying condition should always be sought in this situation, be it Hirschsprung disease, septicaemia, dehydration or cystic fibrosis.

Meconium peritonitis

This form of chemical peritonitis may be followed by bacterial peritonitis after birth as the gut becomes colonised with bacteria from the environment. Meconium peritonitis usually follows antenatal intestinal obstruction and perforation of the bowel proximal to the obstruction. It may occur in bowel atresia, volvulus, meconium ileus and neonatal Hirschsprung disease. Occasionally, the perforation which occurred antenatally may have sealed off and only a chemical peritonitis may be present at birth. This can give rise to numerous small foci of "foreign-body" reactions which may become calcified. The clinical features are those of neonatal intestinal obstruction – bile stained vomiting, abdominal distension and failure to pass meconium. Calcification in the peritoneal cavity may be demonstrated radiographically.

Treatment is by laparotomy, toilet of the peritoneal cavity, relief of the intestinal obstruction and correction of the defect.

Duplications of the gastrointestinal tract

Duplications are spherical or elongated hollow structures lined with some form of alimentary mucous membrane and intimately adherent to the alimentary tube. The duplication is always on the mesenteric border of the gut and the contents are clear, colourless and mucoid in consistency. They may vary in size and shape, being saccular or tubular, and not infrequently may communicate with the bowel. Duplications below the diaphragm may present in four ways:

1 They may grow in size and cause intestinal obstruction.
2 Increase in tension within the cyst may cause abdominal pain.
3 The duplication may encroach on vessels in the mesentery and cause necrosis, sloughing and bleeding in the adjacent bowel.
4 A duplication lined with gastric mucosa may develop peptic ulceration and may perforate into the peritoneal cavity, into the adjoining bowel or into the pleural cavity.

Radiography may demonstrate a space filling shadow and a barium series may show indentation of the lumen. Ultrasound and CAT scan may be required to delineate the lesion. It can be difficult to differentiate duplications from omental and mesenteric cysts.

Treatment

It is usually possible to separate the wall of the bowel from the duplication without injuring the bowel or impairing its blood supply. In most cases the treatment of choice is resection of the duplication with an end-to-end anastomosis. Duplications are associated with vertebral anomalies in about 30% of cases.

Omental cysts

These arise from congenitally misplaced lymphatic tissue very similar to cystic hygromas which occur in the neck. They are in fact lymphangiomas. They vary greatly in size, are thin walled, rounded or lobulated and contain serous lymph fluid. The cysts may be small and lie in the substance of the omentum or they may largely replace this structure.

Clinical features

There is a slowly enlarging abdominal swelling with little associated discomfort. It is usually mobile from side to side since it is attached to the mesentery of the small bowel. Treatment is by excision and presents few difficulties.

Mesenteric cysts

Mesenteric cysts may arise in any part of the mesentery or mesocolon. They are very often due to malformed lymphatic tissues and occur commonly at the jejunum or ileum. The cysts lie between the peritoneal leaves of the mesentery, and may obstruct adjacent intestine.

Meckel diverticulum

A Meckel diverticulum is found in about 2% of all post-mortem examinations in general hospitals. Most of these people have lived their allotted span without any symptoms and it is purely a chance finding. Remnants of the vitello-intestinal tract may, however, lead to dramatic surgical catastrophe in the first few years of life.

In the early weeks of intrauterine life the apex of the midgut loop has a wide communication with the yolk sac. This opening is narrowed to form the vitello-intestinal duct and the duct and its accompanying artery and veins are normally obliterated. Vestiges of the duct or its vessels or cysts within it may persist. A vitello-intestinal fistula is rare and occurs when the vitello-intestinal duct fails to close. Small intestinal contents are discharged at the umbilicus.

In Meckel diverticulum the duct closes at the umbilical end but remains open at the intestinal end. The diverticulum which may be 0.5–2 inches long arises from the antimesenteric border of the ileum 1–3 feet proximal to the ileocaecal valve and may have a small mesentery containing patent remains of the vitelline vessels. It may terminate in a thin cord attached to the umbilicus. The umbilical portion of the duct may remain to form a vitello-intestinal cyst. Although the vitelline duct is embryologically related to the ileum, its remnant is not necessarily lined throughout with ileal mucosa. In 25–30% of diverticulae there is heterotopic tissue – gastric, duodenal, colonic or pancreatic. Complications from a Meckel diverticulum can present in many ways, such as abdominal pain simulating appendicitis, intestinal obstruction, intestinal haemorrhage, intussusception, umbilical fistula, umbilical cysts or polyps, perforation or as an incidental finding at operation. The investigations for this include plain X-ray of the

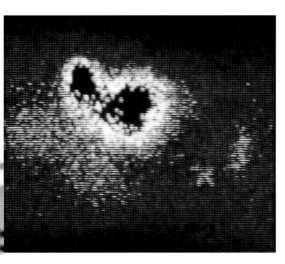

FIGURE 7.14 Meckel scan. ^{99m}Tc pertechnate radionuclide scan showing uptake of radionuclide in the stomach and in a Meckel diverticulum in the right iliac fossa.

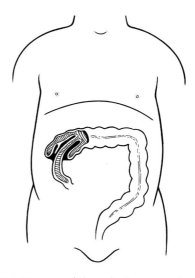

FIGURE 7.15 Diagram of ileo-colic intussusception showing the apex (intussuscipiens) within transverse colon in the right hypochondrium.

abdomen which is rarely helpful and a technetium (Tc) isotope scan which can demonstrate 30% of cases (Fig. 7.14).

Although most textbooks refer to Meckel diverticulitis, this is a rare clinical condition and the signs and symptoms are usually indistinguishable from appendicitis and are diagnosed at operation. Perforation of a Meckel diverticulum may result in peritonitis and haemorrhage. At operation when one is looking for an inflamed appendix and it turns out to be normal then it is routine practice to withdraw the terminal ileum in order to look for the presence of a Meckel diverticulum.

Intestinal obstruction is the most serious complication of a Meckel diverticulum. A volvulus may occur around the fibrous adhesion with loss of viability of the bowel. At operation, it may be necessary to resect the gangrenous portion of bowel and perform an anastomosis after releasing the adhesion.

Intestinal haemorrhage arises from peptic ulceration from the heterotopic gastric mucosa. There may be a sudden passage of blood-stained stool in a young child without previous symptoms. Bleeding may be copious and while the first stool may be dark in colour, subsequent stools are usually bright red. The red cell count may fall to alarmingly low levels in a short space of time. Bleeding from a Meckel diverticulum may be unaccompanied by pain or there may be mild discomfort, in sharp contrast to the colic which accompanies bleeding in intussusception. There are usually scant abdominal signs. The ulcer may perforate soon after the onset of bleeding and there may be evidence of peritonitis. Treatment is by excision of the diverticulum and end-to-end anastomosis.

There are no distinguishing features to intussusception where the lead point is a Meckel diverticulum. As in idiopathic intussusception the clinical picture is one of recurring abdominal colic with pallor, vomiting during paroxysms of pain and the presence of blood and mucus in the stools.

A diverticulum which has not given rise to symptoms but which is discovered at laparotomy is excised if the general condition of the patient is satisfactory. The Meckel diverticulum is a potential source of future trouble and if it can be removed without any risk to the patient this should be done.

Intussusception

Intussusception is a telescoping of one portion of the bowel into the adjacent segment (Fig. 7.15). Most cases of intussusception (over 60%) occur during the first year of life but the condition is rarely seen under the age of 1 month. The peak incidence is between the fourth and ninth months, and boys are more frequently affected than girls (3:2). In infants there is rarely any demonstrable cause and a change from milk to a more solid diet may alter peristalsis in such a way as to initiate an intussusception. Infective causes have been sought but there is no clear pathogen which causes the intussusception. Enlarged mesenteric glands are almost always found at operation and although the glands may be secondary to the intussusception, they may also be associated with a preceding lymphoid hyperplasia from infection. Only rarely is a definite mechanical factor found to be

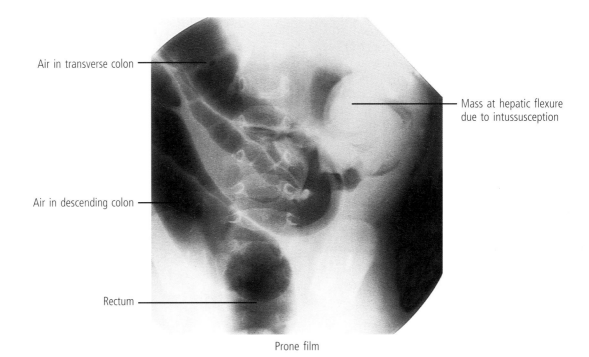

Air in transverse colon

Mass at hepatic flexure
due to intussusception

Air in descending colon

Rectum

Prone film

FIGURE 7.16 Air reduction of intussusception. Air has been pumped into the colon with the infant in the prone position. A filling defect is noted in the splenic flexure due to the intussusception. This was subsequently reduced.

responsible for initiating the invagination. In older children a Meckel diverticulum or a polyp may be the apex or lead point of an intussusception. Other underlying causes include angiomas, lymphoma and intestinal haematoma.

The peak incidence in the UK is in the winter months. There is no relationship between intussusception and seasonal diarrhoea, but upper respiratory infections commonly precede the onset of intussusception. The most common site of the apex (intussuscipiens) is shown in Fig. 7.15. The ileo-ileal and colo-colic are uncommon in childhood and 90% are ileo-colic or ileo-caecal.

Where the mesentery of the caecum and ascending colon has failed to become obliterated, the caecum is mobile and the apex of the intussusception may reach the sigmoid or even the rectum where it may be felt by digital rectal examination. As the ileum advances through the ileocaecal valve its mesentery soon becomes constricted. As a consequence, the venous return is obstructed causing oedema and congestion. The obstruction of blood supply may be followed by gangrene of the intussuscipiens. Obstruction of the lumen of the bowel is a consequence of intussusception but symptoms and signs usually result in the infant or child presenting before intestinal obstruction is clearly established.

Presentation

The patient is usually a healthy vigorous male infant of 3 months or older who was previously well. Onset is dramatic, as the child, without warning, screams, drawing up his knees as though in abdominal pain and becomes pale. The attack ceases as suddenly as it began and in a few minutes the child seems at peace and may even pass a stool and fall asleep. Mother is reassured by the apparent quick recovery and may postpone seeking medical advice. After a short lapse of time, varying from minutes to several hours, a further similar attack of colic occurs. This continues recurring at shorter and shorter intervals. A feature in these children is the pallor during spasms probably due to a vaso-vagal reaction. Vomiting is frequent in these episodes. Pain is not always a constant feature. The other common sign is the passage of mucus and blood per rectum. If the diagnosis is delayed signs of intestinal obstruction supervene.

Abdominal examination often reveals a sausage shaped mass to the right of the umbilicus or in the right hypochondrium. There is no peritonism but tenderness or guarding directly over the mass may make its delineation difficult. Rectal examination demonstrates no faeces in the lumen but blood and/or mucus is often present on the examining finger.

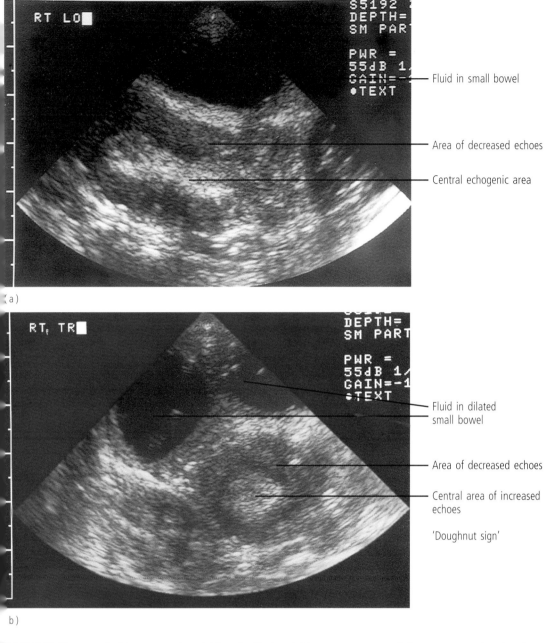

RT LO

Fluid in small bowel

Area of decreased echoes

Central echogenic area

(a)

RT, TR

Fluid in dilated
small bowel

Area of decreased echoes

Central area of increased
echoes

'Doughnut sign'

b)

FIGURE 7.17 Ultrasound of intussusception. (a) Longitudinal and (b) transverse scans of the transverse colon showing a mass with a central area of increased echoes and surrounding rings of reduced echoes (doughnut sign in transverse scan). There are also fluid-filled loops of small bowel due to small bowel obstruction.

The most important factor causing delay in diagnosis is the association of the idea of intestinal obstruction with intussusception. The triad of colic, vomiting and abdominal distension are late signs.

In the older child the picture is less dramatic than in infants. Severe colic is not an outstanding feature and blood may not be passed per rectum for hours or even days after onset. The child usually experi-ences periodic attacks of colic and shows little inter-est in food. Between attacks the abdomen is soft and no mass may be felt.

Diagnosis

Diagnosis can be made on history alone. Plain X-rays of the abdomen may reveal a soft tissue mass with signs of intestinal obstruction such as dilated loops and fluid levels. Ultrasound examination of the abdomen is useful in demonstrating the disorder. An air enema or a barium enema (Fig. 7.16) will confirm the diagnosis and in 60–70% of patients reduction of the intussusception can be successful by the air or fluid pressure which may dilate the bowel and reduce the intussusception. This procedure is both diagnostic and therapeutic. It is important that if this procedure is carried out there is a backflow of barium or air into the small bowel to ensure there is complete reduction of the intussusception.

The differential diagnosis includes volvulus which may present a similar picture but there is seldom remission of pain. Palpation of the abdomen reveals an ill-defined swelling usually in the central area. Ultrasound (Fig. 7.17) and X-ray will differentiate these from intussusception. Gastroenteritis is perhaps the commonest cause of difficulty, but the onset is less dramatic and the colic rarely severe. The rectum in this case contains loose faeces or foul smelling watery stools. Temperature is usually elevated and vomiting may be a prominent feature. Palpation of the abdomen of a child with gastroenteritis reveals no tumour but a generalised tenderness may be present. On auscultation there is increase in bowel sounds. In older children (aged 3 years or more), Henoch–Schönlein purpura may cause difficulty in the differential diagnosis. Blood in the rectum may be accompanied by loose motions and there is evidence of haemorrhagic effusions elsewhere. A child with Henoch–Schönlein purpura may develop haemorrhage in the wall of the bowel and show signs of intussusception and indeed intestinal obstruction.

The management of a child in whom intussusception is suspected should commence with intravenous infusion of dextrose-saline solution and monitoring the peripheral and the core temperature of the child while results of blood investigations are obtained. If there are signs of shock then plasma should be given initially in order to expand the intravascular volume as with acute changes of intussusception, clinical signs of dehydration are not established and are difficult to assess. The blood haematocrit, urea and electrolytes should be checked and constant nursing care given. Many of the children who are entering into the phase of shock no longer exhibit signs of irritability and restlessness, but lie still and uncomplaining between spasms. These children are very vulnerable to rapid deterioration in their clinical condition. Peripheral and core temperature should be measured and a 3°C or greater gap indicates a requirement for more fluid replacement.

If the child has signs of peritonism, then no non-operative attempt should be made at reduction and once resuscitation has been fully achieved, which includes administration of intravenous antibiotics, e.g. metronidazole and either a cephalosporin or aminoglycosides, the child should be taken to theatre. Operative reduction can be achieved in most instances. In some cases where there is delay in diagnosis and the viability of the bowel is impaired or where reduction cannot be achieved, resection of the affected bowel and end-to-end anastomosis should be performed. Once there is a return of peristalsis, then enteral feeds can be started and intravenous infusion reduced. The child who does not require surgery needs to be in hospital for only a day to ensure the intussusception has not recurred.

Recurrent intussusception occurs in 2% of patients with intussusception. The interval between the intussusceptions varies from 24 hours to several years. Peutz–Jegher syndrome, which is the presence of small intestinal polyps associated with pigmentation of the buccal mucosa, may be a cause of recurrent intussusception.

Appendicitis

Acute appendicitis is the most common lesion requiring intra-abdominal surgery in childhood. The disease runs a more rapid course in children and the criteria for establishing a diagnosis and for treatment are different. Under the age of 4 years, the diagnosis is difficult and in 90% the infection has spread transmurally to the peritoneal cavity or the appendix has ruptured.

Pathology

There is marked variation in the anatomy of the appendix. The appendix is attached to the posterior medial quadrant of the caecum. In childhood, the appendix lies in a retrocaecal position in 70% of patients. Obstructive appendicitis is common in childhood, the obstruction being caused by a kink, a faecolith, or the scar of a previous attack of inflammation. When inflammation occurs, there is an accumulation of purulent exudate within the lumen and a closed loop obstruction is established. Blood supply to the organ is diminished by distension or by thrombosis of the vessels and gangrene occurs early in children. Fluid is poured into the peritoneal cavity as a result of irritation, and within a few hours this fluid is invaded by bacteria from the perforated appendix or from organisms translocating the inflamed but still intact appendix. Peritoneal infection may remain localised by adhesions between loops of intestine, caecal wall and parietal peritoneum. There is danger in administering a purgative in these children because it increases intestinal and appendicular peristalsis and perforation and dissemination of infection are more likely to occur.

Appendicitis may present as:

1 Uncomplicated acute appendicitis.
2 Appendicitis with local peritonitis.
3 An appendix abscess or diffuse peritonitis.

The onset of symptoms is vague and initially may be of a general nature. Only a third of younger patients are seen in hospital within 24 hours of onset of abdominal symptoms, and the appendix has ruptured in a high percentage of these young patients before admission. The diagnosis is made late in some cases. One reason for delay in diagnosis is failure to suspect appendicitis in a child under 4 years of age and the other is the poor localisation of pain by the younger child. Although often not severe, the pain appears to come intermittently and irritability, vomiting and diarrhoea may result in the mistaken diagnosis of gastroenteritis. Psoas spasm from irritation of the muscle by the inflamed appendix may cause flexion of the hip resulting in a limp, thus distracting attention from the abdomen and directing it to the hip joint. Vomiting occurs in most patients. The child is usually pyrexial but the temperature is only moderately elevated to between 37°C and 38.5°C. Temperatures higher than this usually suggest upper respiratory tract infections or occasionally diffuse peritonitis from appendicitis. A history of constipation is uncommon and in many patients there is a history of diarrhoea.

The clinical features in the older child are similar to those in the adult. Abdominal pain is usually followed by nausea and vomiting. The pain begins centrally and later shifts to the right iliac fossa. If the appendix is retrocaecal, abdominal pain and tenderness may be slight. If the child has a pelvic appendix then tenderness may again be slight, or absent, or elicited only on rectal examination. Anorexia is a common accompanying sign.

Clinical examination

The child with acute appendicitis is usually anorexic, listless and does not wish to be disturbed. There is often a characteristic fetid odour from the tongue which is furred.

The child is usually irritable, crying and uncooperative. A low-grade pyrexia is usual but the temperature seldom exceeds 38.5°C. Inspection alone may be very informative while attempting to gain the child's confidence. The most important physical sign on abdominal examination is the area of maximum tenderness located in the right iliac fossa and the presence of rebound tenderness. If this is not defined, then a gentle digital rectal examination should be made and tenderness may be elicited or a mass felt in the pelvis in patients with a pelvic appendix.

Urine should be checked for the presence of bacteria or white cells and also to exclude glycosuria or significant proteinuria. Leucocytosis is usually present

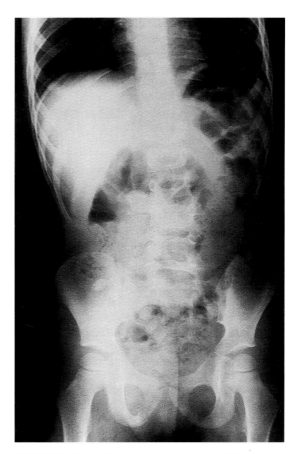

FIGURE 7.18 X-ray of abdomen showing faecolith, scoliosis with psoas spasm, dilated loop of bowel with fluid level and loss of fat line cell.

in children with acute appendicitis but a normal white cell count does not exclude the diagnosis. The child with diffuse peritonitis may have a low white cell count. Plain X-ray of the abdomen often gives useful signs of acute appendicitis (Fig. 7.18).

Differential diagnosis

Differential diagnosis includes numerous other disorders the commonest of which is upper respiratory tract infection. Presence of a common cold, sinusitis, acute tonsillitis, pharyngitis may all be associated with acute non-specific mesenteric lymphadenitis. This is the most common condition to be differentiated from acute appendicitis. The presence of enlarged glands elsewhere in the body accompanied by an upper respiratory tract infection may suggest this condition. Fever may be absent but temperatures can be very high. The presence of abdominal tenderness is not as acute as that in appendicitis. It is usually more generalised and not localised to the right iliac fossa and there is no rebound tenderness. The presence of a cough, increased respiratory rate and runny nose may suggest a respiratory infection. Examination of the chest is mandatory to pick up any signs of consolidation as right lower lobe pneumonia may result in referred pain in the right lower quadrant of the abdomen. Constipation can cause abdominal pain, nausea and vomiting, with tenderness over the distended caecum. It can be easily mistaken for acute appendicitis. Faecal masses may be felt per abdomen or on digital rectal examination. Usually following a suppository, satisfactory evacuation of the colon and rectum will bring rapid relief in patients whose symptoms are caused by constipation.

Pyelonephritis and infection of the kidney and renal pelvis can usually be differentiated by a higher temperature, pus cells in the urine, and tenderness over one or other kidney in the renal angle.

Abdominal trauma, accidental or non-accidental may cause injury to the abdominal viscera. A plain X-ray of the abdomen and a serum amylase should be done to exclude the presence of traumatic or idiopathic pancreatitis and a pneumoperitoneum.

In gastroenteritis and dysentery there may be severe cramping and abdominal pain. The pain and tenderness may be more marked over the distended caecum. Other members of the family may have similar symptoms or diarrhoea. Rectal examination can help differentiate between a pelvic appendicitis and appendicitis with pelvic peritonitis from gastroenteritis.

Infective hepatitis may occur in epidemic form but in an isolated case may simulate appendicitis. The temperature is usually elevated and the child complains of a headache with nausea, vomiting, abdominal pain and tenderness. On examination, the liver is enlarged and tender. The child may or may not be jaundiced depending on whether he is seen in the prodromal phase of the disease. Examination of the urine usually reveals the presence of bile salts, but urobilinogen may be present.

Intestinal obstruction may be due to incarceration of a hernia, secondary to anomalies, e.g. a volvulus around a vitello-intestinal remnant, or adhesions following previous abdominal operations. Vomiting, abdominal colic, abdominal distension and constipation are the usual signs. After a thorough clinical examination plain X-ray of the abdomen in the erect and supine positions should be carried out to differentiate intestinal obstruction from appendicitis.

Primary peritonitis is an uncommon diagnosis and almost always affects the female. There is a diffuse infection of the visceral and parietal peritoneum usually due to a pneumococcus. With the peritonitis there is exudation of fluid to the peritoneal cavity. Mesenteric lymph nodes are swollen. Diffuse abdominal pain, vomiting, dehydration and a high fever are the main features and diarrhoea may be present initially, but is usually followed by constipation.

Rectal examination usually is suggestive of a pelvic appendicitis as there is diffuse tenderness and heat present. The white blood cell count is usually grossly elevated between 20 000 to 50 000 per mm^3. The diagnosis is usually made at laparotomy when peritonitis is found but the appendix is normal.

Severe abdominal pain and vomiting may occur during passage of a renal calculus. Hydronephrosis due to blockage of the pelviureteric junction by stricture, stone or aberrant vessel may present with abdominal pain and nausea. The pain and tenderness are maximal in the flank. Red or white cells may be found in the urine.

Haemolytic uraemic syndrome may present with acute abdominal pain and may be confused with acute appendicitis. The presence of fragmented red blood cells on a blood film and also the presence of oliguria are suggestive of this disease.

Crohn disease is an unusual diagnosis in childhood but the incidence is increasing in western countries. It can present with all the symptoms of acute appendicitis and at operation the terminal ileum is found to be acutely inflamed and thickened. A biopsy reveals the diagnosis and barium meal and follow-through very often indicates the presence of other areas of the affected gut.

In torsion of the right cord or testis confusion with acute appendicitis may occur whereas this is less likely with torsion of the left testis. Routine examination should always include the inguinal regions and the scrotum.

Inflammation of a Meckel diverticulum and intussusception in older children may simulate acute appendicitis. Other medical conditions which should be considered are those of diabetes mellitus, cyclical vomiting and Addison disease. The onset of menstruation may simulate appendicitis and many girls have recurring attacks of lower abdominal pain, sometimes for a year before menstruation actually begins. Pain associated with torsion of an ovary or an ovarian cyst may also present with signs similar to those of acute appendicitis.

It is not uncommon for both adults and children to harbour threadworms (pinworms) without noticeable symptoms. Many symptoms and signs have been ascribed to the presence of threadworms including weight loss, poor appetite, nausea, vomiting and chronic abdominal pain.

Carcinoid tumour in the appendix is rare in childhood but the tumour may obstruct the lumen of the appendix and lead to obstructive appendicitis. It is far more common to find this as an incidental finding on histopathology of the removed appendix. When it is present in the tip of the appendix, no further follow up is necessary in these cases. In older children, if a carcinoid exists in the ileal or caecal region there is a chance of invasive disease with subsequent evidence of the carcinoid syndrome.

Treatment

The treatment of the child with acute appendicitis is early operation. In the toxic child with peritonitis, time may be profitably spent in combating toxaemia and dehydration. It is important to resuscitate the patient and start intravenous antibiotics before surgery is undertaken. In such cases, metronidazole (Flagyl), ceftazidime and cefotaxime should be given intravenously. The institution of intravenous antibiotics given as three doses pre-, per- and post-operatively with peritoneal lavage in children with peritonitis has considerably reduced the incidence of post-operative complications. In children, early appendicectomy is indicated in the child with an appendix abscess. This hastens the recovery period and allows much earlier discharge from hospital.

The best access to the appendix with the minimal disturbance of the peritoneal cavity is through a grid-iron or lance incision and appendicectomy is performed. There is an increasing trend to perform appendicectomy by minimal invasive surgical techniques rather than "open" operation.

Post-operative complications

Wound infection is the most common complication following appendicitis. Since the introduction of metronidazole and cefotaxime given routinely to patients who have appendicectomy, the incidence of wound infection has dropped significantly. Evidence of infection may be obvious within a day or two of the operation or may be delayed for several weeks. There is a rise in temperature, local tenderness of the wound, and redness and swelling. Pus may be released by inserting sinus forceps into the edge of the wound to allow it to be discharged.

Localised intraperitoneal abscesses may form after the subsidence of a diffuse peritonitis, particularly in the pelvis. Fever may fail to resolve and there is usually lower abdominal pain, tenderness and even diarrhoea with increased frequency of micturition. There may also be abdominal distension due to an associated ileus affecting the terminal ileum. On digital rectal examination, a tender swelling is felt anteriorly. Many pelvic collections resolve on intravenous antibiotics, and very occasionally pus may be evacuated spontaneously through the rectum. Alternatively, drainage through the original incision under a general anaesthetic and insertion of a Penrose drain to maintain a route to the surface will help clear the pelvic collection. There is no evidence to substantiate the claim that pelvic peritonitis in the young female may lead to sterility in adult life. Subphrenic collections have become extremely rare in children even in those who have had diffuse peritonitis.

Early post-operative intestinal obstruction is usually due to impaired motility of matted loops of ileum lying in pus in the pelvis. Treatment is by antibiotics, intravenous fluids and continuous nasogastric suction. With this conservative management resolution is usual and very few require surgical intervention. If there is volvulus or a closed loop situation then earlier surgical intervention is mandatory in order to relieve the distension and prevent devascularisation of part of the bowel.

Respiratory complications are seldom severe. Mild atelectasis is not uncommon and infection of a collapsed area should be prevented with help from physiotherapists and breathing exercises. Faecal fistula is rare and may be due to necrosis of part of the caecal wall. The fistula usually closes spontaneously with conservative treatment. Rarely a faecolith may have escaped from the necrotic appendix at the original operation and lie in the peritoneal cavity. This causes persistence of a fistula until the faecolith is removed.

Recurrent abdominal pain

Recurring and unexplained abdominal pain often presents a difficult problem to the family doctor and to both the paediatric physician and surgeon. Organic disorders in this group account for less than 10%. The pain may amount to little more than discomfort. It may be accompanied by nausea and vomiting. It is unusual to find any definite signs on abdominal examination and it may be difficult to assess the severity of the pain. Questions which should be asked of the pain are:

1 What is the duration of each attack?
2 Is the child ever sent home from school because of the pain?
3 Does it interfere with games or does it become worse when there are household chores to be done or errands collected?
4 Does the pain ever waken the child from sleep?

Constipation should always be eliminated in these cases and the presence of dysuria, increased frequency of micturition, pyuria or haematuria call for urological investigation. The presence of threadworms should suggest the possibility of a cause for the abdominal colic. Plain X-rays of the abdomen may be useful to reveal a faecolith in an appendix, calcification in mesenteric glands, or calculus formation in the renal tract. Barium meal or barium enema may reveal lesions such as polyps, peptic ulceration or malrotation which can be a cause of chronic abdominal pain. In the female, recurrent abdominal pain may precede by many months the onset of the first menstrual period (menarche). When organic disease has been reasonably excluded, the proportion of patients who are found to be suffering from emotional disorders is related to the degree of skill and experience in the diagnosis. The term abdominal migraine covers a group of patients who suffer from recurrent attacks of abdominal pain, vomiting and headache. (A child suffering from genuine acute appendicitis very rarely complains of headache.)

Management of the child with recurrent abdominal pain after treatable causes have been excluded is by reassurance to the patient and parents that there is no serious underlying disease and that symptomatic treatment until the child outgrows the problem is indicated.

Colonic atresia

Atresia in the colon is rare, accounting for only 5% of bowel atresias. Presentation and management are similar to the distal small bowel atresia. Some patients presenting with an atresia of the small intestine may in fact have a complicated meconium ileus and a sweat test should be performed at a later date to exclude cystic fibrosis.

Hirschsprung disease

In 1887 Harold Hirschsprung of Copenhagen described the clinical features of the condition which bears his name. The primary pathology is lack of ganglion cells in the bowel for variable lengths from the anus proximally (Fig. 7.19). Aganglionosis is the alternative name for the condition. The proximal normally innervated colon is greatly hypertrophied and dilated as it tries to press the contents through the distal aganglionic bowel which causes a functional obstruction. The rectum and rectosigmoid have a narrow calibre. The narrow segment may be short or long; short segment aganglionosis is where the deficiency extends from the anus proximally into the rectum but not beyond the sigmoid colon; in long segment aganglionosis lack of ganglion cells extends more proximally and occasionally extends into the small bowel.

Clinical features

Although the child appears to be healthy at birth he is likely to have delay in passage of meconium, develop abdominal distension, vomiting and failure to thrive. Constipation is usual and in babies older than 1 month, constipation becomes an increasing problem but in early infancy diarrhoea secondary to entero-colitis may supervene.

Over 95% of term babies pass meconium within the first 24 hours after birth and the remainder pass it within the next 24 hours. Some patients show less well defined clinical signs. There may be intermittent constipation and abdominal distension in the neona-

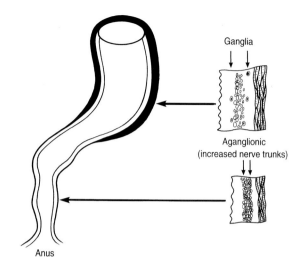

FIGURE 7.19 Diagram of pathology of Hirschsprung disease (aganglionosis).

tal period which is relieved by conservative measures. Gradually, constipation becomes more stubborn and there is marked enlargement of the abdomen. Peristaltic waves may be seen to pass along the dilated and hypertrophied transverse colon going from right to left. Faecal masses are usually palpable through the abdominal wall. Rectal examination may reveal an empty rectum with faeces at its upper limit or there may be a palpable mass of faeces in the sigmoid colon which can be palpated through the rectal wall. There may be faecal incontinence, soiling or spurious diarrhoea. If untreated, growth in these patients is usually retarded and puberty may be delayed. The abdominal distension may be accentu-ated if enterocolitis becomes superimposed and may be relieved by the passage of quantities of foul smelling faeces. Fluid loss may be an acute problem. Another common complication is ulceration of the mucosa and occasionally perforation. Rectal exami-nation by insertion of the little finger into the rectum may reveal meconium present and on removal an explosive evacuation of meconium or faeces and air results in decrease in the abdominal girth. X-ray of the abdomen reveals dilated coils of bowel with lack of gas in the rectum. Clinically and radiologically the condition is a neonatal obstruction.

A barium enema may show the narrow rectum and an expanded rectosigmoid with proximal dilation (Fig. 7.20), but this appearance may not present until the infant is 2–3 weeks of age. Diagnosis is confirmed by a rectal suction biopsy. The rectal biopsy should be performed at least 2 cm above the anal margin since the terminal rectum and anal canal does not have ganglion cells even in the normal individual. A false diagnosis may be made if the biopsy is taken too

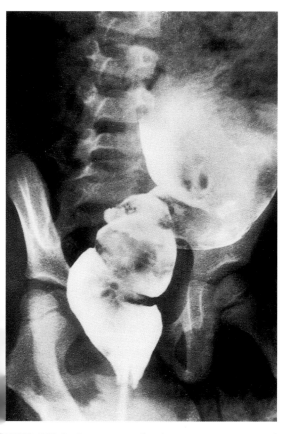

FIGURE 7.20 Barium enema showing narrow rectum and dilated sigmoid colon indicating Hirschsprung disease.

low. The biopsies are usually given directly to the pathologist who, in addition to the above, looks for the presence of increased nerve fibres using acetylcholinesterase staining as a useful adjunct in the histological diagnosis of Hirschsprung disease.

Treatment

Decompression of the bowel is important and can be carried out in the neonatal period in more than 90% of cases by doing daily bowel washouts. This requires a lot of patience and large volumes of saline until the bowel is cleared. Once the infant is thriving a variety of operations may be undertaken. The basis of each is to remove the aganglionic bowel and re-establish continuity. In the older child, bowel washouts are done preoperatively to empty the bowel. If emptying the bowel is unsuccessful or Hirschsprung enterocolitis develops, then a colostomy proximal to the aganglionic zone should be performed. Following resection, most patients have normal sphincter control, take a normal diet and require no laxatives but several years may elapse before full continence is gained. The various operations are known by the surgeons who initially described them, e.g. Swenson, Duhamel, Soave, Rhebein.

Neonatal necrotising enterocolitis (NNEC)

Necrotising enterocolitis (NEC) is a severe disease of the gastrointestinal tract. Prematurity or low birthweight are the most commonly associated factors and occur in 90% of babies with this disease. Term infants are affected to a lesser extent and constitute about 10% of the affected group. Hypovolaemia and hypoxia result in damage within the mucosa cells initiating the NEC. It is often multifactorial in origin, resulting in loss of integrity of the gut mucosal barrier with passage of bacteria into the wall of the bowel.

Prematurity, respiratory distress syndrome (RDS), congenital cardiac malformations, umbilical vessel catheterisation, exchange transfusions, hypoglycaemia, polycythemia, post-operative stress and hyperosmolar feeds have all been implicated in the aetiology. Scholander in 1963 proposed the diving reflex as a mechanism which causes shutdown of visceral blood flow, especially in the superior mesenteric artery, resulting in ischaemic changes in the mucosa. Bacterial infection has been implicated in NEC and from time to time one sees some confirmation of this because of the clustering of the disease in neonatal units. Clostridial infections have been associated with some outbreaks of NEC. There are protective factors in breast milk which decrease the risk but do not completely protect babies from NEC.

The incidence of this disease varies from country to country. There is a very low incidence in Japan and a high incidence in the United States. The severity of the disease is variable from a minor form seen in many cases which are managed entirely in the neonatal units, to a fulminating type of the disease with perforation, peritonitis and death.

Initially, one sees a preterm infant with signs of sepsis, vomiting of feeds, abdominal distension and frequently the passage of blood or mucus in the stools. If the disease continues to progress peritonism develops and this is often appreciated first by nursing staff observing abdominal distension.

Examination of the abdomen may show signs of inflammation, redness, oedema of the abdominal wall with localised or generalised tenderness, and if the baby has a patent processus vaginalis, free fluid or even gas or meconium is occasionally seen in the scrotum. If a perforation has occurred then one loses the area of superficial dullness of the liver on percussion of the abdomen. Palpation may reveal crepitus from the intramural gas which can be palpated among the coils of distended loops of bowel, and this is an important sign of NEC.

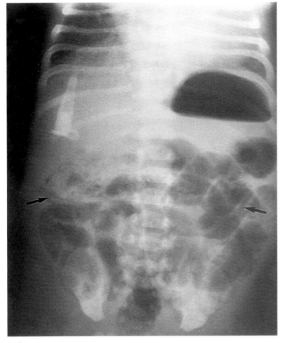

(a)

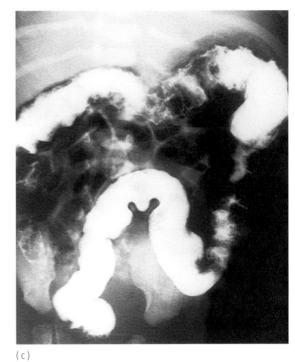

(c)

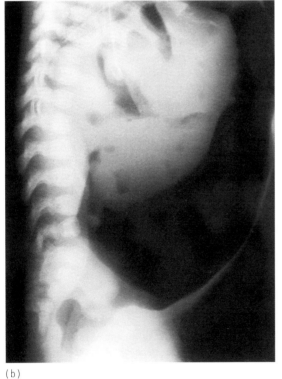

(b)

FIGURE 7.21 (a) Abdominal X-ray of premature infant showing pneumatosis (see arrows). (b) The free air in peritoneal cavity indicates perforation. (c) Barium enema showing extensive pneumatosis coli.

A plain X-ray of the abdomen (Fig. 7.21) may show pneumatosis intestinalis (gas within the bowel wall) and gas in the portal vein and liver. This sign is often an ominous one with a very high mortality. The extent of the NEC may be localised to an area of the bowel, very often the colon, but in extensive disease the whole of the gastrointestinal tract may be involved.

The differential diagnosis early in this disease may be difficult and one should consider the following diagnoses:

1 Septicaemia from other causes.
2 Volvulus neonatorum.
3 Hirschsprung enteritis.
4 Infarction of the bowel.

Management

Most babies with NEC are managed medically and relatively few require surgical care. Management consists of stopping all oral intake, nasogastric aspiration and instituting intravenous fluids to counteract the hypovolaemia, dehydration and acidosis. Infants with NEC tend to lose a lot of fluid which is very rich in protein and electrolytes into the tissues and into the lumen of the bowel. Anaemia, if present, needs to be corrected by blood transfusion and the fluids, electrolytes and protein replaced. The baby must be maintained normovolaemic with a good peripheral perfusion. On the basis that there is a septic element involved, a broad spectrum antibiotic is given. Following stabilisation of circulation and ventilation when indicated, total parenteral nutrition is commenced. When the physical signs have reverted to normal, the oral intake is started and gradually built up over several days until full feeds are again established.

Surgical management

If there is a persistent acidosis which often indicates progressive disease or a perforation of the bowel, then surgical intervention is very often necessary. Perforation is detected by seeing free gas in the peritoneal cavity in an erect or lateral abdominal X-ray. In very low birthweight (under 1500 g) infants percutaneous drainage has been used in preference to laparotomy. This is performed by means of applying a local anaesthetic to the right lower quadrant of the abdomen, and then a 10–12 French gauge catheter is inserted into the abdominal cavity to drain air, meconium and faecal material which has leaked from perforated bowel. In a series of 20 patients, 15 survived and of these eight needed no further operation, whereas seven needed a further laparotomy when they had recovered from the septic episode. Two required bowel resection and anastomosis, whereas the remaining five were left with a temporary stoma after resection of necrotic bowel. This was closed some weeks later. Late development of strictures in the small or large bowel can occur and necessitate resection. The overall mortality in this high risk group was 30%.

CONGENITAL MALFORMATIONS OF THE RECTUM AND ANUS

Embryology

In the 5-week embryo, the urogenital sinus and hindgut empty into a common cavity – the cloaca – separated from the exterior by the cloacal membrane. By the downgrowth of a mesodermic fold (urorectal septum) the separation of the urogenital tract from the rectum is normally completed by the seventh week. For a time there is a small opening between the rectum and the urogenital tract known as the cloacal duct. The urorectal septum also divides the cloacal membrane into the urogenital membrane anteriorly and the anal membrane posteriorly and these become the external openings. A small invagination – the proctodeum – develops in the region of the future anus and the proctodeum and rectum join by rupture of the anal membrane during the eighth week. Rectal and anal anomalies and associated malformations are due to arrests in development in the seventh and eighth weeks of fetal life. A range of anomalies occur in the anorectal region and these will be discussed individually but the subdivisions are not always so clear in practice.

Anal stenosis

The anus is in its normal position but the anal canal shows a degree of stenosis and is less distensible than normal. This condition may be missed at birth and can present weeks, months or even years later with chronic constipation and faecal soiling. There is delay in the passage of meconium and subsequently the infant has to press excessively to defaecate through the narrow canal ribbon-like stools. This condition will be missed completely if rectal examination is omitted. Repeated dilatation is necessary, the size of dilators being gradually increased until the little finger can be inserted. The infant may then be sent home and the mother given a supply of finger cots and instructed to continue dilatation for several months. Failure to continue dilatation may lead to retention of faeces and subsequently to rectal inertia, a secondary megarectum and overflow incontinence. This is very difficult to treat. Rarely some form of anoplasty may be necessary.

Anal membrane

A membrane occludes a normally situated anal canal. Meconium may be seen shining through the membrane which bulges when the infant cries. Division of the membrane followed by supervision over the first few weeks to ensure healing without stenosis results in cure.

Covered anus

This more common anomaly is often described as a low anorectal anomaly as the rectum comes down through the pelvic floor before coming to the malformed part. There is no evidence of the anus in the normal position. In a baby boy a raised ridge of skin or a narrow tract filled with meconium runs forward in the perineal raphe as far as the posterior aspect of the scrotum where a speck of meconium may be seen at the abnormal orifice – the rectoperineal fistula. Treatment is by anoplasty with postoperative follow-up to ensure that stenosis of the new anus does not develop.

Rectal atresia

The anus looks apparently normal but the rectal pouch ends blindly in the hollow of the sacrum. This is a rare anomaly and results in failure to pass meconium, the baby presenting with low intestinal obstruction. Diagnosis is made on rectal examination. Treatment varies from division of a septum to a more major pull-through procedure.

Anorectal anomalies

Anorectal anomalies are a spectrum of malformation from the high to low lesions (Fig. 7.22), the definition of high or low being whether the bowel terminates above the pelvic floor muscles in the high anomalies, or in low lesions the bowel comes through the pelvic floor muscles normally and then terminates by a fistula to the perineum. The latter are more common. High lesions are frequently one of a number of anomalies in the baby and in only one-third is it an isolated defect (*cf.* low anomalies where two-thirds are otherwise normal). There are also less frequent intermediate anomalies where the bowel comes into the pelvic floor muscles and terminates as a fistula to the bulbous urethra in the male and to the vulva in the female. All these lesions should be detected on the initial neonatal examination and the baby referred for investigation and diagnosis of the specific type at a specialist neonatal surgical unit.

Because of the different pelvic anatomy of the male and female, in high lesions the anomalies vary with sex. The boys have a fistula from the rectum to the urethra or bladder and this may result in meconium being passed per urethram. In females the genital tract is interposed between the alimentary and urinary tracts so that the fistulous communication is from the rectum to the vagina. This may be high in the vagina and not visible, but is more often low and may be seen. Low lesions have usually a fistula to the perineum. In the male this may be close to the scrotum or even onto the median raphe of the scrotum whereas in the females it is to the perineum or entroitus. The uncommon intermediate types usually communicate with the

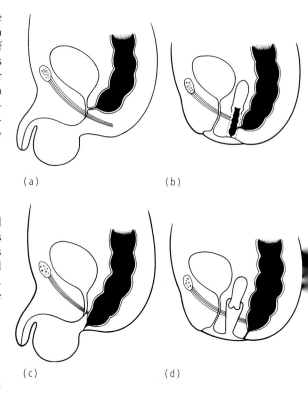

(a)   (b)

(c)   (d)

FIGURE 7.22 Anorectal anomalies: diagrammatic representation of high (a & b) and low (c & d) lesions in male and female.

bulbous urethra in the male and the vestibule in the female.

Investigations of the infant with an imperforate anus should commence with a thorough general examination because of the frequency of other anomalies. Ultrasound examination of the urinary tract and to the perineum should determine whether the infant has a high or a low lesion. At 24 hours of age, once adequate time has allowed air to pass through the bowel to the rectum, X-rays of the abdomen and pelvis, in particular a lateral film with the baby inverted, are taken. If air is present below a line drawn from the pubis to the coccyx, the baby has a low lesion and if above, a high lesion.

Treatment for the high or intermediate varieties in the male is by colostomy and subsequently division of fistula and anoplasty usually through a posterior sagittal approach. The colostomy is then closed. In females, the fistula is usually larger, allowing the baby to spontaneously decompress and pass meconium and faeces, and the posterior sagittal anoplasty may be done without colostomy.

With low lesions perineal operations are performed to establish the anus in the normal site.

The results of the high and low groups are significantly different. With the high group, long-term continence results are much less satisfactory than in the low group where most achieve satisfactory continence. The associated anomalies also significantly affect the outcome, e.g. infants with partial sacral agenesis have poor continence and some may require a permanent colostomy.

Blood per rectum

Passage of blood from the rectum is common in paediatric practice. The diagnosis may be straightforward and the cause obvious, but in many the cause of bleeding is never found even after full investigation including laparotomy. Serious underlying causes have to be excluded.

Most children seen in the outpatient department with rectal bleeding pass only small quantities of blood after defaecation. Anal fissure is the most common cause but it may be due to rectal prolapse or proctitis. Acute anal fissure is the most common cause of rectal bleeding. There is usually a history of constipation and generally pain on defaecation. The bleeding is usually small in amount, bright red, streaked on the outside of the stool and occurs during or just after defaecation. The fissure is usually in the midline posteriorly. Perianal redness and shallow fissures may be the first sign of a granulomatous proctitis sometimes associated with Crohn disease. Most fissures are easily seen and digital rectal examination without anaesthesia, which may be very painful, is unnecessary and should be avoided. Treatment is that of the underlying constipation but at times anal stretch is necessary under a general anaesthetic.

Moderate or extensive bleeding is infrequent but the common lesions are rectal polyps, enteritis or enterocolitis, intussusception, Meckel diverticulum, volvulus, duplication of the alimentary tract, haemangiomas in the bowel, systemic haemorrhagic disorder, trauma (child abuse) and in the neonate, necrotising enterocolitis and haemorrhagic disease of the newborn.

Digital rectal examination, proctoscopy, sigmoidoscopy colonoscopy or barium enema may show up the lesion which can then be treated appropriately. A technetium scan may be necessary to demonstrate a Meckel diverticulum or a duplication of the bowel but a negative scan does not exclude either as it is dependent on the presence of ectopic gastric mucosa.

Rectal prolapse

Prolapse may be partial when the mucous membrane only is prolapsed or complete when there is protrusion of the entire rectal wall (Fig. 7.23). The 1–3-year age group is the usual age. Mucosal prolapse is more common and occurs in children with chronic consti-

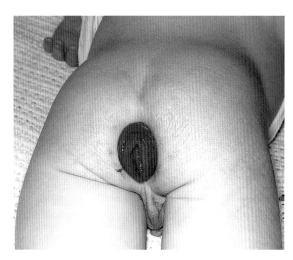

FIGURE 7.23 Rectal prolapse in a child subsequently confirmed as having cystic fibrosis.

pation and is usually initiated by prolonged straining. Prolapse is sometimes the presenting sign of cystic fibrosis. Complete prolapse occurs in debilitated or malnourished children. It is also seen in children with paralysed pelvic floor muscles as in myelomeningocele.

Parents usually notice the red mucosa coming out of the anus after defaecation. The prolapse has usually reduced before the doctor sees the patient. On rectal examination the anal sphincter is found to be very lax and the withdrawn finger is often followed by redundant folds of rectal mucosa. The child presenting for the first time with a rectal prolapse should have a sweat test performed to exclude cystic fibrosis.

To the parent a prolapse may be a terrifying event and it is important that anxious parents are reassured. The prolapse may be reduced by simple pressure or by elevating the foot of the cot, or raising the buttocks on a pillow. Reversion to nappies instead of squatting on the pot should be advised for 3 months from the last prolapse but reassurance that this will not interfere with long-term defaecation control is necessary. For persistent or frequently recurring prolapse the buttocks may be strapped together and the child given a laxative. In most instances once the stool is softened, the prolapse becomes less of a problem and rectal prolapse in children is usually a self-curing condition. Only very rarely is it necessary to treat this surgically with injection of phenol in olive oil into the submucosa of the rectum or by a perianal stitch.

Intestinal polyps

A solitary rectal polyp is a common cause of bleeding from the rectum. This low polyp is easily felt on digital rectal examination. The polyp is a granulomatous hamartoma of the mucous membrane which becomes pedunculated by defaecation and may protrude at the anus like rectal mucosa prolapse. Polyps high in the rectum and lower colon require sigmoidoscopy under general anaesthesia and may be removed by snaring. Occasionally, juvenile polyps are multiple and may be demonstrated by double contrast studies. True familial polyposis is very rare under the age of 12 years, but the rectum and colon can be carpeted with polyps which histologically are papillomas or adenomas of the adult type. This disease is usually carried as a Mendelian dominant and cancer of the colon develops in young adult life. Peutz–Jegher syndrome is a familial condition in which polyps of the small intestine are accompanied by brown pigmentation of the lips, buccal mucosa. Symptoms and signs include repeated episodes of abdominal pain due to transient intussusceptions, blood loss from the intestinal tract and anaemia.

Constipation

Terminology is a problem which causes confusion in communication between doctors and patients. It is important that the doctor be sure of the patient's understanding of the terms used. Constipation may be defined as a difficulty or delay in defaecation that causes distress to the child and the parents. The infrequent passage of stools with no distress does not fall into this category. Encopresis, or faecal soiling, is the frequent passage of faecal matter at socially unacceptable times. This is discussed in Chapter 10. Psychogenic causes are the most frequent. Faecal continence is the ability to retain faeces until delivery is convenient. Ingestion of fluid or food stimulates the gastrocolic reflex and results in two or three mass colonic propulsive activities per day. This process delivers faecal material to a normally empty rectum. On distension of the rectum, stretch receptors start a rectal contraction and a reflex inhibition is sent to the anal canal. This is mediated via the myenteric plexus of nerves in the submucosa and the plexus of nerves between the outer longitudinal and inner circular smooth muscle layers. The process produces sensation since the upper part of the anal canal has sensitive sensory receptors as well as stretch receptors. The motor element of the external sphincter and the puborectalis muscle make up the striated sphincter together with the smooth muscle of the internal sphincter. The striated sphincter is able to contract strongly to prevent the passage of a stool at an inconvenient time. This, however, can only function for 30 seconds, i.e. long enough to contain a rectal contraction wave till it passes. The internal sphincter can maintain persistent tonic activity so preventing leakage of stool between periods of rectal activity by maintaining closure of a resting anal canal. Clinical experience suggests that the external sphincters are of much less importance than the puborectalis sling and the internal sphincter. Defaecation occurs by inhibiting the activity of the puborectalis sling and the sphincter mechanism of the anus, thus allowing faeces to pass from the rectum into the anal canal. This is augmented by voluntarily increasing intra-abdominal pressure using the abdominal wall musculature as well as the diaphragm as accessory muscles for defaecation.

There are two main clinical states, the acute and the chronic state, which must be differentiated.

Acute constipation

Acute constipation usually occurs in a child after a febrile illness with a reduced fluid intake. This situation arises when convalescing after an illness or in the immediate post-operative period. There is a danger that this acute state of constipation may progress to a chronic state if it is not identified early enough. Treatment with a laxative, suppositories or an enema usually correct the problem initially but the child must be encouraged to return to a good diet and adequate fluid intake.

Chronic constipation

Chronic constipation is distressing to the child and the parents. An early diagnosis is essential to prevent a prolonged and persistent problem. In chronic constipation the rectum is overstretched and ballooned. The sensory receptors are inactive and the bowel is flaccid and unable to contract effectively. A greater amount of water is absorbed from the faecal stream. The stool becomes harder, more solid and more difficult and painful to pass. The faecal mass increases in size and spurious diarrhoea can also occur from stercoral ulceration of the distended rectal mucosa.

History is important as failure to pass meconium within 24 hours of birth in the term infant, born normally, makes it likely that there may be some underlying problem. Infants, for whom childbirth has been abnormal, take longer to establish a normal defaecation pattern. The delay in establishing normal stooling may be a sign of other disorders, not only Hirschsprung disease or anal stenosis but also systemic disorders such as hypothyroidism. Psychogenic causes are the commonest origin of constipation in childhood often due to inappropriate toilet training and this aspect is also discussed in Chapter 10.

In older infants and children the distress caused by constipation may be related to pain. There may be abdominal discomfort, usually a dull ache, which may or may not be related to defaecation. Occasionally the pain may be localised to the right iliac fossa due to a distended caecum filled with stool. The pain may be in the anal region, particularly when an anal fissure has occurred, and bleeding may result from the mucosal tear.

There are occasions when there is no complaint of constipation but the parents may notice a distended abdomen, and may even at times feel a mass arising out of the pelvis.

A full dietary history must be obtained. This should include a detailed account of a typical day's breakfast, lunch, supper and any in-between snacks, noting the amount of fluid taken, any dietary fads and the amount of fruit and vegetables and cereals ingested.

An accurate account of drugs given and other remedies tried by the parents before presenting at the clinic is documented.

Examination

A full examination of the child is important noting the presence of any dysmorphic features, height and weight as well as any signs of failure to thrive. Inspection of the abdomen noting any abdominal distension or the presence of local swelling. The abdomen is then palpated in routine fashion, feeling for any abdominal mass. A faecal mass can usually be indented through the abdomen, although at times the impacted mass may be so hard as to make it quite impossible to indent, and may mislead one into thinking it is a malignant mass. A loaded, impacted colon with a megarectum can in turn cause retention of urine resulting in a full bladder which may or may not distress the child if this is a chronic situation.

Digital rectal examination must be carefully explained to the parents and the child before proceeding, explaining the importance of deciding whether constipation is a problem, especially in the presence of diarrhoea which may be spurious in nature. It is helpful to have a nurse in attendance to position the child in the left lateral position with knees bent in the fetal position. It is useful to carry on conversation during this investigation to relax an otherwise tense atmosphere and also explaining to the parent and the child what is being done. While the child is in this position, it is important to examine the spine and the sacrum for any sign of spina bifida occulta. The position of the anus as well as its size should be noted to exclude the possibility of an anterior ectopic anus or an anal stenosis. The skin around the anus should look normal. Erythema may indicate the presence of candida or streptococcal infection or may be due to topical applications by the parents. The presence of puckering of the anus as well as the presence of a skin tag may indicate an underlying anal fissure which could be the result of the vicious cycle of retention of stool, chronic constipation and painful defaecation. The presence of soiling should be noted and the consistency and volume of stool, if it is hard or soft or liquid in form, as well as whether there is any blood present.

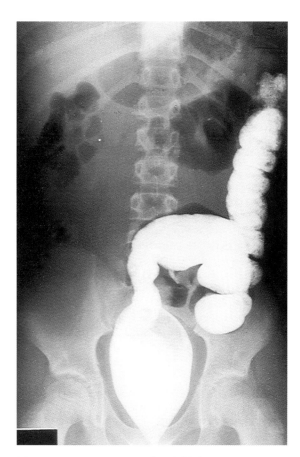

FIGURE 7.24 Barium enema of a child demonstrating gross rectal dilatation and obstruction with mass of faeces ("terminal reservoir").

Investigations

A plain X-ray of the abdomen in a child with a distended abdomen and constipation may indicate the degree of constipation and may also detect underlying bony abnormalities such as spina bifida occulta or sacral abnormalities. Barium enema (Fig. 7.24) may be carried out in a few children with chronic constipation where there is a suspicion of Hirschsprung disease but in most children radiological investigations are not required if an adequate history is taken. These children must not be prepared by bowel washout prior to the barium enema because this will obscure the X-ray appearance.

Management of acute constipation

Acute constipation

It is important to explain the mechanism of acute constipation to the parents and the child and to emphasise the benign nature of this condition. It is treated by increasing the fluid and fibre content of the diet or, if necessary, a bulk agent to restore the normal pattern of defaecation of the child.

Chronic constipation

The management of this condition involves getting the cooperation of the child, the parents, as well as the general practitioner and the nurse. An explanation of the cause of the intractable problem should be given to the parents. Dietary measures with a high fluid intake and an adequate dietary residue should be commenced. Bran should be added to the cereal in the morning. In addition to this it is necessary to dislodge the faecal masses with oral preparations of dioctyl sodium, and lactulose 10–30 ml/day. A phosphate enema (3 ml/kg) is sometimes necessary. During the period of impaction, soiling is often worse and this has to be explained to the parents so that they are not disheartened. The period of regulation of bowel habits to food and fluid intake may take several months to achieve. It may be necessary to give the child, in addition to the above, a stimulant to increase the gastrocolic reflex (Senokot 10–20 ml may be given at bedtime or bisacodyl 5–10 ml/day). Occasionally manual evacuation under general anaesthesia is necessary to dislodge firm impacted faecal masses, before continuing with prolonged dietary and medicinal management.

Rectal inertia results from chronic overdistension of the rectum from chronic constipation rendering it insensitive to the presence of stool. Treatment of this condition involves regular emptying of the rectum and colon if necessary by washouts initially on a daily basis and then extending the period of time between washouts. This must be supplemented by laxatives which include bulk agents and stimulants of the gastrocolic reflex such as Senokot and bisacodyl. Once the rectum has returned to a normal size, then it may be possible to achieve continence but this is a process that may take several months to achieve. Some children require referral for psychological help to treat underlying problems of a psychogenic nature, but this should be only done once other disease processes have been excluded.

GASTROINTESTINAL INFECTIONS

Infantile gastroenteritis

Until 1972 viral enteritis was only a hypothesis. However, with the development of electron microscopy and other techniques it has been found that the rotavirus is the major cause of episodic diarrhoea in infants and young children especially in temperate climates. In the developed world after rotaviruses, group F adenoviruses (serotypes 40 and 41) are the most common viruses associated with infantile gastroenteritis. Seroepidemiology shows that they are common throughout the world and that other viruses can also cause diarrhoea, e.g. parvo-like viruses, astroviruses and caliciviruses.

Most human rotavirus infections occur between the ages of 6 months and 2 years. In temperate climates the incidence of rotavirus infection and disease is much greater in winter than in summer and in the tropics the incidence is probably higher in the cooler and drier parts of the year. It has been shown that human milk and colostrum contain secretory IgA antibodies against rotaviruses which are type specific and that breast fed infants have a lower incidence of rotavirus infection than bottle fed infants.

The incubation period of rotavirus gastroenteritis varies from 48 to 72 hours. Rotavirus disease is usually accompanied by fever, vomiting usually preceeds the diarrhoea and lasts 1–3 days, and the diarrhoea lasts 4–7 days. Rotavirus gastroenteritis is not generally a life threatening disease in temperate climate but the illness can be severe and lead to death from dehydration. Rotavirus particles in stool are most easily detected early in the course of infection. At present, radioimmunoassay and ELISA appear to be the most valuable of the diagnostic techniques.

Bacterial enteritis

Bacterial pathogens that produce diarrhoeal illness in children include shigella, salmonella, *Escherichia coli*, *Campylobacter fetus* subspecies *jejuni* and *Yersinia enterocolitica*. *Vibrio cholerae* does not occur in Britain and infection by *Aeromonas hydrophila* is rare.

Escherichia coli

Only certain strains of *E. coli* seem to be capable of producing diarrhoeal disease in humans. Several mechanisms have been described, many involving enterotoxigenic, enteroinvasive and enteropathogenic *E. coli* which are divided into serotypes of specific agglutinable *E. coli* which are categorised by their somatic (O) antigen. Among the most important are O.111, O.55, O.26, O.119, O.128 and O.114. In spite of their importance the mechanism by which they colonise the small intestine is unknown.

Campylobacter jejuni

Campylobacters are the most frequently identified agents of acute infective diarrhoea in most developed countries. Campylobacter enteritis cannot be differentiated clinically from other acute bacterial diarrhoeas although the intensity and duration of abdominal pain is on average greater in campylobacter enteritis. Treatment with antibiotics is seldom required in the self-limiting infection but for severely affected patients erythromycin or ciprofloxacin is effective.

Yersinia enterocolitica

The true incidence of yersiniosis is unknown but the infection is most prevalent in cooler regions of Europe. In some countries *Yersinia enterocolitica* has surpassed shigella and rivals salmonella as a cause of acute gastroenteritis. In most children there is a mild self-limited illness with fever, vomiting and diarrhoea. Some children have mesenteric adenitis and may present a clinical picture simulating acute appendicitis. Rarely arthritis and erythema nodosum may be associated with yersiniosis.

Shigella

Shigella infection in children is mostly due to *Shigella sonnei* and *Shigella flexneri. Sh. dysenteriae* I infection is less common in Europe and North America but still causes devastating epidemics in developing countries. The infections occur most commonly in the summer months and children usually present with fever and diarrhoeal stools containing blood and mucus.

Salmonella

Although typhoid fever (*S. typhi*) is rare in Europe, salmonella enteritis (*S. paratyphi*) is particularly common in children under 5 years of age. Both present usually with diarrhoea, abdominal cramps, nausea, vomiting and fever. These stools may contain blood and mucus and the diarrhoea is usually self-limiting.

Diarrhoea caused by food borne toxins

Diarrhoea and vomiting can be caused by toxins produced by *Staphylococcus aureas* and *Bacillus cereus* which contaminate foodstuffs such as cooked meat products, cream and reheated rice.

Clinical features of gastroenteritis

Profuse diarrhoea in infants and children can cause serious fluid, acid–base and electrolyte disturbances and these changes can progress with frightening speed to produce circulatory failure. Dehydration may be mild (5% loss of body weight), moderate (5–10% loss of body weight) or severe (10% or more loss of body weight). Table 7.2 summarises the clinical findings. Measurement of actual body weight loss and gain after therapy provides important clinical information. The clinical features can only provide an approximation to the degree of dehydration especially

TABLE 7.2 Clinical assessment of signs of dehydration

% BODY WEIGHT LOST	CLINICAL STATE	CLINICAL SIGNS
< 5%	Not unwell	Thirst, irritable, dry mucous membranes
5–10%	Apathetic	Marked thirst, tachypnoea, oliguria, sunken eyes and fontanelle, decreased skin turgor
> 10%	Shocked	In addition to above – hypotension, cold extremities from peripheral vasoconstriction

in obese or severe malnourished infants. The infant's condition may be further complicated by thrombosis of the renal veins or cerebral venous sinuses.

Types of dehydration

Dehydration may be isotonic, hypotonic or hypertonic. In isotonic dehydration the loss of electrolytes in the diarrhoea and vomit parallel the losses of body water (which comes mostly from the extracellular fluid compartment) and plasma osmolality remains within normal limits (275–295 mmol/kg plasma water). Plasma electrolyte concentrations are not seriously abnormal in the acute stage of isotonic dehydration. Hypotonic dehydration (plasma sodium less than 130 mmol/l) occurs when the loss of electolytes in the diarrhoea exceed the loss of water. When the loss of body water exceeds the loss of electrolytes, this results in hypertonic dehydration (plasma sodium more than 150 mmol/l).

Hypernatraemic dehydration is more common in obese infants fed large amounts of high solute feeds such as undiluted cows' milk or incorrectly prepared powdered milk feeds. Rarely, it is the first indication of nephrogenic or pituitary diabetes. The infant may be irritable, have a normal or full fontanelle tension and a firm doughy feel to the skin. It is important to recognise hypertonic dehydration as the clinical manifestations tend to be less striking than those of isotonic or hypotonic dehydration. This is because the water loss is mainly from the intracellular compartment and the blood pressure and peripheral circulation are maintained until a late stage of dehydration. Its recognition rests largely upon the measurement of the plasma sodium and osmolality.

Haemoconcentration and hypovolaemia are reflected in abnormally high haemoglobin, haematocrit and serum protein values, provided that the infant has not previously been anaemic or severely undernourished. Metabolic acidosis due to excessive loss of stool cation is shown by a reduced plasma bicarbonate and in uncompensated cases by a reduced blood pH. Dimished glomerular filtration rate explains the finding of high blood urea and creatinine.

TABLE 7.3 Composition of recommended rehydration fluids: glucose and electrolyte content (mmol/l)

FLUID	GLUCOSE	Na$^+$	K$^+$	Cl$^-$	ALKALI
WHO oral rehydration powder	111	90	20	80	10 (citrate)
Diorylate oral powder*	90	60	20	60	10 (citrate)
Gluco-lyte oral powder*	200	35	20	37	18 (bicarbonate)
Electrolade oral powder*	111	50	20	40	30 (bicarbonate)
Rehidrat† (+Suc 94 Fruct 2)	91	50	20	50	20 (bicarbonate) 9 (citrate)
Dextrolyte oral solution	200	35	13.4	30.5	17.7 (lactate)
N (0.9%) saline	–	154		154	
1/2 N (0.45%) saline in 5% dextrose	280	77		77	
1/5 N (0.18%0 saline in 4% dextrose	224	30		30	

* Reconstituted as 1 sachet to 200 ml water.
† Reconstituted as 1 sachet to 250 ml water.

Treatment

The principles of treatment for both viral and bacterial gastroenteritis are similar. When dehydration is mild to moderate it is preferable to treat the infant at home. The family doctor must be able to assess the degree of dehydration and be prepared to review frequently the response to treatment. Initially bottle-fed infants and children with acute gastroenteritis should have a period of bowel rest with complete withdrawal of milk and solid foods for 24 hours. During this 24-hour period oral glucose/electrolyte solutions should be given in small frequent amounts. Oral electrolyte solutions have been a matter of controversy but the fluids described in Table 7.3 are suitable. The fluid should be offered freely every 2 hours during the day and every 4 hours during the night. In the first 24 hours the amount given should be equal to the child's maintenance fluid requirement (Table 7.4) with an extra 20% to cover continuing losses. There is also some controversy about the best way in which to reintroduce milk once vomiting has stopped and diarrhoea is rapidly subsiding. One method is to start with half strength formula for 12–24 hours then return to normal feeding. This regimen has been successful in rehydrating most children except for those with severe dehydration requiring intravenous therapy or those who develop secondary disaccharide intolerance. In breast feeding infants the feeding should not be discontinued. The additional glucose/electrolyte solution should be given between feeds.

TABLE 7.4 Maintenance fluids (ml/kg/day) and electrolytes (mmol/kg/day) requirements

AGE (years)	WEIGHT (kg)	H$_2$O	Na	K
< 0.5	< 5	150	3.0	3.0
0.5–1	5–10	120	2.5	2.5
1–3	10–15	100	2.5	2.0
3–5	15–20	80	2.0	2.0

When vomiting or profuse diarrhoea persists or when severe (10%) dehydration or peripheral circulatory failure is present admission to hospital for intravenous therapy is indicated.

The management of severe dehydration using intravenous therapy is based on initial resuscitation to restore the circulation, correction of body water and electrolyte deficit and the provision for maintenance requirements and any ongoing abnormal losses no matter what the underlying cause of the dehydration.

Initial resuscitation

Circulatory failure is treated by the rapid intravenous administration, over 10–15 minutes of 20 ml/kg plasma or plasma equivalent. If these are unavailable, 0.9% saline may be substituted. This should result in a rise in blood pressure, improved pulse volume, a gradual return of warmth to the periphery and improved capillary refill and the establishment of an adequate urine output (greater than 0.5 ml/kg/h). The initial plasma infusion might need to be repeated within 30 minutes if there is no response. Measurement of the peripheral to core temperature differential is a useful indicator of circulatory status and can be used as a guide to the adequacy of volume replacement (differential should be < 2°C)

Subsequent fluid administration

After successful initial resuscitation or in the dehydrated infant without circulatory failure, intravenous fluid requirements in the first 24 hours are calculated as the estimated body fluid deficit (see Table 7.2) or from the known body weight loss. This volume is added to the maintenance fluid requirement (Table 7.4). The fluid deficit is replaced as 0.45% saline in dextrose and the maintenance fluid as 0.18% saline in dextrose. The first half of the total calculated fluids is given in the first 8 hours and the second half in the following 16 hours. It should be emphasised that these methods of calculation are estimates and fluid therapy should be modified dependent upon the child's subsequent clinical progress and serum biochemistry. Continuing abnormal fluid loss through vomiting and diarrhoea and persistent fever may require an increased volume of fluid to be given. Ideally stool and vomit can be collected, measured and replaced as 0.45% saline but an extra 10 ml/kg per 24 hours can be allowed to cover stool loss and maintenance fluids may be increased by 10 ml/kg per 24 hours for each one degree of sustained temperature increase in the child.

Severe hyponatraemia (sodium less than 120 mmol/l) should be corrected by giving the initial rehydration fluid as 0.9% saline until the calculated extracellular sodium deficit (140 – plasma sodium × body weight (kg) × 0.3 mmol) is replaced. Then 0.45% saline and 0.18% saline are given as above. Serum potassium will decrease during rehydration unless renal failure is present. When adequate urine flow is established potassium chloride (20 mmol/l) should be added to the infusion fluids. Plasma electrolytes and body weight should be measured at least 24-hourly and more frequently in the ill child. Stool bicarbonate loss and poor tissue perfusion may cause a metabolic acidosis. If arterial pH is less than 7.1 or plasma bicarbonate less than 10 mmol/l, it is reasonable to half correct the base deficit with 8.4% sodium bicarbonate, using the formula (0.5 × base deficit × body weight (kg) × 0.3 (ml)). When such correction is necessary it should be carried out slowly to avoid the risk of sodium overload and should be avoided in the management of hypernatraemic dehydration.

Hypertonic dehydration, although rare, must be recognised as it requires careful management. Hyperosmolality in the extracellular fluid produces intracellular dehydration and dysfunction with neurological irritability, convulsions and occasionally intracranial haemorrhage and/or thrombosis. Renal function is frequently impaired. Initial resuscitation with plasma will be required if there is circulatory failure but rapid correction of extracellular fluid hyperosmolality will produce cell swelling, brain oedema and cause convulsions. Rehydration must therefore be slow, aiming to correct over a minimum of 48 hours (72 hours if hypernatraemia is greater than 165 mmol/l), and lowering the plasma sodium by no more that 12 mmol per 24 hours. Otherwise the principles of rehydration are similar to other types of dehydration. The deficit volume which will rarely exceed 10% of the body weight is added to maintenance fluids for 48 or 72 hours and is given evenly throughout this period, commencing with 0.45% glucose saline as previously. If seizures do occur during rehydration they should be treated with mannitol 1 g/kg infused over 10–20 minutes. Hyperglycaemia may occur but it should not be treated with insulin as it will resolve spontaneously with rehydration. Hypocalcaemia is also found during the correction of hypernatraemic dehydration and may require treatment with intravenous calcium gluconate.

After a period of 24–26 hours on intravenous fluids the diarrhoea and vomiting of gastroenteritis have usually subsided and milk feeds may be gradually introduced as previously described. As the infant tolerates the oral feeds the volumes of intravenous fluids are correspondingly reduced.

Drugs

Drugs are rarely needed for the treatment of infectious diarrhoea in children. Antimotility drugs do not help acute infectious diarrhoea since it is not motility but transport pathways that are impaired in gastroenteritis. By interfering with transit they may delay the natural flushing action of peristalsis. Other antidiarrhoeal agents e.g. kaolin may improve the appearance of stools but they will not improve the salt and water balance of the child. Antimotility drugs are potentially toxic and other agents should probably be avoided.

FERMENTATIVE DIARRHOEA (DISACCHARIDE INTOLERANCE)

In the healthy child the disaccharide sucrose is split into the monosaccharides, glucose and fructose by small intestinal sucrase-isomaltase enzyme and the disaccharide lactose into the monosaccharides glucose and galactose by the enzyme lactase. Failure of any of these enzyme systems will result in an excess of disaccharide in the intestine where bacteria will ferment the sugars to produce acid and an increased osmotic bowel content. This results in a fermentative diarrhoea with the passage of highly acid watery stools. Symptoms are relieved when the offending disaccharide is removed from the diet. Lactase deficiency inherited as an autosomal recessive disorder causes persistent diarrhoea from birth because both human and cows' milk contain lactose. When there is a delay in the onset of symptoms this suggests a sucrase-isomaltase deficiency as sucrose and starch are not usually added to the diet in the first weeks after birth. In addition to the autosomal recessive inheritance of the deficiency there can be transient disaccharide intolerence acquired secondarily to gastroenteritis or other intestinal mucosal insult. Investigations which help to confirm a disaccharide intolerence include the pH of the fresh stool less than 5.5 and the presence of reducing sugars revealed by the Clinitest and by the identification of faecal sugars

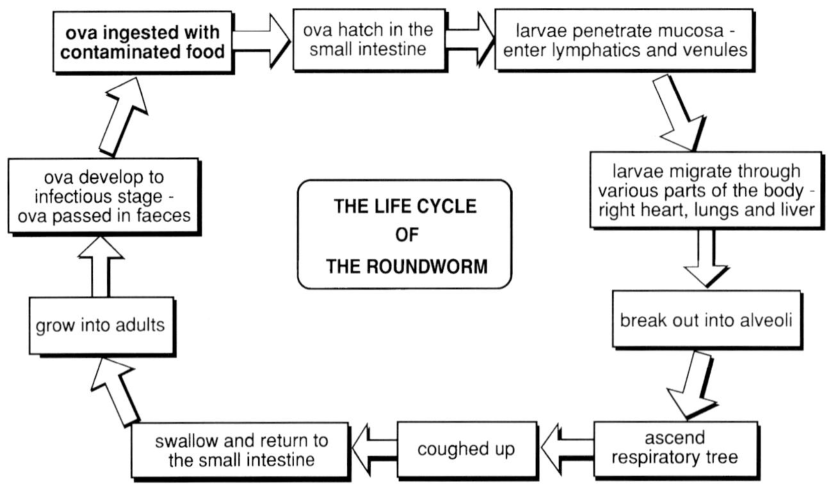

FIGURE 7.25 Life cycle of the roundworm.

on thin-layer chromatography. Removal of all disaccharide from the diet and replacement with monosaccharide will result in a resolution of the diarrhoea. Re-introduction of the disaccharide will result in the return of the diarrhoea and there will be a failure of the normal increase in blood glucose of at least 2.8 mmol/l (50 mg/100 ml) expected in the normal subject. Rarely a monosaccharide malabsorption syndrome (glucose–galactose malabsorption) can occur. Jejunal biopsy will allow direct measurement of enzyme activity in the jejunal mucosa. The diarrhoea in infants with the hereditary forms of the disorder can be abolished by total exclusion from the diet of the offending carbohydrate.

SYSTEMIC ILLNESS

In addition to the acute diarrhoea caused by food poisoning from food toxins or bacterial toxins, viral, bacterial and protozoal bowel infections, there are a number of systemic illnesses which are complicated by acute diarrhoea and vomiting. Septicaemia, meningitis, pneumonia and infectious hepatitis may be accompanied by diarrhoea and vomiting. Abdominal distension with bloody diarrhoea may suggest an acute surgical condition or the haemolytic uraemic sydrome. Hospital admission is indicated if significant dehydration (more than 5%) is present when there is doubt about the diagnosis, when hypernatraemia is suspected, when an underlying medical condition such as adrenogenital syndrome or chronic renal insufficiency is present or when outpatient management has failed or is thought to be inappropriate due to adverse social or other circumstances.

PARASITIC INTESTINAL INFECTION

It is estimated that between 800 million and one thousand million people in the world are suffering from at least one type of worm infection. The most important intestinal worms are nematodes and cestodes.

NEMATODES

These are round elongated, non-segmented worms with differentiation of the sexes.

Roundworm (*Ascaris lumbricoides*)

Mode of infection

Infection arises from swallowing ova from soil contaminated with human excreta. The ova are not embryonated when passed in the faeces but they become infective in soil or water. When swallowed by man the hatched larvae penetrate the intestinal wall and pass via the liver and lungs to the trachea, oesophagus, stomach and intestine where they grow into mature worms (Fig. 7.25).

Clinical effects

A few roundworms in a well fed patient usually produce no ill effects and are not noticed until a

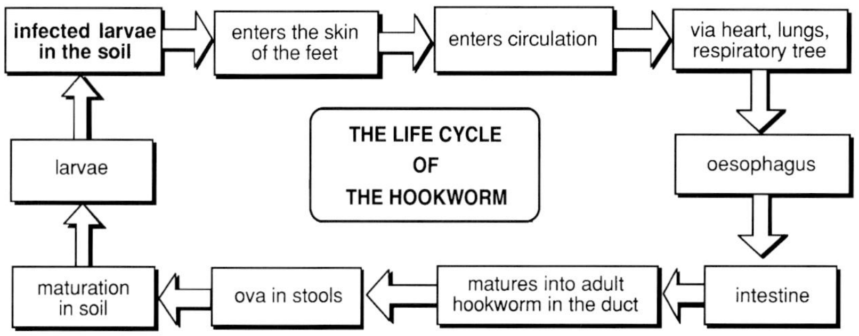

FIGURE 7.26 Life cycle of the hookworm.

worm is either vomited or passed in the stool. Typical clinical features include: a protuberant abdomen, intermittent intestinal colic, digestive disturbance, general debility, loss of appetite and insomnia. In heavy infections worms may migrate into and block the bile duct producing jaundice while similar blocking of the appendix can cause appendicitis. In very heavy infections intestinal obstruction can occur from a tangled ball of roundworms. The presence and extent of roundworm infection is readily detected by microscopical examination of the stools for ova.

Piperazine citrate (Antepar Elixir) in a single oral dose of 75 mg/kg body weight to a maximum single dose of 5 g will clear roundworm from 75% of patients. Two doses on successive days give a marginally higher cure rate. Piperazine citrate has minimum adverse effects, very occasionally unsteadiness and vertigo.

Mebendazole is active against threadworm, whipworm and hookworm as well as roundworm infections and can be safely recommended for children over the age of 2 years. A dose of 100 mg twice daily for 3 days is effective. Pyrantel is also an effective anthelmintic and a single dose of 10 mg/kg (max. 1 g) will usually eradicate Ascaris. It is not recommended under 6 months of age. Levamisole may prove to be the drug of choice in the future but it has not been fully assessed for use in children and is not on the UK market.

Hookworm (*Ancylostoma duodenale; Necator americanus*)

There are two types of hookworm, *Ancylostoma duodenale* being most commonly found in Egypt, Africa, India, Queensland and also in the southern USA, while *Necator americanus* is found in the Americas, the Phillippines and India. These two species differ in small anatomical details but their life cycles are identical (Fig. 7.26). Ancylostomiasis is sometimes encountered in immigrants to the United Kingdom. The male and female worms live chiefly in the jejunum. The worm attaches itself to the intestinal mucosa by its teeth and sucks blood. The ova, passed in the faeces, hatch out in water or damp soil and larvae penetrate the skin of the buttocks or feet. They reach the heart and lungs by the lymph vessels and blood stream, penetrate into the bronchi, are coughed up into the trachea and then pass down the oesophagus to mature in the small intestine.

Clinical effects

The main clinical picture of hookworm disease is caused by prolonged loss of blood. Therefore the clinical manifestations of hookworm infection depend on the number of worms present and the nutritional state of the patient. A few hookworms in a fairly well fed person produce no disease as the small blood loss is constantly being replaced. In children whose diet is inadequate and the worm load heavy severe anaemia may stunt growth, retard mental development and in very severe cases result in death through heart failure. Hookworm infection is diagnosed by microscopical examination of the stools for eggs, the number of which indicates the severity of infection (72 000 ova/g = significant infection).

Treatment

Children with severe anaemia and malnutrition should have blood transfusion and nutritional support before definitive worm therapy is started.

Bephenium hydroxynaphthoate (Alcopar) can be given to children in a single dose of 5 g. Children under 2 years or under 10 kg in weight should receive half the above dosage. Alcopar is given on an empty stomach, thereby ensuring maximum contact between parasite and drug and food is withheld for 2 hours after the dose. To mask the bitter taste of the drug the granules may be added to about a quarter cupful of sweetened water, milk, orange, tomato or other fruit juices. In some cases it may be necessary to continue treatment for 4–7 days to remove infection completely. Residual ova may continue to be excreted for some days after elimination of the adult worms. Therefore, when assessing the effects of Alcopar, ova

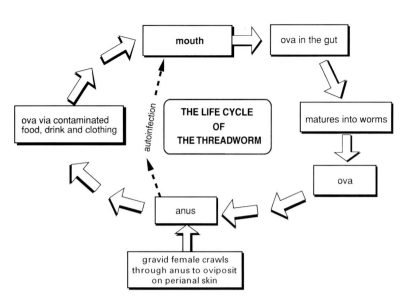

FIGURE 7.27 Life cycle of the thread-worm.

counts should be deferred until 2 or 3 weeks after completion of treatment. *Ancylostoma* is much more susceptible than *Necator* to bephenium.

Other effective agents against hookworm are thiabendazole (Mintezol), mebendazole (Vermox) and pyrantel embonate (Combantrin). These drugs are used only when bephenium is unavailable or has failed to eradicate *Necator* strains.

Strongyloidiasis (*Strongyloides stercoralis*)

These worms are fairly widespread in warmer climates and may be found concurrently with hookworm infection. Incidence is often highest in children and the usual mode of infection is penetration of the skin by infective larvae present in the soil. Migration through the lungs also occurs and can produce respiratory signs and these may be abdominal distension, bloody diarrhoea and anaemia. Creeping eruptions, particularly around the buttocks, can develop as a result of the reinfection. Diagnosis is made by identification of larvae in the faeces.

Thiabendazole (50 mg/kg divided into two doses given morning and evening) is the most effective treatment. Levamisole and pyrantel embonate are effective but their cure rates are lower.

Whipworm (*Trichuris trichiura*)

In mild whipworm infections, which constitute the majority, there are usually no obvious symptoms. In heavy infections abdominal pains, diarrhoea, loss of weight, anaemia and possibly rectal prolapse may occur. Growth retardation and finger clubbing may be found in more chronic infections. Diagnosis is by recognition of characteristic ova in the faeces.

Until recently the treatment of this infection was most unsatisfactory. The effective drugs available today are mebendazole and thiabendazole.

Threadworm (*Enterobius vermicularis-oxyuriasis*; pinworm or seatworm)

The male worm is about 3 mm in length and the female, which looks like a small piece of thread, is about 10 mm. The female lives in the colon. Eggs are deposited on the perianal skin by the female, contaminating the fingers of the child who may then reinfect himself. The ova after ingestion hatch in the small intestine. The male worm also fertilises the female in the small intestine, after which the male dies while the female migrates to the caecum. It is common for this infestation to affect all members of a family because the ova can be found on many household objects. The initial infection may also be acquired from contaminated water or uncooked foodstuffs (Fig. 7.27).

Clinical features of enterobiasis are mainly perianal, perineal and vulval pruritus which can interfere with sleep. Scratching leads to secondarily infected dermatitis and to reinfection through contaminated fingers. Heavy infestations could be associated with episodes of severe abdominal pain. The association of appendicitis with threadworms is exceptionally rare. Diagnosis is made by direct examination of the worms or ova trapped by "sellotape" applied sticky side to the anal skin early in the morning and then stuck on to a glass slide.

Mebendazole 100 mg (one tablet or one 5 ml dose) is usually effective. The treatment can be repeated in 2 weeks to ensure complete eradication. Pyrantel in a single dose of 10 mg/kg is also effective, giving cure rates of 90%. This treatment can also be repeated in 2 weeks if necessary. Measures to break the cycle of reinfection should be taken and these include scrupulous personal hygiene, boiling all infected linen and the wearing of occlusive clothing to prevent scratching. Treatment should also be given to other members of the family and it should be reinstituted when symptoms recur and eggs are again found in the perineal area.

Larva migrans

Cutaneous variety (creeping eruption)

Cutaneous larva migrans is caused by the infective larvae of various dog hookworms. These larvae can penetrate the human skin and, finding themselves in an unsuitable habitat, wander around in the epidermis for several weeks. Their progress is marked by a characteristic itching and a serpiginous urticarial track. The infection is more common in children than in adults and is occasionally seen in people recently returned from tropical countries.

Treatment by freezing the advancing end of the track with dry ice or liquid nitrogen is no longer recommended. Applications of topical 15% thiabendazole powder in water soluble base with or without diethylcarbamazine (Banocide) 5 mg/kg/day for 7 days will eliminate the larvae.

Visceral variety

This is caused by various species of the nematode *Toxocara*, usually *T. canis*, the common roundworm of the dog. The larvae may penetrate the intestinal wall but are unable to migrate to the lungs of their unnatural host and pass through or become encysted in liver, lungs, kidneys, heart, muscle, brain or eye, causing an intense local tissue reaction. The child may fail to thrive, develop anaemia and become pyrexial with a cough, wheeze and hepatosplenomegaly. There is usually a marked eosinophilia and there can be CNS involvement. In addition to this generalised form of the disorder, in the older child (7–9 years old), there may be the isolated loss of sight in one eye associated with ocular toxocariasis. The diagnosis can only be established with certainty from a tissue biopsy, generally taken from the liver and the *Toxocara* ELISA test is a useful screen.

Recently thiabendazole 50 mg/kg body weight for 3–5 days has been shown to kill encysted larvae and

is especially useful for early ocular lesions. Normally the visceral variety is self-limiting and requires no treatment. Regular and routine deworming of puppies and pregnant bitches with mebendazole, prevention of face licking by dogs and the need to wash hands carefully after handling pets are preventative health measures.

CESTODES

Cestodes (tapeworms) of importance to humans are *Taenia saginata* (beef tapeworm), *Taenia solium* (pork tapeworm), *Hymenolepis* species (dwarf tapeworm) and *Taenia echinococcus* (hydatid cyst). The ingestion of raw or inadequately cooked beef or pork can result in human infection. Man is the definitive host for both the beef (*T. saginata*) and pork (*T. solium*) tapeworms. Although the infections may be asymptomatic, epigastric discomfort, increased appetite, dizziness and loss of weight sometimes occur. These features may be more marked in children and debilitated persons. Diagnosis is based on the passage of gravid segments through the anus. The differentiation can be made by a microscopical study of the number of lateral branches in the gravid uterus of each segment, the uterus of *T. solium* having about 10 branches and that of *T. saginata* about 20.

With *T. solium* infection a major danger is the ingestion of eggs from an infected person (heteroinfection) or self ingestion of eggs (autoinfection). This can give rise to cysticercosis where cysticerci develop almost anywhere including brain, skin, muscle and eye.

Taenia echinococcus (hydatid cyst)

The definitive host of *Taenia echinococcus* is the dog, wolf, fox or jackal. Man and sheep may become the intermediate host by swallowing the ova from the dog and this is especially likely in sheep-rearing countries such as Australia. The adult worm in the dog is very small (0.5 cm) but the ingested ovum when swallowed by man liberates a six-hooked onchosphere into the small intestine. This penetrates to the tissues, usually the liver but sometimes lung, bones, kidneys or brain, to form a hydatid cyst. This has a three-layered wall – an outer layer of host fibrous tissue, a laminated middle layer and an inner germinal layer which produces many daughter and granddaughter cysts.

Clinical effects

These are largely due to local pressure effects. The liver may be greatly enlarged and there may be a palpable rounded swelling over which the classical "hydatid thrill" can be elicited. Ultrasound and CT scanning can reveal the cystic nature of the lesions. Eosinophilia may be marked. The diagnosis may be confirmed by complement fixation, haemagglutination or latex-slide agglutination tests but the hydatid ELISA test and improved immunoelectrophoresis tests are likely to prove more specific.

Treatment

The only measure is surgical excision. The cyst must never be tapped as a leakage of hydatid fluid into the tissues can cause shock or death. The outlook is grave if suppuration occurs within the cyst. Spontaneous recovery can occur if the cyst dies, inspissates and calcifies. Medical treatment for this most important tapeworm infecting man is generally unsatisfactory but albendazole 10 mg/kg daily for 8 weeks has been shown to be effective. Successful programmes for the control of hydatid disease in New Zealand and Tasmania include preventing dogs having access to sheep offal and deworming of the dogs with praziquantel.

Hymenolepis (dwarf tapeworm)

Mild infestations due to Hymenolepis (dwarf tapeworm) cause no symptoms, but heavy infestations can sometimes cause diarrhoea, irritability and fits. Diagnosis is made by finding the typical ova in the faeces.

Treatment

Niclosamide (Yomesan) can be given to out-patients without prior preparation. Each tablet of Yomesan contains 500 mg niclosamide BP. It can be used orally in infestation with both large and dwarf tapeworms. For the large tapeworms one single dose is sufficient. For adults and children from 6 years upwards this is four tablets, children from 2 to 6 years 2 tablets, and children under 2 years one tablet. A laxative given 2 hours after the Yomesan dose should ensure a rapid and complete expulsion of the worm. Without purgation the parasite is excreted in pieces during the next few days. In the case of Taenia solium a laxative is essential because worm disintegration may be followed by cysticercosis.

For the infection with the dwarf tapeworm treatment with niclosamide for 7 days is recommended: first day, adults and children from 6 years upwards four tablets; children from 2 to 6 years two tablets; children under 2 years one tablet. For the remaining 6 days: adults and children from 6 years upwards are given two tablets daily; children from 2 to 6 years one tablet daily; and children under 2 years half a tablet daily. Yomesan can be given unhesitatingly to patients with liver, biliary and kidney diseases. There are no known contraindications and no adverse effects have been recorded. Praziquantel is as effective as niclosamide and requires only a single dose of 10–20 mg/kg after a light breakfast but it is not available in the UK. In cysticercosis praziquantel (50 mg kg/day in three divided doses for 14 days) has recently been shown to be effective. Dichlorophen (Anthiphen) is specifically indicated in the treatment of human tapeworm infestation caused by Taenia saginata but is also used for Hymenolepis nana. Each tablet contains 500 mg dichlorophen. It may be administered orally in any one of the following dose regimens:

1 Adults
   (a) 18 tablets in a single dose
   (b) 12 tablets on each of two successive days
   (c) 4–6 tablets three times in 24 hours.
2 Children
   (a) 4–8 tablets on each of two successive days
   (b) 2–4 tablets three times in 24 hours.

No preliminary starvation or additional purgation is necessary but best results are usually obtained if the drug is given in the morning on an empty stomach. No specific or absolute contraindications have been established for Anthiphen but caution should be exercised in the presence of liver disease. Treatment should also be avoided in febrile or severe cardiovascular disease, in pregnancy and in any other condition where purgation is undesirable on general medical grounds.

To assess cure a careful search must be made for the worm's head and if the head has not been passed treatment has failed and should be repeated after a reasonable period. When niclosamide, which disintegrates the worm, has been used it is necessary to examine the stools after 3 months and repeat the treatment if eggs or segments are detected.

PROTOZOAN PARASITIC INFECTION

Giardia intestinalis (Giardia lamblia)

Giardiasis or lambliasis is the only common protozoan intestinal parasitic infection in the United Kingdom apart from the non-pathogenic Entamoeba coli. The parasite may appear as a trophozoite with eight flagella or as an ovoid cyst best seen in a fresh stool suspension by wet film microscopy. Its normal habitat is the upper small bowel. The cystic form is thought to develop in the lower ileum or colon and is excreted in the faeces. The organism is commonly spread by the faecal–oral route.

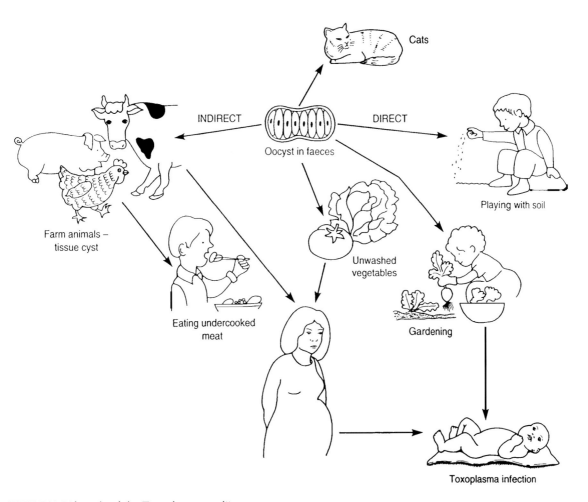

FIGURE 7.28 Life cycle of the *Toxoplasma gondii*.

Symptoms vary according to the degree of infestation, from mild looseness and increase in stool number to frank malabsorption and a clinical picture resembling coeliac disease. If symptomatic it can be readily eradicated with metronidazole 7.5 mg/kg/body weight three times daily. More recently it has been shown that tinidazole (50–60 mg/kg daily for 3 days) appears to be more effective than metronidazole and to have fewer side effects.

Cryptosporidiosis

Cryptosporidiosis is a protozoan and is found in several mammals. The parasite of *Cryptosporidium* appears to be a single species common to all host organisms it infects. The spread is probably both from animals to man and from person to person by the faecal–oral route.

The symptoms comprise diarrhoea without bleeding, abdominal pain, vomiting and sometimes fever. Various complications have also been described including prolonged listlessness, lethargy, loss of appetite, reactive arthritis and failure to thrive.

Diagnosis of cryptosporidiosis is based on demonstration of oocysts in stools.

Healthy immunocompetent children recover spontaneously from their diarrhoea within a few weeks whereas immunodeficient children may need spiramycin to eradicate *Cryptosporidium* from their stools. Otherwise only general measures for maintenance of fluid and electrolyte balance are needed.

Toxoplasmosis

This protozoal disease is now recognised to be a not uncommon cause of illness in humans throughout the world and its congenital form to be one of the causes of severe damage to the brain, eye, cardiac muscle and other organs.

Aetiology

The causal organism *Toxoplasma gondii* is an obligatory intracellular protozoan parasite 4–7 μm in length and half this in width with a crescentic shape.

The primary host is the cat. Excretion of oocysts found only in cat faeces result in widespread infection of many secondary hosts including man. Common sources of infection for children include exposure to toxoplasma oocysts (cat faecal contaminated soil) via sandpits, gardening and eating unwashed vegetables. In addition, both animals and man may become infected by ingesting raw or undercooked meat which contains toxoplasma tissue cysts (Fig. 7.28).

Pathology

In man acquired infections are most often symptomless but if a pregnant women is infected during pregnancy the parasites can cross the placenta to produce severe damage to the fetus. The parasites encyst in various tissues, e.g. brain, eyes, myocardium and lungs. These cysts contain viable toxoplasma which may persist for life.

Clinical features

Congenital toxoplasmosis

Toxoplasma infection acquired during pregnancy is rarely recognised; however, because of maternal parasitaemia, the fetus is always at risk. The severity of congenital toxoplasmosis depends on the age of the fetus at the time of infection – the earlier the more severe. Toxoplasma infection acquired by the mother before pregnancy is no threat to the fetus because of an effective maternal immunity. Fortunately reactivation or reinfection is not usually associated with congenital infection so mothers can be reassured about subsequent pregnancies.

In most instances the affected infant appears healthy at birth and lesions in the brain and eyes become manifest later. The typical triad of congenital toxoplasmosis is choroidoretinitis (Fig. 1.22), hydrocephalus and intracerebral calcification. Other manifestations include generalised purpura, often with thrombocytopenia, heptosplenomegaly, jaundice and erythroblastaemia.

The more typical manifestations cause the parents to seek medical advice usually during the first years because of delayed psychomotor development, convulsions or defective vision.

Acquired toxoplasmosis

Acute acquired toxoplasmosis is usually undiagnosed. The proportion of total cases in whom the infection is asymptomatic is not known. However, symptomatic acquired toxoplasmosis can cause severe illness such as encephalitis, myocarditis, or peripheral neuritis. More frequently in children the illness is relatively benign with fever, generalised lymphadenopathy and splenomegaly. Recrudescent toxoplasmosis and severe primary infections can occur in immunocompromised children with HIV infection and those who are immunosuppressed medically because of transplantation surgery. Most of these children develop encephalitis and a few develop retinochoroiditis (see Fig. 1.22) or myocarditis.

Diagnosis

The isolation of the parasites themselves may occasionally be achieved in active cases by inoculation of animals with cerebrospinal fluid, blood or tissue biopsy material. However, these procedures are not widely available and they take up to 3 weeks for the diagnosis to be confirmed.

The mainstays of diagnosis are the toxoplasma dye test and specific immunoglobulin IgM detection. An increased antibody titre in sequential tests or single high antibody titre are usually diagnostic. The dye test detects immunoglobulins IgG and IgM. In primary infections there is a high dye test result and IgM is present. Usually IgM disappears in 6–12 months but occasionally persists longer.

Treatment

Most children with toxoplasmosis do not require treatment as the illness is self-limiting. The main indications for treatment are severe widespread disease in immunocompromised patients, toxoplasmic uveitis affecting or threatening the macula and neonatal congenital infection. Unfortunately no treatment appears to eradicate all cysts and so reactivation can occur at a later date.

Pyrimethamine, sulphonamides, co-trimoxazole and spiramycin are the most commonly used drugs. Combinations of these drugs are the preferred treatment because of inhibitory effects of each drug becoming synergistic when used together. For generalised and central nervous system infection a combination of pyrimethamine and sulphonamides is indicated.

For pregnant women who seroconvert, toxoplasmacidal therapy is not recommended because of the uncertain benefit and potential hazard to the fetus. Information about toxoplasmosis and how to avoid it should be made available to women planning to become pregnant (see Chapter 1).

At present in the light of current knowledge it is not appropriate to introduce a nationwide routine serological surveillance programme for toxoplasmosis in pregnancy in the United Kingdom

CHRONIC INFLAMMATORY BOWEL DISEASE

The term chronic inflammatory bowel disease includes two clinical conditions in children; ulcerative

TABLE 7.5 Clinical features of ulcerative colitis and Crohn disease

CLINICAL FEATURES	ULCERATIVE COLITIS	CROHN DISEASE
Location	Rectum and colon (variable)	Ileum and right colon
Diarrhoea	Severe	Moderate
Mucus blood	Frequent	Infrequent
Rectal involvement	Always	Infrequent
Fistula *in ano*	Absent	Infrequent
Perirectal abscess	Absent	Infrequent
Abdominal wall fistula	Absent	Infrequent
Toxic megacolon	Infrequent	Absent
Arthritis	Rare	Common
Eye pathology	Rare	Iridocyclitis, granuloma
Proctoscopic appearance	Diffuse, ulceration	Cobblestone
Small bowel involvement	Absent	Frequent
Microscopic appearance	Mucosal ulceration (crypt abscesses)	Transmural granulomas

colitis and Crohn disease (Table 7.5). On the whole the prognosis of chronic inflammatory bowel disease in childhood is good.

Ulcerative colitis

Aetiology

The aetiology in unknown. It is fortunately rare in children. Over the past decade it would appear that there has been little change in the incidence of ulcerative colitis but Crohn disease has increased. The reason for the change is not clear.

Severe behavioural problems in some of the affected children and their families has sometimes led physicians to regard the disease as a psychosomatic disorder, but the evidence in support of this hypothesis is extremely slender. Food allergy has been suspected, but only a small group of patients respond to withdrawal of milk. Boys and girls are equally affected. The mean age of onset is about 10 years. There is no clear cut inheritance pattern but ulcerative colitis is more common in first degree relatives than in the general population.

Pathology

The mucous membrane of part or all of the colon and sometimes of the terminal ileum becomes hyperaemic, oedematous and ulcerated. The lesion is continuous rather than patchy and usually involves only the mucosal and submucosal layers. The earliest lesion in many cases is a crypt abscess (Fig. 7.29). Granuloma formation is rare. In some cases oedema may give rise to pseudopolypoid nodules. Ulceration may extend through the muscularis and perforation of the colon can occur. Usually perforation is preceded by toxic megacolon with dilatation of an ulcerated segment of

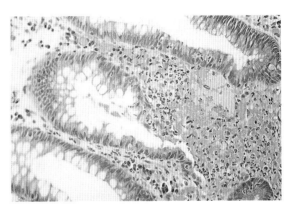

FIGURE 7.29 Ulcerative colitis. Rectal biopsy with crypt abscess formation (obj × 25).

the large bowel. Carcinoma is a common late complication. Hepatic complications such as sclerosing cholangitis and chronic active hepatitis can occur with ulcerative colitis in childhood.

Clinical features

The onset is sudden with diarrhoea and the frequent passage of small stools containing blood and mucus. This tends to be most severe during the early morning but may also be nocturnal. There may be abdominal pain, anorexia, weight loss or poor weight gain. Tenesmus is common.

Hypochromic anaemia due to chronic blood loss is almost invariably present. Hypoproteinaemic oedema may develop. Associated extraintestinal manifestations of the disease are more common in children than in adults. They may include erythema nodosum, aphthous stomatitis, conjunctivitis, iridocyclitis, haemolytic anaemia, arthralgia or arthritis, pyoderma gangrenosum and finger clubbing.

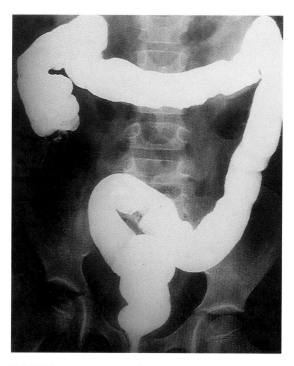

FIGURE 7.30 Barium enema showing loss of normal haustrations (lead-pipe appearance in the colon) in ulcerative colitis.

After exclusion of infective causes of bloody diarrhoea the diagnosis should be confirmed by rectosigmoidoscopy, mucosal biopsy and barium enema. The last shows loss of normal haustrations in the colon and the so called lead-pipe appearance (Fig. 7.30). Colonoscopy may allow the examination of the whole colonic mucosa and thus the extent of the disease. Radiologically differentiation of Crohn disease from ulcerative colitis can be made on the basis that Crohn disease can affect any part of the gastrointestinal tract and is patchy in distribution, whereas ulcerative colitis is a continuous lesion affecting only the rectum, colon and occasionally the terminal ileum ("Backwash ileitis"). It is worth remembering that early in the course of disease no X-ray abnormality may be found.

Ulcerative colitis frequently runs an acute course in the child. The cumulative risk of carcinoma of the colon is 20% per decade after the first decade of the illness. Dysplastic changes in the colonic epithelium are considered to be premalignant.

Treatment

During acute exacerbations bed rest may be required and the child should be encouraged to eat a balanced, palatable and nutritious diet. Anaemia should be corrected by blood transfusion. Remissions can frequently be obtained by daily colonic instillations of hydrocortisone sodium succinate 100 mg or prednisolone disodium phosphate 20 mg in 100 ml of isotonic buffered solution. In severe cases oral or even intravenous prednisolone or intravenous hydrocortisone may be necessary to save the child's life.

Oral prednisolone should be used in a dosage of 1–2 mg/kg/day in two to three divided doses for 3–4 weeks, then gradually reduced to alternate day therapy. Azathioprine (1–2 mg/kg/day) as a single daily dose may be used in those children who do not respond to corticosteroids, although its potentially grave side effects must be kept in mind.

Sulphasalazine is of some benefit during acute attacks but it is of most value in the reduction of risk of exacerbation when taken on a long-term basis. Oral sulphasalazine dosage for both severe and moderate attacks should be 40–60 mg/kg/day in four divided doses and the maintenance dose should be 20–30 mg/kg/day. Another useful drug is mesalazine. Oral disodium cromoglycate has been found useful but it has no significant impact on the course of the disease.

When symptoms are not relieved by medical treatment or if relapses are frequent, the surgeon must be consulted before the child's general condition has deteriorated severely. Total colectomy cures ulcerative colitis but this leaves the child with an ileostomy for life. However, subtotal colectomy with ileostomy with preservation of the rectum in carefully selected cases may be possible. The retained rectal stump can continue to harbour active disease and may develop a carcinoma. Therefore, eventually it must be removed. More recently ileo-anal operations to restore normal continuity of the bowel have become possible. These are often accompanied with a "pouch reservoir".

Crohn disease (regional enteritis)

Aetiology

This disorder like ulcerative colitis is not common in children and it is of unknown cause.

Pathology

Crohn disease may affect any part of the gastrointestinal tract but most commonly the terminal ileum and proximal colon. The lesions are basically chronic granulomatous and inflammatory with a tendency towards remissions and relapses. The histological changes are transmural, i.e. affecting all layers of the bowel wall with oedema and ulceration of the mucosa, fissures, submucosal fibrosis and many inflammatory foci of mononuclear and giant cells (Figs 7.31 and 7.32). Perforation, haemorrhage and fistula formation are uncommon complications in childhood.

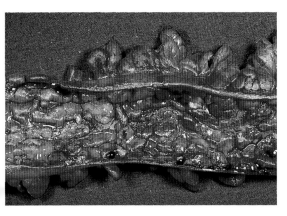

FIGURE 7.31 Crohn disease. Open loop of ileum showing typical cobblestone appearance of the mucosa.

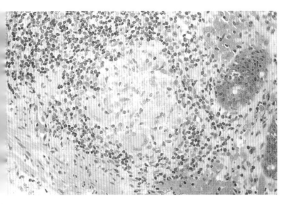

FIGURE 7.32 Crohn disease showing a diagnostic granuloma in the lamina propria of a colonic biopsy with a central collection of epithelioid and multinucleate cells surrounded by a cuff of lymphocytes and plasma cells (obj × 25).

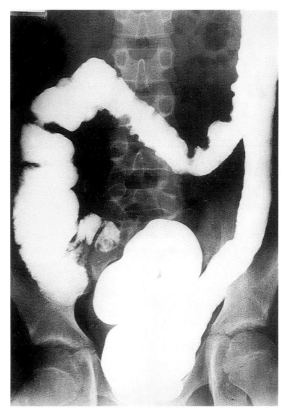

FIGURE 7.33 Barium meal and follow-through illustrating segmental involvement of the same bowel (Crohn disease).

Clinical features

In Crohn disease the diarrhoea is much less severe than in ulcerative colitis; it is often intermittent and there may be little or no obvious blood or mucus in the stools. Crohn disease presents with less specific signs and symptoms than ulcerative colitis, hence the delay in diagnosis often found in Crohn disease.

General manifestations commonly include anaemia, loss of weight, growth failure, pubertal delay, erythematous rashes and a low-grade fever. Other associated features are: erythema nodosum, pyoderma, iridocyclitis, arthralgia or arthritis, spondylitis, finger clubbing, anal skin tags, fissures and fistulae. Quite frequently the disease presents with oral ulceration and this may progress to extensive involvement of the buccal mucosa which becomes oedematous and granulomatous sometimes years before there is evidence of intestinal involvement. Sigmoidoscopy is only helpful when the left side of the colon is involved. A barium meal or enema typically shows segmental involvement of the small bowel and/or colon, sometimes with intervening areas of normal bowel (Fig. 7.33). Crohn disease shows a segmental lesion while ulcerative colitis is diffuse. The appearances vary from a "cobblestone appearance" due to thickened oedematous mucosa to narrowing of the lumen with the so-called "string sign". There may be fistulous tracts to adjacent loops of bowel. Biopsy of a perirectal lesion or even of the involved buccal mucosa may reveal diagnostic granulomatous changes. Colonoscopy and biopsy may provide an immediate diagnosis.

Treatment

There is no entirely satisfactory treatment. A high protein diet and some limitation of physical activity are probably indicated. Anti-inflammatory drugs used are the same as those used for ulcerative colitis.

Sulphasalazine has been shown to benefit patients with colonic Crohn disease but its value for small bowel disease is uncertain.

During acute exacerbations prednisolone (1–2 mg/kg/day) should be given for 4 weeks after which it is slowly reduced over 2–3 months. Azathioprine can be given in non-responsive cases in the dosage of 2 mg/kg/day to the more severe steroid dependent cases. However, the role of immunosuppressive agents is not clearly established. Metronidazole (25–50 mg/kg/day) in three divided doses may benefit patients with perianal disease.

Surgical intervention may be necessitated by intestinal obstruction, fistula formation, growth failure or the complete failure of medical treatment. Unfortunately excision of an affected segment is frequently followed by recurrence some months or years later but may give a prolonged remission. Recent experience indicates a better outlook after total colectomy and ileostomy compared with resection and reanastomosis. Also local surgery is indicated for perianal complications.

Children with persistent activity of the disease can go into remission when treated with a prolonged period of total parenteral nutrition or from overnight feeding with an elemental diet. Crohn disease runs an extremely variable course and the prognosis must always be guarded.

Lymphoid hyperplasia of the colon

Lymphoid hyperplasia of the colon is uncommon in children but can present with recurrent abdominal pain and/or rectal bleeding.

Radiologically the lymphoid hyperplasia is characterised by small uniform umbilicated polypoid lesions involving all or part of the colon. A fleck of barium in the centre of the polyp represents umbilication at the apex of the lymphoid nodule and is unique for lymphoid hyperplasia. This benign lesion probably represents the normal response of lymphoid tissue in children to a variety of stimuli. Biopsy proof of the nature of the nodule is essential. Corticosteroids have led to remission of symptoms in some patients. Long-term prognosis is good but symptoms and signs may take up to 2 years to subside.

MALABSORPTION SYNDROME

The word "malabsorption" is applied to clinical problems arising from a variety of disorders of small intestinal function. Two major causes of small intestinal nutrient malabsorption in children are coeliac disease and cystic fibrosis of the pancreas.

Coeliac disease (gluten enteropathy)

Aetiology

In 1950 Dicke showed that children with coeliac disease improved dramatically when wheat and rye

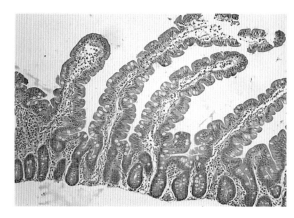

FIGURE 7.34(a) Normal jejunal biopsy: long finger-shaped villi, short crypts, scattered chronic inflammatory cells in the lamina propria and occasional lymphocytes in intraepithelial spaces (obj × 10).

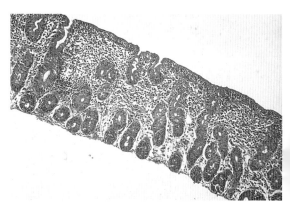

FIGURE 7.34(b) Total villous atrophy with loss of villi, elongated hyperplastic crypts, dense plasmacytic infiltrate in the lamina propria and increased number of surface intraepithelial lymphocytes (obj × 10).

flour were removed from their diet. It soon became apparent that the harmful substance was in the gliadin fraction of gluten in wheat and rye flour. There is also clear evidence of a genetic influence in that there is a high incidence of asymptomatic coeliac disease, as determined by jejunal biopsy in first-degree relatives of index cases. Indeed, this rises to 1 in 4 among first-degree relatives with the HLA-B8 antigen.

Pathology

Histological features have been defined mainly from the study of jejunal biopsy specimens. The most characteristic appearance is called total villous atrophy in which the mucosa is flat and devoid of normal villi but the underlying glandular layer is thickened and shows marked plasma-cell infiltration (Fig. 7.34a,b). Absence of villi has been confirmed by

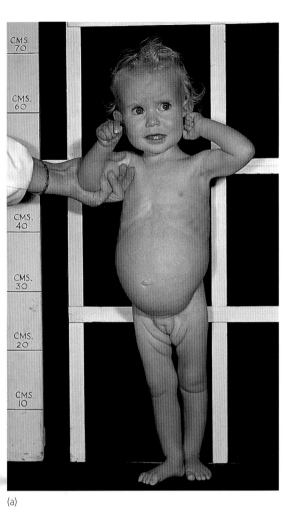
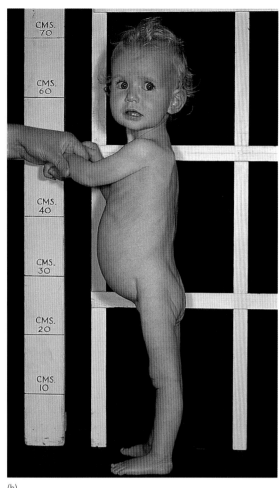

(a)
(b)

FIGURE 7.35 (a) Fourteen-month-old girl with untreated coeliac disease. Note abdominal distension and gross tissue wasting. (b) Lateral view of the same patient.

electron microscopy. In other cases, however, there is subtotal villous atrophy in which short, broad and thickened villi are seen. Although the histology of coeliac disease is characteristic it is not entirely specific. Similar appearances are now recognised to occur in disorders such as secondary disaccharide intolerance after gastroenteritis, cows' milk protein intolerance, giardiasis, intestinal lymphoma and protein calorie malnutrition. Children with dermatitis herpetiformis also have an intestinal lesion similar to that of coeliac disease.

Clinical features

These do not develop until gluten-containing foods are introduced into the infant's diet. In many cases the first signs are noted in the last 3 months of the first year of life, but the child may not be brought to the doctor until the second year. Delayed introduction of wheat containing cereals into the diet of infants in recent years has resulted in the later onset of coeliac disease.

Affected children become fractious and miserable with anorexia and failure to gain weight. Stools are characteristically of porridgy consistency, pale, bulky and foul smelling, but in some children this feature is not very marked. In others, however, the illness may start with vomiting and watery diarrhoea. The abdomen becomes distended as a result of poor musculature, altered peristaltic activity and the accumulation of intestinal secretions and gas. This contrasts with the child's wasted buttocks and thighs and produces the so-called coeliac profile (Fig. 7.35 a, b). A small number of children may be desperately ill with profuse diarrhoea leading to dehydration, acidosis and shock (coeliac crisis). In the worst cases malabsorption of protein can lead to hypoproteinaemic oedema.

Various other defects in absorption may become clinically manifest. Iron deficiency anaemia is common. There is usually diminished absorption of folic acid as revealed by a reduced red cell folate concentration. If there is ileal involvement, serum B_{12} may be decreased. Although deficiency of vitamins A and D is probably always present, rickets is quite rare (due to lack of growth) and xerophthalmia is almost unknown. However, rickets may develop after starting treatment with a gluten free diet if supplements of vitamin D are omitted while active growth continues. Hypoprothrombinaemia is often present.

Diagnostic tests

While the definitive diagnosis of coeliac disease must rest upon jejunal biopsy, the procedure is unpleasant and requires admission to hospital. A variety of screening tests has been developed. These include tests of xylose absorption and for circulating antibodies to food proteins and the measurement of IgA antigliadin antibodies in the serum. The D-xylose absorption test is a good screening test for coeliac disease. A blood xylose concentration of less than 20 mg/dl measured 60 minutes after an oral dose of 5 g xylose would indicate significant malabsorption and be an indication for jejunal biopsy.

Normal values of fat excretion are less than 10% of intake. In infants and children, a fat excretion exceeding 3.5 g/24 hours and 4.5 g/24 hours respectively is considered abnormal. If expressed as percentage of fat intake, an untreated coeliac child usually excretes between 15 and 33% of the fat intake.

A barium meal and follow-through examination will reveal an abnormal coarsening of the mucosal pattern of the small bowel, jejunal dilatation and possibly delay in the passage of barium to the colon. The bones may become osteoporotic and ossification delayed.

Early performance of jejunal biopsy avoids time consuming and discomforting investigations. A second biopsy should be performed after about 12 months on a gluten-free diet to confirm the return of the intestinal mucosa to normal. As gluten intolerance can occasionally be a transient condition the diagnosis should be reconfirmed by a third jejunal biopsy after a gluten challenge, e.g. some 2–3 months after gluten powder, 10–20 g daily has been added to the child's diet. Should this biopsy turn out to be normal a fourth biopsy should be performed after 1–2 years on a normal diet, or earlier if there are indications of a relapse.

Treatment

Coeliac disease is a gluten-induced enteropathy and the results of treatment with a gluten-free diet are impressive. This is first apparent as a striking improvement in personality soon to be followed by rapid growth, while the stools more slowly return to normal. Strict supervision is essential and the child's height and weight should be recorded at regular intervals.

In the United Kingdom a gluten free diet is one from which, in effect, all wheat flour has been excluded. The parents should be supplied with a comprehensive list of the many foodstuffs which contain gluten and are, therefore, forbidden, and also a list of the gluten free foods which are freely permitted. Bread and biscuits made from gluten-free wheat starch are commercially available. It is also possible to home bake gluten-free bread, biscuits and cakes with recipes supplied by dietitians.

An adequate intake of vitamins and especially of vitamin D is important. Iron deficiency anaemia may be corrected with oral preparations such as Sytron 5 ml thrice daily or Ferromyn Elixir 5 ml thrice daily. When the red cell or whole blood folate value is low folic acid should be prescribed in a dose of 5 mg daily.

As long as the child remains on a gluten-free diet growth and development will be entirely satisfactory, and the mortality rate for coeliac disease is nowadays negligible. It is, however, recognised that adults who have been successfully treated for coeliac disease in childhood and who have gone back to an ordinary diet, may later relapse. It is therefore desirable to confirm the persistence of true gluten intolerance in these so-called "coeliac children" before recommending a life-long gluten-free diet. There is in addition the risk that the poorly treated adult coeliac may in time develop a lymphoma or gastrointestinal carcinoma.

The therapeutic trial of a gluten-free diet without a prior biopsy is a dangerous practice and should be abandoned.

Cystic fibrosis

Aetiology

Cystic fibrosis of the pancreas is so named because it was first thought to be primarily a pancreatic disorder. It is now known that the primary defect is in a transmembrane protein of chloride ion channels of all body exocrine glands including sweat, intestinal, mucous and salivary glands and liver. The gene which codes for this protein is located on chromosome 7 and the most common of the over 400 so far described is at the ΔF 508 locus and accounts for about 74% of cases in Caucasians. Transmission of the autosomal recessive gene defects results in an incidence of 1 in 2000 in Caucasian and 1 in 90 000 in Oriental live births.

Pathology

Although the gene defect is present in all nucleated body cells it is only in those cells where the gene requires to be activated for normal cell function that abnormalities are recognised. It is not surprising that the disease has variable clinical manifestations given the range of gene defects. The pancreas is abnormal in over 90% of the cases. A constant change is fibrosis with atrophy of the exocrine parenchyma. Cystic dilatation of acini and ducts is common but not invariable. Islet tissue, however, is rarely involved until later childhood or adolescence. Mucous glands throughout the body are grossly distended and they secrete an abnormal viscid mucus. Stagnation of mucus in the smaller bronchioles usually leads to infection, which in turn stimulates further mucus secretion. Infected sticky secretions spread throughout the bronchial tree leading to a chronic obstructive suppurative lung disease. The liver shows a focal type of biliary cirrhosis, most marked under the capsule, which may progress to produce portal hypertension.

Clinical features

The symptoms tend to occur in a more or less ordered fashion and the diagnosis is not often unduly difficult. In about 10% the illness presents in the neonatal period in the form of meconium ileus in which inspissated meconium causes intestinal obstruction (see Fig. 7.12). The most common presentation, however, is in the form of an intractable respiratory infection dating from the early weeks or months of life. Indeed, cystic fibrosis of the pancreas should always be suspected when a respiratory infection in infancy fails to respond promptly to adequate antibiotic therapy. In the early stages of the disease radiographs of the chest may show only increased translucency of the lung fields; later heavy interstitial markings appear, then multiple soft shadows representing small lung abscesses. In other cases there may be lobar consolidation, empyema or pyopneumothorax. In children who survive the early months of life, the respiratory picture may become that of bronchiectasis, increasing emphysema, and clubbing of the fingers. Sputum culture in such cases will most often show the predominant organisms to be *Staphylococcus aureus* and *Pseudomonas aeruginosa*. Recently the frequency of pulmonary colonisation with *Pseudomonas cepacia* in adults with cystic fibrosis has increased and has been correlated with increased morbidity and mortality rates. Pulmonary colonisation by *Pseudomonas cepacia* is generally refractory to antibiotic treatment and sensible precautions such as avoiding contacts between *Pseudomonas cepacia*-colonised CF individuals and non colonised children should be taken.

In a minority of cases the respiratory infection is less prominent than the presence of semi-formed, greasy, bulky and excessively foul smelling stools. These features coincide with the introduction of mixed feeding. After the first year of life the history of abnormal and frequent stools occurring in association with abdominal distension and generalised tissue-wasting may simulate coeliac disease. The differential diagnosis can, however, almost always be made on clinical grounds alone. In cystic fibrosis a careful history will elicit that signs first appeared in the early weeks of life, whereas coeliac disease rarely presents before the age of 6 months. The excellent, often voracious appetite in cystic fibrosis contrasts sharply with the unhappy anorexia of the coeliac child. Chronic respiratory infection of some degree, often severe, is an invariable accompaniment of cystic fibrosis but it is not a feature of coeliac disease. Furthermore, the diagnosis of cystic fibrosis may be suggested by a history that previous siblings have the disease.

If the affected infant survives the first year, childhood seems often to bring a period of improvement in the chest condition. All too frequently, however, the approach to puberty is associated with cor pulmonale. Less commonly, in about 10% during the second decade, biliary cirrhosis and portal hypertension develop and may lead to massive gastrointestinal haemorrhage. In recent years as an increasing proportion of sufferers from cystic fibrosis survive, insulin-dependent diabetes mellitus has been found in some as they approach puberty. A feature of these cases has been the absence of marked ketoacidosis. A further important manifestation which seems to present in a majority of male survivors into adulthood is aspermia and sterility. This has been shown to be due to absence of the vas deferens. Women have only slightly reduced fertility associated with abnormal tubal ciliary movement and cervical mucus.

Some children with cystic fibrosis can develop distal small bowel obstruction. This disorder is due to viscid mucofaeculent material obstructing the bowel causing recurring episodes of abdominal pain, constipation and acute or subacute intestinal obstruction. The cardinal sign is a soft, mobile, non-tender mass palpable in the right iliac fossa. Mild cases can be treated by increasing the intake of pancreatic enzyme. If the condition is not improved oral N-acetylcysteine 10 ml four times a day or one or two doses of oral Gastrografin 50–100 ml taken with 200–400 ml of water may relieve the patient's discomfort and obstruction. Toddlers with cystic fibrosis may sometime present with rectal prolapse. Also the incidence of nasal polyps in patients with cystic fibrosis is about 70%.

Diagnostic tests

The standard evidence upon which to base a diagnosis of cystic fibrosis in childhood is demonstration of an excessive concentration of sodium and chloride in the sweat. There are various methods of obtaining sweat for analysis but the most accurate and widely used technique is stimulation of local sweating by pilocarpine iontophoresis. One should try to achieve the collection of at least 100 mg of sweat. To minimise diagnostic errors, two reliable sweat tests confirmed in a laboratory used to performing the test should be obtained. Diagnostic levels of sodium and chloride are 70 mmol/kg. Discrepancies of more than 20 mmol between sodium and chloride indicate the need for further testing. The sodium concentration tends to be slightly lower than the chloride in cystic fibrosis patients. Occasionally elevated sweat electrolytes may be found in adrenal insufficiency, diabetes insipidus, ectodermal dysplasia, allergic diseases, type I glycogen storage disease, AIDS and malnutrition.

In the newborn infant later destined to develop the manifestations of cystic fibrosis there is a markedly raised albumin content in the meconium. A simple test strip impregnated with a suitable reagent is available to detect an albumin level in meconium in excess of 20 mg/g (BM-Test Meconium: Boehringer). This method is not sufficiently reliable to serve as a screening test for cystic fibrosis. In neonates, there is a reliable method of screening which is based on the serum concentration of immunoreactive trypsin (IRT). Serum IRT levels are abnormally high (> 80 ng/ml) during the first few months of life, although in older children they fall to subnormal values. Screening for common gene defects using DNA probes for the more common gene defects can now be used for prenatal diagnosis, for carrier detection and for help in diagnosis. Heterozygote identification from DNA analysis on buccal cells obtained by a mouth wash can help to determine whether a couple are at risk of having an affected fetus. Knowledge of the underlying gene defect in the affected child might help guide subsequent gene therapy. Prenatal diagnosis by chorionic villus biopsy obtained at 9–12 weeks post conception will allow termination of affected fetuses.

Tests of pancreatic function on duodenal juice obtained by duodenal intubation have been largely superseded by "the sweat test". In cystic fibrosis all the pancreatic enzyme activities are severely diminished and the volume of pancreatic juice and bicarbonate content obtained after stimulation by secretin and pancreozymin are also reduced. In addition most cystic fibrosis children have an abnormal pancreatic ultrasound after the age of 5 years.

A majority of patients with cystic fibrosis have pancreatic insufficiency which if inadequately treated could result in fat, vitamin and protein malnutrition. The most important factors in the treatment are control of lung infection and maintenance of adequate nutrition; indeed upon the success of these efforts depends the prognosis. Persistent bacterial infection is a major problem for children with cystic fibrosis, the four bacterial pathogens involved being *Staphylococcus aureus, Psuedomonas aeruginosa, Haemophilus influenzae* and *Pseudomonas cepacia.*

For many years *Staphylococcus aureus* was the main respiratory pathogen but since effective antistaphylococcal therapy became available the predominant organism seen is *Pseudomonas aeruginosa* in the mucoid form. Antipseudomonal antibiotics that can be taken by mouth are relatively ineffective. Consequently, treatment has to be given by the intravenous route. Pseudomonas infection is very difficult to eradicate and usually requires repeated courses of intensive intravenous antibiotic therapy. High doses are needed to achieve bactericidal concentrations in the sputum.

At present at a few centres it is recommended that children with cystic fibrosis should be admitted electively for a 14 day course of intravenous antibiotics every 3 months rather than waiting to treat children with cystic fibrosis until they are very ill. The aim is to prevent the gradual progression of lung damage and the elective antibiotics programme appears to be a useful therapeutic advance. However, some centres operate the policy of home treatment with intravenous antibiotics for cystic fibrosis which involves training of the parents and provision of the drugs and equipment.

Inhaled antibiotics administered soon after physiotherapy have proved effective in some young people, but their role is uncertain. Some children develop allergic bronchopulmonary aspergillosis which may respond to inhaled bronchodilators and/or oral steroids.

The current antibiotic policy for cystic fibrosis in children at the Royal Hospital for Sick Children, Glasgow is as follows.

Present antibiotic policy

1 **First year after diagnosis**
   (a) All children should receive oral flucloxacillin 50 mg/kg/day in four divided doses. It should be given half to one hour before food.
   (b) The dosages may be doubled for 2 weeks during episodes of upper respiratory tract infection.

2 **After first year**
   (a) If there are no major respiratory infections; regular oral flucloxacillin should be discontinued.
   (b) However, for episodes of upper respiratory tract infections a 2-week course of oral flucloxacillin 50 mg/kg/day in four divided doses is given.
   (c) If infections are frequent then oral flucloxacillin is given as in (1).

3 **Acute exacerbation of respiratory infections**
   (a) If only *Staphylococcus aureus* – IV flucloxacillin 50 mg/kg/day in four divided doses for 2 weeks.

(b) If *Haemophilus influenzae* – IV augmentin 30 mg/kg/8-hourly for 2 weeks. In more serious infections frequency increased to 6-hourly intervals.

(c) If *Pseudomonas aeruginosa* – a combination of IV ceftazidime and IV tobramycin for 2 weeks.
  (i) ceftazidime doses up to 150 mg/kg/day intravenously in three divided doses should be used (maximum dose 6 g daily).
  (ii) tobramycin 6 mg/kg/day intravenously in three divided doses. Tobramycin clearance varies from one patient to another therefore serum levels should be monitored.

(d) If *Pseudomonas aeruginosa* is resistant to ceftazidime or tobramycin or patient has hypersensitivity to those drugs then use:
  (i) azlocillin intravenously 225 mg/kg/day in three divided doses for 2 weeks OR
  (ii) use ciprofloxacin 5–10 mg/kg/day intravenously in two divided doses for 2 weeks.

If there are frequent exacerbations due to *Pseudomonas aeruginosa*: Colomycin may be added by aerosol inhalation as adjunct therapy for 6 months in a dosage of 50 000 units/kg/day in three divided doses.

All children with cystic fibrosis should receive pertussis, measles, *Haemophilus influenzae* and influenza vaccinations. Polyvalent pseudomonas vaccine has failed to prevent pseudomonas colonisation in children with cystic fibrosis.

A most important adjunct to the management of the pulmonary disease is adequate and consistent physiotherapy. Parents should receive instruction in this from a physiotherapist who is experienced in handling children, and the importance of regular daily physiotherapy cannot be overstated. Children who produce sputum should have physiotherapy at least three times daily. Even those who do not produce sputum should have physiotherapy at least once a day.

The diet should be rich in protein and energy. The goal should be to increase calorie intake to 120–150% of the recommended daily allowance and protein intake to 150% of the daily allowance. All cystic fibrosis children should receive fat soluble vitamin supplements, vitamins A, D, E and K given daily in twice the usual dose.

Pancreatic supplements must be given in a dose sufficient to ensure control of fat malabsorption. Pancreatic enzyme supplements should be adjusted according to the clinical response using enteric coated microsphere pancreatic preparation (Pancrease, Ortho-Cilag; Creon, Duphar Laboratories) which results in significantly greater absorption of ingested fat than that seen in cystic fibrosis patients using conventional pancreatic enzyme preparations. In addition, reduction in the number of dose units required to produce optimal therapeutic effects during treatment with the microsphere preparation results in lessening of the cost of therapy and better compliance.

The services of a surgeon may be required at several stages of the disease, e.g. for meconium ileus in the neonatal period, for distal small bowel obstruction, for lobectomy in bronchiectasis or for portacaval anastomosis if portal hypertension is severe.

There is no doubt that the present day comprehensive treatment of cystic fibrosis patients has dramatically improved their prognosis. The prospect of heart–lung transplantation offers hope for a small number of patients for whom donor organs are available. This has resulted in success over a relatively short term, but the prognosis over decades rather than years is not yet known.

Current research is directed towards gene therapy and early animal and *in vitro* studies suggest that somatic gene therapy using a normal CF gene construct attached to an adenovirus may successfully be applied to correction of the lung defect within the next few years.

JAUNDICE

Jaundice occurs either when there is excess haemolysis increasing the load of bilirubin, when the diseased liver is not able to cope with the normal load or when there is obstruction to excretion of bilirubin. Jaundice can be classified into haemolytic (prehepatic), hepatocellular (hepatic) and (obstructive or post-hepatic) varieties. In this chapter we shall discuss only virus hepatitis, chronic active hepatitis, acute liver failure, cirrhosis of the liver and obstructive jaundice. Neonatal jaundice has been discussed in Chapter 1.

Infective hepatitis

Aetiology

In Caucasians most cases are caused by hepatitis virus A which is acquired by inhalation or ingestion. The incubation period is 24–30 days. Infection by hepatitis-B virus (HBV) is relatively uncommon in Caucasians but has a high prevalence in South-east Asia and parts of Africa where highly infective carriage of HBV is common. The incubation period is 90–120 days. Three antigen–antibody systems are associated with HBV and they have provided researchers with useful markers for epidemiological studies. These are: hepatitis-B surface antigen (HBsAg, Australia antigen) and antibody (anti-HBs); hepatitis-B core antigen (HBcAg) and antibody (anti-HBc); and hepatitis-B e antigen (HBeAg) and antibody (anti-HBe). Individuals who are positive for HBsAg always have antibody to the core component of the virus and this denotes recent or past infection. On the other hand, the presence in blood of the e antigen (HBeAg) indicates the presence of active underlying liver disease and a high degree of infectivity.

HBV is maintained in populations by the existence of symptomless carriers, and in South-east Asia and parts of Africa where there is a high prevalence of e antigenaemia children readily acquire the infection by close contact with other children who are positive for HBeAg. This is called "horizontal" transmission. However, apart from the infrequent syringe-transmitted cases (homologous serum jaundice) the precise mechanisms of transmissions are not known. They may include mosquitoes and other insects and possibly open skin lesions. "Vertical" transmission of HBV can also take place from HBeAg-positive mothers to their infants *in utero* or during the perinatal period when the infants may become carriers of the virus. This is a particular risk among the Chinese and is related not only to high prevalence and infectivity levels but probably also to ethnic characteristics. The distinction between the horizontal and vertical modes of transmission is important because while the former can be prevented by active immunisation with HBV surface antigen vaccine, the latter probably demands both passive immunisation with specific antihepatitis B virus immunoglobulin and active immunisation.

Some cases of infective hepatitis appear to be related to non-A, non-B viruses (NANB hepatitis). Because there are no definite serological markers NANB hepatitis remains a diagnosis of clinical and serological exclusion. Hepatitis-C virus sequences have been detected in children with post-transfusion NANB hepatitis. Other viruses that can cause hepatitis as part of a generalised illness (CMV, herpesvirus, EB virus, rubella and Coxsackie B) will not be discussed here.

Pathology

The principal features are centrilobular parenchymal necrosis of variable severity and periportal cellular infiltration with polymorphonuclears, plasma cells, lymphocytes and macrophages. Bile stasis is also found. In hepatitis-A infection, complete recovery is the rule, although in rare cases acute hepatic necrosis (acute yellow atrophy) causes death. Cirrhosis of the liver is almost unknown. In hepatitis-B infection, however, serious liver disease such as cirrhosis and primary hepatocullular carcinoma may develop after years of symptomless carrier state.

Clinical features

The relative mildness of infectious hepatitis in most children must not lull the physician into an over-

casual approach to what can occasionally be a fatal disease. Jaundice is usually preceded by some days of anorexia, nausea, vomiting and upper abdominal pain. Fever may be absent or quite high. When jaundice develops the stools become clay-coloured. The urine contains an excess of urobilinogen and bile pigments. Pruritus is not a common complaint in children. The liver is enlarged and tender and the spleen may become palpable. Liver function tests reveal abnormal results, e.g. raised levels of plasma glutamic-oxaloacetic and glutamic-pyruvic transaminases as well as raised levels of γ-glutamyltranspeptidase, lactate dehydrogenase and alkaline phosphatase.

Hepatitis-B can be diagnosed on the basis of positive tests for hepatitis-B surface antigen (HBsAg) and the other markers of B virus infection already discussed. It is also possible to detect infection with virus A by means of tests for specific Ig antibody to HAV.

Prevention

Most children infected with HBV by horizontal transmission suffer only a subclinical illness, and as it is not known whether hepatitis-B vaccine will lower the incidence of later cirrhosis or carcinoma the decision to use an expensive vaccine in a poor country is a difficult one. In Britain the infants at risk of vertical transmission are those of non-Caucasian origin, those of the small number of mothers who develop acute hepatitis-B during the last trimester of pregnancy, or those born to mothers found to be positive for HBeAg. At present in Britain supplies of hepatitis-B immunoglobulin are available for such infants and a specific programme has been set up for surveillance and administration of the immunoglobulin. In some areas of South-east Asia, studies are being carried out to test the efficacy of a combination of hepatitis-B immunoglobulin and hepatitis-B vaccine, but the vaccine has not yet been licensed for use in very young infants in Britain, where reliance is being placed on passive immunisation alone. It is already clear that the combination of vaccine and immunoglobulin under the conditions of a randomised controlled trial can offer a high degree of protection to Chinese newborn infants of HBeAg-positive women.

Treatment

The patient should be kept in bed until bile pigment have disappeared from the urine and the appetite ha returned to normal. Thereafter, convalescence take 2–3 weeks. In the acute stage of nausea, light diet with an abundant intake of glucose and fluids is required Later a diet rich in protein and low fat is advised Vomiting can be relieved with a drug of the antihis tamine group which is used for motion sickness Constipation should be treated with a laxative.

Acute liver failure is a rare emergency in childhood. If the hepatitis seems to be getting more severe in spite of bed rest, corticosteroids should be tried. Prednisolone 2 mg/kg/day in four divided doses is continued until liver function tests are at or near normal levels. However, if to persistent vomiting is added mental confusion or abnormal neurological signs, protein must be completely withdrawn from the diet. Glucose, 25% solution, should be given by intragastric drip or by slow infusion into the inferior vena cava (at least 500 g/day). Hypokalaemia should be corrected with potassium chloride, 10 mmol to each 500 ml of 25% glucose solution. Some add insulin, 10 units with each 50 g of glucose to promote the deposition of glycogen in the liver. Neomycin 50 mg/kg/day should be given orally to reduce the ammonia-producing bacterial flora of the gut. Intravenous vitamin B complex (Parentrovite) is indicated on theoretical grounds. Vitamin K 10 mg/day should be given intravenously. Blood clotting factors may be provided by fresh frozen plasma or exchange transfusion. If signs of cerebral oedema develop intracranial pressure monitoring should be instituted and treatment with dexamethasone and mannitol given, together with controlled ventilation. Since increased levels of ammonia may result in hepatic coma, attempts to decrease toxin levels by using various techniques such as plasmapheresis with plasma exchange, charcoal haemoperfusion and haemodialysis have been tried and thought to be beneficial. Two major advances in recent years have given the treatment of severe liver failure and end-stage liver disease a more hopeful prospect: transplantation of the liver and artificial liver support systems.

Cirrhosis of the liver

Aetiology

Hepatic cirrhosis is uncommon in children in the United Kingdom and the histological differentiation into "portal" and biliary" types tends to be less well defined than in adults. A pathological picture similar to that of Laënnec portal cirrhosis may follow neonatal hepatitis, blood group incompatibility, the de Toni–Fanconi syndrome and it may be the form of presentation of Wilson hepatolenticular cirrhosis. Infective hepatitis-B may also lead to hepatic cirrhosis. Other rare causes of cirrhosis of the liver include galactosaemia, Gaucher disease, Niemann–Pick disease and xanthomatosis. Although congenital syphilis can cause a pericellular cirrhosis in stillborn infants it is doubtful if it ever causes postnatal hepatic cirrhosis. Pure biliary cirrhosis is seen invariably in congenital biliary atresia and a focal type is very common in cystic fibrosis of the pancreas. Indian childhood cirrhosis is a common and fatal disease which appears to be restricted to India. It is not found in Indian expatriates in other parts of the world. It usually presents between the ages of 9 months and 5 years and has characteristic histological features in liver biopsy material. These have been called "micro-micronodular cirrhosis" which includes necrosis and vacuolation of liver cells, aggressive fibrosis both intralobular and perilobular and a variable inflammatory infiltrate. The liver contains an exceedingly high copper content and the hepatocytes contain multiple, coarse, dark brown orcein-staining granules which represent copper-associated protein. It is not yet known whether this reflects a metabolic disorder of genetic origin or is due to an excessive intake of copper, but it is possible that the hepatic accumulation of copper is of pathogenic importance. In Jamaica a form of cirrhosis called veno-occlusive disease of the liver, in which there is occlusion of the small hepatic veins, is due to the toxic effects of an alkaloid in bush tea prepared from plants such as *Senecio* and *Crotalaria*.

Chronic active hepatitis is an auto-immune disorder characterised by hepatic necrosis, fibrosis, plasma cell infiltration and disorganisation of the lobular architecture. In the young adult, often female, associated disorders include thyroiditis, fibrosing alveolitis and glomerulonephritis. Some cases are related to chronic virus B hepatitis (positive HBsAg). In chronic active hepatitis smooth muscle antibodies are found in the serum in two-thirds of cases, antinuclear factor in about 50%, and the gammaglobulin level is markedly elevated.

Clinical features

The child usually presents with abdominal swelling due to enlargement of the liver which has a firm edge, sometimes smooth, often nodular. Anorexia, lack of energy and slowing of growth are common complaints. Splenomegaly develops if there is portal hypertension. In most cases jaundice makes its appearance sooner rather than later. Spontaneous bleeding is usually due to hypoprothrombinaemia. Orthochromic anaemia is common. When ascites develops the outlook is grave; it is usually associated with hypoproteinaemia and portal hypertension. The latter may result in massive gastrointestinal haemorrhage. In other cases death occurs from hepatic encephalopathy with flapping tremor, mental confusion, extensor plantar responses and coma. Spider naevi and "liver palms" are uncommon in children, but clubbing of the fingers may develop. Hypersplenism may produce leucopenia and thrombocytopenia. Various derangements of liver function can be demonstrated biochemically, e.g. raised direct bilirubin levels, hypoalbuminaemia, and raised serum gammaglobulin. In hepatic encephalopathy the blood ammonia level is high. Diagnosis should be confirmed by liver biopsy.

Treatment

Specific treatment is available only for the few cases due to metabolic errors such as Wilson disease or galactosaemia. Life can be prolonged with a high protein diet, plus a liberal intake of the B vitamins and oral vitamin K, 10 mg/day. Ascites should be treated with frusemide and a low-sodium diet. Hypokalaemia may require supplements of potassium chloride. In resistant cases diuresis may be improved by giving (along with frusemide) an aldosterone antagonist such as spironolactone, 25 mg four times daily. Paracentesis abdominis should be avoided whenever possible. When signs of hepatic failure supervene protein should be completely eliminated from the diet and the therapeutic regimen already described for this emergency should be started. There is little basis for the use of corticosteroids save in chronic active hepatitis where they do probably slow down the progress of the disease. An alternative but more dangerous therapy is immunosuppression, e.g. with azathioprine.

Obstructive jaundice

In infants investigation of persistent jaundice is necessary in any infant over 4 weeks of age. Biliary atresia is an uncommon disease but is the most important cause of obstructive jaundice in infancy. The history of the baby is important and particular attention has to be focused on the stools – have they been normally pigmented or pale acholic stools since birth? Investigations should include:

1 Haematological and liver function tests.
2 Screening for infection and metabolic causes.
3 Ultrasound examination.
4 Radionuclide studies.
5 Percutaneous liver biopsy.

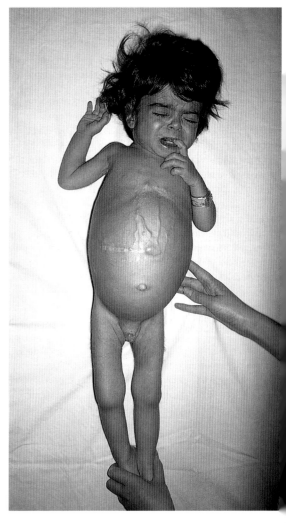

FIGURE 7.36 Infant with ascites secondary to cirrhosis of the liver following biliary atresia.

In addition, some would advise endoscopic retrograde cholangiopancreatography (ERCP), percutaneous transhepatic cholangiography, laparoscopy, duodenal intubation and aspiration, but despite all these tests, laparotomy and exploration may be necessary to establish the diagnosis. At laparotomy, operative cholangiography is performed prior to exploration of the porta hepatis.

The aetiology of biliary atresia has been the subject of much research and speculation. It is not simply a congenital malformation nor an obliterative ascending cholangitis but the end result is obliteration of the bile ducts, progressive fibrosis of the liver and death in the first 2 years of life unless surgical intervention is undertaken. The liver fibrosis results in portal hypertension and oesophageal varices. Ascites becomes a marked feature of the later stages (Fig 7.36). Pruritis can be very distressing.

To achieve adequate drainage the Kasai operation has a much greater chance of longer-term success if performed early, i.e. within the first 2 months of life. The Kasai operation is dissection and excision of the fibrous bile duct remnants and the fibrous "plate" which is often found within the porta hepatis. The exposed portal area is then drained into a Roux-en-Y loop of bowel. With this procedure, two-thirds of infants will achieve satisfactory drainage and long-term adequate drainage will be maintained in half these patients. Where the Kasai operation is unsuccessful and for those who subsequently have progressive liver fibrosis, liver transplantation gives good long-term results. Biliary atresia is the primary pathology in about half of children developing end-stage liver disease and the results of liver transplantation in this group of children are now approaching 90% survival with good quality of life.

Idiopathic dilatation of the common bile duct (choledochal cyst)

This is rare in childhood. Patients present with intermittent abdominal swelling, pain and jaundice. Investigation reveals the cystic dilatation of the hepatic or common bile duct. Treatment in most cases consists of excision of the cyst to prevent long-term complications arising, particularly malignant change in the mucosal lining and anastomosing the bile duct or hepatic ducts to a Roux-en-Y loop of jejunum.

Cholecystitis

Cholecystitis is uncommon in childhood and rarely presents as an acute emergency. Cholelithiasis is rather more common and presents with recurrent upper abdominal pain, nausea and vomiting. It is often associated with congenital spherocytosis. The stones are usually bile pigment stones and should be looked for whenever laparotomy is carried out for removal of the spleen in this condition. Cholecystotomy has been preferred to cholecystectomy when the gall bladder is not diseased.

Pancreas

Pancreatic disorders are uncommon in childhood except that which is part of the generalised disease of cystic fibrosis (mucoviscidosis). Pancreatitis presents as an acute abdominal emergency but the signs and symptoms are less dramatic than in adults. Abdominal pain and vomiting are the most consistent signs. Abdominal tenderness is more marked in the upper abdomen. A high index of suspicion is necessary by the clinician so that blood is taken for serum amylase estimation. In pancreatitis the level is considerably elevated as is the urinary amylase. Ultrasound examination of the abdomen may show the swollen oedematous pancreas. The most common aetiology in Scotland is mumps but many cases are idiopathic. Traumatic pancreatitis is infrequent but may be followed by development of a pancreatic pseudocyst. This can be followed by repeated ultrasound examination and the majority will settle without the necessity of drainage into the stomach or bowel. Familial pancreatitis can affect succeeding generations or siblings. It is a rare disorder of unknown aetiology.

8

The Genitourinary System

Over the past three decades progress has been achieved in the classification of renal diseases and this has been particularly in the realm of glomerular disorders. This has been possible because of electron microscopy and immunofluorescence in the identification within renal tissue of immunoglobulins and complement components. On the basis of experimental work it has been shown that there are mainly two types of immunologically mediated glomerular diseases:

1 due to deposition of antigen antibody complexes (immune complex glomerulonephritis); and
2 due to the action of autoantibodies against constituents of the glomerular basement membrane (anti-GBM disease).

Classification at present is based on a combination of factors, e.g. aetiological agents, association with systemic disease, identification of basic immunopathogenic mechanisms and correlation with clinical findings (Table 8.1). In this chapter only common glomerulonephritides in relation to paediatric practice will be discussed.

RENAL DISORDERS

Acute post-streptococcal glomerulonephritis

In most cases there is a history of a preceding infection 7–21 days before the onset of renal manifestations. In the majority this infection is due to one of the group A

β-haemolytic streptococci, most often type 12. The exact mechanism by which renal injury is produced in this disease is not completely clear. It has been presumed that during the latent period of 7–21 days an

TABLE 8.1 Classification of glomerulonephritis

Primary glomerulonephritis
    Immune complex glomerulonephritis
        Post-infectious acute glomerulonephritis
        Membranous glomerulonephritis
        Membrano-proliferative glomerulonephritis
        Mesangial IgA nephropathy (Berger disease)
    Anti-glomerular basement membrane antibody disease
    (Goodpasture syndrome)
    Glomerulonephritis of uncertain aetiology
        e.g. childhood nephrotic syndrome, minimal lesion
        glomerulonephritis, focal segment glomerulonephritis, etc.
Glomerulonephritis associated with systemic disease
    Immunologically mediated and embolic
        Henoch–Schönlein purpura
        Collagen diseases, e.g. systemic lupus erythematosus and
        scleroderma
        Vasculitides – polyarteritis nodosa, Wegener granulomatosis
        Systemic infections (subacute, bacterial endocarditis; shunt
        nephritis, hepatitis B, malaria, syphilis, toxoplasmosis,
        cytomegalovirus)
Hereditary disorders
    Congenital nephrotic syndrome
    Familial nephritis – Alport syndrome
    Sickle-cell disease
Other conditions
    Diabetes mellitus
    Amyloidosis
    Heavy metal poisoning – mercury
    Drash syndrome – nephrotic syndrome associated with pseudo-
    hermaphroditism and Wilms tumour

ntigen-antibody reaction takes place between the
treptococcal endotoxin and the cells of the glomeru-
is. The latent period may occasionally be as brief as
–5 days with an average of 10 days. Apart from the
ases due to streptococcal pharyngitis, some cases may
ccur following skin infection with streptococci and
ype 49 is most often found in pyoderma related acute
lomerulonephritis (AGN). However, some cases
ppear to be provoked by other bacterial and viral
gents and the clinical signs and symptoms produced
re indistinguishable from those of post-streptococcal
lomerulonephritis. These infectious agents include:
neumococcus, staphylococcus, mycoplasma,
Coxsackie, mumps, ECHO and influenza viruses.

athology

On light microscopy, in the acute stage all glomeruli
how a proliferation of the endothelial cells of the
apillaries and of the mesangial cells. Proliferation of
pithelial cells is seen only in the most severe cases.
here is also polymorphonuclear infiltration. In the
vorst cases there may be fibrinoid necrosis of the
ufts and afferent arterioles. In cases which fail to
esolve and progress rapidly, crescents appear, due to
roliferation of the capsular epithelial cells; some
lomeruli become completely hyalinised and intersti-
ial fibrosis may be marked; the tubules frequently
how dilatation. Thus acute glomerulonephritis may
e predominantly proliferative, exudative or haemor-
hagic. In chronic glomerulonephritis which develops
fter a long latent stage, and is rare in childhood,
here is extensive loss of glomeruli; scar tissue is
rofuse and the arterioles show degenerative
rteriosclerotic changes. On electron microscopy the
nost conspicuous abnormality is the presence of
liscrete electron-dense granular deposits in the subep-
helial space. On immunofluorescence streptococcal
ntigens have been identified only in the earliest
tages of the disease. Also granular deposits of IgG
nd IgM can be demonstrated along the capillary wall
nd C3 is usually present as well.

Clinical features

Usually the child is of school age and the onset is
brupt with fever, malaise, headache, vomiting and
he passage of red or brown coloured urine. The
receding tonsillitis, scarlet fever or other infection
as usually resolved by this time. Examination reveals
nild oedema, most obvious in the face, and hyper-
ension of moderate severity. Urinary output is
educed and the specific gravity is raised. There is
roteinuria (under 2 g/l) and macroscopic haema-
uria. Microscopy shows red blood cells or red blood
ell casts. Hyaline or granular casts are less frequent
luring the acute phase. There may be slight
ardiomegaly and radiographs of the lungs frequently
show central opacities caused by pulmonary oedema.
In many cases, however, constitutional upset is slight
and both oedema and hypertension may be absent.
Haemolytic streptococci are frequently isolated from
the throat swab and in most cases the antistreptolysin-O (ASO) titre is raised within 10–14 days
following a streptococcal infection and will remain
elevated for several months (above 200 units/ml). The
blood urea and serum creatinine concentrations are
frequently raised but a normal level need not invali-
date the diagnosis. It has been known for many years
that the serum complement activity is low in 80–90%
of patients with acute nephritis but a rapid method
of estimation has been developed using the protein
$B1_C$ as a "marker". This serum protein decomposes
after a few days to another protein $B1_A$ but can be
quantitated using $B1_A$ antiserum. The normal $B1_C/B1_A$
concentration in the serum (C3 fraction) is 1.25–1.5
g/l (125–150 mg/100 ml). During the first week or
two of acute post-streptococcal glomerulonephritis
very low levels are found which rise as recovery takes
place. Persistent hypocomplementaemia suggests that
the diagnosis is membranoproliferative glomerulonephritis which has a more serious prognosis.
Ultrasound examination of the kidneys will not reveal
findings specific of AGN.

Complications

Oliguria is almost invariable but fortunately it rarely
goes on to complete anuria in children. When this
does occur peritoneal dialysis may be indicated to
relieve uraemia, metabolic acidosis, hyperkalaemia
and to allow fluid removal so that any anaemia
present can be detected and treated. Left ventricular
failure happens rarely in the severe case and again
immediate peritoneal dialysis is indicated to correct
fluid overload. Hypertensive encephalopathy is rarely
seen because of early use of antihypertensive therapy
but if present can be treated with intravenous beta-
blockers (e.g. labetolol 1–3 mg/kg/h).

Course and prognosis

The prognosis of acute post-streptococcal glomerulonephritis in childhood is excellent. Complete recovery can be expected in about 90% of children without
significant alteration in renal function. A few patients
develop rapidly progressive glomerulonephritis in the
acute stage. Renal biopsy in these patients usually
shows extensive crescent formation. It is important to
clarify the underlying histology as early as possible
because immunosuppressive agents, namely steroid
plus cyclophosphamide or intravenous methylpred-
nisolone may prevent loss of renal function. A few,
however, progress rapidly to end-stage renal disease
and require long-term dialysis with a view to
transplantation. About 10% enter a latent phase

during which they feel well but continue to have persistent proteinuria with red cells and casts in the urine. These patients have chronic glomerulonephritis characterised by excessive thirst and polyuria, hypertension, normocytic/normochromic anaemia and pale urine of fixed specific gravity. They eventually require regular dialysis therapy in later childhood or adult life.

The treatment of acute post-streptococcal glomerulonephritis is symptomatic. There is little that can be done for these children which would alter the course of the disease once it becomes symptomatic. For a long time rest in bed was thought to be essential for patients with post-streptococcal glomerulonephritis. It has now been shown that in the absence of marked hypertension and/or severe oedema, bed rest does not seem to be beneficial. The intake of fluid, sodium and protein should be restricted during the acute stage although physicians vary in the rigidity with which they apply these restrictions. Reasonable intakes are: no added salt to the diet and protein not more than 1 to 1.5 g/kg/day if blood urea nitrogen is increased. Our practice is to limit fluids to an amount equal to insensible water loss (400–500 ml/m² body surface area per day) plus one half of their daily urine output. The calorie intake is augmented with boiled sweets. Fruit juices should be avoided at this stage because of their potassium content. The blood pressure should be measured and urine tested daily. If hypertension is severe or increases this can be treated with intramuscular hydralazine in a dose of 0.15–0.30 mg/kg body weight. This dosage should lower the blood pressure within 30–40 minutes and can be repeated in 4–6 hours if necessary. The loss of oedema is best assessed by daily weighing as measurement of the daily urinary output is not always accurate in young children. When diuresis has occurred and hypertension subsided, cereals, potatoes, vegetables, rice, bread, biscuits and fruit may be allowed. Penicillin should be prescribed at the start of treatment to eradicate any surviving haemolytic streptococci, e.g. oral penicillin V 250 mg four times daily or intravenous benzylpenicillin 500 000 units twice daily for 5–7 days or erythromycin 50 mg/kg/day in four divided doses orally for 10 days for penicillin allergic children. Prolonged penicillin prophylaxis is not of value.

The nephrotic syndrome

This is a clinical syndrome in which gross proteinuria and hypoalbuminaemia are always present. Oedema and hyperlipidaemia are usually severe. Hypertension, azotaemia and haematuria rarely occur in childhood.

Classification

The histological changes in the nephrotic syndrome have been intensively studied in renal biopsy material during recent years using the techniques of both standard light and electron microscopy and immunofluorescent techniques. Even when cases of the nephrotic syndrome which are secondary to systemic lupus erythematosus, amyloidosis, diabetes mellitus, etc. are excluded, the histological changes in the "idiopathic" cases show a wide variety. They have been classified into three main groups and subsequently into four groups. The relation between these groups is not clear and it is not known whether they are variants of a single disorder or represent separate disease entities.

Minimal glomerular changes

Glomeruli appear normal on light microscopy or there is a mild increase in cellularity but no deposition of basement-membrane-like fibrils in the mesangium. Electron microscopy shows fusion of the epithelial cell foot processes. Immunoglobulins and complement components are not demonstrable in the glomeruli. In some cases focal deposits of IgM and/or C3 are found in the mesangium or in the walls of the glomerular arterioles. Basement membrane deposits are not seen. Minimal change disease accounts for 85% of idiopathic nephrotic syndrome presenting in childhood but only 10% of adults and has a very much better prognosis.

Membranous or epimembranous nephropathy

Although very common in the adult this histological change is very unusual as a primary disease in children.

All glomeruli show diffuse capillary wall thickening without cellular proliferation. Preparations stained with periodic acid/silver methenamine (PASM) show spiky projections on the outer aspect of the basement membrane between which lies the subepithelial deposits that form the thickening. Immunofluorescence shows a characteristic diffuse granular stain along capillary loops for IgM and C3. The prognosis is unfavourable.

Proliferative glomerulonephritis (five types)

1. Diffuse proliferative/exudative glomerulonephritis

Many capillary loops are occluded due to swelling of endothelial cytoplasm. There is also marked proliferation of mesangial cells and infiltration by polymophonuclear cells. The capillary walls are normal. This is the picture seen in rapidly progressive post-streptococcal nephritis but it may also occur in the nephrotic syndrome. The prognosis is rarely good but healing sometimes takes place after a prolonged course.

2. With lobular stalk thickening

There is diffuse proliferation of mesangial cells with no endothelial swelling or polymorphonuclear infil-

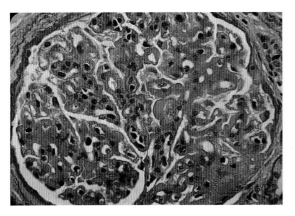

FIGURE 8.1 Membrano-proliferative glomerulonephritis: renal biopsy showing a glomerulus with a coarsely lobular tuft, proliferation of mesangial cells, increase in the amount of mesangial matrix and double contour in capillary loops (obj × 40).

tration. Lobular stalks are thickened due to deposits of basement-membrane-like material. This picture is seen in subsiding post-streptococcal nephritis but also in some cases of the nephrotic syndrome.

3. With crescents

Mesangial proliferation which forms crescents with proliferation of capsular and visceral epithelial cells carries a poor prognosis.

4. Membranoproliferative or mesangiocapillary glomerulonephritis

Mesangial proliferation plus deposition of basement-membrane-like fibrils in the mesangium with pronounced capillary wall thickening are characteristic features (Fig. 8.1). Nephrotic patients with this type of renal histology always show low β,C/β,A levels (low serum C3) and the prognosis is not good.

5. Others

Others show, for example, atypical proliferative changes, thickened capillaries on PAS staining but normal basement membranes on PASM staining.

Focal sclerosing glomerular lesions

Two forms of glomerular sclerosis can be distinguished in patients with idiopathic nephrotic syndrome. These are "focal segmental glomerular sclerosis" and "focal global glomerular sclerosis". In "focal segmental glomerular sclerosis" the striking feature is glomerular sclerosis which is both focal and segmental in distribution. In nephrosis of short duration the glomerular sclerosis may involve only one or two lobules in a few glomeruli. There may also be an associated focal tubular atrophy. In "focal global glomerular sclerosis" sclerotic glomeruli

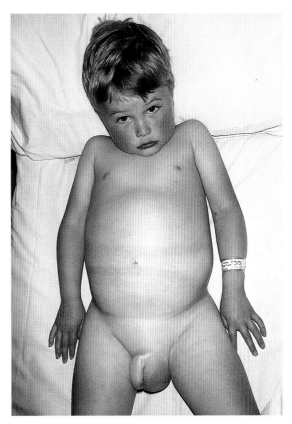

FIGURE 8.2 Typical nephrotic boy showing generalised oedema (including genitalia) and abdominal swelling due to ascites.

containing few cells are scattered throughout the renal cortex. The non-sclerotic glomeruli appear normal or show the same changes as in idiopathic nephrotic syndrome with mesangial changes. These findings should only be considered significant in nephrotic patients when 15–20% of glomeruli are affected. The prognosis is unfavourable.

Clinical features

Although the idiopathic nephrotic syndrome of childhood is seen at all ages the majority of cases occur in preschool children. The first manifestation is oedema which causes swelling of the face, legs and abdomen (Fig. 8.2) often starting after a viral upper respiratory tract infection. Gross ascites is the rule; indeed in some children peripheral oedema may be relatively slight while ascites is massive in amounts. In most, generalised oedema is gross enough to mask the severe underlying tissue wasting which is also a feature of the disease. Hypertension is typically absent. Proteinuria is also very heavy; at least 10 g may be lost each day. Haematuria is uncommon. In the phases of gross oedema and proteinuria the child is anorexic and miserable. Appropriate clinical and laboratory studies establish the correct diagnosis.

Biochemical features

The most characteristic changes in the blood are:

1 gross reduction in the total serum proteins (normal 65–80 g/l);
2 disproportionate reduction in serum albumin (normal 35–45 g/l) with inversion of the albumin/globulin ratio;
3 reduction in gammaglobulin (normal 12% of the total serum proteins);
4 normal or elevated alpha-2- and beta-globulins;
5 high serum cholesterol (normal 4.0–6.5 mmol/l).

These conventional investigations do not permit us to assess whether a child with nephrosis is likely to respond to the lines of treatment described below. This can be done by means of renal biopsy, those children with minimal glomerular changes being very likely to respond to treatment by a complete remission, whereas those with proliferative sclerosing or membranous changes being unlikely to benefit. On the other hand, as 85% of nephrotic children show only minimal change in the glomeruli, routine renal biopsy cannot be justified. Renal biopsy should be reserved for carefully selected cases. In recent years the value of differential protein clearance tests on the urine in assessing the probable response to treatment has been appreciated. These are based upon the fact that in the nephrotic patient the low molecular weight proteins such as albumin and alpha-1-globulins escape through the glomerular filter more readily than high molecular weight proteins but as the glomerular leak becomes more severe proteins of higher molecular weight such as beta-globulin and transferrin begin to appear. Proteins present in nephrotic urine can be determined by a variety of immunological and other techniques.

Hypocomplementaemia (β,C/β,A concentrations below 0.66 g/l) is not a common finding in the nephrotic syndrome in the child. As noted above it is characteristic of membranoproliferative glomerulonephritis and it foretells an absence of response to treatment.

Complications

Many children with the nephrotic syndrome died of intercurrent pyogenic infections in the pre-antibiotic era. This susceptibility was presumably due to the low serum gammaglobulin level in this disease. The most typical infection is primary pneumococcal peritonitis although pneumonia and staphylococcal cellulitis are also common. Pyuria and bacteriuria are not uncommon in nephrotic children who have failed to respond to treatment. Some suffer from bouts of diarrhoea, probably due to malabsorption secondary to oedema of the bowel wall. Death is still more frequently related to infections rather than renal complications.

Course and prognosis

Antibiotics have brought about an abrupt fall in the mortality figures from nephrosis in childhood and they have been further reduced by the therapeutic use of corticosteroids. The prognosis is much better than in the nephrotic syndrome in adults. Indeed, complete recovery may be expected with proper management in 60–70% of cases. Death from intercurrent infection is now rare. The prognosis as well as the likely response to treatment can often be forecast by a study of the differential protein clearance tests and/or the renal biopsy findings. Complete recovery is only likely in those children with a "highly selective" pattern of differential protein clearance and with minimal glomerular changes. Unfortunately, the use of selectivity has its drawbacks. For example, patients with congenital nephrotic syndrome of the Finnish type have selective proteinuria but they do not respond to corticosteroid therapy. Children with proliferative or sclerosing glomerulonephritis or membranous nephropathy are almost certain to progress to renal failure, although a very few with the proliferative type of lesion may ultimately heal. A proportion of nephrotic children initially showing response to steroid therapy later develop resistance to treatment. Renal biopsy at that stage usually confirms the underlying histology to be focal segmental sclerosis and the prognosis is less good.

Treatment

Before the introduction of corticosteroids there was no satisfactory form of therapy. Fortunately it is now possible in the majority of nephrotic children (in contrast to adults) to induce diuresis and complete or partial remission of proteinuria with steroids such as prednisolone, prednisone, or dexamethasone which are comparatively free from sodium-retaining or potassium-losing effects. As relapses also respond favourably the nephrotic child now rarely has to spend long periods in hospital and he can usually attend school and live a normal existence for most of the time. Bed rest is rarely indicated.

The traditional diet of low sodium, high protein is not now accepted as being suitable for the treatment of nephrotic syndrome. The patient should be given a diet which provides the recommended calorie and protein allowance and there should be no added salt. Protein supplements should be used if the appetite is poor and the intake does not meet that recommended. Once steroids are started there is usually a marked increase in appetite and care should be taken to prevent excessive weight gain. Advice should be given to the parents about the use of low calorie products, limiting snacks and preferred cooking methods.

If the patient is very oedematous, oliguric, showing a rise in serum creatinine, intravenous salt-poor albumin infusion in a dose of 1 g/kg given over a 2-hour period is very effective, particularly if supplemented by frusemide 1 mg/kg. These can be repeated every 8–24 hours if necessary until dry weight is attained. This therapy can be continued until the oedema has disappeared. In our experience the steroid of first choice with fewest side effects is prednisolone. Dosage programmes vary from centre to centre and so far there is no convincing evidence that one dosage schedule is better than the other. The programme currently used at the Royal Hospital for Sick Children, Glasgow is that of prednisolone 60 mg/m^2/day in divided doses until the urine is free of protein for three consecutive days when the daily dose is rapidly reduced over a period of 1–3 weeks, then discontinued.

There is little evidence that continuous steroid therapy improves the ultimate prognosis. The remission, as shown by sudden diuresis, rapid loss of proteinuria and reversal towards normal of the blood chemistry, commences between 10 and 14 days after the start of treatment. Eighty-five per cent of responding patients will lose their proteinuria within 4 weeks and 90% within 8 weeks. The same sequence of events is usually to be expected from subsequent courses of steroid when relapses of the nephrotic picture take place. Unfortunately, the prevention of relapses remains an unsolved problem. If relapse does occur it should be treated by the same intensive course of prednisolone, but this should be followed by intermittent treatment for a minimum of 3 months. Various intermittent regimens have been used and we favour the use of prednisolone given at 3 mg/kg as a single morning dose on alternate days. In some cases the child recovers after one or two relapses in the first year or two. In others, repeated and frequent relapses have led to repeated courses of steroids or to continuous therapy with consequent severe steroid side effects, especially arrest of growth, osteoporosis and cushingoid obesity.

The introduction of immunosuppressive drugs such as cyclophosphamide has provided an alternative line of treatment for these frequent relapsers and also the few children who are intolerant of high doses of steroid. Cyclophosphamide is probably the safer and more effective drug although its toxic effects can be unpleasant and dangerous, e.g. alopecia (temporary), haemorrhagic cystitis, marrow depression and chromosomal change. Particularly worrying is the evidence that the drug can cause sterility in adults of both sexes. While it is also capable of damaging the pre-pubertal gonads, it is not yet clear whether this is temporary or sometimes permanent.

It follows, therefore, that the decision to prescribe cyclophosphamide in the nephrotic child cannot be taken lightly and then only when steroids have proved ineffective and productive of unacceptably severe side effects. Parents must always be fully informed of the possible dangers. Cyclophosphamide will either change the frequency or eliminate relapses entirely in 80–90% of frequently relapsing cases of minimal change nephrotic syndrome. The child is brought into remission with prednisolone and this drug is continued in a daily dose of 10–20 mg. A good urinary output is essential. Cyclophosphamide is then given in a daily dose of 3 mg/kg for 6–8 weeks. The prednisolone is slowly withdrawn after completion of the 8-week course of cyclophosphamide. It should be stressed that second courses of cyclophosphamide appear as effective as the first, although long-term side effects may be additive. An important point to remember is that both varicella and measles are highly dangerous to the child who is on either corticosteroids or cyclophosphamide. This risk must be explained to the parents who should report contact with either of these infections promptly to allow the patient to be protected with the appropriate immunoglobulin.

While prophylactic antibiotics are not recommended in children with nephrosis, bacterial infections must be promptly treated. Pneumococcal peritonitis or cellulitis are best dealt with by large intravenous doses of benzylpenicillin. A careful watch must be kept on the renal function with these drug combinations. Intercurrent infections in the urinary tract commonly occur and can be treated with oral drugs chosen according to the bacterial sensitivities.

Congenital nephrotic syndrome

Congenital nephrosis is a rare disorder in which inheritance is probably autosomal recessive. It appears to have a peculiarly high and familial incidence in Finland. The hallmarks of the disease are an abnormally large placenta associated with heavy proteinuria, oedema and ascites. It is unresponsive to steroid therapy and the affected infants die from intercurrent infections or progressive renal failure. The glomeruli show characteristic fusion of the foot processes on electron microscopy and with light microscopy the proximal tubules may show microcystic dilatation with a swan-like neck. Prenatal diagnosis is now possible in families with previously affected children by demonstrating markedly raised levels of α-fetoprotein in the liquor amnii between the 15th and 20th weeks of pregnancy. Indeed, high concentrations of α-fetoprotein have been found in the maternal serum during the 14th week of pregnancy. The only presently hopeful line of management might be to perform bilateral nephrectomy and then to keep the infant alive by peritoneal dialysis or haemodialysis while awaiting a renal transplant.

Shunt nephritis

In the treatment of progressive hydrocephalus ventriculo-atrial shunts were used to reduce intraventricular pressure. Serious infection occurred in between 10% and 30%. Septicaemia and chronic infection with release of multiple septic emboli resulted in nephritis (shunt nephritis) and anaemia, splenomegaly and vasculitic skin rashes associated with complement activation. Most centres now use ventriculoperitoneal shunts but even these may rarely be associated with shunt nephritis.

URINARY TRACT INFECTIONS

It is difficult to write concisely on the subject of urinary tract infections although it is one of the common diseases of paediatric practice. Much remains unknown about its aetiology and natural history. It may involve only a short sharp illness or years of vague ill health which terminate in death from chronic renal failure. The difficulty of accurate localisation of the site of infection in the renal tract has led many physicians to prefer the general term "urinary tract infection".

Aetiology

The most common infecting organism is *E. coli* and the highest incidence of the disease is in the first 2 or 3 years. Less frequently, the organisms are the *Streptococcus faecalis*, *Proteus vulgaris*, *Klebsiella aerogenes* or *Pseudomonas aeruginosa*. Rarely the urinary tract is infected by one of the salmonella group. Renal tuberculosis has become rare in the UK. There has long been controversy as to the route by which the organisms reach the kidney. Haematogenous spread undoubtedly occurs, especially in the newborn, but the present tendency is to attach more importance to ascending infection via the urethral lumen or the lymphatics. There is good evidence that infection often invades the kidneys via the ureters and vesico-ureteric reflux with its associated intrarenal reflux is now recognised to be a common accompaniment of pyelonephritis. Indeed, the relation between vesico-ureteric reflux and renal parenchymal scarring is now firmly established. It is also recognised that the scarring process is initiated in early childhood and is permanent. Urinary stasis due to congenital anomalies of the renal tract or to acquired causes of obstruction such as calculi predisposes to infection. Indeed these conditions most often

present with pyuria and their existence must always be suspected when pyuria proves resistant to treatment or when relapses occur.

Pathology

In the acute stage the inflammation may vary from little more than leucocytic infiltration under the pelvic epithelium to almost complete destruction of the kidney with multiple interstitial abscesses. If the infection is allowed to become chronic extensive scarring and irregular contraction of the kidney may occur. At this stage of chronic pyelonephritis there may be little evidence of active bacterial infection but there can be extensive loss of nephrons and arteriosclerotic changes in the renal arterioles may be severe. In fact the condition is the commonest cause of end-stage renal failure in childhood. It is for this reason that hospital physicians have become increasingly aware of the need for intensive investigations and treatment in every case of acute urinary tract infection and particularly in the under 5-years-old age group.

We remain uninformed as to the frequency with which infections of the urinary tract do progress to chronic pyelonephritis with renal cortical atrophy and scarring. It is clear, however, that early antibacterial treatment in the young child with vesico-ureteric reflux reduces the likelihood of renal scarring.

Clinical features

Urinary tract infections occur four times more frequently in girls than in boys, with the exception of the first 6 months of life. The equal sex incidence in young infants is explicable on the basis of the equal sex incidence of *E. coli* bacteraemias and of congenital anomalies of the urinary tract. The higher female incidence after the early months of life has been attributed to the short female urethra and ascending infections.

The onset of the acute stage is usually sudden with fever, pallor, toxaemia, anorexia, vomiting and tachycardia. Urinary tract infection is one of the few causes of rigor in young children. A bowel upset, constipation or diarrhoea commonly precedes the acute signs. In the young infant meningism or convulsions are common whereas symptoms pointing to the renal tract are often absent. In some cases, however, the mother may have observed that there is frequency of micturition or that the infant screams during the act of urination. Attacks of screaming and drawing up of the legs can simulate an abdominal emergency.

In older children frequency and dysuria make diagnosis easier although their absence does not exclude the diagnosis. Some children may present with new or increased enuresis. In untreated cases of acute urinary tract infection the high fever usually

(a)

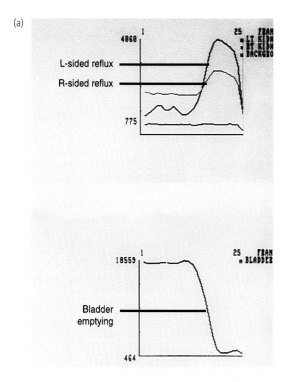

(b)

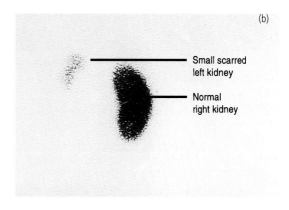

FIGURE 8.3 (a) Indirect voiding radionuclide cystogram using ^{99m}Tc DTPA. The lower graph shows the activity in the child's bladder prior to micturition, the activity falling rapidly during micturition and then the minimal activity present at the end of micturition. During micturition the activity in the kidneys increases markedly particularly on the left due to reflux. (b) A DMSA study was performed 2 days later and shows a normal right kidney despite the presence of reflux. The left kidney is very small with an irregular outline due to severe reflux nephropathy.

subsides spontaneously after 7–10 days but the child remains apathetic, anorexic, has a somewhat characteristic muddy pallor and fails to gain weight. Rarely, death may occur quite rapidly from a combination of toxaemia, dehydration and uraemia.

Diagnosis

In older children symptoms referable to the urinary tract may make the diagnosis comparitively easy but many children and nearly all infants have no localising clinical features. There can be no doubt that pyelonephritis escapes clinical diagnosis in a high percentage of patients and it will continue to do so until doctors make urine analysis part of their routine investigation of every ill infant or child. The diagnosis must be based upon examination of the urine including microscopy and culture. If there is any delay, storage at 4°C will permit accurate diagnosis certainly for 24 hours. Whenever there is clinical suspicion of renal infection a white cell count in the urine should be performed by a quantitative method although there is general agreement that pyuria is absent in 50% of patients with significant bacteriuria. The causal organism and its antibacterial sensitivities must also be determined by culture within 1 hour of their collection of three specimens of urine. Whenever possible midstream specimens should be obtained from the younger child. Clean catch urine specimens are the ideal. Collections in a plastic bag are less reliable. Suprapubic puncture of the bladder can be used to obtain uncontaminated urine for culture from infants and sometimes older children. It is particularly indicated when precise bacteriological diagnosis is urgent, when midstream specimens are contaminated (mixed growth), when bacterial counts of doubtful significance are obtained, or if the perineum is itself unhealthy. The reliability of quantatitive urine culture has been much easier to ensure since the introduction of the dipslide quantitation of bacteriuria.

Significant infection is likely to be present if the white cell count is over 50 per mm^3 in the newborn or 10 per mm^3 in the older child. However, an active infection can be present in the child without a significant pyuria and the final proof must rest upon the presence of a suprapubic bladder specimen or in two or more fresh midstream specimens of a pure growth of more than 100 000 (10^5) pathogenic organisms per ml. However, if there have been no problems in collection and the urine sample has been promptly transported to the laboratory, it is prudent to regard any growth of bacteria as indicating true bacteriuria. Haematuria occurs in about one-third of children with urinary tract infection, particularly in neonates and boys. Although proteinuria occurs in advanced reflux nephropathy it is not diagnostic of acute urinary infection.

Differential diagnosis

In older children acute appendicitis can simulate pyelonephritis and the pelvic appendix in particular

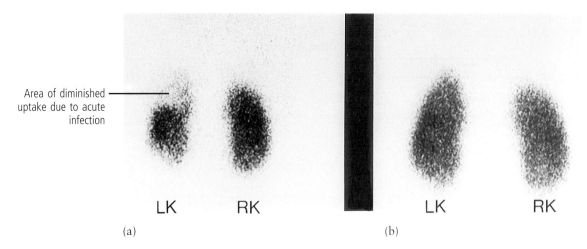

Area of diminished uptake due to acute infection

LK   RK

(a)

LK   RK

(b)

FIGURE 8.4 (a) Tc DMSA scan in acute pyelonephritis. ^{99m}Tc dimercaptosuccinic acid scan showing an area of reduced uptake of the scanning agent in the upper part of the left kidney at the time of an acute urinary tract infection. The function in this kidney was also reduced. (b) The appearance had returned to normal on a follow-up scan 4 months later.

can produce urinary frequency and discomfort. Mistakes will be few if the urine is always examined microscopically before resort to surgery but some pyuria can occur if the inflamed appendix is irritating the bladder. In young infants the presence of meningism may necessitate lumbar puncture to exclude pyogenic meningitis.

Course and prognosis

In the majority of cases of acute urinary tract infections complete recovery occurs with adequate treatment. Failure to achieve a sterile urine or recurrence of pyuria should suggest that there is an anatomical or functional disorder of the urinary tract. About one-third of children in their first attack of pylonephritis have a developmental anomaly in the renal tract, whereas in children with a history of previous attacks such anomalies can be found in two-thirds of the cases. A proven urinary infection in any child is an indication for further investigation and this may include plain radiographs, ultrasonography, intravenous urography, micturating cystography and gamma-camera renography using hippuran-123, ^{99}Tc DTPA (Fig. 8.3a) and DMSA renal scan (Fig. 8.4 a,b). Their use should be tailored to the clinical situation in each case. Inadequately treated urinary tract infection can cause prolonged and vague ill health with pallor, anorexia, failure to grow, febrile episodes and slow renal destruction. If chronic pyelonephritis progresses to end-stage renal failure the child needs to be considered for dialysis and transplantation.

In rare cases chronic pyelonephritis is unilateral, being superimposed upon a hypoplastic or duplex kidney (Fig. 8.5). In a few such cases renal hypertension has been relieved by nephrectomy and every case of renal hypertension encountered in childhood should be regarded as an indication for detailed investigation.

Management

General nursing measures include a large fluid intake, antipyretic agents when there is high fever and a laxative if the patient is constipated. If at all possible antibiotic therapy should not be commenced until the diagnosis has been fully established or at least appropriate urine cultures have been obtained so that the organism and its antibiotic sensitivity can be determined. However, in any unwell child it would be unwise to withhold antibiotic once urine cultures have been taken and treatment should be started with the "best guess" antibacterial agent in full dosage. Full dose antibacterial therapy is given for 7–10 days but a clinical response and sterile urine may be expected within 48 hours. Useful drugs for oral use include trimethoprim (8 mg/kg/day), nitrofurantoin (3 mg/kg/day) given 6-hourly and nalidixic acid (50 mg/kg/day) also given 6-hourly. Ampicillin has lost much of its usefulness due to the high incidence of resistant Gram-negative organisms. In young infants who may have a Gram-negative septicaemia the drug of choice is gentamicin (7.5 mg/kg/day) intravenously at 8–12 hour intervals. Pseudomonas may infect an abnormal renal tract and be combated with gentamicin or carbenicillin (50–100 mg/kg/day). The combination of ampicillin or amoxycillin with a β-lactamase inhibitor restores effectiveness against Gram-negative bacteria. Thus, amoxycillin 125 mg and clavulanic acid 31 mg in 5 ml (Augmentin Paediatric Suspension) can be given orally every 8 hours. When renal function is impaired antibacterial drugs should be prescribed with caution and may need blood level control.

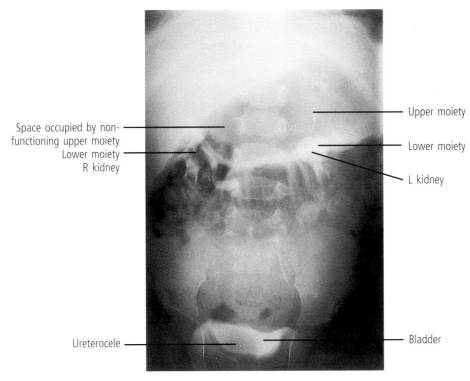

FIGURE 8.5 Duplex kidney with ureterocele. Intravenous urogram showing bilateral duplex kidneys. The upper moiety of the right kidney is not functioning and the pelvicalyceal system of the lower moiety has a "drooping flower appearance". There is a filling defect in the bladder due to a ureterocele at the lower end of the ureter draining the non-functioning upper moiety.

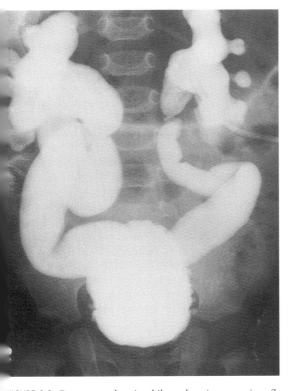

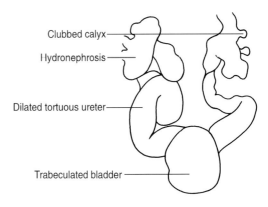

FIGURE 8.6 Cystogram showing bilateral vesico-ureteric reflux.

In view of the risk of renal parenchymal scar formation in the young child with reflux, the appropriate drug, e.g. trimethoprim (2 mg/kg/day) as prophylaxis is given and the child reassessed until he is outwith the vulnerable age group (Fig. 8.6). In children with vesico-ureteric reflux low dose antibacterial prophylaxis may be necessary as long as the reflux persists. If the kidneys are scarred, even if reflux has ceased, it is wise to continue prophylaxis until the kidneys are fully grown. When a renal tract developmental anomaly is not amenable to surgery continuous prophylactic treatment with trimethoprim in half the therapeutic dosage usually prevents reinfections.

The following sequence of initial investigations is suggested:

- 0–2 years
  A plain X-ray of abdomen
  An ultrasound examination of kidneys and bladder
  A DMSA scan to assess individual kidney function
  A cystourethrogram
- 2–5 years
  A plain X-ray of abdomen
  An ultrasound examination of kidneys and bladder
  A DMSA scan
  If toilet trained, a DTPA scan to detect vesico-ureteric reflux
- More than 5 years
  A plain X-ray of abdomen
  An ultrasound examination of kidneys and bladder
  A cystogram is rarely needed in this age group but in some an IVU is necessary.

GENITOURINARY SYSTEM DISORDERS

Many disorders of the genitourinary system are amenable to surgical treatment. The patient usually presents with urinary tract infection, haematuria or disorders of urinary continence. Most disorders of the external genitalia are detected on routine clinical examination and some urinary tract disorders are found by detection of a mass in the abdomen. The remainder of the urinary tract abnormalities are defined by investigation of the urinary tract which includes examination of the urine, examination of the blood, ultrasound examination of the urinary tract, isotope scanning and, less frequently than previously, by intravenous urography and micturating cystourethrography. An anatomical and pathological diagnosis can usually be made without examination by cystourethroscopy which requires general anaesthesia in infants and children. Rarely retrograde pyelography may also be required to define the pathological condition. Renal arteriography is infrequently required to establish the diagnosis.

Disorders of micturition

In infancy micturition has a sharp beginning, quick voiding with a good stream of urine and a decisive ending. Even in the youngest infant there should be dry periods and there should be no straining and no dribbling. When the infant is in nappies and wetting frequently it is only too easy to overlook straining and dribbling. The frequency with which children micturate varies widely from two to 10 times a day.

Increased frequency persisting beyond infancy or returning after micturition has become normal is usually caused by local irritation of the trigone of the bladder, most often by infection – either external (ammoniacal dermatitis, vaginitis) or internal (urethritis or cystitis). Polyuria will cause increased frequency and the fluid intake and output should always be measured when increased frequency persists. Diabetes mellitus and diabetes insipidus must be excluded.

The most common cause of *dysuria* is ammoniacal dermatitis leading to meatal erosion in the male and ammonia burns in the vulva of the female. Cystitis is a less common cause of dysuria in the infant. Pain on micturition often leads to urinary retention as the child will prefer to tolerate a greatly distended bladder rather than suffer the pain of passing urine.

Acute retention of urine is commonly due to pain and spasm caused by local irritation of the foreskin, urethra or bladder. A pelvic appendix abscess irritating the bladder wall will also cause retention. In the newborn, retention may be caused by the tiny ectopic meatus of a hypospadias. Congenital phimosis is extremely rare.

Retention or stasis of urinary flow at various levels in the genitourinary tract is common in the young. Partial obstruction can cause dilatation of varying degree with urinary stasis complicated by secondary infection. Pelviureteric and ureterovesical obstructions may be unilateral or bilateral. Bladder-neck and urethral obstructions due to urethral valves, stricture or diverticulum cause bilateral upper tract obstruction.

Chronic retention presenting with dribbling overflow may be due to an impediment urethra caused by urethral valves, congenital bladder neck obstruction, ureterocele prolapsing into the urethra, congenital or post-traumatic urethral stricture or may accompany the neuropathic bladder associated with developmental anomalies of the spine and the spinal cord such as spina bifida. Infants with the prune-belly syndrome or agenesis of the abdominal muscles almost invariably suffer from chronic urinary reten tion. Retention may occur in some patients with chronic constipation. A digital rectal examination should never be omitted in these cases. Rarely, retention may be caused by a pelvic tumour (sarcoma) which may arise from the bladder, or in the female from the vagina.

Incontinence of urine

Many patients with urinary incontinence appear first with a diagnosis of enuresis. On examination, they fall roughly into three groups:

1 *Dribbling and incontinence.* This may be almost continuous or in tiny infants there may be small squirts of urine every few minutes indicating chronic overflow retention. This type of incontinence is found with posterior urethral obstruction and also in the neuropathic bladder. The bladder in these situations will be very large and well above the level of the umbilicus. It is usually palpable and dull to percussion.

2 *Involuntary voiding.* The involuntary voiding of quantities of urine at intervals occurs with cystitis secondary to infection. It is also found in the neuropathic bladder. Flaccidity of the urinary sphincter occasionally leads to dribbling with retention.

3 *Vertical incontinence.* If there is a urinary leak when the child is upright it is usually diagnostic of an ectopic ureter. This incontinence is constant and persistent and not related to stress.

Pyuria

Cloudiness of urine is commonly due to a phosphatic deposit and indicates alkalinity and lack of fluid intake. Pyuria, which is diagnosed by microscopic examination of the urine, indicates inflammation of the urinary tract. Pyuria is common in children with dilatation of parts of the urinary tract. A child with pyuria should always be thoroughly investigated. Non-specific urethritis is rare in childhood but in girls involvement of the peri-urethral glands may occasionally simulate urinary tract infection.

Haematuria

Unless there is an obvious lesion of the prepuce or meatus, haematuria is almost always of serious significance. At times it can be difficult to differentiate it from bleeding from the bowel or from the vagina. Fear on the part of the mother usually leads to early investigation of haematuria. In little boys bleeding from a meatal ulcer is the most common cause and

this lesion is almost always accompanied by discomfort. The meatus is scabbed over and the child feels miserable. Haematuria may also be accompanied by pain when there is passage of a blood clot. Painless haematuria may be a presenting feature of many patients with glomerulonephritis and in rare instances of Wilms tumour. In the newborn, haematuria and pyuria may be the presenting signs in renal vein thrombosis. Trauma may produce frank blood in the urine and minor trauma which causes haematuria suggests an underlying lesion such as a hydronephrosis. Finally, haematuria can occur in such general diseases as thrombocytopenic purpura and leukaemia. The most important differential diagnosis is from acute haemorrhagic nephritis. In acute nephritis the presence of casts in the urine confirm the diagnosis. In a few children with haematuria no firm diagnosis can be made. In some children attacks are persistent and unaccompanied by any symptoms. This unexplained haematuria may follow violent exercise and ceases when the child is put to bed. On cystoscopy the source of the blood is confirmed from both kidneys and no pyelographic lesions are detectable.

KIDNEY

Renal agenesis

Renal agenesis may be bilateral and be diagnosed prenatally by ultrasound in pregnancies complicated by oligohydramnios. The baby frequently has low set ears and flattened nose (Potter facies), spade-like hands and may have club feet. After birth, respiratory distress due to pulmonary hypoplasia is very common and intubation and intermittent positive-pressure ventilation may be necessary. Unless the infant is maintained by dialysis and subsequent renal transplant the outlook is fatal. Even with full support therapy the respiratory aspect may prove fatal. Where renal agenesis is unilateral the baby should survive normally. Investigation usually shows the compensatory hypertrophy of the remaining kidney with some dilatation of the pelvis and the ureter.

Renal anomalies

The usual position of the kidneys is a high retroperitoneal one, the right kidney being about half a vertebra lower than the left. Kidneys are frequently palpable in the newborn and an assessment of their size can be made. Later the kidneys are not palpable unless they are abnormal or in an abnormal position. An *ectopic kidney* is usually paravertebral but lower in position than normal and may present as a palpable mass in the iliac fossa. The kidney may develop even more caudal and be pelvic in position, being identified by ultrasound or an IVP examination. Rarely the kidney may migrate across the midline and end with both kidneys on one side but with the ureter from the lower kidney (the ectopic one) crossing to enter bladder on the "normal" side. Sometimes the crossed ectopic kidney fuses with the other kidney resulting in a *cross-fused ectopic kidney* but usually with independent drainage systems and the ureters opening into either side of the bladder. These anatomical variations which may never come to light in life may be found by chance investigation of a patient for an unrelated reason, or on investigation of a child with urinary tract infection or other urinary tract signs. The anatomical variation does not in itself require any treatment except in rare cases where there may be obstruction to drainage or urine at the pelviureteric junction or by extrinsic pressure where a ureter traverses behind the inferior vena cava.

Duplex kidney

Duplex kidney is the term given to the condition where the drainage system from the renal parenchyma is double in part or all of its length (Fig. 8.7). This is often an anatomical finding of little functional significance. Urinary tract infection is frequently the reason for the investigation of the urinary tract and the bifid system is found. A duplex kidney is more prone to have a ureterocele (intravesical cystic dilatation) on the distal end of the upper pole ureter which drains into the bladder lower than the normal site or less commonly into the urethra or vagina. The latter can result in constant dampness of a child who also intermittently micturates normally. This wetting occurs more by day and is less troublesome at night when the child is asleep. The lower pole ureter always opens "above" the upper pole ureter – often into the normal site – but this ureter is more prone to have vesico-ureteric reflux. It is only the complications of duplex systems (which may be bilateral) that require treatment. This also applies to horseshoe kidney where the lower poles of the kidneys are in continuity across the midline.

Multicystic kidney

Multicystic kidney is the condition when one kidney is grossly enlarged, is non-functioning and, as the name suggests, replaced by multiple cysts. It is usually associated with ureteric atresia on that side. The disorder presents as a mass in the abdomen which may be detected prenatally or be found on abdominal examination of the infant. The contralateral kidney is usually normal but has to be checked.

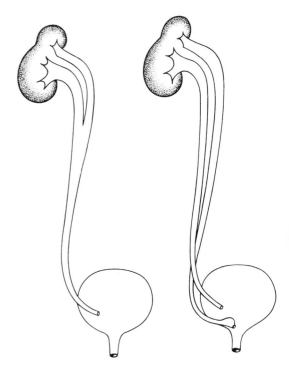

FIGURE 8.7 Duplex kidney with incomplete and complete duplex systems.

Nephrectomy of the multicystic kidney is usually recommended in case of subsequent enlargement of the cysts, infection within the cysts, or later development of hypertension. Some now advise continued supervision without active intervention unless a complication arises and on occasion the kidney may atrophy and disappear.

Polycystic disease

Polycystic disease of the kidneys is a serious autosomal dominant disorder which often has associated cystic disease of the liver. It may be diagnosed prenatally, the infants are often stillborn with massive abdominal distension or early postnatal death. Uncommon in paediatrics is the adult type of polycystic disease with slowly progressive renal failure which is more amenable to treatment by dialysis and transplantation as there is no liver involvement.

Hydronephrosis

Hydronephrosis results from obstruction to the free drainage of urine from the kidney. The hold-up may be at the pelviureteric junction due to an intrinsic stenosis or malfunction at the pelviureteric junction or due to extrinsic pressure from renal vessels passing to the lower pole of the kidney. If the obstruction is more distal at the ureterovesical junction or at the bladder

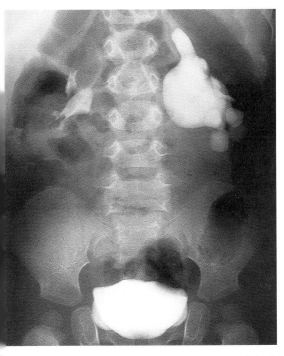

FIGURE 8.8 Left pelviureteric junction obstruction with hydronephrosis.

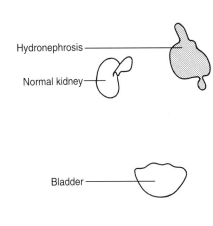

neck, not only will the kidney pelvis be dilated but the ureter will also show dilatation and often tortuosity. Hydronephrosis may present as a mass in one or other side of the abdomen or be detected during the investigation of a urinary tract infection or haematuria. Many infants have hydronephrosis detected *in utero* by ultrasound scanning and in some this dilatation of the renal pelvis disappears by birth or in the postnatal period. In others this obstruction and dilatation increases and ultimately renal function is impaired. Before proceeding to operation it is important to ensure that there is continuing and persistent obstruction at the pelviureteric junction (Fig. 8.8). Correction is usually by a pyeloplasty as shown in the diagram (Fig. 8.9). Post-operatively the urine is drained from the kidney by a nephrostomy tube and once the new anastomosis has healed the tube is clamped for 24 hours prior to removal. The hydronephrotic kidney of the young infant can undergo remarkable improvement following pyeloplasty, whereas the older child who has dilated pelvis and calyces will still have some residual dilatation of the calyces even after successful pyeloplasty.

Renal vein thrombosis

Renal vein thrombosis is a microvascular angiopathy which used to occur more frequently in dehydrated and seriously ill infants. The intravascular coagulation spreads from within the intrarenal vessels into the larger veins and ultimately to the renal vein. In

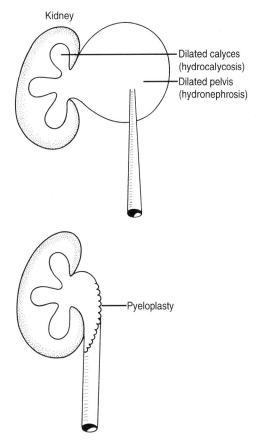

FIGURE 8.9 Showing pyeloplasty.

an ill infant the appearance of gross proteinuria, haematuria and an enlarged kidney suggest the diagnosis. The baby may also have significantly raised blood pressure. Supportive therapy with re-establishment of an adequate circulating volume is most important and treatment of any primary underlying disorder is indicated. The older practice of nephrectomy in the acute stage was successful because of the intensive support therapy in the pre- and post-operative care. The only indication for surgery now is when hypertension is induced by the small shrunken kidney some months or years later.

The relatively common renal tumour of childhood is the nephroblastoma and is considered in Chapter 19.

Renal calculi and nephrocalcinosis

Aetiology

There are three main types of renal calculi in children, i.e. endemic, infective and rare metabolic disorders associated with nephrocalcinosis. The great majority of renal calculi found in children in the UK are secondary to infection of the renal tract especially by *Proteus vulgaris*, which by maintaining a high urinary pH favours the deposition of phosphate in combination with calcium, ammonium and magnesium. The typical "staghorn" calculus fills the renal pelvis and calyces (Fig. 8.10). Calculus formation is especially

likely when there is an obstruction in the renal tract, e.g. at the pelviureteric or vesico-ureteric junction. Nephrocalcinosis is the deposition of calcium salts within the renal parenchyma and it may be associated with urolithiasis. Very rarely calcium phosphate or oxalate stones are a manifestation of primary hyperparathyroidism or hypervitaminosis D. Calculi may also develop after prolonged immobilisation for, e.g. chronic osteitis. *Cystinuria*, one of Garrod's original inborn errors of metabolism, is a rare cause of renal stone. In this condition there is a defect in the tubular reabsorption not only of cystine but also of lysine, arginine and ornithine. In spite of the passage of the typical hexagonal crystals in the urine only a minority of affected children develop calculi. The short stature of some children with cystinuria is related to the presence of similar absorptive defects in the mucosa of the small intestine. This condition must not be confused with the quite separate metabolic error called cystinosis in which cystine is deposited in body tissues. Another exceedingly rare cause of renal lithiasis, also an inborn metabolic error, is primary hyperoxaluria. In addition to calcium oxalate calculi, extrarenal deposits may occur – oxalosis. This rare type of very dense nephrocalcinosis and nephrolithiasis is characterised by the continuous high urinary excretion of oxalate which sufferers from primary hyperoxaluria always show. Other inherited metabolic diseases which increase the excretion of very insoluble substances and thus

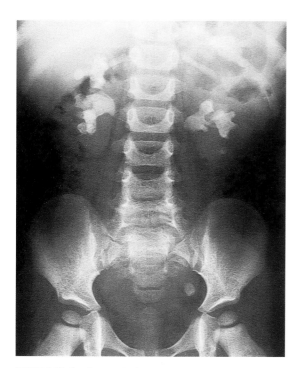

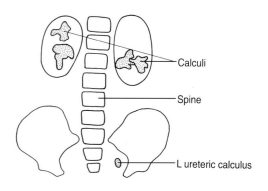

FIGURE 8.10 Staghorn calculus.

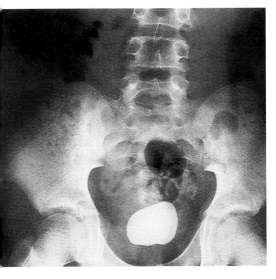

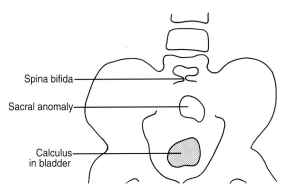

Spina bifida

Sacral anomaly

Calculus
in bladder

FIGURE 8.11 Calculus in bladder.

ormation of renal stones are Lesch–Nyhan syndrome, 2,8–dihydroxy adeninuria, xanthinuria and the orotic acidurias. In certain parts of the world, e.g. India and Thailand, endemic urolithiasis leads to the formation of vesical calculi which are composed of ammonium acid urate. There is evidence implicating dietary factors in their pathogenesis (Fig. 8.11). This used to be seen in England particularly in East Anglia but declined in incidence in the early part of this century.

Clinical features

The majority of children present as cases of urinary tract infection with pyuria. Classical renal colic with haematuria is relatively uncommon in childhood. In a few instances, and especially in primary hyperoxaluria, the infant or child has presented with chronic renal failure sometimes associated with renal osteodystrophy. The presence of a renal calculus can be confirmed by an abdominal X-ray. Calculi cause acoustic shadows and have a characteristic ultrasound appearance therefore nephrocalcinosis and renal calculi can be diagnosed by ultrasound examination. In confirmed cases it is wise to determine the urinary output of calcium, cystine and oxalate so that metabolic disorders are not overlooked.

Treatment

This consists of sterilisation of the urine by appropriate drug therapy and removal of the calculus either by lithotripsy or operation. Previously surgical removal of the calculi was the standard approach to renal calculi but lithotripsy now can fragment the calculi and obtain clearance without a need to operate. In younger patients lithotripsy has been less consistent and successful than it has been in adults but further improvement may occur with greater technical development and experience with the procedure. In unilateral cases nephrectomy may be necessary when the renal parenchyma has been severely damaged provided always that the opposite kidney has been shown to be healthy. The urine should be kept acid in reaction with ammonium chloride in children who have phosphate stones. The formation of stones can be discouraged in cystinuria by alkalinising the urine with sodium bicarbonate and ensuring a large fluid intake. There may be a place for the use of D-penicillamine in the prevention of cystine stones. Hepatorenal transplant for primary hyperoxaluria has been very effective and gene therapy may be available in the near future.

Renal osteodystrophy

The term is used here to denote the bone changes which sometimes develop in cases of chronic glomerular failure or when the life of patients with end stage renal failure is prolonged by long-term haemodialysis. It must be distinguished from the bone changes which may result from renal tubular disorders in which uraemia is not an inevitable accompaniment. The term "renal osteodystrophy" is preferred to "renal rickets", because the bone changes include more than rickets, and to "renal dwarfism" because dwarfism is not invariably present.

Aetiology

Osteodystrophy may develop in slowly progressive glomerular failure from any cause; the most common are bilateral renal hypoplasia, bilateral hydronephrosis, bilateral polycystic disease of the kidneys and chronic pyelonephritis. Dialysis osteodystrophy has been reported due to the presence of a high content of aluminium in the tap water used for preparing dialysate fluid and the incidence falls markedly after the initiation of appropriate water treatment.

Clinical features

In most cases the predominant symptoms are thirst and polyuria which may be extreme. Affected children are usually dwarfed, anaemic and thin. They often have a pale "renal" appearance and the skin around the knees and lower thighs has a curiously mottled look. In some cases deformities are noted first. These are clinically typical of rickets, e.g. enlarged epiphyses and costochondral junctions, knock knees (genu valgum), bowing of the femora and tibiae (genu varum) or pathological fractures. The bone pain of renal osteodystrophy most commonly occurs about the lower back, the hips or the rib cage and less frequently about the knees, ankles and/or feet. Usually the pain is poorly localised.

Biochemical features

The blood urea is increased and there is a metabolic acidosis. In uncompensated cases the pH of the blood will fall below 7.38. This acidosis is due partly to the retention of acid metabolites by the kidney and partly to its inability to manufacture ammonium. Glomerular insufficiency also leads to the retention of phosphate (serum concentrations > 2.1 mmol/l ; 6.5 mg/l00 ml). In some the serum calcium concentration is abnormally low (< 2.2 mmol/l; 9 mg/100 ml). Serum alkaline phosphatase activity is increased. A possible explanation of the hypocalcaemia is excess intestinal excretion of phosphate which combines with calcium in the gut to form calcium phosphate and interferes with calcium absorption. The hypocalcaemia is the cause of secondary hyperparathyroidism which is a characteristic feature of chronic renal failure and a cause of the bone changes. Serum immunoreactive parathyroid hormone (IPTH) activity is almost invariably increased in patients with advanced renal failure.

The rickets is due to a deficiency of circulating 1,25–dihydroxyvitamin D_3 (1,25$(OH)_2D_3$) caused by the failure of the kidney to convert 25-hydroxy vitamin D_3 produced in the liver to the more active 1,25$(OH)_2D_3$.

Radiological changes

These are complex and vary according to the age of the patient and severity of the bone disease. First are the typical appearances of rickets such as cupping and fraying of the metaphyses, deepening of the epiphyseal plates and osteoporosis (Fig. 8.12). There are also in many cases the changes of osteitis fibrosa cystica due to hyperparathyroidism. These include subperiosteal resorption best seen in the terminal phalanges, absence of the lamina dura, a ground-glass or stippled appearance to the skull and a character-

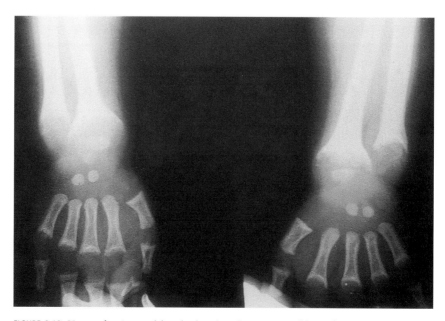

FIGURE 8.12 X-ray of wrists and hands showing changes caused by rickets.

istic irregularly distributed osteosclerosis which is especially obvious at the base of the skull, in the clavicles and in the vertebral bodies which show transverse bands.

Treatment

The renal lesion is always irreversible and the patient is prepared for dialysis and transplantation.

In a few instances the renal tract lesion may be amenable to surgery, e.g. bladder-neck obstruction. However, the main goal of therapy in children with renal osteodystrophy is to correct the biochemical abnormalities, i.e. hyperphosphataemia, hypocalcaemia, high PTH, and also to correct the metabolic acidosis so as to permit healing of the bone disease, correction of the deformities and restoration of normal growth. This is best achieved with a synthetic analogue of $1,25(OH)_2D_3$ called l-alpha-hydroxycholecalciferol (1α-OHD_3) or alfacalcidol which has a short half-life. The only side effect is hypercalcaemia which is rapidly reversed when 1α-OHD_3 is discontinued. An effective maintenance dose is usually 0.05 µg/kg/day although occasional patients may require up to 0.1 µg/kg/day. It usually takes 6–12 months for the bone disease to heal and it can be monitored by plasma calcium, phosphorus and alkaline phosphatase measurements and radiological appearances. Alternatively calcitriol ($1,25(OH)_2D_3$) may be prescribed in similar doses. It is marketed under the trade name Rocaltrol but as it has an even shorter half-life it is probably the drug of second choice because it may provoke marked and undesirable fluctuations in serum calcium values. The serum calcium must be measured regularly since hypercalcaemia may cause further deterioration in renal function. Hyperphosphataemia can be combated with a phosphate binder such as calcium carbonate. The dosage of phosphate binders that is required varies widely from patient to patient. Metabolic acidosis should be relieved with sodium bicarbonate 1–3 mmol/kg daily. Also, calcium deficiency should be prevented by an adequate dietary intake of calcium and an appropriate concentration of calcium in the dialysate.

Aluminium-related renal osteodystrophy can be prevented by reducing the amount of aluminium in dialysis water. Established aluminium-related osteodystrophy can be treated with chelation therapy using desferrioxamine. Surgical removal of hyperplastic parathyroid tissue is rarely indicated.

Familial hypophosphataemic rickets (phosphaturic rickets)

In this disease rickets develops at a later age than is usual in infantile rickets and it is resistant to vitamin D in ordinary doses. It appears to be causally related to a deficiency in the tubular reabsorption of phosphate. In a few cases renal glycosuria has also been reported but the other tubular functions seem to be unimpaired. The disease is usually transmitted by a dominant gene on the X chromosome; affected males have only affected daughters, whereas affected females have equal numbers of affected and healthy children irrespective of sex. The condition is, therefore, more common in girls, but because they have one normal X chromosome the severity of the disorder is less than in affected males. In a few cases an autosomal recessive pattern of inheritance has been reported.

Clinical, biochemical and radiological features

The child develops the classical features of rickets modified from the vitamin D deficient infantile variety only by the patient's age. These include enlargement of epiphyses, rachitic rosary, kyphoscoliosis and deformities of the limbs. Bilateral coxa vara frequently results in a characteristic waddling "penguin" gait. Short stature with disproportionate shortening of the lower limbs is the most important clinical manifestation. Urinary excretion of calcium is small whereas the output of phosphate is excessive. The phosphate reabsorption percentage is less than 85% in spite of low plasma phosphate and normal PTH values. The biochemical findings in the blood are the same as those usually found in infantile rickets, namely, a normal plasma calcium (2.2–2.9 mmol/l; 9–11.5 mg/100 ml), reduced plasma phosphate (less than 1.5 mmol/l; 4.5 mg/100 ml) and increased alkaline phosphatase. The plasma concentration of 25-OHD_3 is usually normal and that of $1,25(OH)_2D_3$ is slightly low or normal. Aminoaciduria which is commonly found in vitamin D related rickets is not a feature of hypophosphataemic rickets. Radiological features are those of uncomplicated rickets, e.g. cupped, frayed and broadened metaphyses, broadened epiphyses, osteoporosis, deformities and pathological fractures.

Differential diagnosis

The age of the child combined with a history of an adequate dietary intake of vitamin D are sufficient to exclude infantile rickets. Coeliac rickets must be excluded by tests of intestinal function and renal failure by tests of glomerular function. The de Toni–Fanconi syndrome is most readily excluded by urinary amino-acid chromatography.

Treatment

The most effective treatment appears to be a combination of 2–3 g of oral elemental phosphate per day with either oral 1,25(OH)$_2$D$_3$ (0.25–0.05 μg/kg/day) or 1α-OHD$_3$ (0.05–0.1 μg/kg/day). Initially, phosphate supplementation may cause diarrhoea but tolerance to the regimen usually develops within 1–2 weeks. Frequent estimations of plasma calcium are necessary to detect hypercalcaemia due to overdosage. Vitamin D therapy alone rarely corrects dwarfism and even if started in early infancy may fail to prevent its development. Patients with residual skeletal deformities may need surgical correction usually after growth has ceased.

The de Toni–Fanconi syndrome (cystinosis)

This syndrome nowadays embraces a group of biochemical disorders resulting from multiple renal tubular defects – glycosuria, aminoaciduria, tubular acidosis, phosphaturia, potassium loss and occasionally sodium loss and uricosuria. Cystine crystals are found throughout the reticulo-endothelial system but there is no gross excess of cystine in the urine as in cystinuria which is a quite separate inborn error of metabolism. The disease is inherited as an autosomal recessive trait.

Clinical features

The physical features usually appear in early infancy and resemble those of hyperchloraemic acidosis. Thus failure to thrive, anorexia, vomiting and severe constipation are constantly present. Thirst and polyuria may also have been noted by the mother. A feature characteristic of cystinosis is photophobia. This is due to the presence of cystine crystals in the cornea and it is not always present. Rickets makes its appearance after some months of illness. Its appearance in a wasted infant is in contrast to infantile rickets which is more commonly found in well grown infants (Fig. 8.13). Severe deformities can develop in some patients. Urine testing usually reveals glycosuria and proteinuria. During the course of a long illness life may be endangered at any time by severe attacks of dehydration and by sudden renal losses of potassium which lead to prostration, muscle weakness and typical electrocardiographic changes. In the later stages of the disease hepatomegaly may develop. Ultimately, glomerular failure with uraemia becomes superimposed. Radiological changes are typical of rickets.

Biochemical features

In additon to glycosuria and proteinuria, chromatography reveals a generalised excess of amino acids in the urine. The renal tubular origin of the aminoaciduria is reflected in normal blood amino-

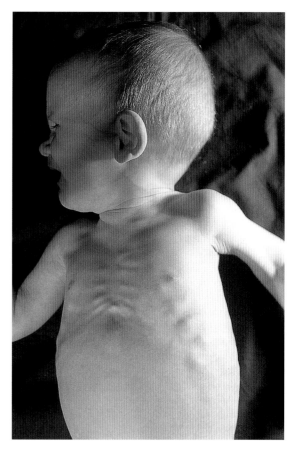

FIGURE 8.13 Rachitic rosary in 7-month-old infant suffering from de Toni–Fanconi syndrome; note generalised wasting.

acid levels. The characteristic changes in the blood are hypophosphataemia, normal serum calcium, increased alkaline phosphatase, decreased plasma bicarbonate and hypokalaemia. In the terminal stages of the disease the onset of glomerular failure may lead to a rise in plasma phosphate and fall in calcium.

Diagnosis

This is based initially on the presence of glycosuria and aminoaciduria. Cystinosis can be confirmed by the detection of cystine crystals in the cornea with a slit lamp, or by finding them in bone marrow or lymph node biopsy material. As cystine crystals are soluble in formalin, tissues to be examined for their presence should always be fixed in alcohol. White cell cystine levels are raised and this is being used increasingly in diagnosis and monitoring treatment. A more reliable and convenient method of confirming the diagnosis of cystinosis is by the demonstration of excess accumulation of cystine in cultured skin fibroblasts, thus it can be diagnosed antenatally.

Treatment

The rickets requires large doses of calciferol for healing (50 000–300 000 units daily). The dose of vitamin D can be kept to a minimum if oral sodium phosphate buffer is also given. Plasma calcium and phosphate values must be carefully monitored on this treatment and the calcium should not be permitted to rise above 3 mmol/l (12 mg/100 ml) Alternatively, 1α-OHD$_3$ (Rocaltrol) may be used in the dosage recommended in renal osteodystrophy. The metabolic acidosis can be corrected with oral sodium bicarbonate 1–3 mmol/kg daily. If hypokalaemia is present some of the sodium salt should be replaced by potassium citrate or potassium bicarbonate. The daily intake of potassium salt may need to be as great as 5 g. The prognosis is poor in spite of the considerable temporary improvement which treatment may bring. Low cystine diets and treatment with dithiothreitol, ascorbic acid and D-pencillamine has not proved to be very efficient in facilitating the elimination of cystine from the body. However, cysteamine and phosphocysteamine have been shown to reduce intracellular cystine levels. Renal transplantation has been successful in children with cystinosis who develop end-stage renal disease.

Nephrogenic diabetes insipidus

This is a very rare condition which must be differentiated from pituitary diabetes insipidus due to failure of production by the posterior pituitary of antidiuretic hormone (ADH). In nephrogenic cases the renal tubules fail to respond to vasopressin and to reabsorb water normally. The condition has been transmitted as an X-linked trait in most of the reported families, only males being affected. The concentrating defect can be partial or complete.

Clinical features

Excessive thirst and polyuria start soon after birth. Failure to thrive, anorexia, constipation and vomiting are common. Infants frequently show hyperelectrolytaemia and azotaemia but these biochemical disturbances become less in those who survive infancy. Deprivation of fluids or a high environmental temperature leads to fever, prostration and hypernatraemic dehydration because these patients cannot produce urine of high specific gravity. This is a particular risk during infancy when the patient is unable to determine his/her own fluid intake. Some children with this disease show signs of organic brain damage which has been attributed to the hypernatraemia and dehydration which frequently exist during the period of infancy. Another clinical feature is that growth may also be retarded. Diagnosis can be confirmed by the failure to respond to vasopressin and by the marked inability to concentrate the urine during water deprivation.

Treatment

In infants it is important to offer water at frequent intervals to avoid the dangers of hyperelectrolytaemia and dehydration. A low sodium diet (sodium 1 mmol/kg/day) and low protein intake (2 g/kg/day) are also helpful. A curious paradox is the useful effect which chlorothiazide and more recent derivatives of this group of diuretics have in reducing urinary output in this disease. The mode of action is unknown but patients on these drugs must at the same time be guarded from the risks of potassium depletion. Also, urine output can be reduced by treating these children with prostaglandin synthetase inhibitors, e.g. indomethacin 2–5 mg/kg/day.

Renal tubular acidosis (RTA)

Two main mechanisms are recognised in renal tubular acidosis. In one mechanism, in the presence of systemic acidosis the kidney is unable to excrete sufficient hydrogen ions to lower the urinary pH below 6. This mechanism is responsible for the classical or distal RTA (type I). In this type giving an ammonium chloride load fails to depress urinary pH below 6.0 and the excretion rates of ammonium and titratable acid are reduced. In the other mechanism, operative in proximal renal tubular acidosis (type II) the proximal tubule is unable to conserve filtered bicarbonate adequately or in other words there is bicarbonate wastage. In this type II RTA the response to ammonium chloride loading test is normal. Type III is a mixture of distal and proximal RTA and type IV is associated with a deficiency of aldosterone production or resistence to its action (pseudohypoaldosteronism).

Distal renal tubular acidosis (type I RTA)

Primary distal renal tubular acidosis is usually sporadic but can be inherited as an autosomal dominant trait.

The classical disorder occurs more frequently in girls and usually presents after the age of 2 years with polyuria and polydipsia. Muscular weakness and flaccid paralysis may result from hypokalaemia. A crisis may be precipitated by vomiting and diarrhoea or by starvation. Often the initial manifestation of the disease is growth failure. Nephrocalcinosis and nephrolithiasis are found in more than two-thirds of the patients.

Laboratory findings consist of hyperchloraemic metabolic acidosis, failure of urinary pH to fall below 6 even in the presence of severe metabolic acidosis. Renal potassium loss is reflected in the persistent hypokalaemia.

Secondary distal renal tubular acidosis can occur in patients with vitamin D intoxication, obstructive uropathy, medullary sponge kidney, Marfan syndrome and after renal transplantation.

Treatment

Treatment is aimed at correcting the metabolic acidosis by using sodium bicarbonate 1–3 mmol/kg/day. Potassium supplementation may also be required to correct the hypokalaemia. Striking improvement in growth can be expected with this regimen.

Proximal renal tubular acidosis (type II RTA)

The primary form of proximal renal tubular acidosis is rare and it may be familial. It appears to be caused by an isolated defect in bicarbonate reabsorption. Most of the reported cases have occurred in boys and present with growth failure and vomiting. Secondary proximal renal tubular acidosis is found in patients with Fanconi syndrome, hyperparathyroidism and vitamin D deficiency rickets and after renal transplantation.

Haemolytic uraemic syndrome of infancy

This condition is much commoner in infants and children than in adults. Also this condition accounts for most children with primary acute renal failure requiring specialist renal care. It is characterised by the triad of microangiopathic haemolytic anaemia, thrombocytopenia and renal failure. The most common findings in the kidneys include thrombi in the glomerular tufts (in fatal cases the glomeruli may be necrotic) and cortical necrosis. The afferent arterioles show fibrinoid necrosis and intraluminal thrombi. In the adult, more commonly than in the child, similar arteriolar thrombi may be found in other organs such as brain and pancreas. The thrombocytopenia of this syndrome may be due to the consumption of platelets by the thrombi in the arterioles and the haemolytic anaemia may result from the destruction of red cells in the diseased small blood vessels – microangiopathic haemolytic anaemia. The aetiology remains obscure but the renal changes resemble those seen in the Shwartzman reaction produced in animals by the injection of bacterial endotoxin. The development of this disease in some infants soon after vaccination or injection of triple antigen may thus be significant. Possible significance may also lie in several reports of small outbreaks of the disease in a community. Haemolytic uraemic syndrome (HUS) has been reported in children with shigella dysentery in Bangladesh. Some authors have reported the association between haemolytic uraemic syndrome and enteric E. coli which produced cytotoxin active on Vero-cells called "verotoxin". While this suggests an association between verotoxin (VT) E. coli and the disease, in some cases it is probable that it is a heterogeneous condition of variable aetiology. It has also been described as occurring after viral infections including Coxsackie, ECHO, adeno and influenza viruses.

Clinical features

There appear to be two subtypes in infants and children, an epidemic form and a sporadic form. The epidemic form is more common in infants and younger children, and occurs more often in the summer months, has an explosive onset with abdominal pain, diarrhoea, vomiting, pallor and is frequently accompanied by convulsions. This group has a better prognosis than the sporadic form which occurs in older children, with a more gradual onset, sometimes with a respiratory rather than diarrhoeal onset. The later features are common to all cases to a variable degree. Oliguria is constantly present but not always appreciated. Hypertension may be severe. The blood shows a severe anaemia, thrombocytopenia, reticulocytosis and increased serum unconjugated bilirubin. Some of the red cells are characteristically misshapen (acanthocytes), a feature which should lead to the correct diagnosis. "Burr cells" have one or several sharp projections along their edges. "Triangular cells" and others with a "broken egg-shell" shape are also common. The blood urea is greatly elevated. The urine shows protein, red cells and granular casts.

It has been recognised that in many of these cases sequential studies of the circulating clotting factors will show evidence of a consumptive coagulopathy due to disseminated intravascular coagulation (DIC).

Treatment

As outlined below the mainstay of treatment for children with HUS is the management of acute renal failure (ARF).

Emergency therapy

Children who have evidence of severe volume depletion should have immediate expansion of circulating volume by giving 20–30 ml/kg body weight of isotonic saline intravenously over 20–60 minutes. During this time blood pressure, heart rate, respiratory status and continuous monitoring of central venous pressure is useful. A low central venous pressure would indicate that more fluid is needed.

Maintenance of fluid therapy

In order to control fluid balance properly the output of urine must be measured and recorded acurately and allowance for insensible losses from skin and lungs must be made. A useful check on the accuracy of fluid balance is weighing the patient daily. The amount of fluid the patient requires should not exceed urinary output plus calculated insensible loss of the previous 24 hours. The insensible loss varies but may safely be set at 350 ml/m^2/24 hours or approximately 20 ml/kg/24 hours for infants, 15 ml/kg in children 3–7 years and 10 ml/kg for older children.

Use of mannitol and diuretics

Children who have their blood volume adequately repleted but continue to have oliguria should have frusemide in increasing doses of 1–5 mg/kg/body weight intravenously. If rapid diuresis does not occur, mannitol 0.5 g/kg (2.5 ml/kg of a 20% solution) over a period of 20 minutes can be given.

Hyperkalaemia is the most serious problem associated with renal failure and causes cardiac dysfunction which may lead to death of the patient. Depending upon rate of tissue breakdown, plasma potassium concentrations may increase rapidly. Hyperkalaemia may also be detected by serial ECGs. Levels about 8 mmol/l almost invariably cause a diminished heart rate with atrioventricular dissociation, widening of the QRS complex, and elevation of T wave and depression of the S-T segment. If ECG changes are present, or if serum potassium rises above 7 mmol/l then emergency treatment is indicated: 10% calcium gluconate 0.5 ml/kg by slow IV infusion over 2–4 minutes to reduce the toxic effect of high potassium on the heart. Infusion of 1 ml/kg solution of 50% glucose containing 1 unit of insulin/ml should then be given. In addition, calcium polystyrene sulphonate (Calcium Resonium) 1 g/kg can be given orally or rectally to expedite the elimination of potassium from the body.

Metabolic acidosis is a uniform and early accompaniment in this condition because of the important role of the kidneys in regulating and maintaining normal body homeostasis. When acidosis is present it should be treated with sodium bicarbonate. Severe metabolic acidosis in an anuric child may warrant dialysis.

Hypocalcaemia is quite common in acute renal failure but it rarely causes symptoms. If symptomatic then calcium can be given by slow intravenous infusion of 10% calcium gluconate 0.5 ml/kg.

Mild to moderate *anaemia* is often present in ARF.

TABLE 8.2 Antihypertensive drugs

Labetalol	1–4 mg/kg/h intravenously
Sodium nitroprusside	0.3–6 µg/min intravenously
Hydralazine	0.15–0.25 mg/kg/dose intravenously
Captopril	0.2–0.5 mg/kg/dose orally
Minoxidil	0.05–0.1 mg/kg/dose orally
Frusemide	1 mg/kg/dose orally or intravenously

Anaemia, when present to a significant degree, may potentiate the complications, especially cardiac failure, and may be beneficial to correct by small transfusions of recently collected packed red cells given slowly.

Severe symptomatic *hypertension* can occur in association with salt and water overload. Treatment of hypertension mainly consists of restriction of fluid and sodium intake and antihypertensive therapy as outlined in Table 8.2. It is vital that it is adequately controlled. Hydralazine or labetalol are the drugs of choice.

Infection is a most serious complication and every effort must be made to prevent it and to treat it if it develops. It can sometimes be secondary to the therapy, e.g. bladder catheterisation. Therefore invasive procedures should be restricted.

Adequate *nutritional intake* is vital for children with ARF. Daily calorie intake should be at least 400 calories/m^2 of body surface. If the patient is not on dialysis then he/she probably will have a protein restriction of 1–1.5 g protein/kg ideal weight. For children who are unable to take oral or enteral feeds, parenteral feeding may be required.

Peritoneal dialysis or *haemodialysis* is frequently indicated and may be life saving. Peritoneal dialysis remains the dialysis treatment of choice and can be more rapidly commenced than is usually possible with haemodialysis. However, although most patients can be managed by peritoneal dialysis, there are a few in whom protein catabolism is so great that uraemia cannot be controlled except by haemodialysis.

Prognosis

In children with haemolytic uraemic syndrome the complete recovery rate is now about 70%, but a small number die in the acute stage of the illness; some die without recovering renal function after weeks on dialysis and other children are left with hypertension and chronic renal failure. In children who develop end-stage renal disease successful renal transplantation has been reported.

The role of prostaglandin infusions and plasmapheresis in children with haemolytic uraemic syndrome need further evaluation and should be used only for children with a bad prognosis.

Hypertension in children

The incidence of hypertension in children is thought to be somewhere between 1 and 3%. In children most cases of hypertension are of secondary aetiology, while in adults most hypertension is idiopathic and secondary forms are uncommon. Also, in the younger hypertensive patient it is more likely that the hypertension is due to a correctable disorder. About 80–90% of cases of severe or sustained hypertension in children are due to some form of renal disease. Causes of hypertension in children are as outlined in Table 8.3. A diagnosis of essential hypertension can be made only after exclusion of all other known causes of hypertension.

As shown in Fig. 8.14 normal blood pressure readings vary according to the age of the child. The most reliable definition is a systolic or diastolic blood pressure above the 95th centile of the expected blood pressure for the child's age.

Clinical features

Children with quite severe hypertension may be asymptomatic and the hypertension is usually detected on routine physical examination. The most common symptoms are headache, nausea, vomiting, polyuria, polydipsia and abdominal pain. Needless to say, blood pressure measurement is essential in a child with headache, in spite of the fact that there is

TABLE 8.3 Causes of hypertension in children

Coarctation of aorta
Renovascular disease
   Renal artery stenosis
   Renal artery aneurysm
   Renal artery thrombosis or embolism
   Renal arterio-venous fistula
   Polyarteritis nodosa
Renal parenchymal disease
   Chronic glomerulonephritis
   Polycystic disease of kidneys
   Haemolytic uraemic syndrome
   Reflux nephropathy
   Obstructive uropathy
Renal tumours
Nephroblastoma
Neuroblastoma
Congenital adrenal hyperplasia
Conn and Cushing syndrome
Essential hypertension

a strong family history of migraine. Some children may present with convulsions, epistaxis, visual disturbances and facial palsy. Symptoms related to catecholamine excess, such as palpitations, sweating and weight loss, may suggest the presence of a phaeochromocytoma.

Physical examination should include careful inspection of optic fundi for evidence of hypertensive retinopathy. Other important findings that

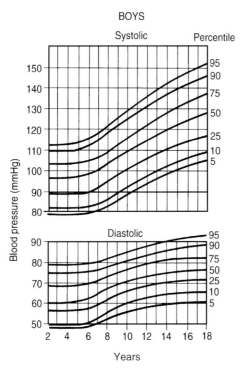
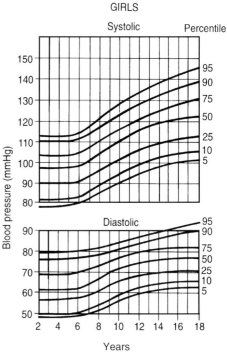

FIGURE 8.14 Normal blood pressure values in children.

suggest renovascular hypertension are cardiomegaly and the presence of an upper abdominal bruit. Physical examination should also include a neurological evaluation, palpation of the abdomen for mass lesions and inspection of skin for *café-au-lait* spots, neuromas and neurofibromas. Cushingoid features or evidence of virilisation suggest disturbances of adrenocortical function. Upper limb hypertension associated with delayed or absent femoral pulses suggests the diagnosis of coarctation of aorta.

Laboratory investigations

It is vital to remember that single high blood pressure values are not reliable. All children with persistent hypertension should have some evaluation but the question arises how intensive it should be. Laboratory investigations should include full blood count, blood urea, electrolytes, creatinine and calcium values, routine urinalysis, ECG, chest X-ray and echocardiography. Renal imaging such as ultrasonography, DMSA and DTPA renal scans and rapid sequence excretory urogram might then be required. Measurement of plasma renin activity, aldosterone concentrations, 24-hour urinary VMA and steroid analysis can confirm the presence of increased pressor activity. If indicated, CT scanning of abdomen and angiographic and digital subtraction vascular imaging should be carried out.

Treatment

Children with severe hypertension should be treated because of the high incidence of morbidity and mortality. Most children with hypertension will require advice regarding diet, exercise and life style.

In children with severe hypertension especially those with retinopathy, encephalopathy, seizures or pulmonary oedema immediate steps should be taken to lower the blood pressure. Drugs that can be used are described in Table 8.2. Labetalol is usually valuable in such a situation. Nitroprusside is indicated in patients who do not respond to labetalol and it allows smooth rapid lowering of blood pressure. Unresponsiveness to nitroprusside is rare. However, when prompt control of blood pressure is required hydralazine may be given by slow intravenous infusion. Any patient with hypertension who has evidence of plasma volume excess should receive diuretics in addition to other antihypertensive agents.

Captopril, the angiotensin converting enzyme inhibitor, is especially useful in patients with a high renin activity associated with renal parenchymal ischaemia as found in renal artery stenosis. Minoxidil is a potent oral vasodilator that may be valuable in severe hypertension, particularly when there is associated renal failure.

The aim of surgical treatment of renovascular disease in children is not only to control hypertension but also to preserve renal function. Over the past decade, because of the advances in microvascular techniques, it has been possible to revascularise renal arteries in most paediatric patients. However, total nephrectomy remains the treatment of choice for patients with complete renal artery occlusion, failed renovascularisation procedure, severe renal atrophy, significant unilateral renal parenchymal disease and other non-correctable renal lesions. Partial nephrectomy is indicated in patients with segmental renal hypoplasia and segmental renal infarction.

Surgical intervention is also indicated in children in whom hypertension is associated with coarctation of aorta, renal artery stenosis, renal tumours, tumours of the adrenal cortex and medulla and localised scarred kidney.

URETERS

Hydroureter

Dilatation of the ureter (hydroureter) is often secondary to obstruction at the ureterovesical junction and less commonly to more distal urinary tract obstruction at the bladder neck or in the urethra, e.g. urethral valves. There is frequent tortuosity of the ureter as well as dilatation. The hydroureter is usually found on investigation of a patient with urinary tract infection. Where there is ureterovesical obstruction this is usually due to a stenotic segment of the distal part of the ureter and this requires excision with reimplantation of the ureter in the bladder. Very dilated ureters should be tapered to reduce to a normal diameter prior to reimplanting the distal end into the bladder.

Vesico-ureteric reflux

Vesico-ureteric reflux is more common in infancy than in childhood. Minor degrees of vesico-ureteric reflux, usually found during investigation of the patient with urinary tract infection, are not of serious consequence. The patient with marked reflux and particularly those with intrarenal reflux are at risk of renal damage. It is probable that the majority who suffer renal damage have also had superimposed infection as well as reflux. The patient who has either gross reflux or who has "breakthrough" infections despite many courses of antibiotic therapy should have reimplantation of ureters in the bladder. This is performed by reinserting the ureter through the bladder muscle at about 4 cm distant and bringing the ureter along a submucosal tunnel to the old site in the bladder (Leadbetter Politano technique) or tunnelling the ureter across the trigone to the opposite side of the bladder (Cohen technique). Alternatively the STING procedure of submucosal injection of Teflon at the ureteric entrance to the bladder has replaced many reimplantation operations in preventing reflux.

Rarely with single ureters but occasionally with the upper pole ureter of a duplex kidney ectopic opening of the ureter into the distal urethra, perineum or vagina results in continuous dribbling incontinence. The diagnosis is suspected in the child who appears to micturate normally but in addition is continuously damp or wet. Investigation reveals the duplex system and the upper pole ureter may have little function and is seldom worth preserving. Hence the upper pole and ureter are excised.

Ureteric calculi

Ureteric calculi occur less commonly in childhood but if they lodge in the ureter then treatment is by performing cystoscopy and passing a dormier basket along the ureter and removing the stone or rarely by open operation.

BLADDER

Ectopia vesicae

This anomaly, obvious at birth, presents a frightening sight to the parents. It is discussed in more detail in Chapter 12.

Neurogenic bladder

A neurogenic bladder may present with incontinence and retention of urine or more rarely as continuous dribbling of urine with retention. The neurogenic bladder is commonly associated with congenital deformities of the spine, myelomeningocele (spina bifida), tethering of the cord, sacral agenesis, trauma, tumours, anorectal anomalies, vascular disorder and in some is idiopathic. In the more common partial sacral agenesis there is little external evidence of a spinal lesion but on X-ray sacral elements are found to be missing.

Clinical presentation

When secondary to spina bifida cystica or sacral agenesis dribbling incontinence is usually a feature

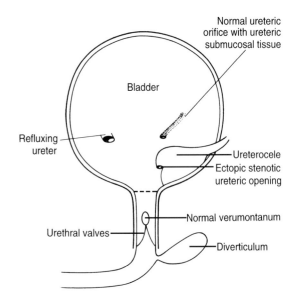

FIGURE 8.15 Pathology of bladder and urethra.

present from birth. Two types of presentation may occur. In the first, there is usually retention of urine with overflow incontinence. A large bladder is palpable and manual expression is possible but if reflux is present damage may occur to the upper renal tract. Urinary infection may occur with further deterioration in function and progressive damage to the renal parenchyma.

Secondary phenomena which develop in a neurogenic bladder include:

1 thickening of the bladder wall with muscular hypertrophy and fibrosis;
2 trabeculation of the bladder;
3 diverticulae formation; and
4 ureterovesical obstruction secondary to pressure on the intramural part of the ureters with an obstructive hydronephrosis.

Pathology of the bladder and urethra is shown in Fig. 8.15.

Treatment

Manual expression of the bladder may achieve complete emptying of the bladder and the child may then be dry for 2 or 3 hours at which time the bladder can then be expressed again. In neonates expression can be performed manually by the mother. Later the child may empty the bladder by abdominal straining and double or triple micturition to achieve complete emptying. Operation on the primary pathology will rarely improve bladder function and at times may make the urological situation worse.

Problems which can ensue are:

1 High pressure in bladder.
2 Stasis with residual urine.

Vesico-ureteric reflux.
Infection.
Incontinence.

he main purpose of treatment is to prevent:

Back pressure in the urinary system.
Stasis of urine which encourages infection.
Incontinence.

High pressure states are deleterious and spasm of
ie bladder neck which is often responsible for this,
eeds to be forcefully overcome by dilatation. Early
itermittent catheterisation to allow free drainage and
revent upper renal tract damage and the prevention
f infection by prophylactic antibiotics is desirable in
ie initial stages and may be continued.

In *low pressure states* there is a risk that the spastic
ladder will become thickened, reduce the bladder
ipacity and cause secondary upper renal tract
bstruction at the ureterovesical junction. Various
rpes of procedures may be carried out to augment
ie bladder with loops of bowel and to tighten the
ladder neck to achieve continence with intermittent
ean catheterisation. If this fails, then other opera-
ons are available to allow continence using a pouch
f bowel which acts as a reservoir and is intermit-
ntly catheterised. Finally, there are operations to
ivert the ureters into one end of an isolated loop of
eum or colon while the other end of the loop is
rought through the abdominal wall as a stoma. A
rinary collecting bag with a tap to allow intermit-
nt emptying is then applied over the stoma to
chieve a dry state.

Bladder diverticulae are out-pouches of the bladder
sually at an area which is congenitally weak and as
result of excessive intraluminal pressure. The poten-
al dangers of diverticulae are that they can enlarge
id grow with time. They can act as a reservoir of
rine with resulting stasis predisposing to infection
id eventually stone formation. In some neurogenic
ladders the bladder is loculated with multiple diver-
culae which may contain more urine than the
adder itself. Another more serious consequence is
iat they can interfere with the normal emptying and
rainage of urine. Para-ureteric diverticulae may be
ie cause of obstructive uropathy or cause ureteric
flux. Incomplete nephro-ureterectomies where the
ump at the lower end of the ureter has not been
xcised may also act as a diverticulum of the bladder
there is reflux into it. This may need to be excised
a separate operation if it is associated with
peated urinary tract infections.

ladder neck obstruction

he bladder responds by muscular hypertrophy and
abeculation and sooner or later bladder distension
ccurs. Back pressure affects the upper urinary tract,

the ureters become dilatated and tortuous and
hydronephrosis may develop. Some patients develop
incompetence of their uretovesical junction resulting
in vesico-ureteric reflux. The onset of renal failure
may be insidious. During fetal life the kidneys
produce urine from the fourth month and the affects
of back pressure may therefore be present even before
birth, the baby being born with distension of the
bladder, ureters and renal pelves. If the obstruction is
complete, oligohydramnios results with deleterious
effect on fetal lung development causing severe
postnatal respiratory problems which may be fatal.
There may also be intrauterine postural deformities
caused by the constrictive effect of the oligohydramnios.

Occasionally no urine may be passed by the
newborn infant in the first 24 hours but this need
cause no alarm if the bladder is not markedly
distended. The external genitalia should be carefully
examined to exclude hypospadias with meatal stenosis.

In the older infant or child acute retention is
usually due to minor causes such as meatal erosion.
If warm baths and sedation do not give relief,
catheterisation or suprapubic stab drainage will.
Chronic retention may also create sufficient pain or
distress to demand immediate drainage but usually
there is time for urological investigations and definitive treatment. Urethral valves, bladder-neck obstruction, and urethral strictures may all be dealt with by
a variety of surgical procedures including diathermy
of valves and dilatation or excision of bladder neck
and urethral dilatation.

URETHRA

Posterior urethral valves

Posterior urethral obstruction may be diagnosed *in
utero* when the dilated posterior urethra, dilated
bladder with hydroureter and hydronephrosis are
detected on ultrasound examination. Otherwise there
is often a delay in the diagnosis because of failure to
suspect the condition. This is especially so in infants
in nappies where dribbling and straining to pass urine
or a poor stream may easily be overlooked.

Clinical features

The infant has difficulty in voiding urine from the
earliest days of life and the act of micturition will
show diminution in the volume and the force of the
urinary stream. There may be only a gentle dribble
from the meatus. Palpation of the abdomen reveals a
distended bladder and this needs to be confirmed by
ultrasound examination. If the urinary tract becomes

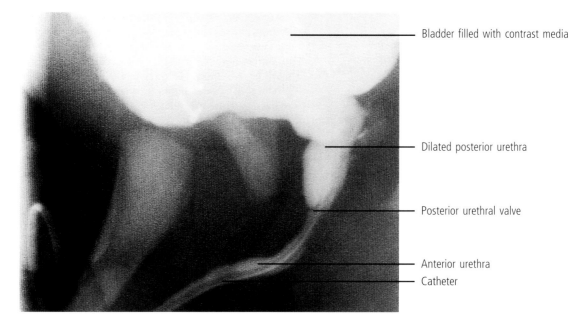

Bladder filled with contrast media

Dilated posterior urethra

Posterior urethral valve

Anterior urethra
Catheter

FIGURE 8.16 Posterior urethral valves. Micturating cystogram showing dilatation of the posterior urethra with the membranous and anterior urethra being of normal calibre. The valve is shown as a tiny anterior filling defect between the posterior and membranous urethra. This neonate also had gross bilateral reflux.

infected early, the infant may show signs of uraemia, vomiting and failure to thrive. The first abnormality to be noticed may be gross enlargement of the abdomen due to the large non-emptying bladder. The older boy may present with persistent wetting due to overflow incontinence.

Management

Full clinical assessment of the infant or child, examination of the urine and biochemical assessment of renal function are necessary. Ultrasound examination should include posterior urethra, bladder, ureters and kidneys. When posterior urethral obstruction is suspected, a small catheter is passed and the bladder partially decompressed. A cystourethrogram should be performed and films taken in the lateral position during micturition or bladder expression after the catheter removal (Fig. 8.16). If the kidneys are enlarged and tense, bilateral nephrostomies or ureterostomies may be preferable to cystostomy. When the child's general condition has improved the posterior urethral obstruction is usually corrected by diathermy of the valves viewed through an operating cystourethroscope. The long-term outlook for these children is generally poor when there is reflux because of severe renal impairment. Unlike many conditions, the earlier the age of diagnosis the worse is the prognosis as the more severe cases present earlier and the mild ones may not present for some years.

Urethral stricture

Uretheral stricture in paediatric practice is almost invariably secondary to previous catheterisation. It can occur after repeated catheterisation or even after a single catheterisation during an acute illness or major surgery. In these children, there has usually been a degree of hypoxia as well as the local trauma. Occasionally stricture may follow trauma or infection in peri-urethral glands. Diagnosis is made by urethrography or urethroscopy and treatment is by dilatation.

Urethral diverticulum

In this rare condition there is penile enlargement and a degree of obstruction to urinary flow. Excision and repair of the urethra are required. Penile anomalies are shown in Fig. 8.17.

Hypospadias

In this condition the urethral meatus does not open on the tip of the glans but opens more proximally on the ventral surface and the degree of hypospadias is defined as glandular, coronal, penile or perineal. In perineal hypospadias the labio-scrotal swellings fail to unite and in extreme cases the presence of a pseudo

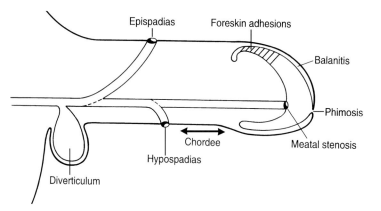

FIGURE 8.17 Diagram showing penile anomalies.

vagina (a persistent Mullerian remnant) may render sex determination difficult. The deformity is always distal to the urinary sphincters and there is rarely any defect in urinary continence.

The origin of this anomaly can be understood easily from the embryological development of the penis and the urethra. Clinical features noted on examination are:

1 The site and size of the urethral meatus may open on the glans (glandular hypospadias), on the coronal sulcus (coronal hypospadias), at any point along the shaft of the penis (penile hypospadias) or in the perineum (perineal hypospadias). The opening may be small and obstruct free discharge of urine, i.e. meatal stenosis.
2 The prepuce has a characteristic hooded appearance due to a ventral defect in the prepuce and a heaping up of skin on the dorsum.
3 Some degree of ventral curvature of the penis (chordee) is present in all but the most minor degrees of the deformity. Chordee is caused by the short urethra and fibrous tissue on the ventral surface distal to the meatus. A blind pit in the glans may be mistaken for the urethral orifice.
4 The median raphe always deviates to one or other side of the midline for some unexplained reason.

Three problems may present in infancy; inadequacy of the urethral orifice, deformity of the penis and in perineal hypospadias doubt about the sex of the child (Chapter 12). Some recommend that all infants with hypospadias should have ultrasound assessment of the urinary tract to exclude undetected anomalies but others restrict investigation to those with a severe form. The infant may not pass urine after birth and a pinhole meatus requires early enlargement by meatotomy. In minor degrees of the deformity the penis is straight and if the orifice is adequate no other treatment is required. In penile hypospadias, where chordee causes the urinary stream to be directed downwards, and in perineal hypospadias surgical correction should be completed before the child goes to school. The chordee is corrected and the penis is straightened before 18 months. The operative repair of the hypospadias is usually completed when the child is 3–4 years old but in some a single operation can be performed. The aim is to achieve a single stream of urine from the glans which will allow the boy to direct his micturition when standing. Although seldom detected and rarely of any functional importance, hypospadias can occur in the female but is rare, while in boys it is a common anomaly.

Epispadias

Epispadias, where the urethral meatus is on the dorsal aspect of the penis, is a rare anomaly often associated with poor bladder neck development. Surgical correction is necessary.

PENIS

The prepuce and circumcision

During the years when the child is incontinent, i.e. in nappies, the glans is protected by the prepuce. Deprived of this protection the glans is easily traumatised by clothes and nappies. Meatal ulceration is almost unknown in Jewish babies circumcised after the first week of life when the urea concentration in urine is very low. The exposed glans rapidly thickens its epithelium at that age and resists subsequent trauma. Therefore, it is advisable to perform circumcision within the first 10 days or to wait until the child is out of nappies. Ritual circumcision is practised in many countries and by one-sixth of the world population. In some instances the procedure is associated with various other forms of tribal markings produced by burning and incision and piercing of prominent skin folds, the lips and the ears.

Reasons given for circumcision include "to reduce sexual desire, to make a better warrior for a tribe, a more faithful husband, and a less frequent disturber of the society in which the native warrior lives". Apart from ritual tribal circumcision the procedure is common only in the English-speaking countries. In the antipodes it is routinely carried out for "social reasons". It is uncommon in continental Europe and in Scandinavia. The earliest Egyptian mummies were circumcised and the practice was introduced into the Roman Empire with Christianity. There is no trace of this operation in mediaeval Europe and apparently it was practised only by adherents of the Jewish faith until the rise of surgery in the nineteenth century when the status changed from a religious rite to a common profitable surgical procedure. The age at which circumcision is performed varies, in Jewish practice it is carried out at the eighth day while in many Africans at puberty.

Circumcision is one of the most common operations performed in this country and most are for ritual or religious reasons, not for medical need. At birth less than 5% of foreskins are retractable and it is only gradually over the next decade that the foreskin becomes freely retractable. In a little more than 50% the external meatus of the urethra or the glans can be displayed but the infant has adequate space to pass urine. This situation can be regarded with equanimity in the preschool child unless the smegma which forms and collects around the coronal sulcus becomes infected, causing acute balanitis with sometimes retention of urine. Treatment with baths, analgesics and antibiotics usually quickly settles the child. If a second attack of balanitis occurs it is more likely that recurrent infection may ensue and then after treatment of the infection, retraction of the foreskin and clearing out retained smegma is performed under anaesthesia. Circumcision may also be performed to guarantee freedom from recurrence.

Phimosis

Another medical indication for circumcision is phimosis. In this condition there is a tight prepuce which does not allow retraction of the foreskin and in severe cases obstructs urinary flow (Fig. 8.18). Forceful retraction of foreskin in early life may cause fissuring of the meatus of the foreskin with scarring and progression to phimosis. True phimosis is rare in early childhood and usually occurs in the 5–10 years of age group. The phimosis is associated with balanitis xerotica obliterans. If such a tight prepuce is retracted this may cause constriction, i.e. paraphimosis resulting in oedema of the glans and mucous membrane. If seen early a cold compress and gentle pressure reduces the swelling and the retracted prepuce can then be drawn forward. A general anaes-

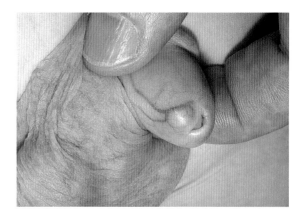

FIGURE 8.18 Phimosis.

thetic may have to be administered and a small dorsal slit performed. Definitive treatment is circumcision.

Meatal ulcer

This lesion is rarely seen in the uncircumcised infant and is best prevented by avoiding circumcision. It can also occur in the child circumcised after the neonatal period and sometimes following instrumentation of the urethra, e.g. intensive care patients who have been catheterised. Treatment is usually that of the associated ammoniacal dermatitis. Local applications of bland ointments may be necessary. If stenosis follows healing, repeated dilatation or rarely meatotomy become necessary.

Balanoposthitis

Inflammation of the glans under the surface of the prepuce may be due to retained smegma, poor

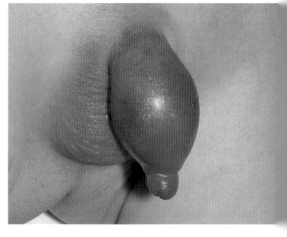

FIGURE 8.19 Balanoposthitis.

hygiene, or it may be associated with an ammoniacal dermatitis. There is redness, pain and swelling and a creamy-purulent discharge from under the prepuce (Fig. 8.19). The condition usually subsides with sitz baths and antibacterial treatment, e.g. Augmentin, but a dorsal slip may be necessary to allow free urinary drainage. Circumcision may be performed after the inflammation has subsided.

Adhesion of the foreskin

Foreskin adhesions to the glans are common and prevent full retraction of the foreskin. Normally most are gone by school age but persistence causes retention of smegma in the coronal sulcus which may cause irritation. If symptomatic, the foreskin is retracted under general anaesthesia and the smegma cleared. This procedure can be carried out in outpatients by the application of a lignocaine cream (Emla, Astra Pharmaceuticals Ltd) which takes an hour to diffuse into the foreskin and then retracting the foreskin gently. This procedure is concluded by the application of Vaseline to prevent the adhesions recurring.

Micropenis

Poor development of the penis sufficient to give rise to later problems is fortunately rare and may occur as an isolated entity or in association with hypoplastic testes. Milder degrees may be improved by application of testosterone cream during the first year of life but the more severe degrees fail to respond to any treatment. In such children, consideration must be given to the sexual identity in which the child is to be reared. It may be preferable to do a modified resection of the penis and create a female perineum. Gonadectomy has subsequently to be performed and the child can be reared as a girl with eventual hormone replacement. In adulthood normal sexual activity may be undertaken but she will be infertile. This is a serious consideration and a decision is only arrived at after consultation among a group of appropriate specialists and the parents. However, a "male" who is impotent may be at a greater handicap than a "female" with ability to have sexual activity although not have children.

Congenital absence of the anterior abdominal muscles (the prune-belly syndrome)

Agenesis of the anterior abdominal muscles is rare and almost invariably occurs in male infants. The muscles may be entirely absent or reduced to a thin fibrous sheath. The abdominal wall is lax, thin and

the outline coils of intestine and even grossly dilated ureters may be seen in the neonatal period. The skin is often wrinkled at birth and lies in redundant folds, hence the term prune-belly syndrome. When the gut distends with swallowed air the "prune" appearance disappears and is replaced with a distended abdomen. In patients with this anomaly there is variable dilatation of the urinary tract but this is not usually due to a high pressure situation. The dilatation usually extends down to the posterior urethra but typical valves are rarely found. Gross dilatation of the urinary tract may be present at birth and many infants with this anomaly die from renal failure in early life but long-term survival can occur. The third anomaly of this triad syndrome is undescended testes.

FEMALE GENITALIA

In the newborn baby girl the external genitals may be swollen, moist and congested, often with prominence of the labia and clitoris which may suggest pseudo-hermaphroditism. Small tags may be present around the inner surface of the labia. These never require surgical interference. There is often vaginal discharge which usually disappears by the seventh day. Occasionally, the vaginal discharge may be blood-stained probably from congestion of the endometrium. In the newborn baby girl the engorged uterus, which has enlarged with maternal hormone stimulation can be palpated on digital rectal examination. The uterus rapidly involutes over the next few weeks making it difficult to palpate thereafter in early childhood.

Adhesion of the labia

At birth the labia rarely may appear to be fused and the infant may not pass urine. In early infancy this is a relatively common and probably acquired condition and the infant's genitalia are otherwise normal. Adhesions are rarely dense and separation can usually be accomplished with finger pressure on a swab held laterally on the labia. Oozing of blood is negligible in this condition. Application of Vaseline at each change of nappies for 72 hours will usually prevent any readhesion. Many are not detected in early infancy and may present later in childhood. Separation of the labia can be achieved using Emla cream as a local anaesthetic or general anaesthesia before separation of the labia and Vaseline application (Fig. 8.20)

Vaginal obstruction

At birth the vagina may be completely occluded by an imperforate hymen or even by vaginal atresia.

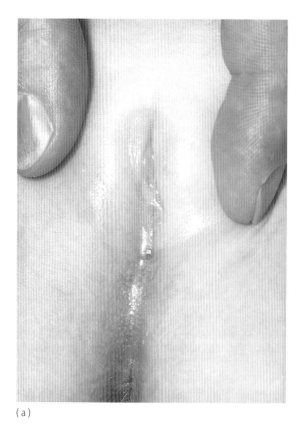

(a)

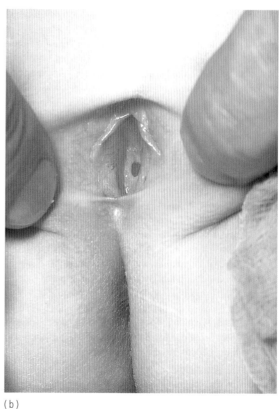

(b)

FIGURE 8.20 Labial adhesions before (a) and after (b) separation.

Maternal oestrogenic hormones may cause excess uterine or vaginal secretion and the vagina is greatly distended with accumulated fluid – hydrocolpos. Occasionally the cervical canal and uterine body may also be stretched – hydrometrocolpos. The cavity is filled with clear or mucoid fluid which tends to become purulent from bacterial invasion and may give rise to a pyocolpos. The ballooned genital tract arises from the pelvic floor into the abdominal cavity and a midline lower abdominal swelling may be present at birth. This mass may cause secondary urinary tract obstruction and bladder enlargement. A digital rectal examination can confirm this physical finding and ultrasound examination delineate it. Differential diagnosis is from an ovarian cyst or a tumour. If the condition is due to an imperforate hymen, gentle separation of the labia will reveal a bulging membrane at or above the hymen. The diagnosis is confirmed by inserting a needle through the membrane and aspirating the entrapped fluid. The hymen should be incised. If not diagnosed in infancy an imperforate hymen may present with a collection of haemorrhagic material within the vagina (haematocolpos) after puberty. There may be abdominal or pelvic pain but rarely nausea or vomiting. There is

tenderness on suprapubic pressure and rectal examination reveals a tender swelling of the vagina. Haematocolpos should be suspected in a girl with pubic hair and enlargement of the breasts who has not yet menstruated. As in the infant, incision of the bulging membrane gives immediate relief.

Vaginal discharge

Vaginitis may occur in young girls sometimes where personal hygiene has been poor either through laziness or lack of adequate toilet facilities. The discharge ceases quickly with local cleanliness and sitz baths two or three times a day. In some girls this discharge is related to deficient defence within the vaginal mucosa and infection occurs. Treatment with appropriate antibiotic may cure this once the presence of a foreign body has been excluded. Occasionally a short course of oestrogen may be necessary to "thicken" the vaginal mucosa. Purulent or haemorrhagic discharge is more often caused by a foreign body present in the vagina and in such cases the vagina should be examined with a speculum. Foreign bodies may be introduced deliberately in older girls although in younger girls fragments from woolly pants can enter during normal daily activities. These fragments may collect in the post-hymenal recess and may be difficult to see or may enter the vagina. They can be demonstrated by looking with a small nasal speculum or the small blade of a laryngoscope.

Very rarely a haemorrhagic discharge may be caused by a highly malignant rhabdomyosarcoma (sarcoma botryoides of the uterus or vagina). In this situation grape like masses may be extruded from the vagina. Vaginal sarcoma has a much better prognosis than the histologically similar tumour in the bladder and is usually cured by excision.

Genital warts may be seen in small children and often need to be treated surgically under a general anaesthetic. Although one's suspicions should be aroused by genital warts there must be other evidence before one can attribute these to child sexual abuse (Fig. 8.21).

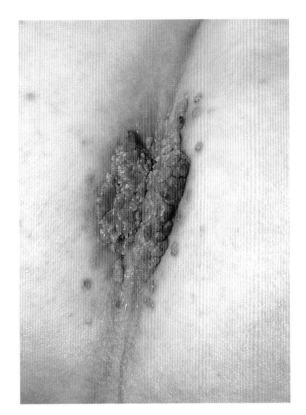

FIGURE 8.21 Genital warts.

MALE GENITALIA

Testes and epididymis

The testis develops from the genital ridge and in the embryo lies on the inner side of the mesonephros in front of the kidney in the lumbar region. Under hormonal control the testis descends through the abdominal wall to its position in the subsequently cooler scrotum in the eighth month of intrauterine life. Fibromuscular bands (the gubernaculum) attached to the lower pole of the testis pulls it through to the scrotal region. In its descent the testis is accompanied by the degenerating mesonephros and its Wolffian duct which form the epididymis and vas deferens. In front of the testis the peritoneum extends as a diverticulum – the processus vaginalis – passing through the muscle layers of the abdominal wall. The lower portion of this processus persists as the tunica vaginalis with the potential of containing a hydrocele or a hernia. The testis may, instead of passing into the scrotum, descend to an abnormal position. Testes found outside the normal path of descent are called ectopic testes. Normal spermatogenesis cannot occur in the human testis retained in the abdominal cavity. The cooler scrotal position for the testes is necessary for this. Variations in the position of the testes may be normal for an age group or may require treatment.

Retractile testes

In the young child the strong cremasteric reflex relative to the small prepubertal testes can pull the testes into the upper scrotum or inguinal region and may be difficult to palpate. This retraction is particularly marked if the child is examined in a cold room or with a cold hand. A gentle examination in the relaxed child enables retractile testes to be brought down into the scrotum and on release often they stay in position for a time. This condition is not pathological and the parents should be reassured that descent will eventually occur spontaneously as the child approaches puberty.

Undescended testes

The cause of defective descent of the testes is unknown although there is an increased incidence of malformation of the testes and epididymis in this group. The scrotum is small and atrophic because it has never contained a testis. The term cryptorchidism is applied to the hidden testis, e.g. the intra-abdominal testes, by some and others use the term for all testes not evident in their normal scrotal position.

Clinical features

Incompletely descended testes must be distinguished from retractile testes. An undescended testis cannot

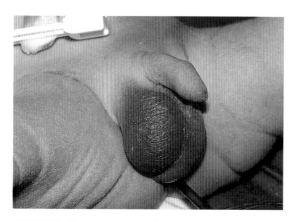
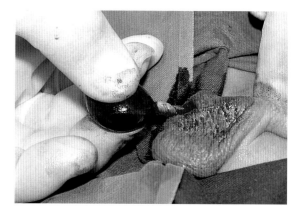

FIGURE 8.22 Neonatal torsion of spermatic cord with necrotic testes.

be palpated while it remains in the abdomen or inguinal canal. It may be milked out at the external inguinal ring but it cannot be brought down to the bottom of the scrotum. The scrotum on the affected side is usually small and atrophic. The condition is commonly right-sided and is bilateral in less than 25%. The diagnosis may be difficult in cases of early male obesity where there is excessive fat and tiny gonads. There is evidence that the testes should be in the scrotum by the second or third year of life in order to prevent further atrophy which would occur if they remained in the peritoneal cavity. Reasons for performing orchidopexy in this age group are:

1 To allow proper development of the testes.
2 Improve the cosmetic appearance.
3 Because of the slight risk of malignancy.

Treatment

There is much discussion of the advantages of early as opposed to late orchidopexy operation for undescended testes. However, the general view is that if there is an associated hernia then a herniotomy should be carried out and an orchidopexy done at the same time. It is desirable that the testes are brought down into the scrotum and a dartos pouch orchidopexy performed before school age. In our practice it is done between the ages of 2 and 5 years in children who have had the diagnosis established. It may not be possible to place a testis in the scrotum without tension on the spermatic vessels and vas and a two-stage operation may be necessary. If the testis is very small and hypoplastic it is essential that the parents are informed prior to the operation that it may be better to excise the remnant of testis. Abnormalities of the testes and vas and epididymis have been reported in 20% of children with undescended testes. Undescended testes are found as

part of a more general underlying condition in syndromes such as Klinefelter and prune-belly.

Ectopic testes

In this condition the testes lie outwith the normal line of descent into the scrotum and come to lie in some adjacent region. Undescended testes within the inguinal canal are difficult or impossible to palpate. A testis palpable over the inguinal canal, lateral to the external inguinal ring is usually ectopic. By firmly pressing the testis medially along the line of the inguinal canal the undescended testis will disappear into the abdomen while an inguinal ectopic testis will become more prominent. The ectopic testis cannot be manipulated into the scrotum. Less common sites of an ectopic testis are in the perineum at the root of the penis or the upper thigh. The testis and epididymis may be atrophic and sometimes completely separate. In some centres, laparoscopy is used to identify an impalpable testis.

Treatment

The only treatment for an ectopic testis is orchidopexy. Through an inguinal incision the testis is freed from its abnormal position and placed within the scrotum. The cord is usually long enough to allow placement without extensive dissection. Microvascular surgery is carried out in some instances where the vessels are extremely short. If a hernia is present a herniotomy is carried out at the same time.

Torsion

Torsion is usually of the spermatic cord but in the infant it may be of the testis within the tunica twisting on the epididymis. In the neonatal period the

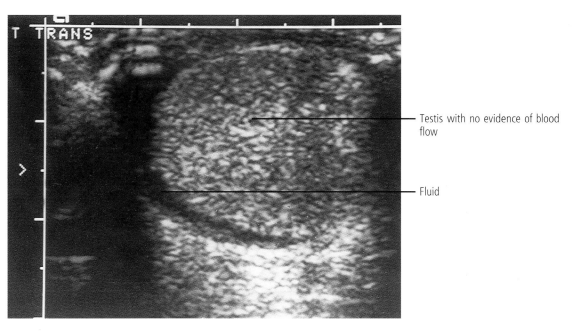

FIGURE 8.23 Testicular torsion. Ultrasound examination showing swelling of the testis with a small hydrocele. There was no blood flow in the testis on colour doppler ultrasound.

presentation is by a large tender mass in the scrotum (Fig. 8.22). Exploration usually shows an infarcted testis. In childhood torsion may occur in the fully descended organ due to a sharp blow or due to some sudden movement as in swimming. Doppler ultrasound examination is very useful to determine whether there is blood flowing into the organ. In a torsion there is no blood going to the testis. Differential diagnosis between torsion and epididymo-orchitis, where there is increased blood flow to the organ is usually clearly differentiated by colour doppler ultrasonic examination (Fig. 8.23).

Clinical features

There is sudden severe pain which may be in the lower abdomen, in the groin, or in the scrotum. Vomiting may occur. Examination reveals marked tenderness of the scrotum. The testis becomes swollen, hard, oedematous and is often in a high position. A hydrocele may develop in the tunica vaginalis. If mechanical relief is delayed, necrosis of the testis and epididymis supervenes and the scrotum becomes discoloured and oedematous with slow resolution and reabsorption of the infarcted testis over 2 or 3 months.

Differential diagnosis

This may be difficult and torsion may be confused with incarcerated hernia, acute epididymo-orchitis, idiopathic scrotal oedema or even torsion of an appendage of the testis, or the vas or epididymis and acute appendicitis. Ultrasound examination is useful in diagnosis and doppler study will show presence or otherwise of circulation to the testis.

Treatment

Treatment is immediate operation. Delay of a few hours may lead to irreparable infarction. At operation the cord is exposed and the testis is dislocated from the scrotum. Reduction of the torsion may permit a return of circulation if the injury is of short duration. In many cases necrosis has already occurred and the testis must be removed. When the testis is retained it is usually fixed to the scrotal musculature to prevent recurrence. It is also wise to fix the contralateral testis in a similar manner through a separate scrotal incision as there is increased risk of torsion of that testis.

Torsion of the appendix testis

The appendix testis or hydatid of Morgagni on the superior aspect of the testis occasionally undergoes torsion on its pedicle. The resulting signs and symptoms are similar to those of torsion of the testes. The condition occurs most commonly between the ages of 5 and 15 years. Rarely there is an appendix of the epididymis or even of the vas which undergoes torsion. The pain is less severe than with testicular torsion and in a co-operative child the testes will be

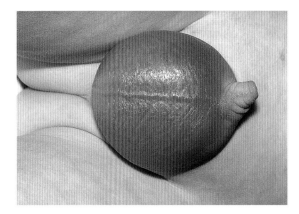

FIGURE 8.24 Idiopathic oedema of the scrotum.

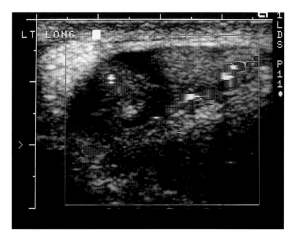

FIGURE 8.25 Doppler ultrasound of epididymitis.

felt and be non-tender with the very tender area at the top of the testis. Ultrasound can confirm this diagnosis. At operation the appendix often looks necrotic and blackened and haemorrhagic when it is exposed and it is excised.

Idiopathic scrotal oedema

This condition is not uncommon and is usually unilateral. The aetiology is obscure but may be caused by allergic phenomena. The scrotum on the affected side is red, swollen and indurated and the redness extends into the groin and into the perineal region (Fig. 8.24). The testis can usually be palpated and is no more tender than the surrounding structures. This condition usually subsides spontaneously within 2–3 days almost as quickly as it appears.

Diseases of the testes and epididymis

Infection of the testes or epididymis is uncommon before puberty and orchitis associated with mumps is rare before the age of 12 years. Orchitis may appear during the course of systemic bacterial infections. Swelling and oedema after torsion or trauma may closely simulate orchitis but with such trauma the onset is sudden. Epididymo-orchitis (Fig. 8.25) is more likely to occur in boys who have an abnormal communication between vas and ureter. An ectopic ureter of a single or duplex kidney may fuse with the vas before entering the bladder or urethra.

Treatment

Having excluded torsion of the testis, treatment consists of bed rest, elevation of the scrotum and antibiotic treatment of any associated systemic infection.

Tumours are discussed in Chapter 19.

9

Diseases of the
Nervous System

Many of the diseases with obvious neurological signs remain somewhat of a mystery from the aetiological point of view. The necropsy findings are not always helpful in determining the primary disturbance, which may have occurred months or years previously. Not surprisingly the treatment of such conditions is usually unsatisfactory. On the other hand, some diseases of infective origin can now be cured provided diagnosis and treatment are established early, and these merit more detailed consideration. One of the most dramatic changes in medicine in the past 40 years has been the ability to cure diseases which used to strike terror into the hearts of parents (e.g. pyogenic and tuberculous meningitis) because of their frightful mortality rates. None the less, deaths and permanent brain damage still occur too frequently due to unnecessary delays in diagnosis or to inadequate treatment. Some of the common diseases of the past, such as otogenic brain abscess, are now rarely encountered in children because of the efficient antibiotic treatment of otitis media.

ACUTE INFECTIONS OF THE NERVOUS SYSTEM

Acute meningitis

The common types of meningitis are pyogenic and aseptic with tuberculous now rare in Britain. Rare forms (not further considered here) are mycotic torulosis, nocardiosis, histoplasmosis), syphilitic and protozoal (malaria and toxoplasmosis).

Bacterial meningitis

Aetiology

Almost every bacterium is capable of infecting the meninges but only a few are common causes of bacterial meningitis. Excluding the neonatal period (Chapter 1) the most common is the meningococcus (*Neisseria meningitidis*). In infants and children a sporadic incidence is usual, but epidemics can occur. The disease is seen most commonly in the late winter and early spring. *Haemophilus influenzae* type b is responsible for almost 80% of cases of meningitis in children from 2 months to 4 years of age. The frequency is expected to change dramatically as a result of the recent availability of highly immunogenic conjugated *H. influenzae* vaccines. The common remaining meningeal infection is due to the pneumococcus (*Streptococcus pneumoniae*); this may be secondary to pneumonia or upper respiratory infection but "primary" meningeal infections are not uncommon. In infants both staphylococcal and streptococcal meningitis are occasionally seen, most often secondary to infection elsewhere, e.g. bone, umbilicus, skin or middle ear. A meningomyelocele may also act as a portal of entry, as may a compound fracture of the skull. Infections of the meninges due to *E. coli*, group B streptococci and to *Listeria monocytogenes* are peculiar to the neonatal period.

In immunosuppressed children and in patients undergoing neurosurgical procedures, including ventriculo-peritoneal shunts, meningitis can be caused by a variety of bacteria such as *Staphylococcus*, *Enterococcus* and *Pseudomonas aeruginosa*.

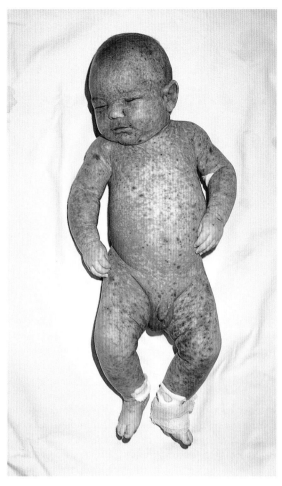

FIGURE 9.1 The typical purpuric and ecchymotic rash of meningococcal septicaemia. Some of the lesions may become necrotic with the formation of slowly healing ulcers.

Clinical features

Symptomatology is common to all types of bacterial meningitis and the causal organism is most often determined by examination of the cerebrospinal fluid. There are a few characteristic signs peculiar to meningococcal infections. The important one from the diagnostic point of view is a generalised purpuric rash although this is seen only in a minority of cases (Fig. 9.1). It is rarely seen in other types of meningitis and may occur in fulminating cases of meningococcal septicaemia without meningitis. It is also characteristic of meningococcal meningitis to develop suddenly and unheralded, whereas there is usually a preceding history of respiratory infection in cases due to the haemophilus or pneumococcus.

The onset of bacterial meningitis is usually sudden with high fever, irritability, headache in older children, vomiting and general malaise. Convulsions are common. Young infants show a tense bulging anterior fontanelle, indicative of increased intracranial pressure, and head retraction is common. The older the child the more likely is there to be nuchal rigidity, but its absence in the baby by no means excludes the diagnosis. The Kernig sign is useful in older children and rarely observed in infants. We have found no value in the Brudzinski sign. Blurring of consciousness of varying degree is the rule and increases in severity as the disease progresses. Focal neurological abnormalities such as paralytic squints, facial palsy or hemiplegia sometimes develop. Extreme restlessness, photophobia and mental confusion are more common in older children and partly caused by the intense headache. Deafness due to damage to the auditory nerve is greatly to be feared because it is usually permanent. Papilloedema is infrequently found.

In infants the disease sometimes has a more insidious onset, especially in meningococcal cases, with diarrhoea and vomiting, irritability and "bogginess" of the anterior fontanelle. The diagnosis is easily missed, sometimes with grave consequences. The state of the anterior fontanelle is the vital clue to most cases in which other characteristic signs are absent.

Diagnosis

Lumbar puncture is usually indicated whenever the possibility of meningitis has crossed the physician's mind and normally treatment should not be started before CSF has been obtained. However, it is reasonable to give intramuscular benzylpenicillin 250 000 units before transfer to hospital for lumbar puncture in a child suspected to have meningococcal meningitis by virtue of the characteristic purpuric or petechial rash seen in meningococcal infection. In pyogenic cases the cerebrospinal fluid will be turbid or frankly purulent. The cell count varies from 1000 to 10 000/mm³. The vast majority of cells are polymorphonuclears. Films of the centifuged deposit may reveal Gram-negative intra- and extracellular diplococci in meningococcal cases, Gram-positive diplococci, often very numerous, in pneumococcal cases, and Gram-negative pleiomorphic coccobacilli in cases due to haemophilus. Rapid identification of bacterial antigen in CSF can be obtained by use of countercurrent immunoelectrophoresis or the more sensitive latex agglutination test. These tests can be helpful in rapidly establishing a diagnosis. The final cause is determined by culture. The protein content of the fluid is raised (above 0.4 g/l; 40 mg/100 ml) and the sugar is greatly reduced (below 2.5 mmol/l; 45 mg/100 ml).

Complications and sequelae

In the acute stage hydrocephalus may first develop and thereafter progress or become arrested

TABLE 9.1 Antibiotic therapy in children with bacterial meningitis

AGE GROUP	DRUG (IV)	DOSE PER DAY
Infants 1–3 months	Ampicillin and	200 mg/kg/day in 4 doses
	cefotaxime	200 mg/kg/day in 4 doses
Older infants and children	1 Cefotaxime or	200 mg/kg/day in 4 doses
	ceftriaxone	100 mg/kg/day in single dose
	2 Ampicillin and	200 mg/kg/day in 4 doses
	chloramphenicol	75–100 mg/kg/day in 4 doses
	3 Benzylpenicillin	250 000 units/kg/day in 4 doses

Permanent brain damage with motor and learning deficits are more common in infants, in part due to the greater difficulties and delay in diagnosis. Symptomatic epilepsy is less common. It may be assumed, however, that after the period of early infancy the persistence of a neurological deficit reflects either a delayed diagnosis or inadequate treatment. The possible exception to this is nerve deafness which can develop early in the illness and unpredictably.

Treatment

Bacterial meningitis ought rarely to be fatal today. Management of bacterial meningitis encompasses many aspects of treatment including antibiotics, correction of fluid and electrolyte imbalance, anticonvulsant medications and possibly dexamethasone therapy.

The major factor in selecting antibiotic therapy for children with bacterial meningitis is the continually changing pattern of antibiotic resistance. Therefore knowledge of local susceptibility patterns is essential. Antibiotic therapy should eventually be aimed against the specific organism causing the meningitis but initial therapy is directed against all usual bacterial pathogens for the age group of the patient.

Recently it has been recommended that children with bacterial meningitis can be effectively treated with third generation cephalosporins alone, or in combination with ampicillin. The recommended antibiotics schedule for initial treatment of bacterial meningitis in different age groups is as shown in Table 9.1.

For infants between the ages of 1 and 3 months a combination of ampicillin and cefotaxime is a prudent choice as this combination would provide cover for age-specific pathogens prior to confirmatory information from culture and susceptibility tests.

For older children a third generation cephalosporin (cefotaxime or ceftriaxone) in preference to the combination of penicillin or ampicillin and chloramphenicol is advisable. Once the organism has been isolated and the antibiotic susceptibility data are available the antibiotic regimen should be modified accordingly. Therefore, intravenous penicillin can be substituted for treating sensitive meningococcal and pneumococcal infections. In those cases of bacterial meningitis where the causative organism cannot be definitely isolated, we suggest that a third generation cepholosporin should be continued. We currently recommend 7 days of treatment for N. meningitis and 10 days for H. influenzae and S. pneumoniae meningitis.

The routine use of dexamethasone for the management of bacterial meningitis is problematical. Recently it has been demonstrated that dexamethasone used as an adjunctive therapeutic agent in dosage of 0.6 mg/kg/day in four doses for 4 days is responsible for a significantly lower incidence of neurological sequelae including hearing impairment.

When treatment is adequate a prompt improvement can usually be expected with subsidence of fever within 48–96 hours. If fever persists with continuing irritability and bulging of the fontanelle the presence of a subdural collection of fluid should be suspected. This is most commonly encountered in cases due to haemophilus. Cranial ultrasound examination should be carried out before tapping the subdural space. Subdural taps should be done through the coronal suture on both sides. Evacuation of fluid may be required on several occasions before the accumulation of the xanthochromic protein-rich fluid stops. A lumbar puncture at the completion of therapy of uncomplicated cases does not provide useful information to determine which patient will develop bacteriological relapse. The child with meningitis requires a high standard of professional nursing and cannot be treated at home or in small, ill-equipped hospitals. Anaemia may have to be corrected by blood transfusions. Convulsions are best controlled with intravenous diazepam, 2–10 mg.

The Waterhouse–Friderichsen syndrome

Acute bilateral adrenal haemorrhage is most commonly seen in fulminating cases of meningococcal septicaemia. Death occurs usually before the meningitis has had time to develop, and may, in fact, take place after an illness of only a few hours' duration. The characteristic clinical picture is seen in an infant who suddenly becomes ill with irritability, vomiting and diarrhoea and tachypnoea or Cheyne–Stokes breathing. The heart rate is very rapid. The infant becomes rapidly drowsy/unconscious. Peripheral cyanosis is associated frequently with a patchy purple mottling of the skin which resembles post-mortem lividity. The child may die at this stage, about 6–8 hours from the onset of the illness. In less fulminating cases a diffuse purpuric and ecchymotic eruption appears which is very characteristic of meningococcal septicaemia. The blood pressure may be so low as to be unrecordable. In the toddler the course of the illness tends on the whole to be less rapid than in the infant. The meningococcus is not always successfully isolated in blood cultures but can sometimes be cultured from the fluid contents of purpuric blebs on the skin. Indeed, we have seen Gram-negative intracellular diplococci in ordinary blood films in a few cases, so overwhelming is the septicaemia. Disseminated intravascular coagulation may also develop in fulminating cases of meningococcal septicaemia and should always be sought by appropriate laboratory tests. Full blood count with platelet count, blood film for fragmentation of red cells, clotting screen including fibrinogen levels, FDPs or D dimers.

Treatment

In cases where the adrenal cortex has been destroyed by haemorrhage, recovery is impossible. In some cases of fulminating meningococcal septicaemia, however, there is intense congestion of the adrenal glands without much haemorrhage. It is in these cases, which are clinically indistinguishable from the fully developed Waterhouse–Friderichsen syndrome, that energetic treatment can save life and lead to complete recovery. A continuous intravenous infusion of 5% dextrose in 0.18% saline should be commenced. Penicillin should be given by direct injection into the infusion as described above. Hydrocortisone hemisuccinate 100 mg should be injected intravenously via the infusion at the start of treatment, to be followed by 50 mg 6-hourly for 24–48 hours; thereafter decreasing doses of prednisone are given orally for another few days.

Tuberculous meningitis

This dreaded complication of primary tuberculosis tends to have an insidious type of onset, with lethargy, fractiousness, anorexia, headache and vomiting. None the less, the mother can usually state the precise day on which the child became ill, and once begun the clinical picture unfolds inexorably and without remission. Rarely, the disease is heralded by a convulsion. A constant feature is constipation.

In the earliest stage of the disease, when correct diagnosis is vitally important, the child's consciousness is unimpaired and neurological signs are absent or minimal. Slight nuchal rigidity, or a full "boggy" fontanelle in an infant, are obviously most significant findings, but their absence in no way excludes the diagnosis. An unusual degree of drowsiness or lethargy should always awaken the suspicion of the alert physician.

If this early stage of the disease is missed, when treatment is most successful, the intermediate stage inevitably ensues. By now there is obvious blurring of consciousness, nuchal rigidity is present, the Kernig sign may be positive and focal neurological signs such as ophthalmoplegia, facial paralysis, hemiparesis and papilloedema ultimately appear. A useful indication of increased intracranial pressure in the child whose fontanelle has not long closed is the "cracked pot sound" obtained when the skull is held in the left hand and percussed by the middle finger of the right. It is due to separation of the sutures. At this stage the patient often lies curled up on his side with his face averted from the light and he resents interference. Choroidal tubercles usually indicate an associated miliary tuberculosis, but their presence is of such diagnostic value that careful ophthalmoscopy is an essential part of the examination of every excessively drowsy child. Most cases in the intermediate state show a good response to treatment, although permanent neurological sequelae sometimes remain.

In the later or terminal stage of the disease, treatment frequently fails to save the child's life, and the incidence of permanent brain damage such as hydrocephalus, blindness, deafness and learning impairment is high. By now the child is comatose. There may be severe head retraction and opisthotonus or decerebrate rigidity. Paralytic squints, unequal or fixed pupils and other neurological signs are obvious. Disturbed vasomotor control is frequently reflected in a characteristic hectic flush on one side of the face, like the paint on the cheek of a toy soldier, and the palms of the hands show a characteristic pink colour. Severe tissue wasting is a further distressing feature of the disease. Convulsions are common. There may be terminal hyperpyrexia, although earlier in the disease there is only a moderate rise in temperature.

Diagnosis

The cerebrospinal fluid total protein content is usually raised above 0.4 g/l (40 mg/100 ml). A low sugar content (below 2.5 mmol/l; 45 mg/100 ml) is very characteristic, but not invariable in the early stage of the disease. The cell count is raised to between 50 and 800/mm^3 and films show a marked preponderance of lymphocytes. The final proof is the isolation of tubercle bacilli. This entails a diligent search in Ziehl–Neelsen films of the spider-web clot which forms in the cerebrospinal fluid when it is allowed to stand overnight, or of the centrifuged deposit. Some of the fluid should also be cultured and inoculated into a guinea-pig. Identification of specific DNA sequences of *Mycobacterium tuberculosis* after polymerase chain reaction (PCR) amplification in the CSF is possible but there are risks of contamination and false positive results. Other evidence of tuberculosis must also be sought. The Mantoux test is usually positive when 1/1000 dilution of Old Tuberculin (OT) is used. Radiographs of the chest may also give valuable supporting evidence. Serial cranial CT scans should be performed on all patients to detect cerebral oedema and the presence or development of hydrocephalus. The efficacy of modern treatment in early cases places a heavy responsibility upon the physician; it is, of course, essential that prolonged drug treatment is not used in cases where the meningitis is non-tuberculous in aetiology.

Differential diagnosis

Tuberculosis meningitis is most likely to be mistaken for aseptic meningitis due to viruses such as those of the poliomyelitis, Coxsackie and ECHO groups. In these cases the onset is usually much more acute than in tuberculous cases, with brisk fever and obvious early rigidity of the neck and spine. The cerebrospinal fluid shows a lymphocytic pleiocytosis in both types, but in viral cases there is no fall in sugar content, the protein content is less markedly raised and a spider-web clot rarely, if ever, forms. There will be no other indications of tuberculosis in viral cases. Human immunodeficiency viral (HIV) infection predisposes children to tuberculous infections including TB meningitis. A rare cause of lymphocytic meningitis is infection by *Leptospira canicola* (from dogs) or *Leptospira icterohaemorrhagiae* (from rats). In those cases proteinuria, conjunctival suffusion and sometimes jaundice should indicate the diagnosis. There is also a polymorphonuclear leucocytosis in leptospirosis. In older children tuberculous meningitis can simulate brain tumour, but the cerebrospinal fluid will reveal the true state of affairs.

Treatment

In tuberculous meningitis the results depend upon the stage at which treatment is started. In Britain today most physicians would elect to treat their patients with some combination of the newer antituberculous drugs, although the mortality rates seem not to be appreciably different from results reported with "classic chemotherapy" (streptomycin, isoniazid, PAS). Even now there is no unanimity of view about the best combination of drugs, the optimal duration of treatment, or the need for intrathecal treatment. However, it would be generally agreed that the treatment of tuberculous meningitis demands the use of a three-drug combination. A suggested regimen is isoniazid (10 mg/kg) and rifampicin (15–20 mg/kg) which are given daily for 9 months, with the addition of pyrazinamide (35 mg/kg/day) for the first 2 months of treatment. Pyrazinamide has a useful role because, like isoniazid, it diffuses readily into the cerebrospinal fluid. For the child who is too ill for oral therapy there is now an intravenous preparation of rifampicin and isoniazid but pyrazinamide is not available for parenteral use.

Rifampicin may cause gastric upset, red coloured urine and a rise in liver transaminases but these side effects are rarely severe. Very rarely the development of thrombocytopenia necessitates withdrawal of the drug. Side effects with isoniazid are rare. They include convulsions in young infants and peripheral neuropathy in older patients. They should be prevented by giving pyridoxine 50 mg daily by mouth.

The authors remain unconvinced of the need for intrathecal treatment which is very stressful for the child. The use of corticosteroids to prevent formation of adhesions and hydrocephalus is of questionable value, but parenteral dexamethasone may be effective in reducing cerebral oedema. In the first week dexamethasone 0.6 mg/kg/day in four divided doses is given, followed by prednisolone (1–2 mg/kg/day) for 2–4 weeks and gradually tailed off.

Aseptic meningitis (including acute poliomyelitis)

This disease presents a perennial problem. Sporadic cases occur throughout the year with annual outbreaks in summer and autumn. From time to time, sizeable epidemics occur. Poliomyelitis is included under this heading because its precise diagnosis requires expert virological investigations, and other viruses can cause a clinically identical illness with meningitis and paralysis. However, poliomyelitis has become a rarity in the UK following the widespread use of live oral polio vaccine.

Aetiology

Many viruses can cause aseptic meningitis. These include poliomyelitis virus (types 1, 2 and 3), Coxsackie virus, ECHO virus, the mouse virus of lymphocytic choriomeningitis, arboviruses such as that of louping-ill, and the viruses of mumps, herpes simplex, herpes zoster, measles, varicella, infective hepatitis and glandular fever. Mumps virus frequently causes meningitis without any of the other manifestations of this disease. Coxsackie virus can cause meningitis and paralysis which is indistinguishable clinically from classical poliomyelitis and this can occur, of course, in persons who have been immunised against polio virus types 1–3. Non-viral agents which can cause aseptic meningitis include *Leptospira (icterohaemorrhagiae* and *canicola), Treponema pallidum, Toxoplasma gondii* and *Trichinella spiralis.*

Clinical features

The onset is usually sudden with headache, muscle pain, anorexia, vomiting, malaise and diarrhoea or constipation. Fever is frequently above 40°C. In some cases, especially of poliomyelitis, there is a preceding illness about 1 week earlier with fever, headache, malaise, sore throat and abdominal pain. The temperature chart in such cases shows two "humps", sometimes called "the dromedary chart". The child may be drowsy, apathetic and irritable when disturbed, but blurring of consciousness is uncommon. Slight nuchal rigidity is usually found. Spinal stiffness is common, especially in poliomyelitis. This may result in the child being unable to kiss his knees when sitting up. Furthermore, he may have to support himself when sitting by placing his hands on the bed behind him, "the tripod sign". The Kernig sign is commonly present. In the infant the anterior fontanelle may be tense and full. In the older child a transient urinary incontinence is sometimes noted. Papilloedema is uncommon.

Lower motor neurone paralysis with loss of power, flaccidity and diminution or loss of deep reflexes may affect any of the voluntary muscle groups, being followed by a variable degree of recovery, or by muscle atrophy and ultimate shortening of the affected extremity. Deformities such as pes cavus, talipes or scoliosis may later become a problem of management. Life is endangered in cases of bulbar paralysis with inability to swallow and obstruction of the airway, and when the muscles of respiration are involved. When encephalitis is also present there may be serious disturbances of cerebration and focal signs such as spasticity, ataxia, intention tremor and sensory disturbances. Paralysis is only likely to develop in cases due to the poliomyelitis or Coxsackie viruses.

Diagnosis

The cerebrospinal fluid is clear or only slightly hazy. The cell count varies from 50 to 5000/mm³ and the predominant cell is the lymphocyte. The total protein content is normal (0.2–0.4 g/l; 20–40 mg/100 ml) in the early stages although increased globulin is revealed by a positive Pandy test. Subsequently there is often a rise in total protein to 2–3 g/l (200–300 mg/100 ml) while the cell count falls, a dissociation between protein and cells which is particularly frequent in poliomyelitis. The sugar and chloride levels are normal and cultures remain sterile. The virus can be identified in the stools. Identification of the viral DNA after PCR amplification in CSF is now possible but there are risks of false positives. The serum (at least two specimens taken with a 10-day interval) may be tested for neutralising antibody or complement fixation in rising titre.

Treatment

In non-paralytic cases, the great majority, spontaneous recovery rapidly follows the diagnostic lumbar puncture. Symptomatic measures to relieve fever, headache or muscle pain are required but there is no specific treatment. The child should be isolated from other patients. A careful watch for paralysis must be maintained.

When there is paralysis the first requirement is to prevent stretching of the muscles by keeping the limb in a neutral position with suitable splinting and padding. Passive movements under expert physiotherapists are helpful, followed soon by carefully graded active movements. In the case with severe muscle spasm, warm compresses and hot packs bring relief. The orthopaedist should be brought into the management at an early stage. When there is bulbar palsy the patient is best placed in the prone position with head lower than feet. Pharyngeal suction should be performed at frequent intervals. In the worst cases tracheostomy followed by intermittent positive-pressure respiration is required. In such cases a broad spectrum antibiotic is also necessary to combat the risks of secondary bacterial infection in the poorly ventilated lungs. The prognosis in bulbar and respiratory cases has been enormously improved in recent years.

Acute encephalitis

The term "encephalitis" is often used to include organic disturbances of the brain which are poorly understood, in addition to its correct use in describing infections affecting the brain substance. The term "encephalopathy" will remain useful until further knowledge is acquired as to the varied noxious influences which can damage the nervous system.

Aetiology

All of the viruses mentioned in connection with aseptic meningitis can cause acute encephalitis. Others include influenza virus, cytomegalic inclusion disease in infancy, and the viruses of rabies, HIV, encephalitis lethargica and the zymotic diseases such as measles and varicella. Special mention must be made of herpes simplex virus. It is an uncommon cause of aseptic meningitis, with a good prognosis, but in the newborn infant can cause a disseminated infection involving many tissues, with a grave rognosis. But it is now known to be the cause of the isease called *acute necrotising encephalitis* which is ssociated with intense neuronal necrosis. As this isease can be specifically treated (see below) its early ecognition is important. In addition to the viral ncephalitis which may occur early in the infectious evers such as measles, rubella and chickenpox an ncephalitic illness of later onset may occur during he period of recovery. This is characterised histolog-ally by extensive demyelination in the brain ibstance and the pathogenesis is probably a vascu-ppathy mediated by immune complexes with lesions ccurring in central nervous tissue myelin. However, et another type of encephalitis produced by measles irus may develop some years after apparent recov-ry from the measles illness itself. This results in the isease which has been long known as *subacute clerosing panencephalitis* or *subacute inclusion body ncephalitis*. The recent work on this disease is so nportant that it is considered separately below.

The term "acute encephalopathy" has to be etained to explain some poorly understood acute erebral disorders associated with convulsions, tupor, coma and abnormalities of muscle tone. In ome cases there has been a recently preceding virus nfection. Rarely it may be related to the administra-on of a vaccine. Occasionally the child may have an nderlying inherited metabolic defect such as maple yrup urine disease, organic aciduria or fatty acid, eroxisomal or mitochondrial metabolic defect. The erebrospinal fluid is usually normal and apart from edema the findings in the brain are remarkably iconspicuous. One distinct clinicopathological entity Reye syndrome. Here an acute encephalopathy /ith fatty degeneration of the viscera in a young child associated with hypoglycaemia, hyperammon-emia, greatly elevated aminotransferases, metabolic cidosis and respiratory alkalosis with prolongation f the prothrombin time. The CSF generally is clear, olourless and acellular with a normal protein oncentration. Demonstration of hyperammonaemia, levated serum transaminases and prolongation of the rothrombin time, coupled with unremarkable ndings on examination of CSF, strengthen the iagnostic impression that the patient suffers from eye syndrome. At autopsy the liver is enlarged and hows gross fatty change, being greasy and pale ellow in colour. The brain shows only oedema. lowever, electron microscopy reveals distinctive itochondrial changes in both hepatocytes and eurones. The aetiology is obscure although various iruses have been isolated in different cases. Two iruses dominate the syndrome – influenzae B and aricella. The evidence to support a possible associa-on between Reye syndrome and aspirin ingestion is ot absolute but sufficient to discourage the use of spirin for children. Treatment remains non-specific n this syndrome because the precise aetiology and

pathogenesis remain obscure. None the less the correction of electrolyte imbalance, bleeding diathe-sis, metabolic disturbances and control of intracranial pressure may suffice in the early cases. The mortality rate is high.

Clinical features

These are extremely protean. The disturbances of cerebration vary from the gradual onset of stupor or coma to the sudden onset of violent convulsions. Headache, fever, irritability, mental confusion or abnormal behaviour may be marked. Focal neuro-logical signs of many kinds are encountered such as cranial nerve palsies, speech disturbances, spastic palsies, cerebellar disturbances and abnormalities in the various reflexes. Spastic paraplegia with urinary incontinence or retention indicates spinal cord involvement. In most cases the cerebrospinal fluid shows a mild pleiocytosis and increase in protein. Virological studies are often successful in determining the causal agent.

The early diagnosis of *acute necrotising encephali-tis* is very difficult and the disease is probably not uncommon. It is most often caused by herpes virus type 1. In addition to the clinical manifestations described above some cases have had neurological signs suggestive of an expanding lesion in the brain, particularly in the temporal lobe. An electroen-cephalogram (EEG) may show gross slow-wave abnormalities over one or other hemisphere and carotid angiography has sometimes revealed a large avascular mass in the temporoparietal area. This can readily be mistaken for an abscess or haematoma but, in fact, represents necrotic brain tissue. A rise in complement-fixing antibody in the serum is strongly suggestive evidence of the disease but this may mean a delay of 10–14 days. A rapid diagnosis is best based on CT scanning followed by a brain biopsy, the speci-men being examined for herpes simplex virus by the immunofluorescent technique, or by electron microscopy. A positive immunofluorescent reaction for the virus may also be obtained in the cerebrospinal fluid. The virus may be cultured from the brain biopsy specimen.

The outcome is always doubtful in every case of encephalitis and especially grave in acute necrotising encephalitis. Death is not uncommon, but many cases end in complete recovery. Others are left with perma-nent disability such as mental deterioration, hemiple-gia or paraplegia, and epilepsy. In some children an apparently good recovery is followed later by learn-ing difficulties or behaviour problems.

Treatment

Apart from general nursing measures it is open to doubt whether any treatment significantly influences the outcome apart from acute necrotising encephalitis. Convulsions must be controlled with intravenous diazepam and the oral use of anticonvulsant drugs. A clear airway must be ensured in the comatose patient by nursing him head lower than feet in the semi-prone position, and by frequent pharyngeal suction. Rarely, tracheal intubation and mechanical ventilation is required. Frequently, tube feeding or intravenous fluids are indicated. The electrolyte balance must be maintained. In post-infectious cases corticosteroids such as prednisolone or dexamethasone are worth a trial on the assumption that this is an allergic form of encephalitis. Their value is, however, difficult to assess in individual patients.

The treatment of *acute necrotising encephalitis* requires the administration of an agent which is active against DNA viruses. Acyclovir is a more effective and safer treatment. It is available as an intravenous injection and in tablet form. It can be given in a dose of 10 mg/kg every 8 hours by bolus injection over 2 minutes for 10 days. Trials of acyclovir treatment have confirmed that the drug is almost completely free of serious toxicity.

Subacute sclerosing panencephalitis (subacute inclusion–body encephalitis)

This subacute form of encephalitis has been known under a variety of names for many years. Its relationship to measles virus was first recognised in 1967 because it was found that there was a very high titre of measles antibody in the serum and cerebrospinal fluid in these cases. Histologically the disease is characterised by intranuclear inclusions, and under the electron microscope these have been shown to resemble measles virus inclusions. Measles antigen has also been demonstrated in the brain by fluorescent-antibody techniques and measles virus itself has been isolated from brain tissue in panencephalitis. However, the initial attack of measles has usually antedated the onset of encephalitic manifestations by several years. The disease has also been reported to follow immunisation with live measles virus vaccine but the risk is very much less than with wild measles virus. Obviously some unusual reaction happens in patients with this disease in which a measles virus infection of the brain spreads inexorably in spite of abnormally large and persisting antibody production. It has been suggested that due to a persisting measles infection of the thymus these patients develop a measles-specific tolerance in thymus-associated immunocytes (responsible for delayed-type hypersensitivity) but retain normal responsiveness in gut-associated immunocytes (responsible for antibodies). On the other hand, an alternative hypothesis has been suggested to the effect that the thymus-dependent lymphocytes are not incompetent immunologically and that the panencephalitis is due to

destructive interaction between these "aggressive" lymphocytes and the host cells of the brain which harbour measles virus. It has been speculated that the measles virus in the brain may have altered its structure to allow it to live in symbiosis with the neurones.

Clinical features

The onset is insidious over a period of months. Intellectual deterioration and behavioural changes, sometimes extreme emotional lability, progress to a state of dementia. Major epileptic seizures may occur. A somewhat characteristic form of myoclonic jerk is commonly seen in which the child makes repetitive stereotyped movements with rhythmic regularity (2–6 per minute); each begins with shock-like abruptness typical of the myoclonic jerk, but then the elevated limb remains "frozen" for a second or two before, and unlike the usual myoclonic jerk, it gradually melts away. Pyramidal and extrapyramidal signs are common. The final state is frequently one of decerebrate rigidity. The cerebrospinal fluid does not often show an increase in cells but a raised globulin content and paretic-type colloidal gold curve are usually found. The EEG at the start of the illness may show only some excess slow-wave activity, and if this is much more marked on one side a space-occupying lesion may be wrongly suspected. Later in the illness bilateral periodic complexes typical of the disease appear. The EEG then shows high-amplitude slow-wave complexes, frequently having the same rhythmicality as the myoclonic jerk, sometimes with a frequency of 6–10 seconds. Death generally occurs within 2 years of the onset. Rarely, clinical arrest or even spontaneous recovery has been reported.

Treatment

None is of proven value.

Acute infective polyneuritis (Guillain–Barré syndrome)

Aetiology

This condition must be distinguished from the polyneuritis of diphtheria and from the rare polyneuritis due to lead poisoning or drug intoxications. The disease is assumed to be precipitated by various virus infections and it is analogous to postviral encephalitis. A similar condition infrequently complicates glandular fever. A preceding upper respiratory infection is common.

Clinical features

After an upper respiratory febrile illness the child develops increasing muscular weakness and tenderness with loss of the deep reflexes. The proximal muscles of the limbs and those of the trunk are more severely affected than the distal musculature. Muscle atrophy is often remarkably slight. Sensory changes tend to be minimal. Their distribution seems to correspond more to the dermatomes than to the peripheral nerves. Intercostal and diaphragmatic paralysis may endanger life. Bilateral facial paralysis is common but bulbar palsy is rare. Tachycardia and cardiomegaly may be present. In the typical Guillain–Barré syndrome the cerebrospinal fluid shows a high protein content with little or no pleiocytosis, but these changes are inconstant and may be late in appearing. If death from respiratory paralysis or intercurrent respiratory infection can be avoided the child usually makes a slow but complete recovery over a period of months. *Landry acute ascending paralysis* is sometimes a variant of this disease, although other cases are due to acute poliomyelitis.

Treatment

Symptomatic treatment is an important part of the management of children with Guillain–Barré syndrome. Respiratory paralysis may necessitate tracheostomy and assisted ventilation. Physiotherapy is useful during convalescence. On the basis of controlled studies corticosteroids seem to be of no beneficial effect. Recently it has been shown that plasmapheresis diminishes morbidity in children. Also high dose IV gammaglobulin therapy (0.4 g/kg/day) administered for 5 days during the initial stages of the disease seem to be as effective as plasmapheresis.

Acute cerebellar ataxia

Aetiology

Cerebellar ataxia is a common phenomenon in young children. There are many clearly defined causes, e.g. infratentorial tumours, post-infective encephalitis, otogenic cerebellar abscess (now very rare) and the various leucodystrophies and hereditary types of cerebellar ataxia. Alcohol ingestion, glue-sniffing, lead encephalopathy, piperazine, and anticonvulsant drugs may also cause ataxia. These are not included under the term "acute cerebellar ataxia", which refers to cases of sudden onset and unknown causation. A virus has been suggested but never proved. The same applies to the idea of an allergic response to a virus infection.

Clinical features

In the typical case the onset of cerebellar signs in a child aged 2–5 years is sudden. There may have been a preceding upper respiratory tract infection but its

significance is difficult to assess. The principal feature is the typical reeling ataxia. There may be a tremor or wobble of the head. Hypotonia is common and the deep reflexes may be diminished. The child may be irritable or abnormal in personality but there is no blurring of consciousness. Other cerebellar signs may be elicited, e.g. nystagmus, intention tremor, dysmetria or disturbance of speech. The optic fundi are normal. Vomiting may occur but there are no other indications of an increase in intracranial pressure. The cerebrospinal fluid is usually normal.

The differential diagnosis from the other causes of cerebellar ataxia is essential and usually possible on careful assessment of the history and physical findings. Computer-axial tomography (CT scanning) should be arranged if there is any suspicion of tumour.

In most instances complete recovery can be expected within a period of weeks. A few cases, often those with an insidious onset, progress steadily but it is likely that they are of different aetiology, possibly in the spinocerebellar ataxia group.

Treatment

Symptomatic measures only are possible.

Acute infantile hemiplegia

This is a characteristic clinical syndrome seen in both infants and children and perhaps better called "acute hemiplegia in childhood". Most cases are associated with a preceding pyrexial illness such as tonsillitis, cervical adenitis, tooth infection or sometimes tonsillectomy. The presence of abnormalities in the internal carotid and first part of the middle cerebral arteries has been clearly demonstrated in cases investigated within a few days of the onset. These have ranged from complete occlusion to very marked narrowing of the lumen of the carotid and its branches and in other cases there have been irregularities of the lumen. A good case is made that this arterial obstruction is the consequence of an inflammatory arteritis of the carotid following throat or neck gland infection. Some of these cases were probably due to the mitochondrial disorder MELAS (Chapter 16).

This syndrome does not, of course, include cases of congenital hemiplegia, brain tumour, otogenic encephalitis (now rarely seen), encephalitis following the infectious fevers or the results of trauma.

Clinical features

The disease may present in one of two ways. In the more common, the child suddenly goes into status epilepticus with high fever and deep coma. The convulsions may be generalised or unilateral. After some hours or days of critical illness, the fits cease and consciousness slowly returns. Hemiplegia is then found to be present, with dysphasia in right-sided cases. The upper motor neurone weakness and spasticity affect principally the face and arm, and recovery in the leg precedes and exceeds that of the arm.

In the second mode of presentation the child, after a recent febrile illness, suddenly develops a hemiplegia, with or without dysphasia; convulsions do not occur and if there is loss of consciousness it is of short duration.

In either type of case signs of recovery are obvious after a week or two, although the hemiplegia rarely completely disappears. Intelligence may be unimpaired, although in some cases serious mental retardation or epilepsy persists permanently. If the hemiplegia remains severe, defective growth and shortening of the arm and leg result.

The cerebrospinal fluid shows no abnormality at the inception of the illness but some days later a slight rise in cells and protein may develop; later, ventricular enlargement occurs on the affected side of the brain with displacement of the ventricular system to that side with enlargement of the sulci. This atrophic change is, in fact, most marked in the territory supplied by the middle cerebral artery, but sometimes it is also seen in the territory of the anterior cerebral artery. The posterior part of the hemisphere is rarely affected. MRI and CT would demonstrate these changes.

Treatment

Other causes of convulsions such as meningitis and encephalitis should be excluded by early lumbar puncture. Status epilepticus is best treated with intravenous diazepam 2–10 mg; maintenance anticonvulsant therapy must be continued indefinitely. Persisting tonsillar or dental sepsis should be treated with an appropriate antibiotic. The consequences of the disease can be so disastrous that careful consideration should be given to the use of anticoagulants although their value in carotid artery disease is unproven. Unfortunately, the clinical syndrome develops so quickly in most cases that maximal damage has already occurred before anticoagulants can be administered. During the stage of recovery physiotherapy is valuable.

PROGRESSIVE DEGENERATIVE DISEASES

This is a "mixed bag" of diseases, most of which are not amenable to treatment. They are uncommon in everyday practice and they will receive only short discussion.

Schilder disease (encephalitis periaxialis diffusa)

The cause of this extensive cerebral demyelinating process is unknown. The onset is usually between the ages of 5 and 13 years and the disease results in progressive dementia and decerebrate rigidity. If the occipital lobes are first affected, visual field defects and later cortical blindness are the initial features. Equally often the onset is with spastic palsies of various distribution but ultimately affecting the whole body and all four limbs. Aphasia, convulsive seizures, dementia, pseudo-bulbar palsy and emotional lability may all develop in varying degree. Increased intracranial pressure with bilateral sixth nerve palsies, papilloedema, and cerebral vomiting are seen in some cases. In others there is a true optic neuritis. The cerebrospinal fluid may be normal or show a mild pleiocytosis and increase of protein. Remissions rarely occur and death takes place within a year or two. Treatment is purely symptomatic. Corticosteroids are not indicated.

The leucodystrophies

This group of diseases are genetic in origin, the mode of inheritance being most often autosomal recessive. They probably should be included with the sphingolipidoses and regarded as inborn errors of metabolism (Chapter 16). Two fairly clear clinical and biochemical entities have been defined and others await further elucidation.

Krabbe globoid body leucodystrophy affects infants in the early months of life. The name derives from the fact that the white matter of the brain contains large globular bodies due to an excess accumulation of neutral ceramide hexosides. The peripheral nerves may also be involved and show the same enzyme abnormality as the brain tissue, namely deficiency of galactocerebroside β-galactosidase. The onset is with incessant crying followed by apathy. Generalised rigidity, seizures, head retraction, blindness, inability to swallow and death may ensue in a year or thereabouts. The involvement of peripheral nerves may be reflected in absent deep reflexes with reduced nerve velocity. The diagnosis can be confirmed by specific-enzyme assay in the blood leucocytes.

Metachromatic leucodystrophy is characterised by the accumulation of cerebroside sulphate (sulphatide) in the white matter of the brain, the peripheral nerves, the dentate nucleus, basal ganglia, and in other organs such as the kidneys. There is widespread demyelination with neuronal and axonal loss. The sulphatide stains metachromatically with basic polychrome dyes. There are two enzyme deficiencies, cerebroside sulphatase and arylsulphatase A, the latter apparently being a component of the former.

Three clinical forms of the disease have been described:

1 Late infantile. This is the most common with its onset between 6 and 24 months. Deterioration in walking due to progressive and mixed pyramidal and cerebellar damage is soon followed by deterioration in speech and social development, loss of the ability to sit or feed without help, fits, misery and withdrawal, finally a decorticate posture leading to death some 5 months or longer from the onset.

2 Intermediate (early juvenile). This has an onset between 4 and 6 years. Disorders of gait, mostly pyramidal with some cerebellar involvement, coincide with educational and social deterioration, convulsions and slow progress to decorticate rigidity and death more than 3 years from the onset.

3 Juvenile. This has an onset between 6 and 10 years. The first signs are educational and behavioural deterioration, followed after some months or years by disorders of gait, mostly extrapyramidal with some pyramidal signs. Progress towards dementia and death may take more than 5 years.

The diagnosis is based on measurements of arylsulphatase A activity in blood leucocytes or skin fibroblasts, confirmed also by demonstrating metachromatic intranuclear material in renal tubular cells shed in the urine. The CSF often shows a raised protein concentration and there is slow motor nerve conduction velocity.

Friedrich ataxia

This disease may be inherited either as a recessive or a dominant trait. It makes its appearance in childhood and before puberty with pes cavus, kyphoscoliosis and some degree of ataxia (e.g. ataxia, nystagmus, intention tremor) and the dorsal columns e.g. absent deep reflexes and loss of vibration and postural sensation). Degeneration of the pyramidal tracts results in extensor plantar responses. Optic atrophy and dysarthria may appear late in the course of the disease and occasionally there is mental deterioration. Cardiac manifestations also occur due to an interstitial myocarditis, e.g. tachycardia, systolic murmurs and S-T changes in the ECG. Death may be delayed for 10–15 years, but it may occur earlier from cardiac failure. There is no specific treatment, but orthopaedic measures may be helpful. Several other rare types of hereditary cerebellar ataxia have also been described.

Hereditary spastic paraplegia

This condition may be inherited as a dominant, recessive or sex-linked recessive disease. It is characterised by the onset during childhood of progressive uncomplicated spastic paraplegia. Severe flexion deformities may develop. The diagnosis rests upon the family history.

Werdnig–Hoffmann progressive spinal paralysis

This is a relatively common disease of infancy inherited as a recessive trait and showing a marked familial incidence. The principal pathological feature is progressive loss of motor neurones in the anterior horns of the spinal cord. The disease may be present at birth or appear within a few weeks. Its onset *in utero* may be recognised by the mother because the previously marked fetal movements suddenly cease. There is flaccidity and weakness of the muscles of the trunk and limbs. The proximal muscles tend to be more severely paralysed than the distal. The deep reflexes are absent or soon disappear. Fasciculation in the muscles of the tongue and limbs is of great diagnostic importance. When the intercostal and other accessory muscles of respiration become affected dyspnoea and inspiratory intercostal recession develop. In due course, involvement of the diaphragm renders the infant extremely prone to respiratory infections, one of which ultimately proves fatal. The loss of power to suck further aggravates the terminal stages of the illness. Life is rarely prolonged beyond the age of 5 years. There is no specific treatment.

A milder type of spinal paralysis which has been increasingly recognised develops at a later age and is compatible with a prolonged course. This is the *Kugelberg–Welander syndrome*. The proximal muscles are mainly involved, the legs may show muscle atrophy before the arms, and skeletal deformities readily develop. The tendon reflexes disappear and the plantar responses are often extensor. In some cases the bulbar muscles become involved ("juvenile amyotrophic lateral sclerosis"). Electromyography shows a denervation pattern and muscle biopsy can also help to confirm the diagnosis. These children may learn to walk, but ultimately become confined to a wheelchair. There is also a third form of spinal muscular atrophy, which in its severity lies somewhere between the classical Werdnig–Hoffmann disease and the Kugelberg–Welander syndrome. In this form the child can sit unsupported but never learns to walk.

The term *amyotonia congenita* is best abandoned. It implies only a "floppy infant" for which there are many causes in addition to Werdnig–Hoffmann disease. These include Tay–Sachs disease, ataxic and flaccid diplegias, infantile myasathenia gravis, idiopathic hypercalcaemia and, most common, mental deficiency with associated hypotonia. None of these conditions should be difficult to distinguish from Werdnig–Hoffmann disease.

The principal difficulty is to differentiate Werdnig–Hoffmann disease from *benign congenital hypotonia*. Here too, extreme hypotonia dates from or soon after birth. The deep reflexes although very sluggish can usually be elicited and muscle fibrillations, commonly seen in Werdnig–Hoffmann disease, do not occur. The true diagnosis in benign congenital hypotonia becomes clear with the passage of time (5–9 years), when slow but not always complete recovery takes place. Muscle biopsy reveals the atrophy of denervation in Werdnig–Hoffmann disease, but the appearances remain normal in benign congenital hypotonia.

A number of rare disorders have been defined in recent years. They should probably be regarded as congenital myopathies and can only be distinguished from each other by means of muscle biopsy and the application of special stains, electron microscopy and biochemical investigation of the mitochondrial respiratory chain complexes. They usually present as the "floppy infant" syndrome, but the muscle weakness may not become apparent until later childhood. They differ markedly from Werdnig–Hoffmann disease in that they run a chronic non-progressive course. Both *central-core disease* and *nemaline myopathy* may be familial with apparently dominant inheritance, whereas there may be a recessive inheritance in *myotubular (centro-nuclear) myopathy*. Two other extremely rare disorders are *megaconial myopathy* in which unusually large mitochondria appear in muscle cells, and *pleioconial myopathy* so called because the cells contain an excessive quantity of mitochondria (Chapter 16).

Charcot–Marie–Tooth peroneal muscular atrophy

This rare disease may be transmitted as a dominant, recessive or sex-linked recessive characteristic. It starts with progressive weakness and lower motor neurone type of flaccid atrophy of the peroneal and tibial muscles and of the small muscles of the feet. The result is paralytic talipes equinovarus. Later, wasting of the calf muscles gives the legs an odd, inverted wine-bottle appearance. At a late stage, weakness and wasting affect the hands and forearms. The disease rarely extends above the knees. The ankle jerks are lost but the knee jerks remain brisk. Some loss of vibration and positional sensation is common. Optic atrophy has been described in adult life.

Dystrophia myotonica (myotonic dystrophy)

This disorder is inherited as an autosomal dominant with the locus being on the long arm of chromosome 19. Affected children nearly always have affected mothers (rather than fathers). It has been regarded as a disease of adult life, characterised by delayed muscle relaxation and atrophy (especially of the hands, masseters and sternomastoids), baldness, cataract and testicular atrophy. It is, however, probable that cases occurring in childhood and even at birth have been missed in the past because clinical manifestations differ greatly from the classical picture in adult life.

The clinical features in the neonate or older infant include hypotonia, facial diplegia and jaw weakness, delayed motor development and speech, talipes and respiratory problems. Mental retardation is relatively common. Clinical evidence of myotonia is absent (although it may be demonstrated by electromyography). Cataracts do not occur. Electromyography is the most helpful investigation. Muscle biopsy with special staining techniques and electron microscopy will confirm the diagnosis. There is no effective treatment.

A variable DNA sequence has been detected in patients with myotonic dystrophy. This finding will assist in accurate diagnosis and genetic counselling of affected families.

Duchenne type (pseudohypertrophic) muscular dystrophy

Most cases are transmitted as a sex-linked recessive trait so that only males are affected, while the disease is transmitted by females.

The onset is usually before the third or fourth years of life, although the significance of the early symptoms is not infrequently overlooked. There may be a history of delay in walking, or a failure of the gait ever to become steady. The child may fall unduly often, or has great difficulty in climbing stairs. Ultimately the gait assumes a characteristic waddle so that the feet are placed too widely apart and there is an exaggerated lumbar lordosis. Weakness of the shoulder muscles may render the child unable to raise his hands above his head. When he is lifted by his armpits he is apt to slide through the examiner's hands because of the weakness of his shoulder girdle muscles. A quite characteristic phenomenon is seen when the child, lying on his back on the floor, is asked to stand up. He will roll to one side, flex his knees and hips so that he is "on all fours" with both knees and both hands on the ground; he then extends his knees and reaches the erect posture by "climbing up his own legs", using his hands to get higher up each leg in alternate steps.

The muscles which first show weakness are those around the shoulders and hips and thighs. Pseudohypertrophy tends to be best seen in the supra- and infraspinati, deltoids, triceps, quadriceps and the muscles of the calves. Tendon reflexes become progressively diminished and finally cannot be elicited as muscle weakness increases. By the age of 10 years the child is usually confined to a wheelchair, although he remains remarkably cheerful. Skeletal and postural deformities may later become severe. Death is usual during adolescence from intercurrent respiratory infection, or the heart may fail from involvement of the myocardium.

In the fully developed case the clinical picture is quite characteristic. The diagnosis can be confirmed in early cases by muscle biopsy. It is possible to identify, shortly after birth, those males who will later manifest the disease. The most useful for diagnostic purposes is the serum creatine kinase which will be elevated much above the normal maximum of about 60 units/l. It will also show a rise in about 70% of the apparently healthy female carriers of the disease, and this correlates with the fact that minor dystrophic changes can be detected in muscle biopsy specimens from known female carriers. Electromyography may also be useful but interpretation is sometimes difficult.

Treatment

There is as yet no satisfactory treatment for muscular dystrophy although many substances such as vitamins, hormones, nucleotides and amino acids have been tested. Myoblast transfer and gene therapy are possible means of correcting the deficiency of muscle dystrophin. An effective treatment may be found in the not too distant future. Physiotherapy is frequently prescribed with beneficial psychological effects upon the child and his parents, in addition to preventing contractures. Lightweight calipers and, later, bracing of the spine may prolong ambulation for several years. Antenatal diagnosis is possible with 100% accuracy for cases in which a DNA deletion is present, especially using cDNA probes.

Facioscapulohumeral muscular dystrophy

This form of dystrophy is transmitted as an autosomal dominant trait and can affect both sexes.

The onset may be in early childhood or early adult life, most often with weakness and lack of expression in the facial muscles. In time the child cannot close his eyes, wrinkle his forehead or purse his mouth. The lips project forwards due to weakness of the orbicu-laris oris to give the appearance of "tapir mouth". Weakness of the shoulder girdle muscles, especially the pectoralis major, serratus magnus, trapezius, spinati, deltoid, triceps and biceps results in winging of the scapulae, inability to raise the arms above the head and looseness of the shoulders. Then the pelvic girdle becomes affected, glutei, quadriceps, hamstrings and iliopsoas, so that there is lumbar lordosis and a broad-based gait. This form of muscular dystrophy usually runs a prolonged and relatively benign course well into adult life. Indeed, the face only may be affected during most of childhood and severe crippling may be long delayed. The diagnosis can be confirmed by muscle biopsy. Elevated levels of serum creatine kinase are found only in some cases.

Treatment

None is available at the present time.

Limb–girdle muscular dystrophy

This form of dystrophy in which pseudohypertrophy is uncommon is probably inherited as an autosomal recessive characteristic. Males and females are equally affected.

This rarely appears during the first decade. Weakness first becomes obvious in the muscles of the shoulder girdle with winging of the scapulae and difficulty in raising the arms. Later the muscles of the pelvic girdle become affected. The facial muscles are never affected. The disease runs a slow course but usually leads to death before the normal age. Serum creatine kinase levels may be normal or moderately raised. Muscle biopsy reveals myopathic changes.

This type of muscular dystrophy is extremely rare in paediatric practice.

Myasthenia gravis

Myasthenia gravis is a disorder of neuromuscular function caused by a reduction of available acetylcholine receptors at the neuromuscular junction. There is good evidence that antibodies to acetylcholine receptors are important in the pathogenesis of the disease, and they can be measured by a radioimmunoassay technique.

Clinical features

Cases of myasthenia gravis have been reported as early in life as the first year, but the onset is rarely before the age of 10 years. Most cases are in girls. The ocular muscles are usually first affected; the child presents with ptosis (Fig. 9.2) or complains of diplopia; the muscle weakness tends to be more

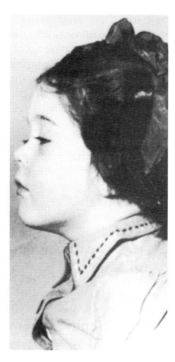

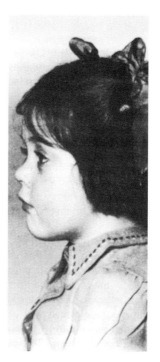

FIGURE 9.2 Bilateral ptosis in a 4-year-old girl suffering from myasthenia gravis.

FIGURE 9.3 Same girl as in Figure 9.2 a few minutes after subcutaneous injection of neostigmine.

severe as the day goes on so that there may be marked ptosis or strabismus, usually bilateral. The bulbar muscles are often next affected although this may not occur for some years. The voice is then weak, swallowing and chewing become difficult, and there may be asphyxial episodes due to the aspiration of upper respiratory secretions and saliva. When the facial muscles are affected a lack of expression is a striking feature and there is inability to blow out the cheeks. In the worst cases the muscles of the limbs and those responsible for respiration are affected. These features are always less obvious, and may totally disappear after a night's rest. Muscle atrophy or fibrillary twitchings do not occur. The deep reflexes are usually present and may even be exaggerated. Although the thymus gland is hyperplastic this is not radiologically obvious unless there is an actual thymoma, when a large opacity may be visible in the superior mediastinum. This is extremely rare in childhood.

An interesting and highly dangerous form of myasthenia gravis is that which can affect the newborn infant of a myasthenic mother and is due to the placental transfer of antibodies to acetylcholine receptors from mother to baby. The manifestations include a weak cry, generalised severe hypotonia, feeble sucking reflex and attacks of choking and cyanosis. They are temporary and disappear within a few weeks, but are not infrequently fatal unless treatment is promptly instituted. Ptosis and paralysis of

the extraocular muscles are apparently uncommon in neonatal myasthenia.

As in the adult, the myasthenic child may run a prolonged course of remissions and relapses, but there is a tendency for the disease to reach a static phase some 5 years from the onset. There is always a risk of death from aspiration of food into the respiratory passages, from respiratory failure if the diaphragm and intercostal muscles are affected, or from intercurrent respiratory infection.

Diagnosis

This should be suspected in the presence of ptosis, strabismus, bulbar palsy or severe muscular hypotonia during infancy or childhood. The manifestations can be immediately relieved by the hypodermic injection of neostigmine salicylic 0.25–1.0 mg along with atropine sulphate 0.3–0.6 mg (Fig. 9.3). In infancy the heart rate should be watched after this test, as occasionally a dangerous degree of bradycardia may require further doses of atropine. A drug of similar action to neostigmine but transient in its effects is to be found in edrophonium (Tensilon). It can be given intravenously in an initial dose of 2 mg. If there is no untoward response and no dramatic relief, a further dose of 4–8 mg, according to age, should be given after a minute or so. The use of one of these drugs will always settle any doubts about the diagnosis.

Treatment

This should be medical in the first instance and many patients can be adequately treated in this fashion. It must be recognised that different muscles show variable sensitivity towards the action of the anticholinesterase drugs. If an overdose is prescribed because certain muscles remain weak on a particular dosage, prolonged depolarisation of muscle end-plates develops and causes transmission failure and paralysis (cholinergic crisis). The short-acting edrophonium may be used to determine whether the dose is optimal. If an intravenous injection fails to increase the efficiency of the respiratory muscles, when given after the drug which is being used as maintenance therapy, of if weakness is increased, the child is already having too much of the anticholinesterase drug. This test should be performed after preparations have been made for assisted respiration.

The most useful drug for continuous treatment is pryidostigmine bromide (Mestinon) given orally in a dosage of 10–60 mg every 3–8 hours according to the child's age and clinical response. Pyridostigmine gives fewer parasympathomimetic effects and smoother control than neostigmine bromide given orally in a dosage of 5–15 mg every 6–8 hours. On the other hand, a more rapid relief of muscular weakness is obtained with neostigmine, and side effects such as colic, sweating and bradycardia can be relieved with atropine sulphate 0.6 mg given orally. In some patients pyridostigmine and neostigmine can with advantage be used in combination.

Apart from such symptomatic treatment with anticholinesterase drugs, immunosuppressive drugs may be employed to reduce antibodies to acetyl-choline receptors. Corticosteroids are indicated for seriously ill patients and in those who are not sufficiently improved by thymectomy. They are also particularly effective where the clinical signs are restricted to the ocular muscles when a small maintenance dose on alternate days may keep the patient in complete remission. As there can be an initial deterioration on steroid therapy, dosage should be low and only increased gradually. A suitable dose of prednisolone is about 1 mg/kg on alternate days. Azathioprine, 2.5 mg/kg/day has produced clinical improvement although usually only after a delay of 6–12 weeks. Its toxic effects limit its use to severe cases and it is doubtful if it should ever be used in children with this disease.

The position of thymectomy in the treatment of myasthenia gravis in childhood is not yet clearly defined because of the relative rarity of the disease, and the reasonably satisfactory results usually obtained from medical treatment. Good results follow thymectomy in 70% of young adults. The indications for operation are a duration of the disease of under 2 years, and inadequate control of the muscular weakness with drugs. Improvement after thymectomy is gradual, and the operation should not be performed as an emergency procedure in a myasthenic crisis.

Yet another therapeutic approach is plasma exchange which can produce dramatic but short-lived improvement by removing anti-acetylcholine esterase antibody. It is only indicated in seriously ill patients while waiting for other forms of treatment to take effect.

Kinnier Wilson disease

Aetiology

This disease, inherited as an autosomal recessive trait, is an inborn error of metabolism in which there is an excessive accumulation of copper in the brain, liver, cornea and other tissues. There is also an increased absorption of copper from the intestine and a lowered level of ceruloplasmin (the copper-binding protein of the serum).

Clinical features

These develop in childhood or adolescence. In many cases they are predominantly neurological, e.g. coarse and sometimes bizarre tremors which may simulate severe chorea, extreme emotional instability with bouts of laughing and weeping, dysarthria, difficulty in swallowing and dementia. A characteristic finding is the Kayser–Fleischer ring, a golden-brown discoloration due to deposition of copper at the corneal limbus. In recent years it has been increasingly recognised that Wilson disease may present with solely or predominantly hepatic manifestations, e.g. jaundice, hepatomegaly, ascites or haematemesis due to portal hypertension. Indeed, Wilson disease should be considered in all children with prolonged jaundice or obscure hepatomegaly. The first presentation may also take the form of a haemolytic anaemia.

Diagnosis

The most characteristic findings are a greatly excessive urinary output of copper and a reduced serum level of ceruloplasmin. Other common findings are disordered liver function tests, aminoaciduria and portal cirrhosis in a liver biopsy.

Treatment

Marked improvement can be achieved by the mobilisation of copper from the tissues with chelating agents. The most useful is D-penicillamine, which is active when given by mouth in doses of 750 mg to

2 g per day. A low-copper diet (excluding cocoa, nuts, liver, shellfish, mushrooms and spinach) is also advised. Copper absorption may be further reduced with potassium sulphide, 20 mg thrice daily, which forms insoluble copper sulphide in the gut. Treatment is best monitored by measuring urinary copper excretion which often increases dramatically at the start of the treatment then returns to normal over a few months.

Ataxia-telangiectasia (Louis–Bar syndrome)

This condition has now been defined as a specific entity transmitted as an autosomal recessive characteristic. The clinical features are diagnostic when fully developed. The first to appear is a progressive cerebellar ataxia in the course of the second or third year of life, occasionally even earlier. There may be, in addition, choreo-athetotic movements and a tendency to turn the eyes upwards when focusing. Telangiectases make their appearance between the ages of 3 and 7 years. Occasionally children present with bleeding from a haemangioma of the bowel. They are found on the bulbar conjuctiva, malar eminences, ears, antecubital fossae and elsewhere. Patches of poorly pigmented skin are often present over the face and neck but the hair is not affected. These children suffer severely from infections of the sinuses and lungs; indeed bronchiectasis is a frequent cause of death. In other cases death has been due to malignant disease (e.g. lymphosarcoma). A constant feature of all the investigated cases, and one which explains the extreme susceptibility to severe sinopulmonary infection, is absence or gross reduction in the serum IgA, normal or low level of IgA and elevated or normal level of IgM. Post-mortem examination has usually revealed hypoplasia of the thymus. There may be reduced responsiveness of cultured lymphocytes to phytohaemagglutinin, suggesting dysfunction of the thymus-dependent lymphocytes. There is no specific treatment yet available. Infection should be controlled with suitable antibiotics. Fetal thymus implants and stimulants of the immunological system have given inconclusive results. Malignant change might be temporarily altered with corticosteroids.

NEUROCUTANEOUS SYNDROMES (THE PHAKOMATOSES)

Tuberous sclerosis (epiloia)

This is a hereditary disease transmitted as a dominant trait with one gene defect identified on chromosome

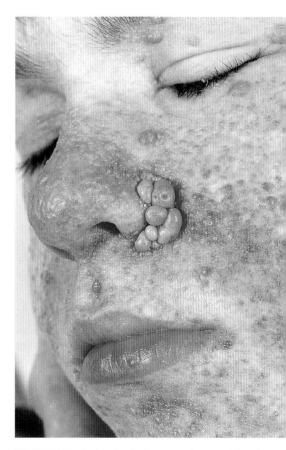

FIGURE 9.4 Typical rash of adenoma sebaceum. Note butterfly distribution of papules.

9 and another probably on chromosome 16. It i characterized in its fully developed form by menta deficiency, epileptic seizures and a rash of butterfly distribution and papular character on the face and nose (adenoma sebaceum) (Fig. 9.4). Seizures are a prominent feature of this disease being reported in 85–93% of cases. Other skin lesions include "shagreen" patches, areas of poor pigmentation and *café-au-lait* spots. Indeed, depigmented areas of skin sometimes assuming an ash-leaf shape, are the earliest manifestations of this disorder. They can best be identified in fair-skinned infants under ultra-violet light which is passed through a Wood's glass. Their detection in an infant presenting with fits or infantile spasms would carry great significance. Ophthalmoscopy may show characteristic yellowish-white phakomata on the retina. In some cases there are teratomata or hamartomata of the kidneys, liver, bone and lung. The heart may be the seat of a rhabdomyoma or a tuberous lesion. Radiologically visible intracranial calcification may be found and is due to the presence of nodular masses in the brain (phakomata). The diagnosis of tuberous sclerosis is based on the combination of characteristic cutaneous

lesions, seizures, intellectual deficit and visceral tumours. There is no specific treatment for tuberous sclerosis. Management is directed at the symptoms of the disorder.

Neurofibromatosis (von Recklinghausen disease)

This hereditary disease is also transmitted as a dominant characteristic. It is characterised by multiple tumours of the peripheral and central nervous system, *café-au-lait* spots, and various lesions of the vascular system and viscera. Two gene defects have been identified; one on chromosome 17 which predisposes to the cutaneous features and peripheral nerve abnormalities and the other on chromosome 22 is associated with central nervous system tumours and acoustic neuromas. In childhood a progressive severe kyphoscoliosis in association with multiple *café-au-lait* spots on the skin is a common mode of presentation. In some cases palpable neurofibromata are to be detected along the course of subcutaneous nerves. The brain may be the site of formation of nodules similar to those found in tuberous sclerosis, and various types of tumour (glioma, ependymoma, meningioma) may occur in the brain, spinal cord or spinal nerve roots. Approximately 10–20% of patients manifest with seizures, intellectual deficit and speech and motor delay.

Treatment

There is no specific treatment and therapy is symptomatic. Neurosurgical intervention is often necessary to remove symptomatic tumours of the central and peripheral nervous system.

The Sturge–Weber syndrome

In this disease there is an association between an extensive cutaneous port-wine haemangioma of the upper face and scalp, which is predominantly limited by the midline, and a similar vascular anomaly of the underlying meninges on the same side. The infant usually starts to have convulsions confined to the contralateral side of the body. The cause is obvious from the distribution of the facial haemangioma. In time a spastic hemiparesis may develop on the contralateral side. Later in childhood, but rarely in infancy, radiographs of the skull show a characteristic double contour or "tramline" type of calcification (Fig. 9.5). Mental deterioration ultimately appears and progresses. Glaucoma may also develop and require surgical intervention. The mode of inheritance of this disease is not clear, but is probably autosomal dominant with a variable penetrance. Treatment is

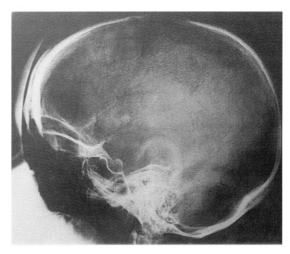

FIGURE 9.5 Radiograph of skull of a child with Sturge–Weber syndrome. Note intracranial calcification in occipital area.

symptomatic and directed at control of seizures and glaucoma. If seizures are refractory to drug therapy, surgical resection of the affected lobe or hemispherectomy may be indicated. In some cases the facial naevus can be corrected by cosmetic laser surgery.

Von Hippel–Lindau disease

This is a rare genetically determined combination of haemangiomatous cystic changes in the retina and cerebellum, sometimes also in kidney, liver and pancreas. It may present with the signs of a cerebellar tumour or with loss of vision due to retinal detachment. Phaeochromocytoma occurs in some patients. Surgical intervention on both the cerebellum and retina is sometimes successful.

NEURAL TUBE DEFECTS

The complex neural tube system which develops from infolding of the dorsum of the fetus is the site of a number of different types of maldevelopment. The global term neural tube defects (NTD) is currently used to encompass the infants who are born with spina bifida and meningocele or myelomeningocele defects and at the cranial end of the neural tube the meningoceles, encephaloceles, iniencephaly and anencephaly (Fig. 9.6 a–d). Hydrocephalus is often associated with NTD and will be considered subsequently as it also occurs due to other causes (Fig. 9.7). There is an interesting geographical variation in the incidence of the different types of NTD with the spinal anomaly of meningocele and myelomeningocele constituting 80% of NTD live-born infants in Europe,

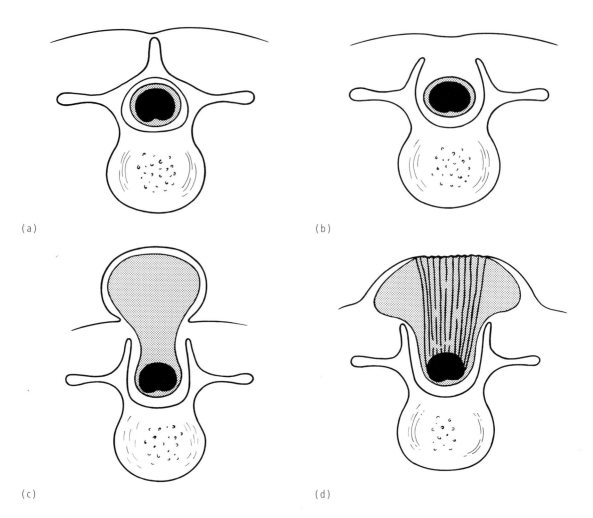

FIGURE 9.6 Line drawings of spina bifida: (a) normal spine; (b) spina bifida occulta; (c) meningocele; (d) myelomeningocele.

North America, Australia and some communities in South Africa. Defects of the cranial end, particularly encephaloceles, are more common in South-east Asia than in Europe and account for 40% of the NTD found there.

Scotland, particularly the west of Scotland, has been an area of high incidence of NTD. For every live-born child with a NTD there has also been a stillbirth or early neonatal death of an infant with anencephaly. Previously, each of these accounted for approximately 3 per 1000 live births, whereas over the last 15 years the incidence of NTD in Scotland has decreased to 1 per 1000 live births. A couple who have a fetus or child affected by a neural tube defect have approximately a 10-fold increased likelihood of subsequent siblings being affected, and if the couple have two siblings affected there is again a further increase by a factor of 3 for subsequent children. In 1992 an expert advisory group of the UK departments of health recommended that to prevent recur-

rence of a neural tube defect women at risk should take a daily folic acid supplement until the 12th week of pregnancy. To prevent a first occurrence of NTD, women who are planning a pregnancy should eat more folate-rich foods and take 4 mg folic acid daily from when they begin trying to conceive until the 12th week of pregnancy. A Medical Research Council study published in 1991 suggested that folic acid offered a protective effect of 72% in the risk of a second affected child.

Detection of elevated maternal serum α-fetoprotein levels and refinement in intrauterine ultrasound diagnosis have resulted in intrauterine diagnosis and pregnancy termination in many cases. A genetic predisposition to the development of neural tube defects may explain the higher incidence in those of Celtic (Irish, Welsh and west of Scotland population) than in those of Anglo-Saxon or Norse origin in the British Isles but folate deficiency is not uncommon in these populations.

Spina bifida occulta

In spina bifida occulta there is failure of fusion of the spinous process posteriorly. In most individuals this is a minor deviation from normal. A few children have an associated haemangiomatous or hairy patch over the site of the spina bifida occulta and in these infants there may be some neurological deficit such as a foot drop or a sudden alteration in continence of urine or problem deep to the lesion. Tethering of the cord is the most common problem and, if producing neurological signs, merits exploration and freeing of the cord. Other variations of the spine include an anomaly where a bony spur protrudes from the posterior aspect of the vertebral bodies and results in splitting of the cord (diastematomyelia). In a few patients this may merit exploration and removal of the bony spur. Visualisation of these has been greatly enhanced with the development of magnetic resonance imaging which can give very much better definition of the intraspinal anatomy than was previously possible.

Spina bifida cystica

The spina bifida defect may result in a *meningocele* in which there is simply a protrusion of the spinal cord coverings to form a sac which contains CSF. This defect accounts for less than 10% of infants born with spina bifida. There are no neurological sequelae from the meningocele itself and treatment is excision of the sac and closure of the dura and overlying structures. Fascial flaps can be brought across the spina bifida defect and no attempt is made to alter the bony structure. The problem which may occur in these infants is the development of progressive hydrocephalus. Some infants already have hydrocephalus at birth and others develop it after excision of the meningocele.

The more severe forms of spina bifida involve neural tissue and range from the *meningomyelocele* (*myelomeningocele*) to the most severe end of the spectrum, myelocele, in which the cord lies exposed with no covering. The most common site of these lesions is the thoraco-lumbar area in which case there is severe impairment of neural function in the lower half of the body. This affects both the motor and the sensory aspects to a level distal to the lesion. The next most common site is the sacral area and affected infants may have much less severe affliction of the lower limbs, but defective neural supply to the bowel and bladder may give rise to serious problems of incontinence.

Effective management of the infant born with spina bifida depends on an initial detailed clinical examination and assessment of level of neurological impairment. Motor and sensory deficits are charted usually by physiotherapists who continue to help parents in managing the lower limb defects. The lack of muscle pull on the bones may leave them weaker than normal and care in handling the infant is necessary to prevent fracture of their fragile bones. In consequence of the intrauterine paralysis which occurs in many of these children, there may be secondary structural problems and deformities such as loss of the normal lumbar lordosis and kyphosis. These problems progress with time as they are secondary to imbalance of muscular activity. Similar imbalanced muscle activity may result in dislocation of the hips, deformities of the knees, or severe feet deformities (talipes). On the initial examination it is also important to assess upper limb function which is normal in the majority of infants, but in a small number, due to further cord problems, upper limb problems become apparent as time goes by. A very common accompaniment of spina bifida is hydrocephalus and this will in many infants be progressive and require active treatment.

Treatment of the infant with spina bifida is to maximise the potential of the child rather than being in any way curative. The neurological problem has been in existence for 6 or 7 months before birth and the exposed neural tissue is irrevocably damaged. However, in some infants early closure of the back defect may be indicated to prevent infection and fibrosis affecting parts of the spinal cord which were not previously damaged. Also closure of the back has an important cosmetic aspect in that it quickly allows the back to be covered by normal skin and is therefore much easier for the parents to manage. The one drawback of early closure of myelomeningocele is that progression of hydrocephalus requiring active treatment is almost invariable, and leaving the larger defects (in which paraplegia is complete) to epithelialise spontaneously can result in the production and reabsorption of CSF becoming balanced so that active intervention is unnecessary. This occurs in one-third of the patients. Decisions have to be made according to the circumstances of each individual child and family.

Encephalocele

Protrusions at the cranial end of the neural tube are usually in the occipital region. These defects are occasionally simply meningoceles, but very much more commonly they contain brain tissue – cerebellum or cerebrum, i.e. encephalocele. There is frequently malformation of the brain in addition to the posterior protrusion which can result in a significant impairment of the intelligence of the child despite the fact that there is no neurological deficit affecting the trunk or limbs. The protruding neural tissue is rarely of any functional value to the infant and is usually excised and closure of the dura over

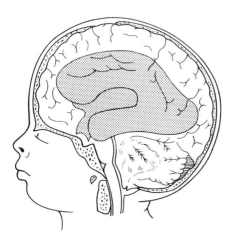

FIGURE 9.7 Hydrocephalus.

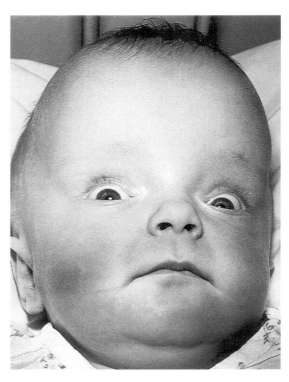

FIGURE 9.8 "Sunsetting sign" due to loss of upward gaze.

the defect is achieved. This leaves a bony defect which may or may not close as the child grows. Hydrocephalus may also complicate this condition and require treatment.

Hydrocephalus

In hydrocephalus secondary to spina bifida there is increased CSF within the ventricular system and dilatation usually of the lateral ventricles, but the third and fourth ventricles may be affected (Fig. 9.7). It is very much more usual that there is enlargement of the head in infants with hydrocephalus. Examination of the head reveals enlarged fontanelles and there may be separation of the cranial bones. Early eye signs are lid retraction followed by failure of upward gaze and ultimately a picture of sunsetting of the eyes (Fig. 9.8). Subsequently there may be sixth nerve palsy with paralysis of lateral rectus giving an internal turning of the eyes (squint). The occipito frontal circumference (OFC) should be measured and charted, taking account of the infant's gestational age. Serial measurements are necessary to establish the diagnosis of progressive hydrocephalus.

Neural tube defects are the most common cause of hydrocephalus but with the survival of an increasing number of small, preterm infants an increasing cause of hydrocephalus is intraventricular or intracerebral haemorrhage. It is a relatively common occurrence particularly in those who have respiratory problems and hypoxic episodes. Intraventricular haemorrhage can occur in term infants. Obstruction to the normal CSF circulation can be associated with structural anomalies of the brain, tumours of the brain or brain stem and post-meningitic states. Most post-infective hydrocephalus is the result of postnatal bacterial infection but on occasion may be due to prenatal

infection, e.g. toxoplasmosis. An infrequent cause of hydrocephalus is the genetically determined X-linked hydrocephalus.

Investigation

A careful history of the family, the pregnancy, delivery and the postnatal course of the infant will usually allow identification of the likely cause of the hydrocephalus. After a full clinical examination has been performed transillumination of the head in a darkened room will demonstrate severe degrees of hydrocephalus. Cranial ultrasound examination can clearly delineate abnormalities of intracranial anatomy and while the fontanelle remains open can be repeated frequently without any risk to the child. In the older patient with a closed fontanelle computerised tomography (CT) has replaced previous methods of ventriculography (Fig. 9.9). For spinal definition magnetic resonance imaging (MRI) is more useful and for individual unusual patients there is a range of highly specialised isotope imaging techniques which give further definition.

Infants with neural tube defects and hydrocephalus have almost always an associated Arnold–Chiari malformation which is a secondary phenomenom and not the cause of the hydrocephalus. In this malformation part of the cerebellum and the medulla extend through the foramen magnum into the upper cervical spinal space. The presence of hydrocephalus does not.

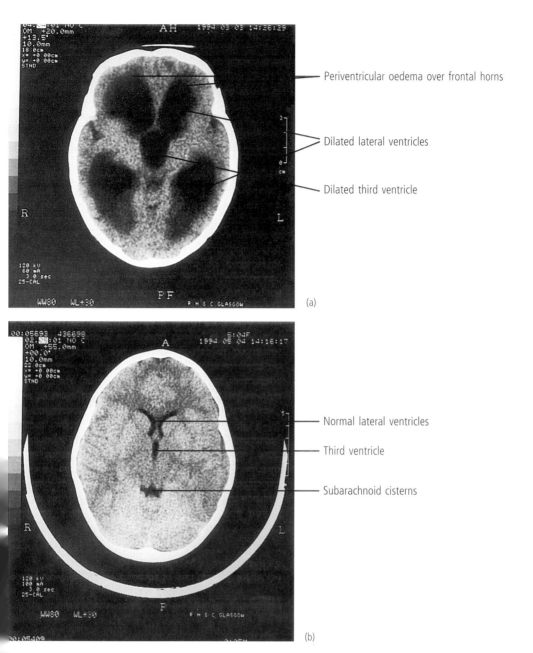

Periventricular oedema over frontal horns

Dilated lateral ventricles

Dilated third ventricle

(a)

Normal lateral ventricles

Third ventricle

Subarachnoid cisterns

(b)

FIGURE 9.9 Acute hydrocephalus. (a) Unenhanced CT scan showing marked dilatation of the third and fourth ventricles due to aqueduct stensosis. There is some oedema in the white matter adjacent to the anterior horns of the lateral ventricles. A normal CT scan (b) taken at the same level is shown for comparison.

n itself, indicate the necessity for any intervention. Hydrocephalus with raised intracranial pressure will cause fullness or bulging of the fontanelle or the progressive enlargement of the head circumference and deviation of head growth away from the normal centiles and will require treatment.

Treatment may be tried with drugs such as isosorbide (up to 2 g/kg body weight × 4/day, i.e. g/kg/day which decreases CSF production and causes diuresis. Sometimes this will give temporary arrest of progressive hydrocephalus but in the majority of infants with associated neural tube defects surgical drainage of hydrocephalus is necessary. The current methods of drainage of hydrocephalus stem from the introduction of the Holter valve which was designed by John Holter, an engineer who had a child with hydrocephalus. In the last three decades there have been many variations of the system originally devised and patented by Holter. These entail insertion of a catheter into a lateral ventricle and then

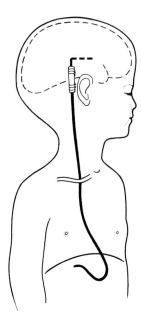

FIGURE 9.10 Ventriculo-peritoneal shunt with one-way valve.

CT scanning will show increased dilatation of the ventricles and periventricular oedema. In such a situation it is not always easy to be certain whether the block is proximal or distal. If the valve is still palpable, pumping the valve will give clinical guidance as to whether there is a proximal or distal block. Early revision of a blocked system returns the child to a normal state and even repeated episodes of block and raised intracranial pressure do not, in the long term, significantly damage the child. In contrast to this, recurrent ventriculitis results in further intellectual impairment.

The outcome for children with hydrocephalus depends on the primary cause of the hydrocephalus. In general, children who have neural tube defects have a spectrum of intellectual ability but the average level is below that of the normal population. Hydrocephalus secondary to intraventricular haemorrhage may result in no detectable impairment of the child's abilities but if there has been significant intracerebral haemorrhage then, depending on the site of the haemorrhage, there will be neurological sequelae.

drained subcutaneously into the peritoneal cavity (Fig. 9.10) or directly into the right atrium via a jugular vein. Incorporated within the system is a valvular mechanism which allows only one-way flow of CSF and these valves are manufactured to function at different pressures. The Holter valve had two one-way valves in series with a compression or pumping chamber between. However, despite considerable refinements in the valves it has not yet been possible to design the perfect valve which will take account of factors such as the temporary increases in intracranial pressure, which occurs when the child is fretful and screaming. With time, some infants progress into a stable situation and do not continue to require their drainage but others continue to be shunt dependent. Blockage may occur at the proximal or distal end of the drainage tube and bacteria may colonise the valve or cause ventriculitis. Blockage produces a rise in intracranial pressure which may cause fits, headache, vomiting, neck stiffness or the child may progress rapidly to an unconscious state and "coning" with cardiorespiratory arrest can occur. Most parents and subsequently the child are the best judge of whether the patient has raised intracranial pressure. Initial changes may be very subtle and the parents, though not always correct, are more often so than inexperienced, or, on occasion, experienced doctors. In a few children, raised pressure may produce very few symptoms and a dangerous sign is impairment of vision. Examination may reveal papilloedema which, if the blockage is promptly corrected, may regress and vision return to normal, but if there is delay, permanent blindness may follow.

THE AUTONOMIC NERVOUS SYSTEM

Pink disease (infantile acrodynia)

This once common and distressing disease of infancy has become extremely rare since mercury (in the form of grey powder or calomel) was removed from the proprietary "teething" or "soothing" powders, so beloved of mothers and so completely lacking any rational justification.

Aetiology

There is strong evidence that the ingestion of mercury in small amounts is closely connected with pink disease. Only a minority of the many infants given mercury developed pink disease and the disease can occur in babies who have apparently never ingested mercury and in whose urine no traces of the metal can be found. It may be that factors or causes other than an unusual sensitivity to mercury explain some cases.

Clinical features

The onset is most often during the early "teething" period with increasing irritability and sleeplessness, severe anorexia, failure to gain weight, and excessive sweating especially over the head and neck. There is often a severe hypotonia although the deep reflexes are retained. Photophobia is striking and the infant often adopts a characteristic knee–elbow position with his face buried in the pillow. The hands and feet look swollen and grossly hyperaemic although they feel cold to the touch. The palms and soles may desquamate. The nose and cheeks may also be unduly red. Generalised but fleeting erythematous rashes may be seen. The invariable tachycardia is marked and its absence excludes the diagnosis. The teeth may become loose and the gums swollen and hyperaemic. Hypertension is common. The children are highly susceptible to respiratory infections which can be dangerous to life or produce permanent bronchiectasis. In their absence complete recovery can be predicted, but only after 3–6 months of a miserable and trying illness.

Treatment

There is no effective specific treatment. Chelating agents such as dimercaprol (BAL) proved to be disappointing. Symptomatic measures include encouraging the infant to take milk, ensuring an adequate intake of vitamins and treating intercurrent infections.

Prevention

It should be accepted by all medical practitioners that there is no place in the paediatric pharmacopoeia for mercurial preparations of any kind.

Familial dysautonomia (Riley–Day syndrome)

This is a rare familial, probably autosomal recessive disease, seen more commonly in Askhenazi Jewish children.

Aetiology

The aetiology remains obscure. There may be some form of faulty neurotransmission.

Clinical features

In severe cases the diagnosis is usually made in infancy but milder cases can remain undetected for years. The striking features are severe hypotonia and muscle weakness with absence of the deep reflexes, excessive salivation, continual sweating and an inability to produce tears. The corneal reflex is usually absent. Difficulty in swallowing is common. There may be markedly delayed psychomotor development. Recurrent pyrexial attacks unassociated with signs of infection may cause anxiety. Periodic erythematous blotching of the skin may occur. Transient episodes of arterial hypertension have been reported, whereas in some cases there has been postural hypotension. In the older child attacks of cyclical vomiting are not infrequent. Another feature is an apparent indifference to pain. Urinary frequency has also been a symptom in some patients; in others inco-ordination can be demonstrated.

Treatment

No specific treatment is available. Behaviour disturbances in some affected children require expert psychiatric attention. The most severely affected children may die in infancy of severe pulmonary complications related to the excessive production of mucus and saliva. In these episodes antibiotics may prove to be life saving.

CONVULSIONS IN INFANCY AND CHILDHOOD

We have considered convulsions of all sorts and from many causes together in this chapter. This is not only because epilepsy is common in children, but also because the nature of other types of infantile convulsions and the extent to which they are fundamentally epileptic are inseparable problems. Some would regard all convulsions as denoting "epilepsy". Most paediatricians would prefer to reserve the term "epilepsy" for the child who is subject to recurring convulsions or lapses of consciousness as a result of a brain disorder producing recurrent paroxysmal discharges and to exclude from this group those convulsions which are not repeated over a prolonged period of time and for which a substantial localised or generalised "provoking" cause can be determined.

Aetiology

Although there was a tendency in the past to regard almost any preceding event as a cause of convulsions, and although today no one would accept such minor peripheral irritations as threadworms, constipation or teething as causative, the majority of convulsions in infancy can be related to a specific provocation. These include perinatal damage, hypoglycaemia, neonatal tetany, the tetany of rickets, intracranial infections, tumours and injuries, inherited metabolic disorders and developmental anomalies of the brain. In the preschool child the common provoking cause for a generalised convulsion is the fever of an acute infection. The speed and height of the temperature rise are more important than the precise nature of the infection which may be otitis media, tonsillitis, pyelonephritis, pneumonia, bacillary dysentery or any of the common infectious fevers. Indeed, the high incidence of convulsions in childhood is largely due to the high incidence of infections.

On the other hand, none of the factors cited above invariably provokes a convulsion in every infant and child. We must, therefore, postulate a convulsive tendency, variable in degree, in some subjects. It is tempting to suggest that in its highest degree it results in idiopathic epilepsy, whereas in those who possess the tendency in a lesser degree a convulsion will occur only when provoked by some specific stimulus and that further convulsions will probably not occur in the absence of the stimulus. It is probably best to restrict the term "epilepsy" to spontaneously occurring losses of consciousness which are entirely dependent upon inherited or inborn convulsive tendencies, and to prefer the word "convulsion", suitably prefixed, for the provoked attacks. But the close inter-relationship between the two groups, which overlap each other, must never be forgotten. It should be stressed further that in a high proportion of epileptic children and in a similar proportion with provoked convulsions a family history of epileptic seizures or of infantile convulsions is obtainable.

Whereas there is a 1 in 200 risk of any child or adolescent experiencing an epileptic seizure, approximately one-third of children and adolescents with learning disabilities, cerebral palsy and autistic disorders will develop epileptic seizures. Such seizures are difficult to treat. The Ohtahara syndrome presents with focal or generalised seizures in the first days or weeks of life, idiopathic infantile spasms (West syndrome) presents with clusters of seizures between 4–6 months of age and Lennox–Gastaut syndrome begins after the first year of life; all are associated with a high risk of severe learning disability.

In some infants repeated seizures are due to an inborn error of brain metabolism, whereby the daily requirements of pyridoxine greatly exceed that in a normal diet. This state is known as *pyridoxine dependency* and it is rapidly amenable to treatment. Various other metabolic disturbances, in addition to hypoglycaemia already mentioned, can cause convulsions: these include hyponatraemia from water intoxication or from retention of water, acute infections of the brain tissues, hypernatraemia from disease of the hypothalamus or frontal lobes or from severe hypertonic dehydration, and lead poisoning. Finally, hypertensive encephalopathy as a cause of convulsions in childhood is not excessively rare.

Clinical types

Various clinical types of epileptic seizures are well recognised and the international classification of seizures is shown in Table 9.2. The electroencephalographic changes are frequently characteristic in the different clinical types but this correlation is by no means firm and a good deal of interlap and mixing of types exist.

TABLE 9.2 International classification of seizures

Primary generalised
   Tonic–clonic (grand mal)
   Myoclonic
   Infantile spasms
   Absences (petit mal)
Partial seizures
   Simple partial
   Complex partial
   Partial with secondary generalisations

Tonic–clonic seizures (grand mal)

This is the commonest clinical manifestation of epilepsy and the only form which provoked seizures take. In children with grand mal seizures, seizures may be precipitated by excessive fatigue or lack of sleep, infectious illness with fever and by withdrawal from anticonvulsant medication. Its features include sudden loss of consciousness, possible injury from falling, tonic followed by clonic spasms, tongue biting, possible urinary or faecal incontinence, frothing at the mouth. It is followed by post-ictal sleep, or a period of confusion or automatism. A careful examination is essential to exclude a provoking cause which requires specific treatment. In febrile attacks the convulsion is short, solitary and occurs at the onset of the illness. A prolonged or recurrent convulsion in a febrile child may well herald idiopathic epilepsy and the physician should be guarded in his prognosis in these circumstances. In grand mal epilepsy the EEG shows most often frequent high-voltage spikes, but there may instead, or in addition, be spike-and-wave or slow-wave patterns. Even a normal EEG is not uncommon in major epilepsy and in no sense excludes such a diagnosis when the history is typical. Evaluation with cranial CT or MR scan for children with generalised tonic–clonic seizures is not routinely required.

Seizures in the newborn rarely follow the classical course of grand mal. The most common manifestation is twitching, often focal, sometimes generalised or there may be generalised tonic contraction with cyanosis, and possibly staring eyes. Convulsion during the first 48 hours of life are usually due to birth trauma, asphyxia or hypoglycaemia. However when convulsions develop in a previously healthy neonate who has had an uneventful birth some 6–8 days previously the most likely cause in artificially fed infants is *neonatal (hypocalcaemic) tetany*. This condition is never found in the wholly breast fed baby, and it has been attributed to the high phosphate content of cows' milk. Another factor in the aetiology of neonatal hypoglycaemia may be degree of vitamin D deficiency in the mothers, who tend to be of higher parity and lower social class. Neonatal tetany is more common in male infants.

especially in late winter and early spring. The diagnosis is confirmed by finding a low serum calcium (below 2 mmol/l; 8 mg/100 ml) and a high serum phosphate (above 2.6 mmol/l; 8 mg/100 ml). Fortunately, brain damage is rare from this cause. There is often an associated hypomagnesaemia and in a very few cases the cause has been hypomagnesaemia without hypocalcaemia.

When clonic seizures occur in early infancy due to *pyridoxine dependency* there are usually some additional and characteristic clinical features which should alert the physician to the underlying cause. These are an extreme irritability and a sensitivity to small noises that indicates true hyperacusis; a remarkable fluttering of the eyelids and upward rolling of the eyes; and repetitive convulsive twitchings. Both the clinical and electroencephalographic abnormalities can be abolished completely with one intravenous injection of pyridoxine hydrochloride 100 mg, although continued oral medication will be required to keep the infant well and to prevent permanent mental impairment.

Myoclonic attacks

These may occur as the sole manifestation of epilepsy or in children who also have grand mal seizures. The attacks are quite transient and consist of a sudden convulsive jerk of the head and neck, or of a limb, without loss of consciousness. The muscular contractions may be sufficiently violent to throw the child to the ground, and repeated soft tissue injuries may occur. The EEG frequently shows atypical slow spike-and-wave or polyspike discharges which are more or less symmetrical.

Akinetic seizures

In these attacks the child suddenly drops to the floor with transient unconsciousness. There may also be other types of epileptic episode and akinetic seizures are commonly seen in children with severe learning difficulties.

Infantile spasms

These have also been called "salaam fits", "flexion spasms", "jack-knife seizures" and "lightning fits". There are three main types of infantile spasms: flexor, extensor and mixed flexor–extensor. Mixed spasms are the most common type followed by flexor spasms; extensor spasms are the least common. The onset is usually between the ages of 3 and 9 months. Mental impairment is a distressingly frequent and irreversible accompaniment of infantile spasms. In about half the children this has been present before the onset of the fits and attributable to such perinatal insults as hypoxia, hypoglycaemia and intracranial haemorrhage, or to prenatal causes such as developmental malformations, toxoplasmosis and tuberous sclerosis, or to an inborn metabolic error such as phenylke-

tonuria. Other infants have appeared to develop quite normally until the onset of the attacks. In some of these the aetiology is known, e.g. encephalitis. Others are "cryptogenic", but a few affected infants have shown evidence of recently acquired cytomegalovirus infection. There is no evidence that pertussis vaccine can cause infantile spasms. The attacks, which are often extremely numerous each day, consist of a series of sudden jerks of the whole body, head and limbs. Most often the head and trunk flex ("jack-knife") suddenly forward while the arms jump forwards or up alongside the head, but the spasms may also be opisthotonic in nature. The fits often become less frequent with the passage of time and may cease spontaneously. They are poorly responsive to the customary anticonvulsant drugs. The EEG always shows gross abnormalities; the most severe and characteristic has been termed "hypsarrhythmia". This amounts to total chaos with asynchrony, high amplitude irregular spike-and-wave activity, no organised discharges and no formal background activity. The triad of infantile spasms, retardation and hypsarrhythmia has become known as the West syndrome. The seizures usually are refractory to standard anticonvulsants. Long-term mental and developmental outcome of patients with infantile spasms is poor.

Absences (petit mal)

This diagnosis should be reserved for those children who show brief, often frequent, lapses of consciousness unassociated with twitching or loss of balance in whom the EEG shows a characteristic 3 per second spike-and-wave pattern. Consciousness and activity are resumed suddenly after a few seconds. There is no post-ictal confusion or drowsiness. Activation, particularly hyperventilation, often can precipitate electrical and clinical seizures. Having the patient take about 60 deep breaths per minute for 3–4 minutes often precipitates a typical attack. Petit mal must not be confused with abortive grand mal or temporal lobe seizures. These may be very brief but there is usually loss of balance or posture, and frequently the eyelids twitch or there are other muscle movements never seen in true petit mal. The distinction is important in treatment. Petit mal attacks may be very frequent in childhood and show a tendency to disappear towards puberty (pyknolepsy). Unfortunately they are not infrequently replaced by grand mal.

Simple partial seizures

In the typical case twitching or jerking starts in one area, arm or limb, and spreads in an orderly fashion until one half or the whole body is affected. The site of the organic lesion may thus be localised. Conjugate deviation of the head and eyes to one side may indicate a lesion in the opposite frontal lobe. Tingling in a foot incriminates the opposite lobe. A visual aura points to the temporal or occipital lobe. However, in children it is not uncommon to have Jacksonian attacks in the absence of a focal lesion in the brain. When one half of the body is affected the attack may be followed by a transient hemiparesis – *Todd paralysis*. A simple partial seizure may progress to a generalised tonic–clonic seizure.

Complex partial or psychomotor seizures (temporal lobe epilepsy)

This type of epilepsy is often difficult to diagnose in childhood because the young child is unable to describe the emotional or sensory elements of the seizures. It may take various forms, each rather bizarre and their epileptic basis should be indicated by their continued recurrence without obvious cause. There is an aura in psychomotor attacks more often than other types of epilepsy in childhood. It may take many forms, e.g. sudden fear, unpleasant smells or tastes, abdominal pain or tinnitus. The attack itself frequently consists of abnormal repetitive movements, e.g. jaw movements, smacking the lips, eye fluttering or blinking, or staring, clasping or fumbling with the hands. Sudden difficulty in speaking or incoherence is common. The most distressing features involve mental disturbances, e.g. violent tantrums, dream-like states or the *déjà vu* phenomenon. Various types of visual, auditory or olfactory hallucinations may occur. There may be post-ictal confusion or sleepiness. The EEG typically shows a focal discharge from the temporal lobe, slow wave or spike-and-wave. Not all cases of psychomotor epilepsy have a temporal lobe discharge and not every case with a temporal lobe focus is associated with psychomotor attacks. Temporal lobe epilepsy is to be regarded always as due to a focal lesion in the brain. It is not idiopathic. Various lesions such as hamartoma have been discovered in young adults undergoing surgery for its treatment. The most common, however, is mesotemporal sclerosis in the region of Ammon's horn. This may be a sequel to perinatal hypoxia, but status epilepticus itself may be the asphyxial incident which is followed by temporal lobe seizures. This observation reinforces the fact that the prevention or treatment of prolonged grand mal seizures is a vitally important matter.

Febrile seizures

The most common convulsive disorder of early childhood is febrile seizures. A febrile seizure is an event in infancy or childhood usually occurring between 3 months and 5 years of age associated with fever but without evidence of intracranial infection or defined cause. Most often febrile seizures are generalised tonic–clonic convulsions and are usually brief and self-limited. There is a genetic predisposition to febrile seizures but the exact pattern of heredity is unknown. Infections are usually of the upper respiratory tract, otitis media and gastrointestinal. In approximately two-thirds of children who experience febrile seizures there is only one febrile seizure.

The value of the EEG in the management of the child with a febrile seizure is doubtful. No investigations are routinely necessary in children after a febrile convulsion. In general children with febrile seizures have a good prognosis and only a small minority of children go on to become epileptic.

Status epilepticus

This dangerous state, which involves a series of grand mal seizures between which the child does not regain consciousness has been described as the sword of Damocles which hangs over every epileptic head. It may develop suddenly, but is a particular danger if anticonvulsant treatment is suddenly withdrawn; parents must be carefully warned against this. For practical purposes status epilepticus is any seizure that lasts more than 30 minutes.

Diagnosis

The first task of the physician must be to exclude an organic cause for the convulsions, by careful history taking and complete clinical examination. When convulsions recur, radiography of the skull and electroencephalography are essential. Lumbar puncture should only be performed when there is a reasonable suspicion of an organic basis, because this minor operation is unpleasant for the child and not wholly devoid of risk. In exceptional cases computerised tomography, magnetic resonance imaging or cerebral angiography will be required. We prefer not to label a child "epileptic" before the age of 2 years.

Prognosis

"Idiopathic" convulsions in infancy frequently herald mental retardation. Poorly controlled epilepsy is often associated with a slow mental deterioration through the years. Severe EEG abnormalities, frequent akinetic or myoclonic seizures, and infantile spasms all augur a gloomy prognosis. On the other hand solitary "febrile" convulsions, hypocalcaemic tetany and epileptic seizures which can be well controlled by drugs are most often associated with normal psychomotor development and they are not incompatible with a high intellectual performance.

Treatment

General

In the case of provoked convulsions it is obvious that early diagnosis followed by specific treatment is essential. The treatment appropriate to many causes such as meningitis, hypertensive encephalopathy, intracranial tumour, etc. is discussed in the appropriate chapters. The common "febrile" convulsion is best treated by tepid sponging to lower the temperature and the infection itself may be amenable to specific therapy. The use of an antipyretic drug is effective and paracetamol is recommended. The best treatment for a prolonged convulsion (over 10 minutes) or for status epilepticus is diazepam, in a dose of 0.1 mg/kg body weight, given by slow intravenous injection. Diazepam 0.5 mg/kg body weight given rectally acts almost as rapidly as when the intravenous route is used and is a completely satisfactory alternative. This drug has largely replaced paraldehyde in the immediate treatment of prolonged grand mal. If the status epilepticus is not rapidly controlled by diazepam resort may be had to intravenous thiopentone, but this should always be administered in an intensive care unit with facilities for assisted ventilation. The deeply comatose child should be nursed in the prone position and the pharynx kept clear by frequent suction. Cyanosis should be relieved by oxygen.

Neonatal tetany can be quickly relieved with oral calcium chloride in solution, 300 mg 4-hourly for 3 days; the calcium is poorly absorbed but the chloride ion enters the blood to produce a metabolic acidosis. Alternatively, the serum calcium level may be raised with 10% calcium gluconate, 5 ml intravenously (slow injection). As hypocalcaemia is often associated with hypomagnesaemia it is recommended that a 50% solution of magnesium sulphate 0.2 ml/kg be given intramuscularly on two or three occasions at 12 hourly intervals. With this, both hypocalcaemia and hypomagnesaemia are corrected. Convulsions related to relative deficiency of pyridoxine will stop after 100 mg pyridoxine given intravenously. Thereafter oral pyridoxine should be given continuously in a dosage of 50–100 mg/day. A test dose of pyridoxine given intravenously is worth a trial in every case of "idiopathic" convulsions in infancy which does not respond to anticonvulsants, preferably with EEG monitoring.

Anticonvulsants

The aim of treatment is to control, or prevent if possible, the recurring seizures of the epileptic, and to achieve this with one drug. A combination of anticonvulsants is only rarely to the epileptic child's advantage. There may be value in estimating the serum concentrations of the anticonvulsants, particularly indicated when the response to treatment is poor, when adverse reactions develop, or when suspicion arises that administration of the drug is irregular. The therapeutic ranges for some of the more commonly used drugs are: phenobarbitone 80–100 µmol/l (15–40 µg/ml), phenytoin 40–80 µmol/l (10–20 µg/ml), carbamazepine 25–50 µmol/l (6–12 µg/l), sodium valproate 350–700 µmol/l (50–100 µg/ml), ethosuximide 300–750 µmol/l (40–100 µg/ml) These ranges are only guidelines and the optimal values for an individual may lie well outside these ranges. The dose of the anti-epileptic drug is optimal when the child is seizure free and experiencing no (or acceptable) side effects.

Phenobarbitone has had a long history as the drug of first choice for tonic–clonic seizures. However, it has considerable disadvantages in children. These include drowsiness, restlessness and behaviour disorders in a fair proportion of patients. Most paediatricians prefer *phenytoin*, which is a highly effective anticonvulsant, less inclined to cause drowsiness, and reasonably inexpensive. A suitable dose is 30–50 mg twice daily, increasing to 100 mg thrice daily if necessary. Overdosage results in ataxia and it is helpful to monitor serum concentrations. An unwelcome although reversible side effect is hypertrophy of the gums, seen in a sizeable proportion of patients. Furthermore, prolonged medication can result in hirsutism, coarsening of the facies towards an acromegaloid appearance and acne. Very rarely the appearance of a rash is an imperative indication for withdrawal of the drug because of the danger of agranulocytosis. *Carbamazepine* has now become the preferred drug by many paediatricians because it rarely causes drowsiness, and is almost free from the adverse effects of phenobartitone and phenytoin. It has considerable advantages for children and adolescents, in whom learning ability is extremely important. Not only is it effective in grand mal epilepsy but it is the drug of choice for temporal lobe seizures. It may cause ataxia if started in full doses too abruptly. A suitable initial dosage is 100 mg twice daily, increasing gradually to 200 mg three times daily as required. *Sodium valproate* is highly effective in grand mal epilepsy but, unlike any of the other drugs mentioned above, it is also effective against petit mal or "absence attacks" and myoclonic jerks. It has very little sedative action. Adverse reactions include mild nausea and transient alopecia, but they are rare. The dosage is 20–30 mg/kg/day, but the value of estimating the serum concentrations is less than for other drugs as it seems to have a longer action than its half-life (4–14 hours) would suggest. It is often effective with a twice-daily dose. In a very few children it has caused acute liver failure or pancreatitis and some might regard this as an unjustifiable risk in a disorder which is itself unlikely to threaten life. Another drug effective against grand mal is *primidone*. Its usefulness is limited by the frequency with which it causes ataxia, although this usually disappears if small doses are persisted with for a few weeks. The initial dose should not exceed 125 mg twice daily increasing gradually to 250 mg thrice daily. Primidone is partially metabolised to phenobarbitone and occasionally causes drowsiness and behaviour problems. On the other hand, it is inexpensive. Both primidone and phenytoin can cause megaloblastic anaemia, but only very rarely in children. The anaemia responds to folic acid but not vitamin B_{12}.

In petit mal or absence seizures alone the drug of choice is ethosuximide, in a dosage of 125–250 mg twice or thrice daily. Adverse reactions are uncommon; they include nausea, drowsiness and ataxia. However, if petit mal is accompanied by grand mal, ethosuximide alone is inadequate and may even aggravate the latter. In this situation the drug of choice is probably sodium valproate despite the small risk involved. Myoclonic attacks are much more difficult to control. Sodium valproate would be our first choice, although an alternative is *clonazepam*. It should be started with a single evening dose of 250–500 µg gradually increasing to a daily dose of 1–6 mg in three to four divided doses. It should be noted, however, that clonazepam can cause quite severe behaviour disorders in some children, particularly those of an aggressive nature. Finally, the point should be made that brain-damaged children respond much less favourably to all the anticonvulsant drugs than those with "idiopathic" epilepsy.

Infantile spasms are remarkably unresponsive to any of the anticonvulsant drugs although they sometimes cease spontaneously with time. At present, the only known effective treatment for infantile spasms is ACTH or corticosteroids. The therapeutic efficacy of these two drugs is relatively equal and one may be effective if the other drug fails. In many cases the fits can be stopped or markedly reduced in frequency with ACTH (corticotrophin) given intramuscularly in doses of 40 units/day, or with prednisolone given orally in doses of 20–30 mg/day. A 21-day course of treatment is usually sufficient, although in some cases prolonged but reduced dosage is necessary. Unfortunately control of the fits is rarely accompanied by significant intellectual improvement although "cryptogenic" cases may not suffer intellectual impairment if diagnosis and treatment are sufficiently prompt.

Social management

The epileptic child whose convulsions can be prevented or rendered infrequent should attend an ordinary school and live as normal a life as possible. The physician must by explanation and advice bring the parents to accept the need for an unrestricted existence and even to accept a few risks. Certain restrictions such as riding a bicycle in the city streets or mountain climbing are clearly unavoidable, but they should be reduced to the minimum. For many children and their families, social and psychological factors far outweigh those problems associated with the prevention and control of seizures. A multidisciplinary approach, provided within a specialist clinic, with support and advice from a clinical nurse specialist, with help from relevant voluntary support organisations and occasionally from psychologists and psychiatrists has proved helpful to some families. Special schooling may be necessary for the learning-impaired epileptic. The assistance of voluntary agencies devoted to the problems in society of the epileptic should be sought if later difficulties of social adjustment or employment arise. It is an unfortunate fact that the epileptic adult often proves "difficult" with his fellows in industrial rehabilitation units, sheltered workshops and vocational training centres so that he derives less benefit than he might. It is also sad to relate that members of the general public, including non-medical professional people, are often ill-informed about epilepsy so that they are less helpful towards the epileptic than they would be towards other handicapped persons. None the less, the majority of epileptics who are of normal intelligence are today enabled to live valuable and normal lives in a wide variety of professions and trades.

Breath-holding attacks

These occur not infrequently in infants or toddlers and they are usually precipitated by pain, indignation or frustration. Shortly after the onset of a fit of loud crying, the infant suddenly stops breathing in expiration and becomes cyanosed. If inspiration does not quickly follow the infant loses consciousness and goes rigid with back arched and extended limbs. He may have a few convulsive twitches. Respiration always starts again with rapid recovery and there is no danger to life. The susceptibility to breath-holding attacks is usually short-lived and they cease spontaneously as the child matures. The EEG shows no abnormality between or during attacks. These attacks are not epileptic and they do not require any treatment. Their differentiation from epileptic seizures, in the absence of personal observation, rests upon good history from an observant mother. When there is doubt an EEG should be advised.

Reflex anoxic seizures

Reflex anoxic seizures are not uncommon and occur in infants and children who have exaggerated vagal cardiac reflexes. Attacks may be precipitated by pain which causes reflex cardiac asystole with sudden onset of extreme pallor, loss of posture and muscular hypotonia. Recovery takes place as quickly as the onset with the resumption of ventricular contractions.

CEREBRAL PALSY

The term "cerebral palsy" is used here to denote "a disorder of movement and posture resulting from a permanent, non-progressive defect or lesion of the immature brain". An enormous amount of interest in the problems of cerebral palsy (CP) has been generated in the past 30 years. Some of this has been so emotionally charged that it has at times been misdirected. Some workers have been led to make unrealistic claims for various therapeutic and educational methods. Even now, we are a long way from understanding the problem sufficiently to plan a completely rational and reasonable economic system of diagnostic, therapeutic and educational help for affected children. The incidence of CP is in the region of 2.5 per 1000 in childhood. Figures have always varied from one country to another. The problem is, therefore, a large one. It is essential to stress, also, that children who suffer from CP frequently have other severe handicaps. Approximately 50% of cerebral palsied children have an intelligence quotient (IQ) below 70, as compared with 3% of the general population. Furthermore, while 75% of the general population have IQs above 90 this applies to only 25% of the CP group. Epileptic seizures are common in cerebral palsied children and speech defects occur in about 50%. Most commonly the problem is simply one of retarded speech development which tends to parallel the degree of learning disorder. Speech dysrhythmias and different forms of dysarthria also occur in spastic, ataxic and athetoid children. In the athetoid group in particular, retardation of speech is commonly due to impairment of hearing. Squints occur in almost one-half of all affected children. Refractive errors are common, especially degenerative myopia in children of low birthweight. Blindness is not uncommon, especially in the severely spastic group. Other ophthalmological abnormalities include defects of the choroid, retina and optic nerve. Visual field defects are especially common in hemiplegics. Deafness, frequently unsuspected, is common, especially in athetoid cases when it is of high-tone distribution. It should be looked for in every affected child. Dental problems are common, such as gingivitis due to defective chewing, tooth grinding and malocclusion. Enough has been said to justify the view that the results of treatment in the cerebral palsied group should be stated with reserve. Some of the highly optimistic claims in this field can apply only to a very small minority of children.

Aetiology

It is frequently impossible to determine the precise cause of CP in individual patients. None the less, a good deal is known about the various causative factors and their varying influence in the different clinical types of CP. In some cases there are *prenatal* influences as in cerebral agenesis due to clear genetic factors or unknown origins, rubella in the first trimester of pregnancy, toxoplasmosis transmitted across the placenta, and X-irradiation. Some cases of spastic tetraplegia with severe learning disorders belong to this group. On the other hand, milder cases of spastic tetraplegia and of paraplegia, a group sometimes called "diplegics", show a remarkably high incidence of premature birth and low birthweight. Approximately half of all cases of CP are associated with preterm delivery and birthweights of less than 2500 g although only 7% of the population are of low birthweight. The precise nature of this relationship is not clear although hypoxia and hypotension are important factors. Hypoxia and hypoglycaemia in the preterm infant predisposes to athetoid CP. Another cause of athetosis is kernicterus due to blood group incompatibility or to the hyperbilirubinaemia of prematurity, although phototherapy and the widespread use of replacement transfusion has greatly reduced the incidence of these cases. Other *postnatal* causes of CP include biochemical disturbances such as hypernatraemia or hypoglycaemia, acute infantile hemiplegia, meningitis, subdural haematoma and virus encephalitis. Birth trauma, apart from anoxia, has become relatively uncommon in modern obstetric practice.

Classification of cerebral palsy

There have been several different types of classification, but the problem is difficult due to the frequent occurrence of "mixed" neurological abnormalities in individual patients and because of our inability to determine the aetiology in many cases. The classification shown in Table 9.3 is a modification of that approved by the American Academy for Cerebral Palsy. This divides cases according to the functional disorder present, its anatomical distribution and its severity.

TABLE 9.3 Classification of cerebral palsy

Type of motor disorder
Spasticity
Athetosis
Rigidity
Ataxia
Tremor
Hypotonia
Mixed
Anatomical distribution
Tetraplegia
Paraplegia
Triplegia
Double hemiplegia
Hemiplegia
Monoplegia
Degree of severity
Mild
Moderate
Severe

Spasticity

The spastic group shows the features of lesions of the pyramidal tracts such as muscle spasm which may be of the "clasp-knife" variety, spastic postures of the limbs, exaggerated deep reflexes, ankle clonus, and after the age of 2–3 years an extensor plantar response. The most common type is *spastic tetraplegia* in which all four limbs are involved. This group is subdivided into types I and II. In the common type I spastic tetraplegia the legs are more severely involved than the arms. Variants of this group are *spastic paraplegia* in which the arms are apparently unaffected by ordinary clinical standards, and *spastic triplegia* (which is rare) in which one arm appears to be normal. This group is traditionally called "cerebral diplegia". It is often associated with premature birth; cyanotic attacks or convulsive twitching are common soon after birth and the intelligence is usually only moderately reduced. The degree of motor dysfunction is frequently symmetrical. In the much less common type II spastic tetraplegia the spasticity is extremely severe in all four limbs so that the contractures develop early and disuse muscle atrophy may be marked. Epileptic seizures are common. Pregnancy and birth have usually appeared to be normal which, when considered alongside the not infrequent presence of microcephaly and of other major or minor physical abnormalities, suggests a prenatal failure of development. These children invariably have severe learning difficulties. They have frequently shown abnormal neonatal behaviour such as lethargy, reluctance to feed or convulsions in spite of an uneventful birth, and it is difficult to decide whether these abnormalities occur in the individual baby from adverse perinatal events or because of an abnormally formed brain. The term *double hemiplegia* is reserved for a few children with spastic tetraplegia in which the arms are manifestly more severely affected than the legs. A prenatal defect is often suggested by a family history of mental abnormality or of epilepsy. *Spastic hemiplegia* is a remarkably "pure" type of CP. Approximately two-thirds of the children so affected have congenital hemiplegia. In a few of these there is a developmental malformation of the brain such as hypoplasia or agenesis of a hemisphere. In most, however, the birth details suggest the probability of perinatal hypoxia or trauma during labour or delivery. In the remaining third of hemiplegic children the cause is disease or trauma affecting the brain after birth but within the first few years of life, e.g. acute infantile hemiplegia, meningitis, cerebral thrombophlebitis, encephalitis of various types and subdural haematoma. The right side is more often affected than the left, and the arm more severely than the leg. Sensory loss is common, e.g. impairment of kinaesthetic and two-point discrimination with some loss of postural sense, but the appreciation of light touch, pin prick and temperature is often normal. Hemianopia is not infrequent. Convulsions are common and only sometimes confined to the affected side. Some of these children are of normal or even high intelligence but many are retarded in varying degree. Finally, *spastic monoplegia* implies involvement of one limb only. This is probably a group of mixed aetiology. Thus brachial monoplegia is likely to represent a partial hemiplegia, whereas crural monoplegia may represent a partial paraplegia and fall into the "cerebral diplegia" category.

Athetosis

Various clinical subtypes of athetosis have been described although their neuro-anatomical basis cannot be differentiated. The most common type involves the limbs, trunk and face in irregular, slow, writhing or rotating movements which are, of course, involuntary. The term "choreo-athetosis" has been used for cases in which the writhing athetotic movements have a quick jerkiness which somewhat stimulates the movements of Sydenham chorea. In very young children who are later destined to have persistent athetoid movements there may be a hypotonic phase during which involuntary movements of writhing type are slight and easily overlooked. In others, hypertonicity with opisthotonic spasms or writhing movements of the trunk occur, sometimes called "dystonic athetosis". In some athetoid children there is a marked degree of muscle tension which inhibits the involuntary movements to some degree although the disability is severe. This type is sometimes referred to as "tension athetosis". When athetosis has been caused by kernicterus there is often a high-tone deafness and unless this fact is recognised the degree of learning capacity may be seriously underestimated. It is important to remember that in the athetoid group the degree of learning difficulty may be quite unrelated to the severity of the athetosis.

Rigidity

It is unfortunate that the word "rigidity" has been used with different meanings by different workers. As used here it is not intended to include the contracted muscles of the spastic child nor the tension sometimes accompanying athetosis. The term is used to describe the "lead-pipe" or "cogwheel" muscle stiffness seen typically in lesions of the extrapyramidal system. This amounts to an uneven resistance experienced by the physician when he flexes or extends the patient's limbs. It is, in practice, a distinctly uncommon variety of CP and always accompanied by significant learning disorder.

Ataxia

In a small proportion of children with CP, the clinical manifestations indicate a cerebellar defect, e.g. ataxia reeling gait, intention tremor and past pointing, dysdiadochokinesis, hypotonia and diminished deep reflexes. Nystagmus and positive Romberg sign are comparatively uncommon in ataxic CP. Most of these cases are congenital in origin and due to malformations of the cerebellum. The birth is usually normal. Early diagnosis may be difficult. The early signs are lethargy, relative immobility and hypotonia. Indeed, congenital ataxic cerebral palsy is one of the important causes of the "floppy baby syndrome". In a few cases of ataxic cerebral palsy the onset is postnatal and due to such causes as meningitis, encephalitis and trauma.

Tremor

This type of CP is rare and characterised by a constant, severe coarse tremor. Spasticity and athetosis are rare but true extrapyramidal rigidity is not infrequently also present.

Hypotonia

In a few children CP takes the form of a hypotonic tetraplegia without any spasticity or overactivity of the deep reflexes. This group has sometimes been called "flaccid diplegia". Many infants destined to develop typical spastic tetraplegia pass through a flaccid or hypotonic phase. The true situation is usually revealed by adductor muscle spasm, but in some cases differentiation from flaccid diplegia depends upon continued observation. In benign congenital hypotonia there has usually been a normal birth and later normal development, whereas in flaccid diplegia there has often been perinatal asphyxia and is associated with severe learning difficulties.

The early diagnosis of cerebral palsy

In very severe cases the diagnosis is easy from the early weeks of life, e.g. in type II spastic tetraplegia with severe generalised spasticity and gross developmental delay. In cases of typical kernicterus which survive the acute stage of hyperbilirubinaemia, the certainty of brain damage makes subsequent interpretation of the neurological signs easy. In many cases, however, early diagnosis is extremely difficult and, on occasion, impossible. It can be beyond the skill of the most experienced to decide just when adductor muscle tone is outside normal limits or when the knee jerks are pathologically brisk. The authors freely admit to having been confused rather than assisted by attempts to elicit and interpret most of the primitive reflexes described in the literature, although persistence of the Moro reflex beyond the age of 8–10 weeks is good cause for suspicion of CP. Undue persistence of the stepping reflex, so that the legs may make "cycling movements", is another common finding in infants who have CP. The Landau reflex is also of some value. It is seen normally in infants between the age of 3 months and 1½ years. When the baby is held in the air in the prone position with the examiner's hand under the lower part of the anterior wall of the chest there is extension of the head, arching (to a variable degree) of the spine, and some extention of the hip joints. The Landau reflex is absent in most cases of CP, lower motor neurone disease and severe developmental delay. Valuable indications of spastic cerebral palsy in the young infant are poverty of movement and facial expression, extended or crossed legs when the infant is suspended by the armpits, marked adductor spasm, exaggerated deep reflexes and in the upper limbs a persistently clenched hand with thumb adducted after the first 3 months. At a later age the child may walk on his toes with a typical spastic gait and the plantar responses will by then be extensor. There may be a dissociation in his various developmental stages when mental progress may run ahead of motor skills.

In cases of hemiplegia the contrast between the spastic and normal sides of the body is obvious at an early age to the careful and unhurried observer. Athetosis may only become obvious after the age of 2 years. The child who is later to develop athetotic movements shows delayed motor development in infancy. Opisthotonic spasms with intervening periods of generalised hypotonia, poverty of movement and "floppiness" have frequently been reported in infants who later developed frank athetosis. The Moro reflex persists for several months, as does the asymmetrical tonic neck reflex. In early infancy it may be impossible to distinguish between the developmentally delayed child and the CP child who is also developmentally delayed but the true situation will become clear as time passes. It is always important to keep in mind that delay in speech in cerebral palsied children may be due to spasticity or athetosis of the tongue, or to high-tone deafness. Such delay when associated with athetotic grimacing of the face may lead to an erroneous diagnosis of developmental delay. This can only be avoided by taking a careful history from the time of conception and when doubt remains by formal intelligence testing which must be performed by an experienced psychologist.

Management

The management of children with CP has many facets such as physiotherapy, play therapy, orthopaedic surgery, speech therapy, hearing aids, orthoptic care and education. It is the responsibility of the paediatricians to co-ordinate the whole management as far as possible. The earlier in the child's life treatment can be begun the better will be the result. In many cases of CP the general facilities available from the School Health Service in the United Kingdom are quite adequate. Thus the spastic child with mild learning disorder and with only slight physical disability can be quite well educated at an ordinary school, although he may receive some physiotherapy at a local clinic or hospital. The child with severe learning disorder and with slight physical disability can be managed well enough in a special school for the learning disordered. On the other hand, the spastic or athetotic child who is severely crippled but of normal intelligence is best educated in a special school (day or residential) for cerebral palsied children. Such schools are extremely expensive because they must carry a large and highly trained staff of physiotherapists, occupational therapist, speech therapists, educational psychologists, and specially trained teachers. They must also be visited regularly by paediatrician, otorhinolaryngologist, orthopaedic surgeon, audiometrician and other specialists. There is no doubt that special schools for spastic children achieve some impressive results in the fields of both general and physical education. The residential type of school can also serve a most useful function in difficult cases by admitting children for a short period of weeks during which a much more accurate assessment of the learning and physical disabilities can be made. In the individual child this may then allow his future management at home or at a day school to be more usefully planned. It should be realised that the child who is severely damaged both mentally and physically can never be taught to live an independent and useful existence within the general community. He can be considerably helped in a special school provided his learning disorder is not too severe. In adult life he will require hostel or institutional care. If his intellectual deficits are severe and he cannot be adequately cared for at home admission to a caring institution may be the only reasonable course to advise.

Perhaps the most difficult problem of all, although it is not a common one, is the spastic child of high intelligence who is severely handicapped physically. Although he has the ability to learn, his physical defects, e.g. speech and motor functions, frequently make a real higher education impossible. None the less, if he can be found a place in one of the few highly specialised schools, where he can receive expert physical treatment as well as an advanced education, even a university course may be within his grasp. In the few exceptional successes of this sort which the authors have personally encountered, they have been impressed by the vital element for success in the form of quite outstanding, almost obsessional, parents who had made the most remarkable efforts and self sacrifices on behalf of their child.

It is obvious that for a physical disability such as cerebral palsy physiotherapy has an important part to play, along with general education, speech training, and the amelioration of other physical defects of hearing, vision etc. The physiotherapy must be conducted by workers who have a special interest in the cerebral palsied, and supervised by paediatricians, orthopaedists or neurologists similarly motivated. The results are difficult to assess objectively. They appear to be best in children with moderately severe spasticity and poorest in those with athetosis. They must be accepted as of limited value, but when added to other measures such as special education the results are in some instances highly gratifying. Even more difficult to assess is the place of orthopaedic surgery in cerebral palsy. Ill-conceived operations have frequently done the patient more harm than good. Increasing realisation of this fact has greatly reduced the number of spastic children submitted to surgery, although the orthopaedic surgeon can frequently assist by fitting special leg-irons, boots and the like. The need for the correction of deformities, such as flexion contractures of the thighs and knees, would be diminished if all spastic children had their tight muscles stretched by parents or physiotherapists at frequent intervals each day. All severely palsied children should have the benefit of expert orthopaedic opinion at regular intervals.

A word must be said of the vital part to be played by the parents, especially the mothers, of cerebral palsied children and of the guidance which they should receive. Simple inexpensive equipment for use in the home is available or can be cheaply constructed. Thus a special chair that will allow the spastic child to sit upright can be made for him by a suitable manufacturer. These are available in the UK made to order, at the local Limb-fitting and Appliance Centre. Walking aids of various types can be obtained on the advice of the orthopaedic surgeon. Special handles for feeding utensils, wide-based cups, and suction discs to hold plates in position can be extremely useful. The mother will have to spend much time helping her child to feed himself with a spoon because in this simple way muscle control and co-ordination are encouraged. Some of the difficulties of the cerebral palsied child are probably due to a defective "body image", so that sense of position in space is faulty and incomplete. This makes dressing and undressing difficult, and here again much patience and encouragement are required. The problems can be simplified somewhat by the use of zip and "Velcro" fasteners, slip-on shoes and simple forms of clothing which do not involve the use of buttons. Various forms of help for parents are available from the National Health Service and various voluntary bodies in the community. Finally it should be stated that there is a very limited place for drugs in cerebral palsy. Baclofen has been found useful in reducing the severity of spasticity and the increased muscle tone of dynamic deformities. It will not affect fixed contractures for which some form of orthopaedic surgery is usually required. It has been claimed that levodopa will occasionally produce dramatic results in children with athetoid cerebral palsy. Anticonvulsant drugs are indicated in epilepsy but their effects are frequently disappointing in brain-damaged children. In a few older children or adolescents with congenital hemiplegia complicated by frequent and uncontrollable epileptic seizures, the operation of hemispherectomy has abolished the seizures. The hemiplegia is apparently not much worsened and cerebration may be improved.

LEARNING DISORDERS

The literature on this subject is vast in its extent and in some measure reflects the magnitude of the problem. Indeed, this increases numerically year by year as modern therapeutics keep alive individuals who would in the past have died in childhood of intercurrent infections; and also relatively, as our increasingly complex society makes it more and more difficult to find a niche for the intellectually or socially handicapped. Within recent years there has occurred a change of outlook in enlightened members of the community towards the handling of the mentally subnormal. Instead of a tendency to hide them away from sight at home or in institutions, and an attitude of hopelessness, there is a growing realisation that the learning disordered child is as entitled to education and the opportunity to develop his capabilities as the normal child. Local authorities and education authorities have steadily improved their services. Various voluntary bodies, such as the Society for Mentally Handicapped Children, have done excellent work in initiating services which have not so far been supplied from public funds. They have also done good work in an educative capacity to enlighten public opinion. One of the biggest problems, as yet unsolved, is how to make it possible in a complex society for the mentally subnormal adult to be accorded the right to work. It is obvious that this problem cannot be resolved within the rigid framework of economics and "profit and loss" accounting. The viewpoint that mental handicap is as much a social as a biological problem is one which our society is only now beginning to take seriously.

Definitions

As a group these children have in common learning difficulty. The severely affected have difficulty learning to walk, feed, dress and communicate. The more mildly affected have difficulty in acquiring social and physical skills to enable them to earn a living and cope with the demands of society.

Words used to describe individuals with learning disorders such as the terms mental deficiency, mental, mental retardation or mental handicap are taken to mean a failure of development of the mind. This is in contrast to dementia which means a disintegration of the fully developed mind. These words and others used to describe the severity of the learning difficulty (e.g. idiot = IQ 0–25; imbecile = IQ 25–50; feeble-minded (moron) IQ = 50–70) have become terms of abuse and even the terms mental retardation and handicap are being abandoned. The WHO classification of mental handicap is 0–20 IQ, profound; 20–50 severe; and 50–70, moderate handicap. Although IQ measurement is a rather too broad assessment on which to base specialised educational input for the child, a rough educational classification is that children with an IQ of less than 50 are severely educationally subnormal (ESN) and those between 50 and 70 have moderate ESN. There are, of course, varying degrees of severity of learning difficulty. Those with an IQ below 50 are likely always to need care and attention and unlikely to be educable in any formal sense. Those with an IQ between 70 and 90 are not included within the group of learning disordered children, but they are likely to be educationally backward and to be placed in the lower educational stream of a normal school. Some, in fact, require the facilities and specially trained staff of a special school.

Aetiology

The vast majority of cases of learning disorder can be placed in one of two broad aetiological groups, *primary amentia* which is due to inheritance or defects in the child's genetic material; and *secondary* in which the brain, derived from a normal germ plasm, has been damaged by environmental influences which may be operative prenatally, perinatally or postnatally. In the few cases both genetic and environmental factors combine to result in brain damage. It must be stressed, however, that in individual patients it is quite often impossible to determine the precise cause of the mental retardation. For example, in the case of a severely retarded child apnoeic and cyanotic attacks in the first week of life could indicate brain damage resulting from anoxia or respiratory difficulties due to malfunctioning of an abnormally formed brain.

Inheritance

A large number of single gene defects have been uncovered as causes of learning disorder. Many of these fall into the category of inborn errors of metabolism. They are now numerous and include phenylketonuria, maple syrup urine disease, the organic acidurias, homocystinuria, argininosuccinic aciduria, Hartnup disease, galactosaemia, pyridoxine dependency, Niemann–Pick disease, Gaucher disease, Tay–Sachs disease, mucopolysaccharidoses and others such as Sturge–Weber syndrome, tuberous sclerosis and neurofibromatosis. Some cases of sporadic cretinism and all cases of non-endemic familial goitrous cretinism are also due to single gene defects. Another rare example is familial dysautonomia (Riley–Day syndrome). While the single gene defects cited above are each relatively rare, it has been recognised more recently that X-linked genes are quite frequently responsible for non-specific mental retardation. In many of the affected males a marker X-chromosome has been identified. The marker in this *"fragile X syndrome"* is a *"fragile site"* occurring at band q27 or q28 (i.e. towards the end of the long arm) of the X chromosome. However, not all males with X-linked non-specific mental retardation have this fragile site on the X chromosome. At least three distinct forms of X-linked mental retardation have been described which seem to breed true within families. The most clearly definable is found in males with the marker X chromosome and macro-orchidism. The enlarged testes become obvious after puberty and are only occasionally noticeable at birth. The degree of learning difficulty is usually severe but may be mild. Specific speech delay is common and is associated with a characteristic rhythmic quality of "litany speech". Epilepsy may be a feature in some severely affected boys. In another group of families both the marker X chromosome and macro-orchidism are absent but the other clinical features are indistinguishable from those described above. In the third type of X-linked mental retardation there is no marker chromosome but the affected boys show microcephaly, severe retardation and small testes. The female carriers of the marker X chromosome are generally of normal intelligence although some have been mildly retarded, possibly related to non-random X-inactivation in the central nervous system. Chromosome analysis of boys with non-specific learning disorder is essential for genetic counselling. When the characteristic clinical features described above are present in a boy with no family history the recurrence risk seems to be about 10%.

Some types of mental retardation have been clearly related to gross chromosomal abnormalities. The most severe degrees are usually produced by non-dysjunction during gametogenesis in the mother, leading to trisomy for one of the small acrocentric autosomes. In these conditions the long-recognised correlation with advancing maternal age has been explained on the assumption that the ageing ovum is more prone to favour non-dysjunction. Down syndrome is the most common of the trisomies (about 1.8 per 1000 live births) and is a major cause of profound and severe learning disorder. Only a rare case falls into the moderate category. The incidence of trisomy 21 is about 1.8 per 1000 live births, and it accounts for about one-third of all severely subnormal (IQ of 50 or less) children in the United Kingdom (see Chapter 1).

The next most common autosomal trisomies in live-born children are trisomy 13 (Patau syndrome) and trisomy 18 (Edward syndrome) with frequencies of about 0.5 and 0.1 per 1000 live births respectively. Each causes such severe and multiple abnormalities including profound learning disorders that those affected rarely survive infancy.

A variety of structural chromosome anomalies have also been found associated with severe learning disability. The best defined of these is the *cri-du-chat syndrome*, which is due to partial deletion of the short arm of chromosome 5. About two-thirds of the patients have been females and its frequency at birth is 1/50 000 to 1/100 000 or less. The name of this syndrome derives from the characteristic mewing-like cry which is present from the neonatal period. The birthweight is low. Both physical and mental development are markedly retarded. In *Wolf syndrome* many similar features to the *cri-du-chat* syndrome occur, although the cat-like cry is often absent. It is due to partial deletion of the short arm of chromosome 4.

Rett syndrome

In 1966 Rett described 22 mentally handicapped children, all of them girls, who had a history of regression in development and displayed striking repetitive hand movements. It is now evident that this clinical disorder affects between 1 in 10 000 to 1 in 30 000 female infants, with signs of developmental regression appearing during the first year of life and accelerating during the second year of life. At the onset of the regression in locomotion, manipulation and speech, screaming attacks are common. Rhythmic hand movements with fingers usually adducted and partly extended are characteristic with patting or lightly clapping them, banging the mouth or wringing and squeezing intertwined fingers. In some girls there are choreiform trunk and limb movements and dystonia. As they grow older the girls become more placid, their lower limbs progressively stiff with wasting, scoliosis and respiratory dysrhythmias, hyperventilation and apnoeic episodes. The cause is unknown although a defective gene on the X chromosome has been proposed.

Most of the genetically determined types of disordered mental function discussed so far have been of severe to moderate degree. On the other hand, rather more than 75% of all learning disordered fall into the moderate learning difficulty category (IQ 50–70) and cannot be attributed to single gene or gross chromosomal abnormalities. None the less, it is accepted that genetic influences play the major part in determining the child's intelligence. It is commonplace that persons of high intelligence marry others of high intelligence and that their children are mostly of superior intelligence. Similarly the children born into families of lower than average intelligence tend also to be of somewhat poor intellectual calibre. The dullest of these children will have IQs between 50 and 70. This type of learning disorder has sometimes been called "*simple primary amentia*" and it is due to multifactorial inheritance. There is good evidence that environmental influences also affect intelligence and, of course, the children of highly intelligent parents normally enjoy a much better and more stimulating environment than the children of dull or backward parents. None the less, although a good environment can improve a child's intellectual performance while a bad influence such as emotional deprivation or insecurity in early life can retard him, potential ability is almost wholly derived from inheritance.

Environment

In some cases learning disorder has resulted from damage to a normally developing brain by some noxious environmental influence. They may operate at various periods in the stage of development. Microbial causes of brain damage account for about 10% of all cases of learning disorder associated with microcephaly.

Prenatal

Rubella during the first 12 weeks of pregnancy can certainly damage the fetal brain. Toxoplasmosis may also be associated with mental retardation. Cytomegaloviris is the commonest known viral cause of mental retardation. About 40% of women enter pregnancy without antibodies, about twice the number who are susceptible to rubella. It has been estimated that about 1% of pregnant women in London undergo primary infection and that half of their infants are infected *in utero*. While most of these congenital infections are asymptomatic and only a few exhibit the severe illness, a proportion are subsequently found to have learning disorders or to suffer other neurological deficits. Maternal irradiation has been shown to result in mental retardation with microcephaly, and sometimes microphthalmia as in the survivors of the Hiroshima and Nagasaki atomic attacks. Congenital syphilis is very rare in the United Kingdom today. The effect upon a child's intelligence of adverse environmental factors during the mother's pregnancy, such as poverty, malnutrition, excessive smoking and emotional stress are difficult to assess. They might increase the risk of learning disorder by their association with intrauterine fetal malnutrition. The effects on the fetus of chronic alcoholism in the mother are described on page 291.

Perinatal

There is a well documented association between some of the complications of pregnancy and abnormalities of the brain including mental retardation. These complications such as antepartum haemorrhage, pre-eclampsia, breech presentation and complicated or instrumental delivery are frequently associated with intrapartum fetal anoxia. It is, however, extremely difficult to assess the importance of intrapartum or neonatal anoxia as a cause of later neurological disability.

Postnatal

Postnatal causes of mental retardation include meningitis, encephalitis, hypoglycaemia, bilirubin encephalopathy, subdural haematoma, hypernatraemia and head injury. Lead encephalopathy is a rare but undoubted cause of permanent brain damage. It remains uncertain whether low level lead exposures, with blood levels below 1.9 μmol/l (40 μg/100 ml) may cause some cognitive impairment and possibly behavioural abnormalities.

Diagnosis

In most cases the diagnosis of disordered learning ability can be made in the first year of life, provided the physician is familiar with the stages of development in the normal baby and that he realises the variations which may occur in perfectly normal babies. It is essential that a thoughtful history be obtained from the parents, to be followed by a detailed physical examination of the child. Frequently the child must be seen on several occasions before a final conclusion is possible. There may be factors which indicate that the child is "at risk" and more likely to be retarded than others. These include prematurity, complications of pregnancy or labour, a history of asphyxia neonatorum, intra or periventricular haemorrhage, jaundice in the newborn period, convulsions or cyanotic attacks, maternal rubella or a family history of learning disorder. The basis of the diagnosis of learning disorder may be conveniently discussed under four headings.

Physical abnormalities

Certain physical features are undoubted evidence of associated mental defect. These include the characteristic signs of Down syndrome, microcephaly, cretinism and gargoylism. Other physical abnormalities are often, although not invariably, associated with learning disorder. In this group are cerebral palsy, the bilateral macular choroidoretinitis of toxoplasmosis, Turner syndrome and hydrocephalus. Certain other physical "stigmata" are seen more commonly in learning disordered than in normal people, but in themselves they can do no more than direct the physician's attention towards a more careful assessment of the child's intellectual development. Such peculiarities are a high narrow (saddle-shaped) palate, abnormally simple ears, hypertelorism, marked epicanthic folds and short, curved fifth fingers.

TABLE 9.4 Developmental steps in the normal child

AGE	DEVELOPMENT	AGE	DEVELOPMENT
4 weeks	Head flops back when lifted from supine to sitting position		Points to three or four parts of body on request
	Sits with rounded back while supported		Indicates need for toilet
	Grasp reflex elicited by placing object in palm		Lifts and controls drinking cup
	Responds to sudden noise		Feeds himself with spoon: only slight spilling
	Sucks vigorously		Points to three to five objects or animals in picture book
8 weeks	Almost no head lag when pulled into sitting position	2 years	Runs safely on whole foot: can avoid obstacles
	Sits with almost straight back and head only nods occasionally		Can kick a ball without losing balance
			Can walk upstairs: holding rail coming downstairs
	Grasp reflex slight or absent		Turns door handles
	Smiles readily: vocalises when talked to		Forms short sentences: vocabulary of 50 words
	Follows objects with head and eyes		Spoon-feeds without spilling
12 weeks	No head lag when pulled into sitting position		Can put on hat, shoes and pants
	Sits supported with straight back: head almost steady		Demands constant adult attention
	No grasp reflex: holds objects in hand for short time		Dry most nights if "lifted" at 11 p.m.
	Watches own hand movements	3 years	Walks upstairs with alternating feet
	Turns head towards sounds		Washes and dries hands with supervision
	Recognises feeding bottle placed before eyes		Rides tricycle
6 months	Lifts head from pillow		Draws a man on request – head, trunk and one or two
	Sits unsupported when placed in position		other parts
	Rolls from supine to prone position		Can count up to ten
	Holds feeding bottle. Grasps objects when offered		Discusses a picture
	Drinks from cup		Asks frequent questions
	Transfers objects from one hand to the other		Listens to and demands stories
	Responds to name		Likes to help mother in house, father in garden
	Held standing can bear weight on legs and bounces up and down		Eats with fork and spoon
		4 years	Can dress and undress
	No more hand regard: finds feet interesting		Asks incessant questions
12 months	Understands simple sentences and commands		Climbs ladders and trees
	Can rise to sitting from supine position		Engages in imitative play, e.g. doctor or nurse
	Pulls to standing position by holding on to cot side		Uses proper sentences to describe recent experiences
	Walks holding hand or furniture		Can give name, age and address
	Speaks a few recognisable words		Draws man with features and extremities
	Points to objects which are desired		Matches four primary colours correctly
	Throws objects out of pram in play		Plays with other children
15 months	Walks unsteadily with feet wide apart: falls at corners		Alternately cooperative and aggressive with adults or
	Can get into standing position alone		other children
	Tries untidily to feed himself with spoon	5 years	Runs quickly on toes: skips on alternate feet
	Plays with cubes: places one on top of another		Can tie shoelaces
	Indicates wet pants		Can name common coins
	Now seldom puts toys in mouth		Draws recognisable complete man
	Shows curiosity and requires protection from dangers		Names four primary colours: matches 10–12 colours
18 months	Can walk upstairs holding on to hand or rail		Uses knife and fork
	Can carry or pull toy when walking		Cooperates more with friends: accepts rules in games
	Can throw ball without falling		Protective towards younger children and pets
			May know letters of alphabet and read simple words

Delayed psychomotor development

It is characteristic of the learning disordered child that his development is delayed in all its parameters. He is slow in showing an interest in his surroundings, slow in attempting to handle or play with objects, slow to sit or stand unsupported or to walk on his own, late in speaking, late in acquiring bladder or bowel control. A lack of concentration or sustained interest is also obvious. Thus, after handling a new toy or object for a minute or two he loses interes and throws it down. His lack of interest in thing around him may raise the suspicion of defectiv vision, just as his lack of response to sounds is apt t lead to a mistaken impression of deafness. Infantil practices tend to persist beyond the normal perio e.g. putting objects into his mouth, excessive an prolonged posturing of his hands and fingers befor his eyes, drooling and slobbering. The physician mus obviously be familiar with the various developmenta stages of normal infants and children before he is in a position to make a judicious assessment of an individual patient. A brief outline of the more positive developmental steps is shown in Table 9.4. The best assessment is to be expected from the doctor who has had long and intimate contact with normal children in the Child Health Clinic or in their family practice, provided that during their undergraduate period they have developed the capacity to observe, and to appreciate the significance of their observations.

Abnormal behaviour and gestures

Learning disordered children frequently engage in types of behaviour and mannerisms which are obviously abnormal for their age. Thus, in early infancy the retarded baby may be excessively "good" in that he will lie in his pram for long periods without crying or showing restlessness, interest in surroundings, or boredom. In other cases there is constant or prolonged and apparently purposeless crying. Teeth grinding when awake is a common and distressing habit of many with profound learning disorders. The older child may exhaust his mother by his aimless overactivity which may at times endanger his life. Certain rhythmic movements although by no means confined to learning disordered children are more commonly indulged in by them and for more prolonged periods. These include head-banging, body-rocking to-and-fro, and head-rolling. Profoundly disordered children frequently lack the normal capacity for affection, they may be prone to sudden rages, and they may assault other younger children.

Convulsions

Most epileptics are of normal intelligence. None the less, epileptic seizures occur more frequently among mentally retarded children than those who are normal. Frequently repeated generalised seizures lead to slowly progressive intellectual deterioration. The association of infantile spasms (hypsarrhythmia) with severe learning difficulties has been described previously.

Differential diagnosis

The diagnosis of learning disorder is obviously one in which the physician must not be wrong or he will cause the parents unjustifiable and unnecessary grief and anxiety. Some infants have a "slow start" but catch up later, and in the absence of manifest physical signs, such as microcephaly or Down syndrome, a firm diagnosis of learning disorder should only be made after a period of observation during which the rate of development is assessed. There are now available developmental screening protocols in which a child's development can be charted in a longitudinal fashion, making it easier for the less experienced

doctor to detect early departures from the normal. It is easy to confuse learning disorder with cerebral palsy. Indeed the two frequently coexist. Careful neurological examination, repeated on several occasions, will reveal the motor handicaps of cerebral palsy. The deaf child has frequently been diagnosed as mentally retarded, sometimes with tragic results. This mistake should not occur when the physician takes a detailed history and follows it with a careful physical examination. The deaf child will, of course, show a lively visual interest and his motor skills will develop normally. A difficult if not very common problem is the child who fails to develop speech (developmental dysphasia). He is readily confused with the learning disordered child although here too a careful history and period of observation will reveal that in other respects his psychomotor development is proceeding normally. Particular caution is required in the intellectual assessment of the child who has been emotionally deprived by the break-up of his home, death of his mother, or who has been otherwise bereft of normal security. It may require a long period outside an institution before he can be assessed.

Until recently many autistic children were wrongly labelled mentally defective. In a sense such children are defective because they cannot be normally educated and the prognosis is not good. None the less, the autistic child has often a revealing intelligent expression, and in his reactions to objects and various test materials shows considerable innate ability to the careful observer. The most characteristic features of infantile autism are a complete lack of interest in personal relationships which contrasts with an interest in inanimate objects; frequently a preoccupation with parts of objects but not in their real functions; abnormal posturings, as with the hands and fingers, or abnormal interest in the parts of the body; a tendency to react violently and unhappily to changes in environment; loss of speech or failure to acquire it, or the meaningless use of words or phrases; grossly abnormal mannerisms such as rocking, spinning or immobility (catatonia). The most outstanding feature of the autistic child is the way he rejects social contacts. None the less, although he is aloof, does not respond to a greeting with a smile, does not wave goodbye and so forth, he is yet aware of social contact. Thus, he may engage furiously in one of his more irritating mannerisms when someone enters his presence and cease whenever he is left alone. There is an odd high incidence of professional and educated people among the parents of autistic children. Such children, of course, are wrongly placed in institutions for profound and severe learning disorders. Some have responded considerably to psychotherapy as outpatients or inpatients in departments of child psychiatry. None probably becomes a normal child. (See Chapter 10.)

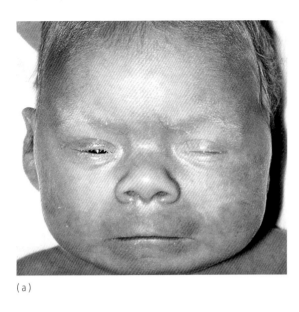

(a)

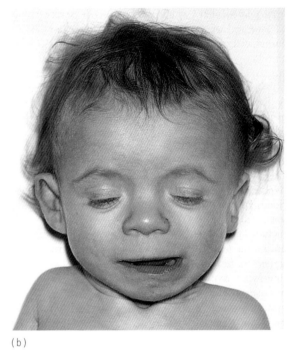

(b)

FIGURE 9.11 (a) Newborn infant with fetal alcohol syndrome. Note absence of philtrum, short palpebral fissures, upturned nose and broad nasal bridge. (b) Same child aged 1 year. Dysmorphic features have become more marked.

Intelligence tests

Psychological testing and evaluations are of considerable although limited value in providing an estimate of a child's probable potential ability. They cannot, naturally, take into account the influence of such variables as zeal, ambition, interest, encouragement or the lack of it, good or bad teaching and so forth. There are many aspects of intelligence and personality and the various tests assess these in different degrees. It is not proposed here to describe these tests in detail; they are reliable only in the hands of the expert. The most commonly used are: the Gesell tests for infants and the modifications of Cattell and Griffiths; for older children the Stanford–Binet scale and the revised test of Terman and Merrill, also the Wechsler Intelligence Scale for Children; for adolescents and adults the Wechsler Adult Intelligence Scale and Raven's Progressive Matrices. There are also several useful personality tests of which the best for the mentally retarded are the Rorschach test and the Goodenough "Draw-a-Man" test. In the case of the school child it is also important to enquire as to educational progress. An evaluation of the results of various tests competently performed is of great value in planning suitable education or training for the mentally handicapped child.

Specific types of learning disorder

Some types of retardation have already been described in previous chapters. Phenylketonuria, galactosaemia, maple syrup urine disease and cretinism are especially important in that timely diagnosis and treatment can often prevent or ameliorate the mental subnormality.

Microcephalus

Severe microcephaly is recognisable in the neonatal period. It is frequently genetically determined (autosomal recessive) and may be familial. Apart from its smallness the head has a characteristic shape with narrow forehead, slanting frontoparietal areas, pointed vertex and flat occiput. The neck is short and the sudden movements of the head give the child a bird-like appearance. The ears are often large and abnormally formed. There may be a receding chin. Generalised muscular hypertonicity is a common feature. Convulsions frequently develop. These children have profound learning disorder, are often devoid of the capacity for affection and sometimes dangerous to younger children.

These genetic conditions which probably have underlying biochemical abnormalities can be distinguished from microcephaly which is secondary to severe brain damage such as toxoplasmosis, encephalitis and maternal irradiation during pregnancy.

The fetal alcohol syndrome

A distinctive pattern of altered growth and morphogenesis can be recognised in the children of mothers who consume large quantities of alcohol during pregnancy. They exhibit both pre- and postnatal growth failure involving weight, length and head circumference. Neurological abnormalities include hypotonia, irritability and jitteriness, poor co-ordination, hyperkinesis, and learning difficulties which may vary from severe to mild. Dysmorphic features include short palpebral fissures (canthus to canthus), epicanthic folds, hypoplastic or absent philtrum, thin upper lip, broad nasal bridge with upturned nose and mid-facial hypoplasia (Fig. 9.11). Other congenital anomalies may involve the heart, genitourinary system, eyes, ears, mouth or skeleton. Haemangiomata and herniae are not uncommon. Abnormal palmar creases and hirsutism have also been recorded. A review of the problem in the west of Scotland showed that the mothers of the 40 affected infants drank heavily while pregnant and most were socially deprived. Apart from the clearly identifiable syndrome produced in the fetuses of women who drink heavily there is increasing concern that even moderate drinking during pregnancy may adversely affect fetal growth and development and subsequent learning ability. Until the situation is clarified it would seem prudent to advise total abstinence from alcohol during pregnancy and possibly even before conception.

The prevention of learning disorders

The prevention of neurological disorder has become increasingly possible in recent years. Indeed, the more efficient application of knowledge which has been available to us for some years would considerably reduce the present incidence of brain damage from such disturbances as perinatal hypoxia, hypoglycaemia, kernicterus and hypernatraemia and the prevalence of maternal rubella by the institution of anti-rubella vaccination. Screening programmes during the neonatal period for several of the treatable inborn errors of metabolism such as phenylketonuria, homocystinuria, maple syrup urine disease, galactosaemia as well as congenital hypothyroidism are making some impact upon the number of learning impaired children in the United Kingdom.

A most important development in the field of prevention is to be found in *prenatal diagnosis*. This is most often based upon examination of the amniotic fluid obtained by transabdominal amniocentesis between the 14th and 16th weeks of pregnancy and supported by ultrasonography. Sampling of chorionic villi or fetal blood or tissue may also be employed in selected cases. Chromosome analysis of amniotic cell cultures may reveal abnormalities such as trisomies 21, 13 and 18, or trisomy affecting the sex chromosomes (XXX and XXY). It may, on the other hand, lead to a diagnosis of 21/14 translocation in the fetus when one of the parents is known to be a translocation carrier and other more complex translocations have also been demonstrated. The sex of the fetus can also be determined when there is a known sex-linked inherited disease in a family, and where the risk to male progeny is 50:50. While most of the X-linked disorders are not associated with learning disorder (e.g. haemophilia) a few, such as Hunter syndrome (Chapter 16) do lead to progressive mental deficiency.

Recent years have seen a rapid increase in the number of inborn errors of metabolism which are capable of prenatal diagnosis. A considerable number of these are associated with progressive neurological deterioration. Most are autosomal recessives although a few are X-linked. The laboratory techniques involved include enzyme assays on cultured amniotic fluid cells, measurement of stored metabolites, and biochemical analysis of the liquor. The increase in the list of inborn errors involved is too rapid for any textbook to keep up to date but in Britain the highly sophisticated techniques employed are confined to a small number of specialised laboratories from which the latest information on both pre- and postnatal diagnosis can be obtained.

Analysis of fetal blood obtained at fetoscopy has also been applied in the prenatal diagnosis of the haemoglobinopathies. Molecular genetic techniques will allow earlier diagnosis and intervention.

When severe and irreversible disorders of the fetus are recognised prenatally therapeutic abortion may be advised. This is a complex problem with ethical, legal and religious implications, but for most people in Britain termination of pregnancy is a preferred alternative to having a severely handicapped child. Occasionally, prenatal testing will reveal a treatable disease, as when congenital adrenal hyperplasia due to 21–hydroxylase deficiency is confirmed by a high level of 17–hydroxyprogesterone in the amniotic fluid, when no delay should arise in instituting appropriate treatment from the time of the infant's birth. *In practice it has been found that in the majority of cases involving prenatal diagnosis the extreme parental anxiety which is common in this situation is relieved because in most instances the fetus is found not to be carrying the chromosomal or enzyme abnormality.*

Prenatal diagnosis demands careful selection of patients as the techniques are not entirely devoid of risk and there can be no absolute guarantee of success. Not only must there be full discussion and investigation of the family problems, but there must also be close liaison between the clinicians, geneticists and the laboratories. This should preferably be undertaken before and not after the female partner has become pregnant. Suitable indications for prenatal diagnosis include:

1 Advancing maternal age, where the risk of chromosome abnormalities, particularly trisomy, is increased.
2 When either parent is a translocation carrier or has chromosomal mosaicism with a high risk of an abnormal fetus.
3 When there has previously been a child with a chromosomal abnormality such as Down syndrome.
4 In families with X-linked and certain autosomal recessive diseases.

Management of children with learning impairment

The concept of management rather than treatment is central to the care of the learning disordered child. Treatment involves measures aimed at curing or improving a disorder or disability. Management is the continuing totality of all treatments of all the patient's dimensions – somatic, intellectual, emotional and social.

It must first be stated that with the exception of cretinism, phenylketonuria, galactosaemia, and a few other rare inborn errors of metabolism there is at the present time no specific treatment for the learning disordered. The only drugs of value are anticonvulsants for children who also have epileptic seizures, and sedatives for restless hyperkinetic children.

Secondly, the authors would state their opinion that once the physician has reached a definite diagnosis of developmental delay in a child, but not before, he must impart this information to the parents. This task requires time, tact, abundant sympathy and understanding, but it must be discharged in simple unambiguous phrases. In the case of the very young child, the doctor would be wise not to commit himself too firmly or too soon to an assessment of degree or to a forecast as to educability. These matters can be resolved with time, and it is the physician's duty to see the child and his parents regularly, and to be prepared to give of his time to answer their many questions. In particular, the irrational feelings of guilt which many parents have on hearing that their child has a significant learning disorder must be assuaged by quiet discussion and explanation. Some parents will refuse to accept the situation at first. They may "go the rounds" of the specialists seeking a happier diagnosis. This is completely understandable. At the end of the day they will still require and

merit all the help which their personal physician can offer. This is often particularly necessary when the child is at home with normal brothers and sisters where many different stresses and strains can arise. Genetic counselling will frequently be indicated, and the physician should also consider discussing contraception with the parents. They may well need guidance as to where these services can be obtained.

The child with an IQ between 50 and 70 is usually educable at a special school (day or boarding). His progress there will depend not only upon his innate ability but on the support and training he receives, and has earlier received, from his parents. The child who proves unable to benefit from formal education at a special school, can be placed in an occupation or training centre. Here he is taught social behaviour and simple manual skills. While the child whose IQ is around 50 is never likely to be educable to the extent that he can be self-supporting, it is a considerable advantage to him to become socially acceptable. It is undesirable that a mentally retarded child should be sent to an ordinary school if he is intellectually quite unable to benefit from such education. Suitable placement at the beginning will frequently avoid the behaviour problems and frustrations from which the retarded child must suffer if he is kept for long in an ordinary school competing with children of normal intelligence. The ability of a child to benefit from education at a special school or his suitability only for a training centre is not solely dependent on his IQ. Some children who do well at special schools have lower IQs than others who have to be transferred to training centres. Important factors are the child's personality and behaviour patterns, his home environment, and his willingness to learn. In preparation for school or training centre it is an advantage if the retarded child can be admitted to a suitable day nursery from the age of 2–3 years. This helps him to make social contact with other children while also relieving the mother of some of her load.

Children with profound learning disorder may require placement in small units specially adapted to their needs. Very few such units are available in the UK. As a general rule the earlier this category of child is placed the better, because a prolonged stay at home may cause the parents to neglect their normal children or the parents of a first-born learning disordered child to deny themselves further children. However, each case must be assessed on its merit with due regard for the parents' wishes, the home and financial circumstances, the ages and reactions of the other children in the family, and the behaviour and general condition of the child. Some of the voluntary societies run short-stay homes in which the child can stay while the parents have a holiday on their own or during illness or pregnancy in the mother. The Down syndrome child is more often kept at home because he is happy and good natured. The child with aggressive or destructive tendencies is likely to be placed in an institution at an earlier age. Some retarded children find their way into institutions because they break the law and prove to be out of control, although they may be less severely retarded than other children who remain happily at home. There is, furthermore, a shortage of accommodation in suitable units in the UK and severely affected children too frequently have to spend several years on a waiting list before a place can be found for them. This can result in great distress in some homes and it is in such circumstances that voluntary bodies can often help the parents and the child. Paediatricians in the hospitals of the National Health Service can also help in emergency situations by admitting the child for a limited period to the ordinary paediatric ward or respite unit.

The paediatrician is frequently asked about the employment prospects of children, although it is not strictly a paediatric problem. Provided the child is physically fit he will be capable in many instances of simple manual work. Many jobs in modern industry are repetitive and do not require a great deal of intelligence. It must be realised, however, that the learning disordered adult is incapable of forethought, of planning their future financial or marital arrangements, even although they may be capable of efficiently performing a repetitive type of skill. This fact makes their future prospects unpredictable and not a matter for optimism. There has recently grown up the idea that hostels for the learning disordered could allow them to become economically self-supporting, while still having available constant advice and a measure of supervision. In practice, it will be a long time before suitable hostels can be built and before there is a sufficiency of trained staff and social workers. It may take even longer to educate the general public to see the desirability of such provisions.

10

Disorders of Emotion and Behaviour: An Introduction to Child and Adolescent Psychiatry

The contents of this chapter are different in many ways from those which have preceded it. The disturbances to be discussed are not usually based upon an "organic" disease. Although the techniques of brain scanning and knowledge of neurochemistry are becoming more sophisticated, it is only in the minority of these disorders that laboratory investigations yield useful information. While there has been some improvement in the measurement of symptoms like depression and some attempts to quantify some parameters of family disturbances, these data rely on questionnaires or rating scales which are less objective than most laboratory or clinical tests. When a diagnostic formulation is reached, the treatment or management still varies in the hands of different physicians or psychiatrists. Finally, in organic disease there is usually a primary cause such as an infective agent, the mutant gene or the immaturity of an enzyme system, whereas in psychological disturbances the interplay between the patient and his parents or siblings or school teachers, the conflicts between him and his cultural surroundings and the relative importance of his heredity versus his environment all go to make up a complex situation where at least some of the variables are difficult to change.

It will be seen that it is difficult to make a diagnosis of a behavioural/emotional disorder using the usual medical model. Diagnosis in medicine depends partly on a collection of symptoms and physical signs fitting into a pattern that is recognised, but the quality of diagnosis improves when the aetiology can be proven. For example, there may be disagreement about a pain of acute onset in the left upper abdomen or lower chest where a patient may be in a state of collapse. One may vote for a myocardial infarct, and another may claim an exacerbation or early perforation of a peptic ulcer. Once the ECG is done or the abdomen opened, opposing views will be reconciled. It is seldom possible to get further than the grouping of presenting signs and symptoms with emotional and behavioural difficulties, but some attempt to deal with the complexity of the aetiology is to be found in multi-axial classification systems. Most child and adolescent psychiatrists will soon be using six-axial classification. The first axis is usually phenomenological and labels the presenting symptoms, e.g. encopresis or hyperkinesis. The second axis offers a range of developmental delays, e.g. specific reading retardations or developmental speech/language disorder. Axis 3 deals with grades of mental handicap. Axis 4 labels any associated physical disorder in the child, e.g. asthma, epilepsy, chronic renal failure. Axis 5 lists categories of psychosocial difficulty including mental disturbances in other family members, discordant intrafamilial relationships, inadequate or inconsistent parental control and familial over-involvement. The list also includes social transplantation, stresses in school or work environment and other wider social problems including persecution or adverse discrimination.

This five-axial classification has been in regular use for a number of years but with the 10th revision of the International Classification of Disease, a sixth axis is included which enables a rating to be made for the degree of social disability caused.

It is only when all these categories have been accounted for that a meaningful jigsaw of inter-relating factors is produced. The skill of the clinician comes to the fore when it is decided which of these factors are amenable to change and what is the best way of bringing these changes about.

While the more serious disorders require the involvement of a child psychiatrist, many can be dealt with by an interested family doctor or paediatrician. Many of the problems presented are normal stages of child development which are ill understood by overanxious or depressed parents, and frequently the more severe and intractable symptoms in the child require a more detailed look at why the parent is mishandling the situation. A critical or moralistic approach has little to offer and if the parent is angry, distressed or limited, he/she may be unable to take in and implement "good advice" until the therapist is seen to empathise and understand the parent's difficulties. Much of this process of listening and building up an understanding of the family relationships can be done by non-medical professionals. The child psychiatric team usually includes social workers, a psychologist, frequently an occupational therapist and psychiatrically trained nurse therapists, as well as a psychotherapist.

The style of taking the initial history is important in making the shift from the child's presenting symptom to finding out what has actually gone wrong in the family relationships. The traditional psychiatric interview allows considerable time for the parents to express their concern.

An attitude of non-judgemental empathy will often enable the parent to move on from describing the complaint to feelings of hopelessness and anger and then perhaps how unhelpful other members of the family can be. It is not uncommon for the parents of the child with psychogenic pain to move on to their own feelings of despair and depression and at the end of half-an-hour or 40 minutes, they may be in floods of tears about their marital difficulties. Although the first part of the initial interview can be time-consuming, it may save hours on unnecessary further investigations for the child. Having allowed this time for free association, the psychiatrist would ask a wide range of questions including details of the child's eating, digestive upsets, problems with elimination, pain, levels of activity, details about temperament and relationships, antisocial behaviour, sexual difficulties, attack disorders and school progress. The usual run through the systems, cardio-vascular, respiratory, gastrointestinal, motor and urogenital, is included. The personal history pays particular attention to pregnancy, birth and postnatal period, as well as details of development and the relationship between child and parents during these stages. The family and social history may take more than one interview to complete and it is important to know about the parents or the child's carers, and also to obtain details about the child's grandparents so that cultural patterns and the parents' own childhood experiences can be ascertained. Parents, like children, have their own social values and models from their own families of origin. Social factors include details of the housing, neighbourhood and finance, and an understanding of relationships within the family needs to be built up.

Apart from the physical examination determined by the complaint, it is important to assess the child's emotional state. One notes the child's speech, mood and self-esteem. Children are not always told why they are attending the clinic and can often be put at their ease if this is addressed early in the interview.

Sometimes youngsters have been threatened with the hospital because the issue of behaviour has been fudged, they may sit in trepidation awaiting surgery or some imagined painful procedure. The child will usually talk about his or her interests, friends, family, school and about relationships at home. At the end of such an interview the six-axial classification can be completed and a plan of action made which may involve further assessment, either physical, neurological, psychometric or, more usually, of family relationships.

As there are frequently difficulties in family relationships even when there is an obvious physical component to the disorder, some child and adolescent psychiatrists begin with a family therapy interview. In this situation all members of the family living at home are invited to attend. The therapist leaves the safety of his/her position behind the desk and joins the family, occupying one of a circle of easy chairs. The initial explanation involves an acceptance that the presenting problem of the child or adolescent in one way or another involves all members of the family. The aim is to help the family discover where the difficulties are so that the therapist can plan with them what changes are needed to bring about the resolution of the difficulties. While family therapy techniques require special training, it is worth bearing in mind that involving more than just one parent in the interview can often yield here and now information about the style of communication and the degree of mutual support available. Much psychopathology in youngsters has its roots in conflict between the parents. As will be seen, disharmony leads to inconsistent methods of discipline which predispose to behavioural difficulty in the children. Children and adolescents can so easily be blamed or blame themselves for one or other parent's unhappiness; this over-concern and guilt in a young person can lead to anxiety and depression, school phobia and other psychogenic symptoms.

TODDLER MANAGEMENT PROBLEMS

Most people readily understand and accept the bodily changes as children gain in height and weight with the passage of time. Perhaps less easily understood are the cognitive changes of intellectual development and the growth of understanding. The development of speech, language and skills of communication is crucial to further learning and developing skills of social interaction. A massive amount of learning takes place during the toddler years. By the time a normal child enters school he has a good grasp of language. Although physical growth and development of intelligence are accepted, the growth of social and emotional behaviour is often less well understood by parents. Although adverse environmental circumstances can certainly retard physical growth and hold back children who function intellectually below their potential, the effects of adverse family relationships and social difficulties can have devastating effects on children's feelings and behaviour. The first year of life or infancy is largely to do with the relationship between the mother or caring person and the child. The infant needs to be kept warm, fed, clean and cuddled and talked to. The beginning of shaping up vocalisation into speech involves eye-to-eye contact and social interaction. There can be problems during this stage of the development. The initial bonding may be adversely affected by maternal depression, handicap or early illness in the child requiring long hospitalisation. The preschool behaviour problems usually start during the next phase of emotional development often referred to as "negativism". During this phase children are rude, defiant, self-opinionated and irascibly demanding. Temper tantrums are normal and made worse by the parents' lack of awareness of what to expect at this developmental stage. Whereas the infant can be "put away" for periods of time in a cot or playpen the toddler becomes mobile. Cognitive development takes a rapid spurt so he/she is hugely interested in exploring an environment that was previously inaccessible.

The toddler's time sense is poorly developed and the ability to tolerate frustration, do it later, or wait until tomorrow has not yet occurred. There is little biological maturity to suffer anger and the toddler thinks everything in the world revolves around him, and there is little awareness of the needs of others. Under these developmental conditions it is often a full-time job for the mother to keep the toddler physically safe and usefully involved in learning social skills. Tablecloths are pulled down, taps left running, gas switched on and electrical sockets interfered with. Mechanical gadgets are to be taken apart to see how they work, and as speech develops there is a need to constantly ask unanswerable questions, sing loudly and be offended if visitors, grandparents or siblings interfere with activities or social discourse with the parent. Where the parent is feeling below par and perhaps depressed, living in a high flat where there is no where to go out to play or in an area which is clearly unsafe for youngsters to go out alone, the tension mounts. The patient may not be the only preschool child, and where two or three youngsters are vying for attention, in a single room apartment, the parent may be reduced to shouting, smacking or ignoring behaviour that requires attention or correction.

Discipline

Discipline should be firm, kind, reasonable and consistent. It should relate to the developmental stage that the child has reached so the child can understand what is expected of him. Obedience based on repression is never permanent and rules should be few, easily understood and always kept. Positive reinforcement with respect, praise and love is important and bribes lead to inflation. The more frequent the punishment the less tends to be its effect.

Repeated threats do not work and punishment should be meted out when the child behaves badly and not merely saved until inappropriate behaviour causes damage or an accident. For younger children punishment should be immediate and, most important, parents must not be split, one colluding with behaviour which the other is trying to correct.

A number of behaviour disorders can arise – namely food fads, temper tantrums, difficulty going to sleep and battles over the potty. By the time professional help is sought, mothers have usually become quite inconsistent in their management of the problem and they have usually "tried everything".

If the child will not go to sleep he may be told a story and then he calls out, a reprimand is given and a testing cry tinged with uncertainty follows. Perhaps he will be given a drink and put back to bed. Opportunistically he cries again only to be given a severe telling-off by a mother who is beginning to be irate and exhausted. She makes some threat or says that she will go away if he is not good, so he cries again. Eventually after further loss of temper the mother feels guilty or is upset that the child's shrieking will invite criticism from others and brings the child back into the living area to watch the television, or a scary video, and another attempt is made to go to bed. The crying starts again and night after night the situation worsens. Mothers have confided that they put a pillow over the child's head momentarily and then became overwhelmed with guilt so they take the child to bed with them. The same theme is repeated with food fads. Children can raise the parent's anxiety by refusing to eat and can manipulate the situation so that their favourite baked beans or digestive biscuits have to be eaten for breakfast, lunch and tea. Again all kinds of bribes, punishments and ultimata are given while the toddler resolutely refuses to comply with normal meals. The inconsistency between anxiety that the child may become ill or even not survive, coupled with temper loss and sometimes severe smackings and episodes of rejection are the order of the day.

Distraught parents require a sympathetic ear, some explanation of why this stage of development is difficult and reassurance that the child will not grow up delinquent or anorexic. Where possible the principles of appropriate discipline should be enforced.

ENURESIS

Enuresis refers to the persistent involuntary or inappropriate voiding of urine. This can occur while the child is asleep (nocturnal) or in the daytime (diurnal). The disorder may have been life long (primary) or come on at a later stage (secondary). Nocturnal enuresis is a commonly occurring disorder which affects approximately 10% of children at the age of 5 and 5% at the age of 10 with 1 or 2% continuing to wet throughout the teens. I would not consider nocturnal enuresis to be primarily a child psychiatric problem and it occurs with similar prevalence as all the rest of the psychiatric disorders put together. There is frequently a family history and it is usually a mono-symptom with family discord and emotional factors being secondary to the inconvenient and undesirable symptom. There is an increased incidence of wetting amongst populations of children with child psychiatric problems, but the correlation is not with any specific disorder. While it is assumed enuresis is associated with anxiety, it more often occurs in children in poor social circumstances where early training has not been established. Some children have had disturbing life events at the time when night-time bladder control should be acquired and the symptom is more frequent in children with other developmental delays and with encopresis, one mechanism being that the faecal impaction fills the space occupying the pelvis and presses on the bladder neck, giving rise to incomplete voiding of urine.

Associated urinary tract problems and other medical problems are unusual but should be kept in mind when a new case is seen. Structural anomalies including urethral valves and reflux into mega-ureters are associated with incomplete bladder emptying and a reduction in the amount of urine voided at any one time. Although it is easy to test for urinary infections, most children with urinary infections do not bed wet and most bed wetters are not infected. Uncommonly children may pass urine during nocturnal seizures while disorders involving a high output of urine, including some kidney disorders and diabetes, may be relevant. Very occasionally neurological disorders affecting the spine may affect bladder emptying. It therefore seems pertinent to ask about the nature of the stream during voiding. Structural anomalies and incomplete bladder emptying are frequently associated with dribbling and frequency and also with daytime wetting. It is also useful to ask about the child's fluid intake because high output of urine involves an excessive thirst. There is little difficulty in testing for abnormal constituents by the Stix method and sending a sample of urine for bacterial count. While infection is unlikely to present as long-standing enuresis, infected urine may suggest the need for further investigation of the urinary tract.

It appears that the all or none reflex, associated with voiding, sparks off at an earlier stage in children with enuresis than in children not so affected. There are various ways of improving bladder capacity. Tricyclic antidepressants imipramine and amitriptyline are sometimes used, although their mode of action is uncertain. It may be the atropine-like effect or possibly a central effect of these drugs which gives relief of symptoms when they are prescribed. I seldom use tricyclics for bed wetters as these drugs are dangerous and not always carefully given. I have known neighbour's children treated to a dose from well-meaning mothers of enuretics with little regard to their body weight. The bed wetting usually recurs when the drug is stopped unless the child has grown out of the problem during the time the prescription has been given. An occasional exception can be made with an adolescent who is upset or possibly depressed, and who needs treatment to go away from home with a group of other youngsters. Medication should then be tried in advance of the holiday so that side effects can be established.

Antidiuretic hormone, in the form of desmopressin nasal spray, has been recently introduced. A symptomatic improvement may occur but the disorder may relapse when the medication is stopped after 1 or 2 months. While there should be concern that children may overload their circulation with water while this drug is acting, this does not seem to occur in practice although one should be cautious if there is any renal or cardiac problems.

The most effective treatment is the pad and buzzer, which is designed to wake the child when voiding commences. Great care is needed in securing the cooperation of child, his/her parents and siblings. Attention to detail is important so that false alarms caused by inadequate cleaning of the pad, excess sweating or the pad folding over on itself are avoided. The time of voiding may move from midnight until 3 a.m. then to 5 a.m. over some weeks. In all cases there is still a wet bed, but progressive lengthening of the dry spell indicates that the conditioning apparatus is working. If there is no progress after 2 or 3 months, it is better to withdraw the apparatus for another 6 months or a year, assuming the child is not developmentally ready to benefit.

The simple technique of "lifting" a child when the parents go to bed sometimes solves the problem at a practical level. Those doctors who practice medical hypnosis may achieve good results with enuretics. The use of star charts should be reserved for those children who wish to fill them in. All too often there is an expectation that the star chart will work and if it does not there is loss of face for the child, the parent or for the doctor. Where angry feelings underly the problem the chart will merely emphasise the extent of the difficulties which may please the youngster. If the child has regressed the chart will be meaningless. Either way the chart implies that the child has voluntary control; to be dry is "good" and to have accidents is "bad". Some children who wet are quite depressed and therefore it feels appropriate to be smelly wet and to be chastised; it is not until their self-esteem is improved that they take more interest in attempting to become dry.

I would therefore avoid a set treatment package for enuretic children but check out the feelings, attitudes and family relationships before deciding whether a family therapy or psychodynamic approach is needed before using the pad and bell technique.

ENCOPRESIS

The international classification of disease in its definition of encopresis refers to the persistent voluntary or involuntary passage of formed motions of normal or near-normal consistency into places not intended for that purpose in the individual's socio-cultural setting. Two different types are described by one author:

1 *Continuous soiling* where the soiling has always been present. These children usually come from families with low expectations concerning their development, poor motivation and inconsistent attempts to enter into a toilet training situation. Often these families have other social difficulties and the caring person, usually the mother, may have acquired poor models of parenting from her own background or be depressed and preoccupied with relationship problems in the family.

2 *Discontinuous soilers* may have been satisfactorily trained or may have been especially early trained in bowel control. The soiling occurs in response to rigorous and demanding potting regimens from parents with high aspirations who apply coercive pressure and expect early bowel control. Unlike the continuous soilers, many of the discontinuous soilers come from families where the parents at least superficially appear confident, in step and driven.

Perhaps a more useful way of looking at the psychogenic mechanisms and family attitudes of soiling children is to look for signs of *inconsistent training*, *regressive behaviour* or an *aggressive toileting situation*. Children with *inconsistent training* resemble the continuous soilers. The child has never received appropriate praise for being clean although sometimes has been subjected to angry responses. These families are chaotic and disorganised and sometimes the child may have been in and out of children's homes, with foster families and for periods of time with relatives. The continuity of picking up the child's cues and continuing appropriate rewards has therefore been destroyed. Not all families in this category are necessarily unkind or abusive to their children. Sometimes an attitude of friendly tolerance prevails.

Regressive soilers are usually reacting to stress and anxiety. The soiling may not be the only developmental milestone that has slipped back as the youngster may be anxious, clingy, tearful, exhibiting toddler-like temper tantrums, and sometimes psychogenic pains. These youngsters are often difficult to engage in play therapy and sit dull, poorly motivated and emotionally flat. Discussions about their bowel problem or an attempt to use a star chart are useless at first as the mental mechanism of regression switches them off from any apparent understanding of the disorder. Many nurses have been surprised when changing a child with loaded pants at the apparent unawarenesss and indifference to a situation which is all too obvious to others in the vicinity. Usually these stresses are from within the family, and many of these children are criticised and scapegoated and some have been harshly disciplined when they are soiled. One family admitted that they had held the child up by his feet, put his head down the toilet and activated the flush.

Aggressive soilers often resemble discontinuous soilers. The parent may at first describe reasonable attempts to toilet train, but if sufficient interview time is allowed, one becomes aware of considerable tension and anger regarding the soiling. All too often the youngster is expected to perform as an angry mother becomes tense so that placid painless potting does not occur. The child may respond negatively and retain faeces either voluntarily or sometimes involuntarily and all too often retention results in a megacolon situation.

Although many retentive soilers have angry relationships with their main caring person, children with all the above psychogenic mechanisms can present with chronic constipation and dilatation of the rectum and/or descending colon. In extreme cases the accumulation can be massive and readily ballottable. More usually rocks and lumps can be palpated in the descending colon, and sometimes the accumulation of putty-like or hard faeces can almost avoid detection behind the pelvic brim, but becomes all too obvious on rectal examination. Any child with a history of intermittent, runny stools, often with a fusty acrid smell, must be suspected of overflow incontinence, especially if there is an intermittent history of extremely large bowel evacuations which are often graphically described. It is difficult to understand why some children are seen with a large degree of bowel dilatation and little psychopathology and conversely some youngsters have only mild bowel dysfunction despite enormous emotional pressures. Similarly it is difficult to explain why some children who are extremely loaded and dilated can respond rapidly to treatment while others go on amassing faeces around the transverse colon and into the ascending colon long after good-enough family relationships have been established.

Where a megacolon situation exists, it is usually best to try and empty the bowel. Enemata or suppositories are given followed by a prescription for laxatives. Lactulose is in vogue as a faecal softener, but does not always tone up a flaccid bowel. Senna (Senokot), docusate sodium (Dioctyl Paediatric) and other laxatives may be used alone or with a softener. Methycellulose is sometimes helpful and dietary advice often including the use of bran may be helpful where families have the capacity to act on advice. As daily laxatives often lose their effect, we have recently tried weekly or twice weekly doses of stronger laxatives on intractable cases. Drugs like bisacodyl should only be started when the bowel has been emptied of marked faecal accumulation. Future research mau show some value in cisapride which stimulates bowel motility. At the time of writing there is insufficient data to recommend its use and it is not yet licensed for this purpose or for children under 12. There seems little value in using laxatives where there is no megacolon and the child passes a normal consistency stool at regular intervals, even although this may result in soiling.

A behavioural approach with the use of a star chart may be helpful to an untrained child and sometimes the angry relationship of an aggressive soiler can be helped if the chart recognises success but not failure. Positive reinforcement is always more acceptable than a programme that increases the parents' anger or discourages the child. Where the child is under considerable stress as in the regressive group, or where there is too much anger for mutual cooperation with a behavioural regimen, there is no substitute for looking at the wider issues of family relationships. This always takes time and in some cases the social worker, the health visitor, educational psychologist or child psychiatrist may need to become involved. It should be remembered that some sexually abused children soil and this should be borne in mind when a rectal examination and/or use of a suppository or enema is clinically indicated. Where the child and parents can fully understand the need for rectal intervention the procedure should be talked through beforehand and my own practice is usually to offer that the procedure be carried out by a doctor or nurse of the same sex as the patient.

Where the child is preschool or has difficulty in understanding what is required it is sometimes best to introduce the child to the clinical room and explain what needs to be done, then allow the child to return home so that the parent can prepare the child, possibly involving dolls or other toys. If the soiling has a strong psychogenic component and on-going psychotherapy or play therapy is needed, it is often best to delegate physical aspects of the treatment to another member of the team or a separate paediatric or paediatric surgical clinic. The same applies for older children involved in on-going psychotherapy, especially where transference occurs where the child begins to relate to the therapist as a parent or other significant person controlling his/her life events. Feelings of anger and anxiety are shared but this process can be sabotaged if the therapist plays the dual role of doctor and psychotherapist. A preschool toddler, who soiled in anger, attacked a daddy doll during therapy, buried him in the sand and beat the sand down with a shovel. The mother doll was also given a hard time for sending the daddy away. Having empathised with 30 minutes of this distressing anger it would not feel right for the therapist, let alone the child, for the session to have been followed by the therapist giving the child an enema against his/her will. Where the faecal impaction is severe or requires dealing with urgently, it is often best to admit the child and the parent (if the child is young) to a paediatric ward where enemas can be given after the procedure has been explained and the child can be calmed and comforted by experienced nurses. Sometimes enemas can be given on an outpatient basis, especially if the child is familiar with the hospital and the faecal loading is likely to resolve with a single enema or suppository. Where regular enemas are required, they can be given at home by the community nurse. Some mothers can give the enemas at home, but this is seldom satisfactory if the faecal retention has a psychogenic cause.

On rare occasions the author has resorted to a straight X-ray of abdomen to find out the extent of faecal impaction where a child is particularly scared of rectal examination and very occasionally has requested that a child be disimpacted under a general anaesthetic for the same reason. It is hard to justify subjecting a child to irradiation or to a general anaesthetic for these procedures. There is no substitute for building up trust, explaining what will happen to the child and helping him through the painful and difficult stages of intervention, then being around to answer questions and consolidate the relationship afterwards. Very few children appear to bear malice, unless the emotional need to continue to soil is unresolved.

COMMUNICATION DISORDER

Normal children are taught language by a two-way process of interaction with an adequately responsive mother or other caring adults. It is a pleasure to watch the intense eye-to-eye contact as the infant sits on the mother's knee while producing baby vocalisations which are praised as they approximate to some simple, wellknown word like "mum". As the noises approximate to the word "mum" the mother responds, the baby excites and the dialogue slowly and surely proceeds into a basic vocabulary where the child develops some understanding of the meaning of words as well as being able to articulate them. For this process to occur the hearing must be intact, the auditory nerve functioning and the incoming stimuli from the input side of the brain must work in harmony with a memory store so that messages can be devised in the output or expressive part of the brain and these coded into impulses going down the motor nerves to the larynx and pharynx. If a child presents with defective speech or language it is worth being satisfied that there is no deafness or even high tone deafness. Some children can imitate the alarm of a fire engine but the higher frequencies needed to imitate the human voice may not be received, in which case incoming language can only be perceived as distorted. If the hearing is alright and there are no anatomical or neurological problems of the sound producing organs, one can assume that the disorder is in the brain. It is useful to think of language disorders as receptive, mixed or expressive. The most benign of these disorders is the delay in expressive speech where the child clearly understands what is being said and will obey verbal instructions but has a hesitancy in finding words to express himself. Children with this problem are invariably irritable and demanding, as they live in a frustrating world of adults moving on to the next topic before they have been able to join in and make their own wishes

understood. There is frequent gesticulating, pulling parents over to indicate their wishes by body language and general frustration. Providing the child is socially aware and develops an understanding of language the problem usually corrects itself with support and possibly speech and language therapy.

Much more sinister is the receptive language disorder where impulses coming along the auditory nerve cannot be decoded into anything meaningful. Sometimes children appear to repress language in the same way that children with a squint can repress vision, and on occasions it requires an audiogram to be performed where the child is fixed to an EEG machine set to give evoked response readings. In this way it can be deduced that noises coming into the child's ear are decoded by the brain. If little meaningful sense can be made of the spoken word the child becomes seriously socially disadvantaged and may begin to withdraw in a world which increasingly depends on social interaction through language. Children with severe receptive disorders require special educational means so that a language can be built up in the memory with stimuli being presented through the visual or tactile route.

In practice most language disorders are not clearly defined, mixed or central language disorders, with some receptive and some expressive difficulties, are often seen.

Infantile autism appears to have much in common with severe receptive language disorder but other routes through the brain may also be affected. The symptoms usually present within the first 30 months with abnormal responses to both auditory and sometimes visual stimuli. Speech is delayed and if it begins to develop it tends to be echolalic and lacking in ability to use abstract terms. Autistic children appear detached socially and classically there is an impairment of eye-to-eye contact and lack of ability to relate meaningfully to parents or age-mates. Autistic children frequently resist change and may have catastrophic screaming attacks if some small item in a room has been moved or if their transport to school goes by an unusual route. Routines, rituals and obsessional behaviour are commonplace and as the disorder improves patterns of logically concrete thinking emerge with a lack of social empathy. The resulting behaviour can appear somewhat eccentric.

There are a number of theories of possible aetiology. The disorder is male predominant in a ratio of 4 : 1. Whereas in the past family influence and the quality of parenting was suspect, it now seems more likely that biological disorders of the brain, e.g. fetal rubella, and genetic factors may be more relevant. The prognosis depends on the return of speech and approximately half of these children end up with measured IQ levels of below 50, although many will require on-going family and community support with only a minority becoming gifted eccentrics or gifted musicians.

LEARNING DIFFICULTIES

There are many reasons why children may be behind in their school attainments. The child may be mentally handicapped and therefore retarded in all areas of cognitive development. The disorder may be recognised to have a genetic cause, e.g. Down syndrome. There are a number of disorders where an inborn area of metabolism can be proven; for example, Wilson disease which is a defect of copper metabolism and the mucopolysaccaride disorders which are progressive. The child may look dysmorphic or have an associated movement disorder, e.g. Huntington chorea. Some children are born with neurological damage, such as spastic hemiplegia or microcephaly, and frequently have learning difficulties. All children are screened at birth for phenylketonuria, and the insidious mental retardation resulting from hypothyroidism should be borne in mind. The effects of severe head injury, cerebral tumours and other forms of major brain damage will also take their toll, although it is remarkable how intellectual abilities can remain remarkably intact after marked anatomical damage has occurred, especially if early in the child's life. The field widens when the side effects of certain medications are taken into consideration. Anticonvulsants, especially when used in a high dose, can impair learning although carbamazepine and sodium valproate are less likely to cause problems than the more old fashioned drugs. A child with a chronic or relapsing illness may find learning difficult because of malaise, pain, repeated, time-consuming or traumatic medical treatments and because of time lost from school.

Many of the disorders referred to in this chapter can directly or indirectly affect school potential. Children with emotional disorders are frequently anxious and depressed. They find it difficult to concentrate in class if they are preoccupied by feelings of worthlessness and are worrying that their mother or father may be unwell or in the process of separation. The distress and falling off of attainments may be missed by the teacher who is more preoccupied by the disruptive behaviour of behaviourally disturbed children. Somatic symptoms including abdominal pains and headache or stress-induced illness like asthma lead to frequent school absence and the continuity of learning is lost.

Attainments are frequently poor in conduct disordered children. The causes are multifactorial. First, most of these youngsters come from areas of social deprivation where the attitudes of parents towards education is not always positive, homework is not encouraged, nor is there peace and a quiet space for academic pursuits in overcrowded, noisy, disorganised households. Truanting may be regarded as fun and a youngster who becomes behind with his attainments is frequently criticised by irate teachers. If the child accepts that he is an idiot, no use and a waste of space, his motivation will be adversely affected as he feels angry and hurt.

The mental process of guarding against depression and poor self-esteem is to blame the system that is being undermining to one's confidence. It is safer to reject the school and consider the teachers to be rubbish than to accept the criticism. This attitude can become the group norm and self-respect can be better preserved by outshining truanting colleagues with antisocial behaviour than being ridiculed by increasingly hostile teachers. Under these conditions school attainments fall further and further behind.

An important epidemiological survey referred to in the conduct disorder section of this chapter showed that one-third of children with conduct disorder were more than 2 years retarded in reading, and children with reading retardation had an increased incidence of conduct problems. Of particular interest was the suggestion that in a number of cases learning difficulties preceded the behavioural difficulties. Where learning difficulties are not discovered and where appropriate educational help is not given, a child's self-esteem and motivation worsens and the situation escalates. Many children underfunction for the reasons described above, but others fail because of specific learning difficulties often labelled as dyslexia.

Dyslexia

Dyslexia is a term much in vogue which is really synonymous with *specific learning difficulty*. One of the early descriptions referred to the disorder as "word blindness" and an early textbook on the subject gives an account of a boy who electrocuted himself on an electric railway because he could not make sense of the warning notices advising all and sundry to keep off the line. There has been enormous pressure from certain professional groups and parents of children with specific learning difficulties to get these problems increasingly recognised by teachers.

The term "dyslexia" can give rise to confusion. Worried parents can be fearful that dyslexia is some frightful illness while other more sophisticated families may push dyslexia as an explanation for their child's school failure which may turn out to have its roots in poor family relationships and motivational problems.

The increased awareness of specific learning difficulties is to be welcomed. The problem may present with depression or conduct disorder. The psychiatrist may be immediately impressed by a youngster's unhappiness or suicidal ideas and when dealing with the emergency it is all too easy to miss the underlying stress of a child trying his/her hardest and never being able to succeed at school. Unfortunately, the response in some learning situations is that the child is subjected to more of the same. If he does not have the underlying innate ability to cope with learning tables it is often wrongly assumed that mass practice, perhaps being made to write them out several times over, will improve the situation when so often the converse is true.

The problem about using "dyslexia" as a label is that it does not describe the precise nature of the underlying learning difficulty. Many professionals prefer to describe the nature of the problem in functional terms. There are three cognitive processes which are often found to be affected. The first is the problem of short-term memory or sequencing difficulty. This may be associated with difficulty of recall of information obtained through the auditory route, or the problem may be in recalling material which has recently been read from writing or print.

A person can be told a telephone number and this may not be recalled whereas the same number read from a book can be more easily retained and vice versa. The second major difficulty is with spatial ability or orientation. Some children have enormous difficulty in learning left from right. Cross-laterality, being right-handed, right-eyed and left-footed or some other combination are thought to be related to spatial difficulties, although careful research shows that most people with cross-laterality do not suffer significant spatial ability problems. The third common specific difficulty is with visuo-motor or perceptual difficulties. This is often associated with problems of putting thoughts into legible writing and decoding information from the written page. In some instances a child may acknowledge that his written page is full of mistakes but be unable to correct them. Even the process of copying may be severely impaired.

Severe dyslexic problems may overlap with mild communication disorder difficulties and specific learning difficulties can be found in association with hyperkinesis or in children who are clumsy with poor motor control. These three disorders, namely hyperkinesis, specific learning difficulty (dyslexia) and clumsiness can be grouped together under the umbrella of minimal cerebral dysfunction. The aetiological theories of cerebral dysfunction are covered in the section on hyperkinesis.

HYPERKINESIS

Many people believe that hyperactivity is a straightforward condition manifested by motor restlessness, distractibility, poor concentration, impulsivity and labile mood. The simple explanation that this disorder is caused by minimal brain dysfunction and elegantly responds to methylphenidate (Ritalin) is much too neat and tidy a concept which bears little

relationship to the hordes of badly behaved, inappropriately controlled, understimulated children who are referred to paediatricians and child psychiatrists. It has been stated that as knowledge of developmental neuropsychiatry has increased, so the simple story has seen to be fatally flawed. The most important aspect of this has been the realisation that hyperactivity is not simply a manifestation of brain impairment. It is unlikely that hyperkinesis is a unitary condition and the following are some of the aetiological theories that have been put forward. Very occasionally hyperkinesis may follow brain damage, and more commonly there may be some evidence for "cerebral dysfunction" as some hyperkinetic children are clumsy and others have specific learning difficulties not explained by global retardation. While it is sometimes assumed that difficulties in the pregnancy, delivery or neonatal period correlate with cerebral dysfunction, this is a dangerous assumption when dealing with individuals as the majority of children with low Apgar scores at birth do not exhibit these problems later on. Having made a plea for caution in arguing from early trauma to present behaviour, one must acknowledge that there is sometimes a link. The infant brain is both vulnerable and plastic with an enormous capacity for function to develop in spite of areas of damage. Such damage will often be generalised rather than localised, e.g. by anoxia, or the effect of low blood sugar so that it is reasonable that some years on the effects of damage will be manifest by impulsivity and labile mood.

Studies of family history show that the parents of hyperkinetic children have increased rates of alcoholism, sociopathy and hysteria when compared with the relatives of normal children. One study showed that a significant number of hyperkinetic children developed alcoholism, sociopathy and hysteria when they grew up. Theories of disorders of monoamine metabolism have been proposed and there are theories that hyperkinesis is a result of cortical under-arousal or of cortical over-arousal. At the present time the concept of food allergy is polarised by those who feel diet is nearly always to blame to those who consider allergy to be synonymous with neurosis. Unfortunately some of the additive-free diets are complicated, expensive and difficult to follow and are handed out often with the goodwill of a supportive voluntary organisation to a mother who would be unlikely to put the diet into operation. If there is some evidence that certain foods seem to upset the child, it may be valuable to enlist the opinion of a dietitian who can devise a trial diet which is sensible, within the grasp of the parent and unlikely to deprive the child of essential nutritional substances. Sometimes helpful results are obtained, although it is not always clear what is due to support and what is due to diet. It appears reasonable to keep an open mind and carefully accumulate data. While coeliac disease is considered a respectable paediatric diagnosis, the possibility of wheat allergy is often discounted. There is little doubt that some children are irritable and restless when they are itchy with eczema or frustrated by coryza and nasal stuffiness. Whether or not there may be underlying constitutional disturbances there always needs to be an emphasis on consistent and appropriate management. If there is a constitutional problem the child will usually not cope with a classroom situation at school without receiving criticism and negative reinforcements which alienate him from teachers and sometimes classmates.

This kind of arousal makes the concentration and distractibility worse and the youngster rapidly develops a feeling of poor self-esteem. The child may then present with unhappy depressive feelings which further reduce motivation, or alternatively cause a reaction formation defence: "that teacher is always bugging me" or "I am not working for him".

In so many cases it is difficult to sort out cause and effect when the parents are tired, angry and depressed. As the cycle of events winds up, the parents become inconsistent, being either inappropriately angry or at other times too negative and exhausted to intervene.

Hyperkinesis is viewed differently in different countries and indeed by different paediatricians. Undoubtedly stimulants like methylphenidate are sometimes a useful adjunct to a wider treatment programme, but their use can cause sleeplessness, retarded physical growth and occasionally psychosis. In cities where social deprivation may be a factor in the aetiology, stimulants are likely to be abused by others or could be sold for financial gain. It may be useful to consider a period of admission to a child psychiatric unit or paediatric ward to see how much of the claimed hyperkinesis melts away with consistent care before embarking on years of pharmacotherapy. Other medications that control hyperkinesis include phenothiazines and haloperidol but these drugs have numerous side effects including the long-term danger of tardive dyskinesia. There is some evidence that tricyclic antidepressants may have a useful effect in proven cases although they have not been widely used for this purpose and carry an enormous risk if overdose occurs.

Hyperkinetic children should have a tailor-made treatment plan often involving the educational psychologist and sometimes the family's local social work department.

CONDUCT DISORDER

Although the management of children with aggressive and destructive behaviour giving rise to social disapproval usually falls to other professionals, the paediatrician is bound to become involved as one-third of children falling into the psychiatric disorder category will exhibit these problems. The incidence of these antisocial disorders varies from around 2–10% of the mid-childhood years depending on the kind of population being served.

Some of these difficulties arise from unresolved behaviour disorders previously described. There are two principles underpinning the learning of social behaviour: first, the behavioural model where consistent rewards and reprimands are needed to learn appropriate responses; second, the psychodynamic approach which concentrates on the quality of relationship between the child and the parent or authority figure. Where the relationship is sound and the adult responds to meet the child's needs, the child will model his or her behaviour on the style of the adult and will want to behave in a way that pleases and gets acclaim from that person. Anything that interferes with the consistency of responses or anything that interferes with the warm and caring relationship can impede social learning. Difficulties can arise in the family. The family norms may not be acceptable to society: many delinquent children have fathers and sometimes mothers with a criminal record. Some families issue no clear guidelines and throw their children into confusion by being very punitive on one occasion and amused at a different time when the youngster does something inappropriate. Some families have unclear roles with perhaps the elder sister taking over when the mother is not coping, and the impact of personality disorder of the parent or parents and social difficulties must also be taken into account.

Apart from difficulties in the family, antisocial behaviour can be fostered by the mores of the community. Many housing departments work on a point system so that families with social difficulties can only be housed in unpopular housing schemes so that their children are immediately exposed to a peer group with high delinquency rates and neighbours that help to potentate this downward cycle. The effect of the school can make or break a youngster who is not well supported at home. One-third of children with conduct disorder living on the Isle of Wight were found to be more than 2 years retarded in reading; conversely children with learning difficulties had an increased rate of conduct problems. If the child is encouraged and made to feel an important individual in his own right within school, identification with the school system and certain teachers will exert a positive influence, whereas if the child does not succeed academically and is humiliated further in the school setting he is much more likely to get recognition from other antisocial youngsters who themselves undermine educational values and gain prowess from delinquent behaviour.

The medical skill lies in picking out conditions within the child himself that predispose to antisocial difficulties. Children vary in their innate temperamental traits. Parents who have successfully reared one or more "easy" children may find that their methods do not succeed with a more wilful child. Children who are hyperkinetic with poor concentration and sometimes clumsiness are difficult to discipline. They easily get discouraged with repeated failure or develop negative ways of opposing those putting pressure upon them (see Hyperkinesis). Specific learning difficulties are sometimes missed in school and the child who is probably of at least average intelligence is labelled as lazy or not trying in the area of his disability. Once again motivation can fail because of a depressive or angry attitude towards school.

Depression in childhood as in adulthood can sometimes give rise to stealing and underfunctioning as the "I am bad" guilt is sometimes acted out or the object stolen may be held for comfort. The effects of early deprivation lead to continuing temper tantrums and toddler-like behaviour sometimes for many years, even though a child may be in an improved home situation. Lastly, some children with long-term illness or handicap who are feeling vulnerable may need to over-react to show their friends and teachers they are a force to be reckoned with.

EMOTIONAL DISORDER/CHILDHOOD NEUROSIS

It is helpful to understand the difference between psychosomatic disorders and the neuroses. Psychosomatic disorders are known physical illness where there are changes in tissue structure or function but where the disorder or exacerbations of the disorder are partly or mainly induced by stress. A number of illnesses can be included in this category, for example some cases of asthma, skin disorders or bowel problems ranging from ulcerative colitis to acquired megacolon. The neuroses are predominantly psychiatric disorders which nevertheless cause a number of worrying and at first apparently "physical" symptoms including abdominal pain, headaches and limb pains. These so-called psychogenic regional pains are accompanied by negative laboratory findings but the symptoms can be severe and disabling.

The symptoms of *anxiety* and *depression* usually coexist in primary school children and present in the following ways. Psychogenic pains are commonly occurring. Abdominal pain can at times be apparently severe and although there should be no real guarding or tenderness, some of the children appear exquisitely tender or find it difficult to relax to have their

abdomens palpated. It is surprising how pain can become localised to the right iliac fossa or epigastrium when various doctors have made repeated examinations querying acute appendicitis or peptic ulceration. Headaches often lack a specific site or quality, although the "tight-band" or "heavy weight" described by adult patients can be described on occasions. Tension and depression does not exclude true migraine which is sometimes seen in children especially where there is a family history.

The concept of abdominal migraine or the periodic syndrome is sometimes useful where cyclical attacks of prostrating vomiting occasionally needing intravenous fluids can last for 1 or 2 days and as the child gets older visual disturbance, photophobia and pulsating headache become more apparent and the vomiting less obvious. Children with true migraine are often normal between the episodes and we would regard this disorder as organic or psychosomatic and not neurotic. Nausea and vomiting can be symptoms of anxiety and emotional disturbance and children under stress can appear pale, lethargic and tired. Sleep difficulty with anxious or depressing thoughts keeping the child awake or preventing him/her going to bed is a common symptom of anxiety, while early wakening, usually regarded as a symptom of endogenous depression, can also occur, especially in older children who are depressed. Poor concentration is nearly always present and this may have gone unnoticed in school as children with emotional disorders do not usually present a behavioural problem in the classroom. Tearfulness, oversensitivity, agitation and irritability frequently occur. Anxious toddlers and young children are unsettled and on-the-go and may be thought to be hyperkinetic. Where depression predominates the youngster will admit to feeling bad and guilty and sometimes the overwhelming feelings of wretchedness can be associated with stealing, tearing up promising work, being unable to accept praise and wanting to die. While it may be difficult to understand these symptoms, some children are so frequently undermined and put down by their parents, teachers and potential friends that they can only see themselves as useless, inadequate and hopeless.

Anyone trying to be nice to them must be a phoney, and they feel so bad that somehow it feels right for them to indulge in self-deprecatory behaviour. Children often exhibit their feelings in the way they behave. A happy child will dance, sing and be spontaneously bright. A child in pain will cry and hold up an injured limb for inspection or for comfort and the child who is feeling bad will sometimes be unable to stop him/herself from doing bad things.

School phobia is the term used for children who develop psychogenic symptoms in the morning before school. The symptoms ameliorate either when they have been at school for a while or when the decision is made that they are too ill to attend. Sometimes the symptoms are not a true phobia to the school itself but are caused by separation anxiety about leaving home and parents. School phobic children are often intelligent and good achievers, and although they may try to go to school, symptoms occur to prevent this happening. The parent or parents are much in evidence with worrying about the child's pains, vomiting, or else being angry that he/she has failed to leave the home for school. These patterns of behaviour are totally different to truancy. The truant frequently underachieves, comes from a family who, rather than being overinvolved with the non-attendance at school, are unconcerned or unaware of the situation until the authorities make contact. There are no psychogenic symptoms associated with the truant who frequently goes off to join his friends in conduct disordered activity, whereas it is frequently found that the school phobic child is depressed.

In preschool and young primary children the ultimate depressive thought seems to be separation and abandonment from the parents or those looking after them. Feelings of guilt leading to suicidal ideas have to be checked out in the older primary school child and certainly in the adolescent. It is helpful to ask: "Do you sometimes feel so bad or unhappy that you would like to run away from home or have a bad accident or die?" A reply in the affirmative must be taken seriously and it is a myth that children who talk about harming themselves would not do so.

Phobic anxiety presents where there is a specific anxiety in certain situations, e.g. thunderstorms, fear of dogs and being upset by insects. Often these fears are not generalised into other situations and the youngsters may in other ways be quite emotionally robust. In my experience these phobias in primary school children are often learnt from a parent, friend or relative. This is not always volunteered until asked about during a detailed history taking. It is then useful to try and help the affected parent to try and overcome their own difficulties.

Obsessive/compulsive disorder

The outstanding symptom here is a feeling of compulsion to carry out some action or repeatedly dwell on an idea which is difficult to resist. This leads to repetitive rituals, e.g. handwashing which has to be performed time and time again, despite the child and the parent wishing this not to happen. In older children and adolescents this disorder resembles the adult form which is sometimes difficult to treat and may have an uncertain long-term prognosis. In primary school children, however, the rituals can sometimes be seen as a way of reducing anxiety which may have its roots in disturbed family relationships, school work which is too hard, or pressure

from friends. Toddlers and young children can exhibit ritualistic behaviour as part of normal development, e.g. needing to go round every lamp post twice. Toddlers love repetitive games and songs. These preoccupations are usually short-lived unless reinforced by an anxious parent; after all, which of us has not walked along a pavement avoiding the cracks in the flagstones.

Conversion hysteria

Examples of hysteria include psychogenic regional pain, disorders of movement, apparent paralysis of limbs, blindness and pseudo-seizures. Hysteria in this sense of the word does not refer to the shallow self-centred attention-seeking behaviour of the hysterical personality, but involves the psychological mechanism of dissociation whereby the patient is at first unaware that the symptom is other than organic. Children presenting with these disorders are usually in some kind of an emotional trap. Where conversion hysteria is suspected one should look at all aspects of the child's life situation and find out what purpose the symptom is serving or how it is protecting the child from whatever happens if the symptom goes away. A severe cough or episodes of vomiting may keep parents together who are on the verge of separating. A girl's sore tummy may be stopping her highly esteemed father from trying to have sexual intercourse with her. The astute clinician sometimes sees something symbolic in the presenting complaint as it is not just chance that certain symptoms are unconsciously selected. There are two pitfalls in dealing with these disorders. First some symptoms can be frankly manipulative where there is conscious awareness of the gain involved, but for a diagnosis of hysteria there must be an element of dissociation or unawareness. Second, many cases of so-called hysteria turn out to have an organic basis when the case is followed up. Most psychiatrists are only ever certain of a diagnosis of hysteria after a satisfactory formulation of the child's difficulty has been made, and when attempts to ameliorate that situation bring about a considerable improvement in the disorder. Often there is dual pathology, e.g. psychogenic seizures are often found in children with epilepsy. One should never agree that the diagnosis is hysteria just because there are no physical findings. Unusual presentations of common disorder and sometimes extremely unusual disorders can appear within the course of time. Peculiar panic attacks can be temporal lobe tumours, dystonias are frequently initially thought to be hysterical and peptic ulcers are a more common cause of intermittent abdominal pain than perhaps one would expect.

The aetiology of childhood emotional disorders is usually to be found in the family relationships. In many cases the mother of the affected child is frankly depressed or very anxious. In the seclusion of a one-to-one interview, mothers will often begin to cry and disclose morbid ideas. Doctors are thought to be missing a fatal disorder in the child and depressive thoughts become unwittingly projected onto the youngster. Where school phobia occurs, the parent feels worn out by the daily decision whether to send the child to school after being reassured he is physically well. Sometimes if you ask, "Have you ever felt that you could not go on any longer with this", the mother will disclose feelings of total hopelessness and frustration. If you then ask the child if he/she worries that his/her illness upsets the mother, the child may burst into tears, and on questioning it emerges that he/she is worried that the mother may go away and not cope with their illness. Occasionally the mother has announced she can go on no longer and she may leave home or try to "end it all". Separation anxiety is then only too real, the child is afraid to allow the depressed parent out of his/her sight, and the parent requires the child to be around to help her get through the day.

Frequently there are associated marital problems as the father resents the over-enmeshment of the child and his spouse. Emotional disorders can also arise because of other stresses affecting the child, especially in school or with friends. Some youngsters have specific learning difficulties which are seen by the teachers as laziness or lack of application. The stress is increased if the child is ridiculed or punished when trying to do his best. Other losses and separations can cause depression. The illness or death of an important family member may cause a bereavement reaction in the parent for many months. The parent is reluctant to discuss this and the child patient feels to blame when his carer is irritable and unresponsive.

Emotional disorders occur in at least 2% of the population of late primary school children. A small proportion of these children have a *mixed conduct and neurotic disorder*. These children are often brought up in disorganised, delinquent and socially deprived families with patterns of antisocial behaviour. If they become depressed by their life events, the symptoms are more likely to be difficult to contain and control. Outbursts of self-destructive behaviour and anger are exhibited by children with extreme sadness, guilt and feelings of hopelessness.

Sometimes the mixed conduct and neurotically disordered youngster will have trouble in trusting adults and needs to be contained and controlled because of the disturbed risk-taking aspects of their behaviour. Some of these youngsters are best admitted to well supervised secure units where their outbursts can be contained and longer-term treatment plans established.

ANOREXIA NERVOSA

Minor degrees of anorexia in teenage girls are commonplace. Some of the most difficult cases to treat by the child and adolescent psychiatrist are young people with a more severe degree of this disorder. Anorexia nervosa still carries a significant mortality, approximately one-third make a full recovery while many remain vulnerable, psychiatrically disturbed and requiring repeated periods of hospitalisation.

Patients are extremely thin with spindly limbs, apparently deep set eyes and a sharpness of facial features that goes with extreme weight loss. The degree of weight loss is often disguised by their tendency to wear big woolly pullovers and baggy clothes. It is only when one has sight of the protruding ribs, scapulae, clavicles and the scaphoid abdomen with the iliac crests sticking out that the degree of starvation becomes apparent. Anorexic patients usually remain active and alert and are frequently hyperactive despite their appalling nutritional state. The disorder sometimes develops from dieting and there is a selective rejection of carbohydrate food. The anorexic adolescent is often elsewhere at mealtimes or frankly refuses to eat, other than perhaps a few lettuce leaves, tomatoes and thin vegetable soup. Considerable deviance is displayed with various tactics to lose weight, the most common of which is vomiting. Anorexic patients have a habit of sliding out of the room imperceptibly to the toilet where they learn to vomit quietly and with remarkable ease. Bursts of frantic exercise occur either openly or behind locked doors while increasing quantities of laxatives and purgatives are sometimes secretly consumed. Girls develop amenorrhea and the disorder is typified by bradycardia, hypotension, a growth of fine hair, and an increase in melanin pigmentation. Sometimes the parotid glands are swollen and the back teeth decayed because of constant acid reflux from the vomiting.

The emotional state is adversely affected often with severe depressive, self-abusive and suicidal thoughts. The business of starving becomes linked with guilt. Other youngsters show hysterical attention seeking and confrontational behaviour which involves the families, the therapists or work colleagues who become fearful for the fate of the patient and also angry with them. Anorexic patients are extremely difficult to nurse with their oppositional, manipulative and self-destructive behaviour. Severe cases are often best dealt with by total bed rest for a few days, which enables total control and 24-hour nursing care to be given, including close supervision of using the bathroom and lavatory. While dietary supplements can be used it is as well to work with a dietitian and insist that prescribed food is taken regularly and nurses have the exhausting task of sitting with the patient until prescribed food has been finished and not allowing them to go to the toilet for at least another hour. Most nurses require time out themselves for a cup of coffee and an opportunity to regain equilibrium after one of these feeding sessions.

Sometimes antidepressants or major tranquillisers are used, but as with the diet, increase in dosage should be gradually built up if the patient is frail. Most of the drugs in these categories can produce hypotension while very severe cases which have been re-fed too rapidly (usually with a stomach tube) can develop acute gastric dilatation, which on occasions has been fatal. Although the dietary intake should be built up progressively it is important finally to aim the calorie intake on the youngster's expected weight and not on weight at admission.

Some workers have adopted a confronting family therapy approach, making the parents aware that their child has a limited time to survive unless they take greater control of the feeding situation and some very difficult cases have been managed by this approach. Some psychiatrists who specialise in treating this disorder are now moving to an intensive day-patient programme of care where group dynamics are used to instil a greater responsibility for the youngsters to enforce their own dietary control. This approach appears successful in the hands of skilled therapists. Patients remain less stuck in the angry oppositional approach to their carers and there is less scope for secondary gain and regression to childish patterns of dependency if the realistic limits are set by other patients who are not in authoritarian or parental positions.

Aetiology remains a topic for debate. The disorder is more common in girls than boys and appears often during adolescence. Some youngsters are parented by rigid overprotecting mothers and fathers, often, but by no means always, in higher income brackets. It is interesting that psychotherapists described a fear of oral pregnancy and now that information of sexual abuse is more openly sought, it appears that at least a minority of anorexic girls have had this experience. There are obvious hormonal and physical changes but most of these appear secondary to starvation. Those who pursue a relapsing course often develop bulimia nervosa, where there is intermittent gorging and food forcing often with very large amounts eaten in a single binge. The guilt which follows involves self-induced vomiting or purging. As with anorexia, treatment plans must be clear often with contracts drawn up so that the scheme of therapy is underpinned with behavioural objectives.

WORKING WITH PHYSICALLY ILL CHILDREN

an adult becomes unwell the therapeutic task is to store normal health as far as possible, bearing in mind the nature of the disease. If children become unwell for significant periods of time the task is not only to get them as well as possible but to enable them to be placed back on the escalator of development. Children grow in three ways: they become taller, heavier and sexually mature; they increase in cognitive abilities so they become more intelligent; and lastly, there is the less straightforward area of emotional development. As children become older and more mature they are better able to handle extremes of feelings and to give and take in interpersonal relationships and finally to cope with the tasks of adolescence involving separation and dependency issues as well as coping with more adult value systems and developing sexual maturity.

The work of a child psychiatrist is much involved with the pathology of interpersonal relationships within families and any disability, inborn or acquired, will increase the risk of harmful attitudes in other family members, e.g. overprotection, rejection and that curiously martyrish approach of parents called compensatory overprotection, where the parents need to overindulge the child, is often based on usually irrational feelings of guilt about the nature of the disorder.

Hospitals, like families, sometimes contain potentially harmful sick systems where doctors, nurses and other therapists in professional networks may have their own anxieties, frustrations and interpersonal difficulties. It is therefore the aim of the liaison psychiatrist to put the child back on the moving stairs of development to climb towards maturity in the best possible way, while acknowledging fully the limitations of the underlying disorder.

Technical advances in treatment subject children of all ages to horrendous situations where they are kept alive by stressful regimens. Family disruption with frequent attendances, transport problems, the effects of boredom, pain and tiredness take their toll. The stresses can decompensate families which are already vulnerable. Preschool children do not always understand why they are being hurt or why their parents sometimes have to leave when they are scared and in pain and for many years the sequence of angry protest followed by despair and then an emotional detachment from the parents has been recognised. Although children's hospitals lead the field in user-friendliness with a welcoming approach to parents who are encouraged to look after the essential caring needs of their children, mothers sometimes have to go home to look after the rest of the family and one can observe the harmful, albeit temporary, effect on bonding which results from this kind of separation. A young child noted to be perplexed when the mother visited at first, turned to run towards the mother but halted in her tracks, and did an about turn to run to the comfort of the ward sister.

Children think in concrete practical terms and can be confused about illness and occasionally the possibility of dying. Death is seen as a reversible phenomenon by the very young. One young child almost died from a very deliberate overdose of several tablets which had been put on a high shelf. His grandfather had died and it appeared the only way to visit him was to go to heaven, and the only way to heaven was to become dead. Having been told the tablets were poisonous he forced the contents of several bottles of pills down and waited for a "sort of aeroplane ride" to get to heaven. When it was explained that there was no way back and he would not be able to see any of his friends and relatives again, he decided that he had been unwise. The child can often accept handicaps or painful treatments as long as all is explained honestly and at a level that can be understood. Anxiety increases if the parents do not appear to be at ease with the situation or if the child is told untruths or let down. Essentially one has to be available to listen to the child's worries and questions and then discuss with the parents how the questions should be answered. While it may well be unnecessary to trouble a child with details of a poor prognosis it can be very cruel to fob him off with platitudes. Anxious children can be told not to be silly or "let's see a smile" so that the anxieties which are worrying them are deflected and not dealt with.

How does the family cope?

There are predictable patterns, coping with bad news for example – the mild malaise is actually renal failure and a transplant is required. Or the anaemia is really a cancer of the blood, or his intelligence will be seriously impaired and there is no treatment for this disorder. *Denial* where there is disbelief must be present in all of us. The effect of this is that potentially successful treatment regimens may not be adhered to, or second or third opinions may be sought. *Reaction formation* is where there is opposition to the underlying feeling so that there may be overcompensation which might put pressure on an ill child to achieve more than he/she is easily able to do. *Anger* is also very common. Some professionals find the anger of parents hard to take. This anger should not be taken personally as it is a response to the loss of function in the child. If someone buys a new washing machine and it leaks or ceases to function it is usual to be angry with the manufacturer or the supplier. Such an event is trivial compared with serious loss of function in a child and the anger will pass, as long as it is not reciprocated by staff who take on board the criticisms of distraught parents. *Guilt* is really anger turned inwards and there is always soul-searching as to how the disease or accident could have been avoided. Sometimes this turns into *depression* where there is an escalation of guilt with sleep and appetite disturbance and

sometimes morbid thoughts in the parent. The *marital situation* can deteriorate where one parent, often the mother, spends a long time in hospital while the father may be marginalised. The exhaustion and the disruption of routine cause irritability and sometimes disagreements at the way the child is managed. The *siblings* are also compromised in that their basic emotional needs are not always met by the parents. One little girl with a urinary infection was reassured that she would not need dialysis like her sister. She took an instant temper tantrum, slammed out of the office in anger, saying "does that mean I am not getting the machine as well then". The *child* may show similar defences and adolescents with *denial* may not cooperate with treatment regimens.

Although denial is in many ways an excellent defence, it becomes unhelpful when insulin injections penetrate the arm of the settee rather than the youngster's subcutaneous tissues. Small vulnerable children may need to be big and tough, which is an example of *reaction formation* while others may *regress* to infantile, whiny and dependent behaviour. Some youngsters develop rituals before treatment regimens and others dispel their anxiety in fantasy. There are a lot of bandaged teddies in Yorkhill hospital. Adolescents sometimes identify with medical staff by taking an intellectual interest in their disorder. All these mental defence mechanisms can be helpful as well as destructive and if these defences fail too rapidly the patient may be overcome with *anxiety* become *severely depressed* or on occasion curl up in a fetal position and *withdraw* from all therapy which includes pulling out lines, catheters, gastric feeds and refuse to eat.

The predicament of a sick child affects the whole family and the patient and the family member should end up with a realistic acceptance of the disorder so that the child is not overprotected or expected to do more than he is able. It is best to see both parents together, and for the same person to see the parents on a number of occasions, finding out what they took away from the previous interview. The aim is to achieve realistic acceptance of the child's loss of function. A conspiracy of silence and non-communication should be avoided and the child's questions answered directly and honestly. School attainment should be considered important as long-term disorders can interrupt education. If the child remains physically unwell he will be employed for his thinking ability rather than for his capacity to do physical work. Staff must not bear hostility personally and team approach is necessary in a ward of a specialised unit so that communications between team members is strong enough to avoid anxious parents inadvertently setting one professional up against another. The parents should be given their place although strong relationships will build up between children and nurses. Nurses should be encouraged where they need, to set limits. Chronically ill children need discipline as well as care and anxious parents make nurses feel ill at ease. With chronically ill children the work is multidisciplinary and all members of the team should feel appropriately useful and valued. Work will be stressful especially when children do not recover. Most hospital units have excellent morale. There is a place for regular discussion, both case centred and more informally, so that anxieties are shared and treatment goals are established.

CHILD ABUSE

Fractures, scalds, burns, lacerations, cuts, head injuries, poisoning with medications or ingestion of damaging substances provide the everyday work of the Accident and Emergency Department. Damage around the mouth and ears and bruising in unusual places, e.g. between the thighs, around the genitalia, or in the centre of the back or abdomen, should raise a degree of suspicion. Bruising, taking the form of finger prints, where a child has been too forcefully held or shaken, is even more worrying, especially if fingertip bruising or lacerations occur on the face or on the trunk of babies. While children who are mobile frequently fall over and bump into things, babies who are too young to walk or crawl are much less likely to have these kind of accidents.

The signs that arouse suspicion of sexual abuse are now legion. Apart from obvious trauma around the genitalia or anal region, recurrent urinary tract infections and vaginal infections or pregnancy in older girls should be considered. There is an increased incidence of psychogenic pains, often abdominal, and other symptoms amounting to conversion hysteria. For example, partial loss of function in a limb, may indicate that a child is under stress which is too difficult to go on tolerating and too difficult to be disclosed. Some cases of anorexia nervosa, psychogenic vomiting, soiling, sleep disturbance, anxiety, depression and absconding from home may also occur.

The way in which the child behaves should also be noted. Abused children may be particularly fearful of adults, especially of the same sex as the abuser and appear apprehensive or withdrawn. If a child is taken to a playroom and immediately cowers in the corner when the therapist closes the door this can be very revealing. Children often replicate confusing worrying accidents in their play. Children's drawings may also indicate fears of sexual objects or sexual knowledge beyond what is age-appropriate. Most of all, it is important to listen to what the child has to say. Although children can be regarded as manipulative troublemakers, it is very unusual for children to disclose abuse which has not actually occurred. They are more likely to remain mute or ill at ease in order to protect their perpetrators.

Lastly, one should take careful account of the way in which the cause of an accident is described by the parents. Explanations which are doubtful and inconsistent, or where the visit to the casualty department has been delayed should give rise for concern. Conversely, too frequent attendance with injuries should also cause concern. It should also be remembered that one of the causes of "failure to thrive", including the so-called deprivation dwarfism, can be the result of lack of food.

Working with social workers and police

It is important that doctors familiarise themselves with the social arrangements and statutory procedures for liaison with social work departments (or their equivalents) and where necessary appropriate links with the police, juvenile courts, reporters to children's panels and other legal bodies are made. Careful notes should be kept of interviews and physical examinations. If sexual abuse is suspected, it is important that special local arrangements for examining children are adhered to. In some situations examinations are carried out jointly by a paediatrician trained in sexual abuse work and the police surgeon so that only one examination is performed. The provision of special units with quietness and appropriately comfortable chairs is to be welcomed. In this kind of setting full explanations can be given and trust built up between the child and the examining doctor. The skills of being frank and open at a level the child can understand, seeking the child's permission and talking him/her through the examination goes some way to reducing the secondary emotional damage from the fear resulting from disclosure. Any attempts to tussle with the child to perform the examination must increase the horror of further abuse. If a parent or relative has been the perpetrator and then doctors remove the child's clothes and intrude into the child's personal space, it must seem to the child as if no adult in authority can ever be trusted again.

Physical abuse is often relatively easy to recognise and prove, while *sexual abuse* may be devoid of physical findings. Although dialogue with the child or interpretation of his/her behaviour sometimes leaves little doubt to the clinician that abuse has occurred, the legal system is not always well equipped to cope so that a number of cases are not proven with resulting further difficulties for those managing the case.

Perhaps most difficult of all is the category of *emotional abuse* and *failure to thrive* where the parents contest the need for intervention. Close cooperation is required with social workers and the appropriate legal networks. Mention must also be made of the *Munchausen by proxy (Meadows syndrome)* where children are repeatedly brought to hospital with symptoms which tempt the physician or surgeon to subject the child to numerous investigations, sometimes of an increasingly intrusive, traumatic and expensive form. Sometimes surgical intervention or complex treatment regimens are set up and still the problem fails to resolve. Mothers have been known to dip their tampons into their child's urine specimen to precipitate investigations for haematuria, drinks can be doctored to make the child unwell or present with abdominal pain, and anoxic seizures have been produced by mothers attempting to suffocate their children and then nursing staff are summoned to deal with the convulsion that has again mysteriously occurred despite normal ECGs, EEGs, X-rays, scans and biochemical assessments. It is well recognised that many depressed mothers of Munchausen by proxy children are usually suffering from much more long-standing disorders of personality. These are often the result of severe early deprivation and physical and sometimes sexual abuse at periods of time throughout important stages in their own emotional development. The mothers are often most cooperative and adapt well into the ward routine. It is not unusual for them to have nursing experience so that they are acquainted with hospital life. Often they spend many hours in hospital with their children, "taking in" the concern and caring of doctors and nurses.

It is difficult to empathise with their psychopathology and the concept of dissociation must be understood. The ability to role-play the competent caring mother and yet to behave destructively in order to gain the interest and emotional input from doctors and nurses can only be understood by hearing these mothers describing their past and their feelings at the present time. Obviously confrontation is not always met by an honest admission of guilt and it is important that appropriate care and protection orders are sought if the symptoms appear life-threatening to the child. If a confrontation is made either by the clinician or after what is sometimes a long and arduous court hearing, the parent may decompensate. The needy, distraught mother once again in her life is shown to have failed. Psychiatric intervention may be necessary as the depressive self-destruction feelings are mobilised when the mechanism of dissociation is broken down. While many anxious parents unwittingly subject their children to the effects of their anxiety and over-concern, in the Munchausen by proxy situation the problem is of a different order because the parent is usually doing something actively thought out to produce the child's symptoms.

11

The Skin

SKIN DISORDERS

In this chapter we will discuss only some common skin disorders of childhood which differ in important respects from those of adult life. The history from the parents must be taken carefully and it should not be restricted to the skin alone. The aims of the dermatological/physical examination are to determine as accurately as possible the distribution, size and arrangement of the components of the eruption and to define the morphology of the individual lesions. The whole surface area of skin of the unclothed child should be examined, including the hair, nails and mucosae. In most children with skin disorders a diagnosis can be made just by inspection and palpation, as in cases of atopic eczema, warts, impetigo, psoriasis and Henoch–Schönlein purpura. It is only occasionally that a histopathological examination of the skin, bacterial, viral and fungal investigations and allergic skin testing are required to clarify the clinical diagnosis. Before turning to common skin disorders it would be useful to think about cutaneous manifestations in relation to general systemic disorders. There are rare inherited disorders, involving many systems which manifest by their skin lesions.

Tuberous sclerosis

Tuberous sclerosis (epiloia) is one of the phakomatoses with manifestations in the skin, central nervous system, and eye as well as hamartomas of internal organs such as kidney, heart, lung and bone. In most cases, ash leaf spots are present at birth but they may appear in infancy and childhood. Ash leaf spots occur most commonly on the posterior trunk. These hypopigmented lesions can be best seen with the help of a Wood's light which accentuates areas of hypopigmentation. Other cutaneous features of tuberous sclerosis include angiofibromas of the face (adenoma sebaceum), peri-ungual fibromas and shagreen patches (like rough leather) may be present on other parts of the body (see Fig. 9.4).

Neurofibromatosis (von Recklinghausen disease)

Neurofibromatosis is another phakomatosis with manifestations in the skin, eye, bone, soft tissues and the central nervous system. As in tuberous sclerosis the earliest sign of neurofibromatosis is pigmentary change on the skin. *Café-au-lait* spots or patches are

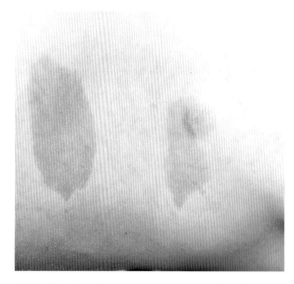

FIGURE 11.1 Neurofibromatosis, showing *café-au-lait* spots on the trunk.

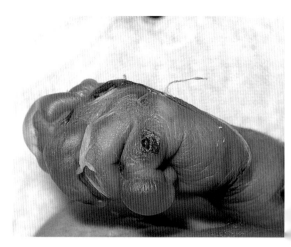

FIGURE 11.2 Epidermolysis bullosa, showing blisters on fingers.

irregularly shaped macules and are often present at or shortly after birth and may increase in size and number with age (Fig. 11.1). This cutaneous manifestation is virtually pathognomonic of neurofibromatosis. Therefore a diagnosis of neurofibromatosis should be considered in children who have six or more *café-au-lait* spots greater than 0.5 cm in diameter. Other cutaneous manifestations are the presence of pedunculated neurofibromas.

Extracutaneous manifestations of tuberous sclerosis and neurofibromatosis are discussed in Chapter 9.

Epidermolysis bullosa

Epidermolysis bullosa comprises of a group of inherited disorders of skin characterised by an abnormal susceptibility to blister formation at the site of mechanical trauma. There are three main types of epidermolysis bullosa depending upon the anatomical site of splitting at which blistering occurs.

Epidermolysis bullosa simplex is the most superficial type with splitting of the epidermis within the basal layer. The junctional type has splitting within the lamina lucida and the dystrophic type has a split within the dermis, below the lamina densa. Epidermolysis bullosa usually presents in the neonatal period with blisters caused by trauma from delivery or trauma from handling in the first few days of life (Fig. 11.2). Treatment is essentially supportive care, but even with this blistering and adhesion of fingers with secondary syndactyly may occur. Prophylaxis against trauma is crucial and infants may benefit from padding over the sites of friction. Other treatment modalities at present being studied are cultured epidermal allografts and synthetic skin allografts. Prenatal diagnosis is available.

CONNECTIVE TISSUE DISORDERS

The skin manifestations of connective tissue disease are often characteristic and sometimes specific for one particular clinical entity or they may simply indicate the presence of a connective tissue disease. The degree of cutaneous involvement is not proportional to the extent of visceral involvement and sometimes there may be no skin lesions. The cutaneous manifestations of acute rheumatic fever and Henoch–Schönlein purpura are well known and present no problems in diagnosis (see Chapter 15). The rash of systemic onset type juvenile chronic arthritis consists of small macular lesions with a slightly irregular margin which often show central pallor. The rash may be slightly raised, especially when it first appears, but does not itch. In colour, the rash is bright salmon pink and is usually encircled by a narrow areola of normal skin which is paler than its surroundings. The rash is characteristically fleeting, tending to appear in association with raised skin temperature (e.g. after a hot bath).

Of all the connective tissue disorders the skin manifestations of scleroderma are probably the easiest to diagnose. There are two broad classes of scleroderma: localised and systemic. In the systemic form of scleroderma the well known atrophy and tightening of the skin gives a characteristic appearance of pinched nose and pursed lips. The hands become shiny with tapered fingertips and restricted movement. There may also be subcutaneous calcification and occasional ulceration. Raynaud phenomenon is not uncommon and may be severe with resultant gangrene. The localised type of sclero-derma has three main variants, guttate morphoea, generalised morphoea and linear scleroderma. Guttate morphoea usually presents with multiple, small, ivory coloured lesions with minimal sclerosis. The neck, anterior chest and shoulders are the most common sites. Children with generalised morphoea have more of these sclerotic patches involving a greater surface area. Linear scleroderma occurs as a linear band of hypopigmentation and sclerosis occur-ring most commonly on one leg.

In dermatomyositis the face is commonly involved. There may be a violaceous colour of the eyelids and some dilatation of the capillaries over the malar bones, the eyelids, the knuckles, various pressure points and the dorsum of the hands. There is no correlation between the extent of skin markings and the degree of muscle involvement in dermatomyosi-tis.

In systemic lupus erythematosus the classic cutaneous feature is an eruption on both cheeks spreading over the bridge of the nose. In acute systemic lupus erythematosus cutaneous lesions may appear on the face, trunk and limbs. The erythema-tous rash may be transient or long-standing. It is often revealed or exacerbated by sunlight or other ultraviolet radiation. Alopecia is often an early sign of systemic lupus erythematosus in young teenage girls but is uncommon in younger children. Vasculitic lesions are rare but have been reported on mucous membranes of the mouth and nose.

ERYTHEMA NODOSUM

In children it is associated with streptococcal infec-tion and primary tuberculosis and rarely due to sarcoidosis, ulcerative colitis, Crohn disease and drugs, in particular sulphonamides. Erythema nodosum is characterised by red tender nodular lesions, usually present on shins, though the lesions may be found on other parts of the body (Fig. 11.3).

GLANDULAR FEVER (INFECTIOUS MONONUCLEOSIS)

Glandular fever is caused by the Epstein–Barr (EB) virus. Antibodies to this EB virus can be demon-strated in the serum of 100% of patients with glandu-lar fever. They persist for long periods and can be clearly distinguished from the heterophil antibodies of the Paul–Bunnell test which disappear within a few months. The mode of transmission of glandular fever is most often by intimate oral contact.

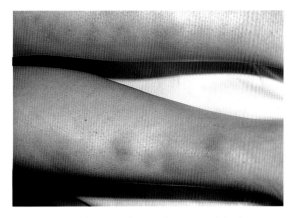

FIGURE 11.3 Erythema nodosum, showing nodular lesions on shins.

The incubation period has usually been stated to be 10–15 days but a much longer interval of 30–45 days has been postulated. Children are usually less ill than adults, and severe anginose cases with membra-nous pharyngitis are rare. The onset is acute with fever, malaise, headache and anorexia. The pharynx is inflamed but the young child may not complain of a sore throat. The fever may last only a few days, or for a few weeks. A characteristic finding in many cases and of diagnostic value is the presence of petechiae over the soft palate and other areas of the buccal mucosa. Generalised enlargement of the super-ficial lymph nodes is characteristic, although it may not develop for a week or more after the onset. Splenomegaly is almost invariable. In some cases jaundice and hepatomegaly occur. A rubelliform rash is not infrequent. Rarely, a child with glandular fever develops meningism and a lymphocytic reaction in the cerebrospinal fluid. Peripheral blood examination in glandular fever reveals a marked excess of mononuclear cells. Most of these are abnormal with deep blue staining cytoplasm which often contains vacuoles. The nucleus is frequently eccentric and the cell margin may appear to be lobulated, as if pseudopodia were forming. Some of the cells closely simulate lymphoblasts when the suspicion of leukaemia can be aroused. Proof of the diagnosis rests upon the Paul–Bunnell test for heterophil antibodies to sheep red cells. This becomes positive after 1 week. False positive results, such as may develop after an injection of horse serum, can be excluded by absorp-tion techniques using guinea-pig kidney and beef red cells. A titre of 1 in 64 is considered to be diagnos-tic. A rapid slide test, the "monospot" test, is also available and is based on the presence in the serum of agglutinins to horse red cells.

There is no specific treatment. Rest in bed is indicated until the fever has disappeared and the lymphadenopathy has subsided. Relapses occasionally

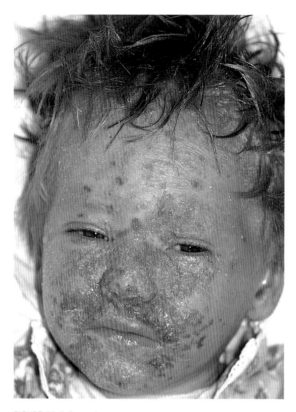

FIGURE 11.4 Impetigo.

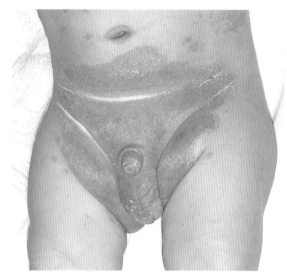

FIGURE 11.5 Seborrhoeic dermatitis.

occur and convalescence should be gradual. Complete recovery is assured.

IMPETIGO

It is a superficial infection usually caused by staphylococci and/or streptococci. It is usually associated with poor hygiene, undernutrition and overcrowding. It starts as a vesicle which ruptures, releasing a yellow exudate that dries and forms a crust (Fig. 11.4). A skin swab should be taken to determine the causative organisms and sensitivity. The treatment of choice is with topical antibiotic preparations. Systemic antibiotics are indicated only when the child has constitutional symptoms.

SEBORRHOEIC DERMATITIS

This is common from birth to 18 months of age but uncommon afterwards. The aetiology is unknown. In infants it may present as scaly, crusted, greasy patches over the scalp (cradle cap), sometimes reaching behind the ears or onto forehead or eyebrows (Fig. 11.5). Infants with seborrhoeic dermatitis do not

usually scratch and this would help in distinguishing it from atopic dermatitis in which pruritis is usually present. It may get secondarily infected. The prognosis is excellent and in most cases it will clear within a few weeks. Seborrhoeic dermatitis usually responds quickly to topical corticosteroids in combination with an imidazole agent (Daktacort or Canesten HC). Cradle cap can be treated with coconut or arachis oil massaged into the scalp prior to washing with a mild baby shampoo. Salicylic acid preparations should be avoided because of their irritant effect and the risk of percutaneous absorption.

ATOPIC ECZEMA (ATOPIC DERMATITIS)

There is a recognised genetic predisposition and the majority of children have a family history of atopy. Atopic eczema does not start until the infant is at least 2 or 3 months old, when it usually affects the face, trunk and extensor surfaces of the limbs. Between 2 and 4 years of age a change may occur in distribution. In older children the face often is spared, the trunk is minimally involved and the lesions on arms and legs are predominantly flexor (Fig. 11.6). In the chronic stages of eczema there is scaling, thickening and lichenification. Bacterial infection with staphylococci is common and aggravates the eczema. In contrast to infantile seborrhoeic dermatitis there is marked irritation with scratching and loss of sleep.

Herpetic eczema or Kaposi varicelliform eruption is due to infection with herpes virus. Prompt treatment with intravenous acyclovir is indicated in these seriously ill children. Children with eczema should

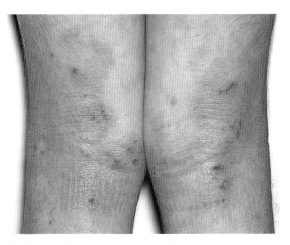

FIGURE 11.6 Flexural eczema in popliteal fossae.

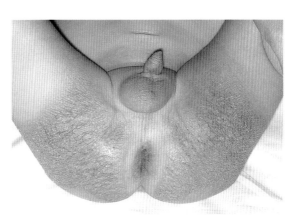

FIGURE 11.7 Napkin dermatitis.

avoid contact with individuals who have active "cold sores".

Children with atopic eczema usually have increased plasma IgE values and often produce multiple positive prick tests to a variety of common allergens. There is also evidence of a defect in cell-mediated immunity with a reduction of suppressor T lymphocytes.

The prognosis of children with eczema is good. If asthma is going to develop in these children it usually does so in the first 5 years. A child with acute eczema may need admission to hospital for a short period, perhaps to control secondary infection, or habit scratching and possibly to give the parents a rest. Emollients using a bath oil reduces the pruritis and helps the dry skin. Application of 1% hydrocortisone is usually sufficient although sometimes a potent topical steroid may be necessary. Occlusive medicated bandages, e.g. zinc paste and icthammol underneath a dry elasticated bandage, are useful for treating excoriated lichenified eczema of the limbs.

NAPKIN DERMATITIS (DIAPER DERMATITIS, NAPPY RASH)

The most common form of napkin rash is an irritant contact dermatitis due to the contact of urine and faeces with the skin. The rash is usually limited by the margins of nappy with sparing of the inguinal folds (Fig. 11.7). It should be remembered that secondary infection due to *Monilia* and bacteria can occur.

Napkins should be changed as soon as they are wet or soiled by stools. A protective covering of zinc and castor oil, zinc cream or petroleum jelly is usually all that is required. Secondary bacterial or monilial infections should be treated if present.

URTICARIA

Urticaria may be acute or chronic. Urticarial lesions may occur on any area of the body. They usually have raised erythematous edges and blanched centres. These lesions are intensely pruritic. Urticaria may be associated with angio-oedema. Angio-oedema occurs in deeper subcutaneous layers as areas of oedema that may or may not be pruritic. In angio-oedema the oedema occurs on the face (lips, tongue, perioral and periorbital areas) and extremities. In the majority of cases no cause is found. However, in a small number of cases the causes of urticaria include allergy to foods (e.g. fish, eggs, chocolate), drugs (e.g. aspirin, penicillin) and sensitivity to bites by insects. Immunoglobulin E-mediated release is often responsible for acute episodes of urticaria, especially those associated with food sensitivity and animal contact. In hereditary angio-oedema the absence of functional C1 esterase inhibitor results in complement activation and repeated episodes of angio-oedema. The best treatment is to remove the cause but it is not always discoverable. Systemic antihistamines remain the treatment of choice.

Urticaria pigmentosa (cutaneous mastocytosis)

Urticaria pigmentosa in children presents as red brown papules or nodules found mainly on the trunk. These lesions are foci of mast cells and become urticarial when rubbed. Most affected children develop lesions by 2 years of age. Long-standing lesions show increased pigmentation. Skin biopsy can confirm the diagnosis as it will show collections of mast cells in the dermis and subcutaneous tissue.

A small number of children may show systemic involvement, i.e. flushing, headaches, tachycardia, hypotension and coagulation abnormalities. In the systemic form mast cells may infiltrate bone marrow, liver, spleen and gastrointestinal tract.

In the majority of children with cutaneous masto-cytosis the lesions resolve spontaneously by puberty.

SCABIES

Scabies is caused by the *Sarcoptes scabiei*. The fertilised female mite lives and lays eggs in burrows in the outer layers of the skin. The burrows in older children and adults are usually found in the interdig-ital spaces. Lesions of scabies in infants and young children are frequently vesicular and are distributed more widely with the head, neck, palms and soles particularly affected. Children become sensitised to the scabies mite and develop an intense itch at the affected areas. Secondary bacterial infections commonly complicate scabies. It is very contagious and is transmitted by close personal contact.

It is vital that all members of the family and close contacts should be treated simultaneously. It is crucial that any treatment of scabies be applied to the whole body from the head downward, with special atten-tion to the hands, feet, soles of the feet and under the finger nails. Benzyl benzoate is an effective treatment although it is irritant to the skin. Scabicides such as malathion and permethrin can be applied with care to the hair and body, avoiding the face.

PEDICULOSIS CAPITIS (LOUSE INFESTATION)

The condition may be asymptomatic in early stages. Sooner or later sensitisation to insect allergen occurs and itching develops. Secondary infection of the scalp lesions is common and is an important cause of impetigo of the scalp in children. The eggs (nits) are readily detected as minute oval structures firmly attached to the hair shaft. They are usually found in the post-auricular and occipital areas where infesta-tion tends to be heaviest.

Treatment consists of application of a pediculoci-dal shampoo or lotion such as malathion or perme-thrin, taking care to avoid the eyes. Treatment should be repeated in 10 days.

CANDIDIASIS

Oral candidiasis, called thrush, is common in child-hood and is characterised by white, elevated lesions

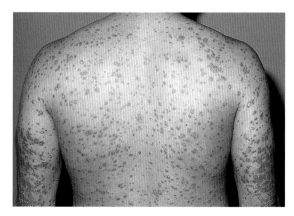

FIGURE 11.8 Guttate psoriasis.

that adhere to the mucosa. Removal of the lesions may leave superficial erosions. The treatment of choice for thrush is the application of nystatin suspension to the lesions four times daily for 7 days.

Secondary infection of napkin dermatitis with candida is a common clinical problem. This presents as confluent areas of intense erythema often with small satellite areas with red centres and white flakey margins near and beyond the border of confluent areas. Areas infected with candida may become extremely inflamed and swollen. Nystatin ointment may be applied four times daily and is ordinarily effective. Oral nystatin will reduce or eradicate the population of candida in the gastrointestinal tract and this has been recommended in difficult to eradicate infections.

Cutaneous candidiasis may occur on any warm or moist part of the body especially in immunosup-pressed children. The clinical appearance and treat-ment are essentially the same as that of candidiasis affecting the napkin area.

Chronic mucocutaneous candidiasis is a rare syndrome whose prominent manifestation is chronic infection of skin, nails and mucous membranes with candida without systemic infection. The onset of skin lesions occurs in infancy. Most patients have defects in cell-mediated immunity and may have associated deficiencies in humoral immunity. Also some children with chronic mucocutaneous candidiasis are associ-ated with various endocrinopathies. As regards the treatment, ketoconazole is the most effective drug available for chronic mucocutaneous candidiasis. For systemic candidiasis see page 46.

PSORIASIS

Psoriasis is a chronic relapsing inflammatory skin disorder. A family history of psoriasis is common. The typical lesions are plaques of silvery scales capping a

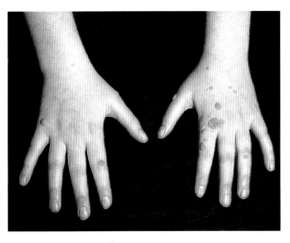

FIGURE 11.9 Warts on fingers.

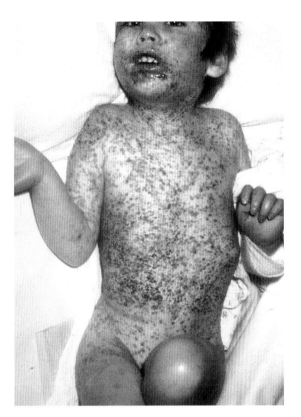

FIGURE 11.10 Chicken pox.

sharply edged salmon-red base. They occur most commonly on extensor surfaces of limbs, but also on the scalp and trunk. A special form of guttate psoriasis is typically seen in children aged between 5 and 12 years after a streptococcal infection (Fig. 11.8).

Crude coal tar remains a most effective treatment for psoriasis. Initially 1% tar in zinc ointment should be applied to the involved areas twice daily, the strength of tar being gradually increased to 15% if required. Alternatively, dithranol in zinc and salicylic acid paste can be used.

COMMON WARTS (VERRUCAE)

These are the result of hyperplasia of epithelial cells due to the human papilloma virus. Children who are immunosuppressed are especially susceptible to warts. The commonest appearance is that of a small raised painless lesion with a rough dry surface (Fig. 11.9). Warts are very contagious and the child may autoinoculate in different places. Plantar warts can be very painful and are difficult to treat. Genital and perianal warts are not uncommon and when found the possibility of sexual abuse has to be considered. Many common warts disappear spontaneously although this can take a few months. However, they can be treated with keratolytics such as salicylic acid and glutaraldehyde. Warts can be treated by diathermy or by freezing with liquid nitrogen or carbon dioxide snow (cryotherapy).

HERPES SIMPLEX INFECTIONS

Cutaneous infections with herpes simplex virus are not uncommon in children. Primary herpes gingivos-

tomatitis is the most common clinically apparent herpes infection. It is characterised by fever, malaise, headache and small eroded vesicles on the lips and oral mucosa. Herpetic infections of the fingers and thumb may occur during the course of herpetic gingivostomatitis if children put them in their mouths. Herpetic genital infections are much less common in children than they are in adults. Sexual abuse should be considered a possibility in children with herpes genitalis.

No effective therapy is available for herpetic gingivostomatitis or any other herpes infection though oral acyclovir can be used for disseminated herpes infections. In children with gingivostomatitis healing usually occurs in 7–10 days.

CHICKEN POX (VARICELLA)

Chicken pox is a disease mainly of childhood. The virus of chicken pox belongs to the herpes group and it is identical to that of herpes zoster. The incubation period varies from 14 to 21 days. The disease is highly contagious. It is characterised by a rash with centripetal distribution. The lesions appear in successive crops, initially as papules, and passing through the stages of vesiculation, pustulation and crust formation (Fig. 11.10). The virus can pass through the placenta and thus a baby may be born with congenital chicken pox or develop it in the early neonatal period. Complications such as chicken pox pneumonia, encephalitis and encephalomyelitis with cerebellar involvement are rare. However, patients who are on long-term corticosteroid therapy can develop intercurrent infections with chicken pox virus which may result in a severe or fatal illness. These children should be given zoster or varicella immune globulin.

In a typical case of chicken pox the diagnosis rarely causes any real clinical difficulty. There is no specific therapy. An attack of chicken pox confers long-lasting immunity to varicella but not to herpes zoster.

MEASLES

Measles is caused by a paramyxovirus, an RNA virus closely related to the canine distemper virus. The virus enters the body by droplet spread. The incubation period to the commencement of the catarrhal stage is 10–11 days.

The clinical manifestations are sufficiently distinctive so that a specific clinical diagnosis can be made in most cases. Usually the infection starts like a common cold, with a rise in temperature, dry or croupy cough, conjunctivitis and photophobia. On the second day Koplik spots (tiny bluish white specks upon a red base) appear on the buccal mucosa and these are thought to be pathognomonic of measles. On the third or fourth day a maculopapular rash starts behind the ears, face, neck and upper chest. The child is miserable, irritable and resists examination. The temperature falls by lysis as the rash fades. Pneumonia in undernourished children is a dreadful complication. The other serious complication is post-infectious encephalomyelitis which occurs 7–14 days after rash is subsiding. Subacute sclerosing panencephalitis is an extremely rare later complication. Gammaglobulin given intramuscularly to contacts within 6 days of exposure to measles usually achieves either prevention or modification of the attack of measles. Routine immunisation with MMR (measles, mumps and rubella) vaccine at the age of 12–18 months should be carried out.

RUBELLA

The disease is caused by a single stranded RNA virus. It is disseminated by droplet spread. The incubation period varies from 14 to 19 days. A variable prodrome of malaise, cough, sore throat, fever, headache and eye pain may occur. In children there may be no prodro-

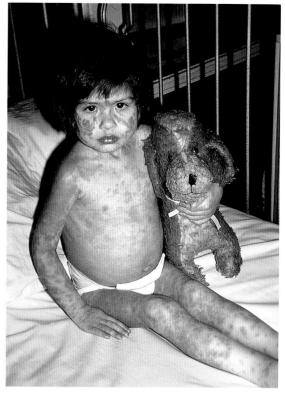

FIGURE 11.11 Drug rash.

mal symptoms and the first sign of the disease is the rash which is usually light in colour and less confluent than the rash of measles. The rash first appears behind the ears then spreads to involve the neck, face, trunk and limbs. Enlargement of lymph nodes is a very constant finding in rubella, and it is usually the suboccipital glands that are enlarged, but occasionally other groups of glands may be affected. Complications are rare. If the virus infects the fetus during the first 4 months of pregnancy the infant may be born with microcephalus, cerebral damage, cataracts, congenital heart disease, deafness and thrombocytopenia.

No specific therapy for rubella is available. Treatment is mainly symptomatic. Immunity following rubella is life long. Children should receive MMR (measles, mumps and rubella) vaccine at 12–18 months of age.

DRUG RASHES

These are less common in children than in adults. Any drug may produce nearly any type of cutaneous reaction but most commonly cause a macular erythematous rash (Fig. 11.11). Drug rashes are usually sudden in onset. The diagnosis of drug rash is made by having a high index of suspicion and by obtaining

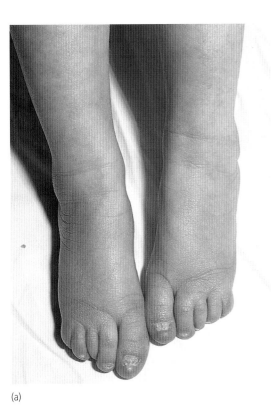

(a)

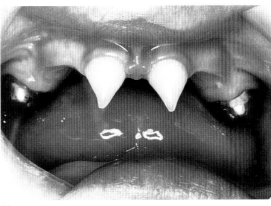

(b)

FIGURE 11.12 Ectodermal dysplasia. (a) Dysplastic nails. (b) Conical teeth.

a careful drug history. Treatment in a suspected case is to withdraw the drug. A soothing calamine lotion can be applied and antihistamines may help.

ALOPECIA AREATA

Alopecia areata usually presents as one or two well circumscribed smooth bald areas of the scalp. The aetiology of this condition is not clear. The diagnosis of trichotillomania is made in children who develop the habit of twisting and pulling out hair. In these children the bald patches are usually found on the frontal and temporal areas of the scalp. Fortunately in most affected children hair growth will recover with or without treatment. Occasionally some children may need psychiatric help.

ECTODERMAL DYSPLASIA

There are two main types of ectodermal dysplasia: the anhidrotic and hidrotic type. In anhidrotic-type affected children have a characteristic facial appearance with soft dry wrinkled skin, sparse hair, conical teeth, nails which are often thin and ridged and unexplained hyperpyrexia (Fig. 11.12). The mode of inheritance is X-linked recessive. The hidrotic-type

ectodermal dysplasia is autosomal dominant in inheritance. It is less disabling than the anhidrotic form.

APLASIA

Congenital skin defects are most often found on the scalp but occasionally an infant may have lesions on the trunk and these are often bilateral. Rarely they are of a size which benefits by skin grafting but more commonly cicatrise and heal spontaneously.

HAEMANGIOMA

Birth marks may be unsightly and cause great distress to both the patient and parents. Haemangiomas are developmental malformations of proliferating blood vessels. They commonly occur in the skin but may occur in any organ.

Clinical classification

The spider naevus

These lesions may appear after birth or later in association with cirrhosis of the liver. Usually they

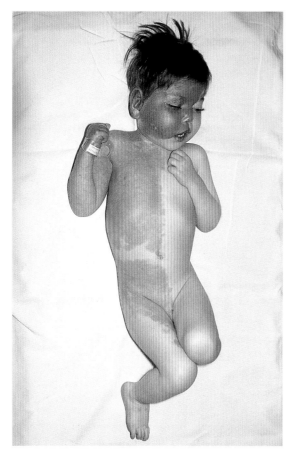

FIGURE 11.13 Sturge–Weber syndrome, showing facial haemangioma.

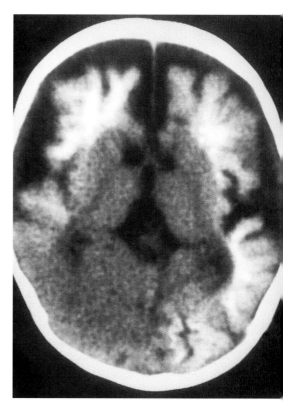

FIGURE 11.14 Sturge–Weber syndrome, cranial CAT showing calcification.

are isolated and have a bright red central core with intradermal vessels radiating for a few millimetres and blanch on pressure.

Treatment

These may disappear spontaneously but if they do not they can be treated by point diathermy under a general anaesthetic.

Salmon-patch (stork marks)

The salmon-patch or stork marks are superficial capilliary haemangiomata which are light pink in colour, most commonly seen in young infants on the nape of the neck and forehead, bridge of the nose and upper eyelids. The colour varies with temperature changes and deepens when the child cries or strains.

Treatment

Most lesions have almost disappeared by school age. If they are unsightly they may be treated with carbon dioxide snow which may improve the cosmetic appearance.

The port wine stain

These lesions are entirely in the dermis and produce a flat red lesion. There is a thin layer of capilliary tissue in the dermis causing a purplish discoloration which does not blanch readily on pressure. On the face, these lesions are very unsightly. They may affect the hemiface and scalp and be associated with intracranial vascular malformation which may cause convulsions (Sturge–Weber syndrome).

Treatment

This type seldom regresses but disfigurement can be concealed by cosmetic make-up and many lesions respond to targeted laser therapy.

The Sturge–Weber syndrome

In this disease there is an association between extensive cutaneous port wine haemangioma of the upper face and scalp, which is limited by the midline, and a similar vascular anomaly of the underlying meninges on the same side. The infant usually starts to have convulsions confined to the contralateral side of the body. The cause is obvious from the distribution of the facial haemangioma (Fig. 11.13). In time a spastic hemiparesis develops on the contralateral

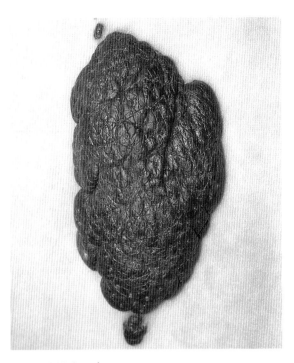

FIGURE 11.15 Strawberry naevus.

side. Later in childhood, but rarely in infancy, radiographs of the skull show a characteristic double contour of "tramline" type of calcification (see Figs 9.5 and 11.14). Mental deterioration ultimately appears and progresses. Glaucoma may also develop and require surgical intervention.

Raised haemangiomas – superficial

The *capillary tissue* with subcutaneous extensions forms a bright red, raised mass – *strawberry birth mark* (Fig. 11.15). These lesions may be very small and not obvious at birth but then may enlarge rapidly in infancy. Rarely they may ulcerate and may also become septic. The resulting scarring may be unsightly. There is also a risk of haemorrhage. They are most common around the face and scalp but may occur anywhere on the skin surface.

Strawberry birth marks usually grow in size from birth onward and they usually increase in size during the first year of life; they then stop growing and subsequently regress spontaneously. At the age of 6 or 7 years they usually disappear leaving little or no blemish.

Treatment

It is important to resist surgical intervention in all except those around the eyes until this phase of spontaneous resolution occurs. Surgical intervention may be necessary to debulk the lesion and to allow normal binocular vision to be developed. Treatment with steroids and interferon-α is being evaluated. Other treatments sometimes tried include hypertonic saline injections and carbon dioxide snow applied locally.

Cavernous haemangiomas

Cavernous haemangiomas consist of deep proliferative vascular channels and are more common than the capilliary ones. At birth, there is usually a small lesion which is hardly visible. Over the ensuing months it increases in size but may disappear again without treatment. Clinically they are raised with a light bluish discoloration. It is possible to squeeze the blood out of them and make them blanch using extrinsic pressure. Therapy is usually reserved for those areas where they may occur such as the lip, the subglottic region, and the eyelid. Because of complications such as bleeding and amblyopia, it may be necessary to treat these conditions early on.

Diffuse haemangiomatous gigantism

The vessels in these lesions are of adult type and hypertrophy of the affected part of the body, usually a limb, may involve all components including the bones. There is often a combination of lymphangiomatous and arteriovenous elements. Heart failure can result from some large arteriovenous shunts. Abnormal blood flow within the tissues may result in platelet trapping and thrombocytopenia as in the Kasabach–Merritt syndrome.

Treatment

No form of treatment is completely satisfactory. Surgical excision can prove hazardous. In special situations radiotherapy, despite the potential carcinogenesis consequent on its use, may have a place. Embolisation of feeding vessels with superglue is another form of aggressive therapy in a clinically threatening situation. Treatment with steroids and with interferon-α may be of value.

Multiple familial telangiectasis (Osler disease)

This consists of multiple capillary haemangiomata affecting chiefly the mucosa of the nose, throat and intestine. There are often spider naevi in the skin. These children may present with a massive unexplained haematemesis or melaena.

Complications of haemangiomas

Complications of haemangiomas include:

1 Infection.
2 Bleeding.
3 Pressure effects with loss of function; obstruction to airway, vision, vascular obliteration.

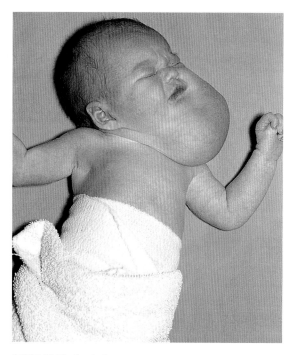

FIGURE 11.16 Cystic hygroma.

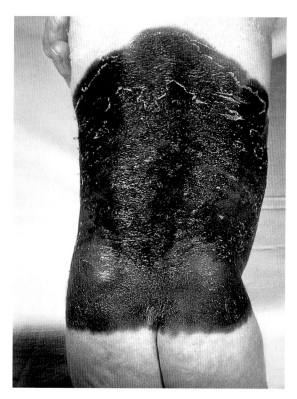

FIGURE 11.17 Pigmented naevus.

4 Thrombocytopenia from platelet trapping in a giant cavernous haemangioma.
5 Shunting (arteriovenous) which can cause high output failure.

LYMPHANGIOMA

Lymphangioma (cystic hygroma)

These present as a soft multicystic fluctuating mass that is transilluminable. They arise as a result of disordered lymphatic vessel development resulting in inadequate lymphatic drainage of the affected area. The head and neck is the most common site. Lymphangiomas may occur in the lips and tongue and may cause macroglossia. The size and number of cystic spaces vary from being single or few in number to massive numbers of minute cysts many of which only open up as years pass. Occasionally, they may form part of a haemolymphangioma where both haemangiomatous and lymphangiomatous elements are present.

Clinical features

Most cystic hygromata appear in the posterior triangle of the neck but are not confined to a single area

(Fig. 11.16). They may extend into the axilla and the swelling may be present at birth, although many increase in size during the first year of life. They usually enlarge during an upper respiratory tract infection, and become more tense after trauma and when haemorrhage occurs into them. The overlying skin is normal in texture and there is a bluish tint from the underlying fluid. The whole mass transilluminates and the presence of haemorrhage or infection may alter the size and consistency of the swelling. The main complaint is disfigurement but rarely it may cause pressure on the trachea or other structures in the neck. When it infiltrates the normal tissues it may cause enlargement of the affected organ and the child may present with a macrocheilia or a macroglossia when the tongue protrudes from the mouth. These conditions are, from the pathological aspect benign, but do not regress as do the haemangiomas. They all require surgical excision, injecting with sclerosants, e.g. hypertonic saline 30%, OK432 or bleomycin. Radiotherapy has no place in the treatment and should be positively discouraged because of the risk of later thyroid cancer. Surgical treatment should involve the complete excision of the lesion, if technically possible, otherwise it recurs and many previously flattened endothelial lined spaces fill up with lymphatic fluid, i.e. clinically there is recurrence of the lymphangioma.

Antenatal diagnosis of hygromas

Hygromas may be detected in the antenatal period on ultrasound examination and have to be differentiated from the transient oedema seen in Turner syndrome. Very occasionally a lymphangioma may present as a thoracic or an abdominal mass which on investigation is diagnosed as lymphangioma and these are discussed in the section relating to thoracic and abdominal pathology.

Pigmented and hairy mole (naevus)

These common lesions vary from small brown moles (benign melanomata) to hairy pigmented areas which may cover large areas of the face, limb or trunk (Fig. 11.17).

Treatment

This is rarely indicated for removal of a pigmented naevus which has been present since birth. If the area is subject to constant trauma, wide surgical removal may be undertaken. Large pigmented areas can be treated by serial excision or by complete excision and skin grafting. There is a risk of malignant change in childhood. Lesions which affect the palms of the hands or the soles of the feet should be followed up by an experienced dermatologist in order to pick up any early change which might indicate malignancy.

12

The Endocrine System

In recent years there has been a much improved understanding of the chemical messengers (hormones) which control the metabolic activities of our tissues. It is most important for paediatricians to have a knowledge of the endocrine system and its constituent hormones because of their critical influence on growth, development and response to stress of the child.

THE PITUITARY GLAND

Disturbances of pituitary function are uncommon in children. The release of the pituitary trophic hormones is dependent upon hypophysiotrophic or "releasing" hormones which are present in the distal part (median eminence) of the hypothalamus. Thyrotrophin-releasing hormone (TRH) stimulates release of thyrotrophin or thyroid-stimulating hormone (TSH) from the pituitary, and luteinising-hormone-releasing hormone (LHRH) promotes the release of luteinising hormone (LH) and follicle-stimulating hormone (FSH). The search for the growth-hormone-releasing-hormone or factor (GHRF) took a great step forwards when a growth-hormone-releasing factor was found in a rare type of human pancreatic tumour. This is a large molecule of around 40 amino acids in length (hpGRF-40) and the same material has now been demonstrated

in the hypothalamus. Intravenous administration of hpGRF-40 to man results in an immediate and massive release of growth hormone and, more importantly, an increase in somatomedin C, which is the peripheral mediator of the effect of growth hormone.

Sermorelin, a synthetic peptide consisting of the 1–29 amino-acid sequence of natural GHRF is now available for the evaluation of GH deficiency.

HYPOPITUITARISM

Aetiology

The incidence of hypopituitarism is not precisely known. Idiopathic hypopituitarism remains the most common cause of growth hormone deficiency. Perinatal insults may be responsible for some of the cases: growth hormone deficiency in idiopathic hypopituitarism is probably secondary to hypothalamic dysfunction because most of these children secrete growth hormone in response to GHRF.

Clinical features

The usual presenting feature is short stature but its pituitary origin is only clinically obvious when there

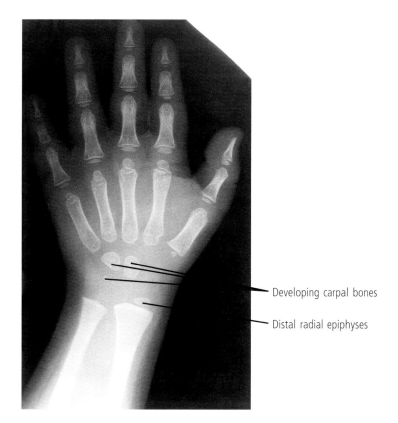

Developing carpal bones

Distal radial epiphyses

FIGURE 12.1 Bone age. X-ray of left hand and wrist of a boy aged 4 years, 3 months. The bone age using the TWII 20 bone score (Tanner and Whitehouse) is 3.8 years which is just below the 50th centile for his age.

is a demonstrable local lesion such as a cranio-pharyngioma with radiographic changes in the region of the sella turcica, visual field defects, "bursting" headaches, and other abnormal neurological signs such as those indicating increased intracranial pressure. Visual field defects and papilloedema in a short child often indicate an optic or hypothalamic tumour. In many instances the clinical diagnosis rests upon the exclusion of other types of short stature, e.g. hypothyroid, primordial, and those due to bone diseases or renal, cardiac or intestinal disorders. The pituitary deficient child is usually of normal birth-weight. In fact, deceleration of linear growth only becomes apparent after a year or thereabouts. The pituitary deficient child of short stature has normal body proportions but looks much younger than his years. He has very small hands and feet and often protruding frontal bones with a saddle nose. Children with disproportionate short stature generally have a skeletal dysplasia syndrome or rickets. A tendency to spontaneous hypoglycaemia may cause episodes of sweating and tremor and convulsive seizures. A rare but important clue to congenital panhypopituitarism is the occurrence of micropenis in association with neonatal hypoglycaemia and prolonged jaundice.

Bone age is retarded and becomes more so in relation to height age as chronological age advances. Puberty is usually delayed and in adolescence there is an absence of sexual hair, the testes remain underde-veloped and gonadotrophins are not detectable in the urine. For some reason pituitary dwarfism is much commoner in boys. In a minority of cases there are signs of functional failure of target glands such as the thyroid and adrenal. Gonadal hypofunction is not demonstrable before the normal age of puberty.

The diagnosis of short stature requires accurate measurements of height, including the charting of height velocity and taking note of the parents' heights. It is also important to determine bone age from a radiograph of the left hand and wrist because a normal bone age may be reassuring evidence of normality (Fig. 12.1). However, if successive height measurements over 6–12 months cross the centile lines downwards, or deviate progressively below the third centile and if the height velocity falls below the 25th centile over a full year, tests for growth hormone are indicated. During much of the day plasma GH is low and spontaneous peaks are often and unpredictable. Therefore measurement of GH in a random blood sample is not a satisfactory screening test for GH deficiency. The presently accepted method for diagnosing GH deficiency is based on eliciting a growth hormone peak in response to pharmacological stimulus. Measurements after physiological stimuli such as 20 minutes of exercise or after 1 hour of sleep are not considered adequate. The pharmacological stimulation tests, e.g. propranolol, clonidine, insulin and growth-hormone-releasing hormone, are useful in identifying GH deficiency. Propranolol should not be used if the patient has asthma, congenital heart disease or hypoglycaemia. Although severe insulin reactions are rarely a problem, an intravenous line must be in place for glucose infusion when performing the insulin stimulation test. Since clonidine can cause sleepiness or mild hypotension the child should be lying down during the test. All of these tests can be performed in an outpatient setting after an overnight fast. A growth hormone concentration of less than 7 ng/ml after a stimulation test is generally considered indicative of impaired pituitary function.

Differential diagnosis

In many types of short stature the diagnosis can be so firmly established that hypopituitarism is thereby excluded. These include metabolic disorders such as intestinal malabsorption, chronic renal failure, chronic anaemia, cardiopulmonary diseases, hypothyroidism, malnutrition, hypogonadism, Turner syndrome and primary bone disorders such as rickets, achondroplasia and Morquio disease. It is important to separate the pituitary short stature from the primordial short stature and the dwarfism arising from constitutional slow growth with delayed adolescence. Yet another clinical situation is growth retardation due to emotional deprivation, psychosocial dwarfism, which may closely mimic hypopituitarism. There may even be reduced responses of GH to insulin-induced hypoglycaemia. These unfortunate children who have been rejected or otherwise deprived of mother love frequently show a depressed or depraved appetite, a remarkable apathy and disinterest and abnormal behaviour such as pulling out their hair or catatonia. After admission to hospital they often eat voraciously, begin to gain weight rapidly and to grow, and soon become friendly and responsive. Their pituitary function tests also return to normal. The diagnosis is reached by enquiries directed towards discovering the disturbed parent–child relationships, but their correction is usually a difficult business.

Treatment

Recombinant human growth hormone (rhGH) has been available for treatment since 1985. It is physiologically indistinguishable from the naturally occurring pituitary hormone. It is indicated for the treatment of short stature and/or growth failure due to growth hormone insufficiency (isolated or with other pituitary hormone deficit) and Turner syndrome. The linear growth response to an initial year of therapy with GH appears to depend on a number of pretreatment variables. These include: chronological age, height, weight and bone age. In general young children respond better than adolescent children, obese children respond better than thin children and severely growth hormone deficient children appear to respond better than those with partial deficiency. It is also used to treat short stature of other aetiologies, skeletal dysplasias, chronic renal failure, inflammatory bowel disease, intrauterine retardation. There are, however, three other brands of growth hormone available: Norditropin (Novo Nordisk), Saizen (Serono) and Humatrope (Eli Lilly) which are used for selected diagnostic categories of patients. Growth hormone must be administered parenterally. This is most convenient and painlessly achieved by subcutaneous injection. Several factors influence the effectiveness of growth hormone replacement therapy including dose and frequency of injections. The optimal weekly dose of growth hormone for prepubertal children is 15 International Units (IU) per square metre. This is increased to 20 IU/m²/week during puberty. Rotation of injection sites is essential to prevent lipoatrophy.

Contraindications to growth hormone therapy include epiphyseal fusion, malignant disease, pregnancy and lactation. Growth hormone affects glucose metabolism, hence patients with diabetes mellitus or with a family history of this disease should be monitored carefully. Hypothyroidism may develop during growth hormone treatment, which, if untreated, may inhibit the growth response. Regular monitoring of thyroid function is therefore essential. Side effects include the development of antibodies to growth hormone or bacterial protein and local reaction at the injection sites, e.g. pain, itching, lipoatrophy and oedema.

During the first year of treatment dramatic results are often observed. This is the initial period of catch-up growth, when height velocity may increase two- to fourfold, the most rapid growth being observed in the first 3–6 months when a marked decrease in subcutaneous fat is usually seen. As treatment is continued there follows a gradual decline in height velocity towards normal values as one might expect to see in any type of "catch-up" growth.

Constitutional slow growth and delayed adolescence

In this type of short stature there is often a family history of the same growth pattern in which both linear and skeletal growth lag behind in a parallel fashion. This contrasts with the increasingly delayed skeletal maturation in relation to height of hypopituitarism or hypothyroidism. Puberty is also delayed but normal sexual development ultimately takes place. It is, of course, important in such cases to exclude any endocrine disorder.

Treatment

Many children with constitutional delay can be managed with an explanation of their natural growth pattern and reassurance that they will develop fully and naturally in time. In some cases delayed sexual maturation is associated with significant psychosocial difficulties. In these cases a brief course of androgen therapy is effective in inducing the rapid development of secondary sexual characteristics.

PRIMORDIAL DWARFISM

This "label" undoubtedly includes several distinct entities which cannot yet be clearly distinguished. They all have in common a history of low birthweight and dwarfism which dates from early infancy. The dwarfism may be of extreme degree but it is usually associated with a normal bone age, normal sexual development and the capacity for procreation. In many cases radiographs show pseudo-epiphyses at the proximal ends of the metacarpals and there may be other minor bone abnormalities. The term Lorain–Lévi dwarfism, often given to such cases, is best avoided because the precise nature of the cases described by Lorain and Lévi is not certain. Some types of primordial dwarfism are undoubtedly genetic in origin; in others an environmental influence has seemed more probable. These patients do not respond to hGH.

Two principal types of primordial dwarfism can be recognised. In the symmetrical type, which may be inherited as a dominant or recessive trait, the characteristics are low birthweight, normal sexual development and the ability to reproduce. In the asymmetrical type the characteristics are disproportionate growth and minor skeletal abnormalities. There may also be congenital heart disease or mental deficiency. One group is distinguished by slender bodies, small heads and old-looking features ("bird-headed dwarfs"); another by a stocky build and flattened nose ("snub-nosed dwarfs"). Both these types are probably genetic in origin, but some cases of primordial dwarfism seem to be related to disturbances in early or late pregnancy.

Treatment

None is available.

PROGERIA

The remarkable onset of premature senility in a 3–5-year-old child characterises this rare condition. There have been a few reports of a familial recurrence suggesting an autosomal recessive inheritance. The cause is unknown and there is no effective therapy at present.

HYPERPITUITARISM

Aetiology

Overactivity of the anterior pituitary is very rare in childhood. The commonest type involves overproduction of growth hormone. This is often related to tumour or hyperplasia of the eosinophil cells although it has also been reported with a chromophobe adenoma. In childhood it results in gigantism, and after the epiphyses have united, in acromegaly. In both gigantism and acromegaly there is an elevated serum hGH level in the fasting state (>30 mU/l) which is not suppressed by intravenous glucose, a raised serum phosphate, and abnormally high blood glucose and hyperinsulinism with insulin resistance. Cushing disease was first related to tumour or hyperplasia of the pituitary basophil cells, but in children it is more often a result of adrenocortical overactivity.

Clinical features

In gigantism an excessive rate of growth starts in early childhood and continues for longer than normal due to a delayed puberty and epiphyseal closure. Hypogonadism is sometimes added to the picture in adult life. When the epiphyses begin to unite, acromegalic features are frequently added, e.g. hypertrophy of the mandible (prognathism), coarse facial features due to nasal and maxillary overgrowth, thickening of the skin, huge spade-like hands and feet. Diabetes mellitus develops in some cases. A pituitary tumour may also produce local pressure effects on the optic chiasma and increased intracranial pressure.

Differential diagnosis

Pituitary gigantism must be distinguished from hereditary tallness. In the latter the body proportions are normal, the bones show normal development and there is a family history of large stature. Fasting hGH levels are normal. It is also important to differentiate cerebral gigantism (Sotos syndrome) thought to be related to excessive production of fetal growth factors. There is an abnormally large head with broad forehead, receding hairline, antimongoloid eyes and some degree of intellectual impairment. The child is abnormally long from birth and growth velocity is high for the first 4 years or more. Bone age is advanced. The hands and feet are large. Fasting hGH levels are normal.

Treatment

Surgical removal of a pituitary adenoma has become less hazardous since the introduction of both the binocular operating microscope and the X-ray image intensifier made the trans-sphenoidal approach a routine neurological procedure. Bromocriptine inhibits the release of growth hormone and can also be used in treatment. Side effects such as nausea, vomiting, dizziness and headaches may be troublesome. Dosage should start at 1.25 mg/day increasing gradually to 20–40 mg/day until the fasting level of hGH falls to below 15 mU/l. Recently a long-acting analogue of somatostatin has been proved successful in reducing the excessive GH secretion seen in acromegaly with resolution of some of the clinical features.

DIABETES INSIPIDUS

Aetiology

This disease is due to deficient production of antidiuretic hormone (ADH; vasopressin) by the neurosecretory system, which includes the posterior lobe of the pituitary and also the supraoptic and paraventricular nuclei of the hypothalamus. This system also secretes oxytocin and possibly other hormones. The function of ADH is to promote reabsorption of water by the renal tubules. It may also cause hypertension by its effects on vascular smooth muscle. The output of ADH is reduced by a fall in plasma osmolality which explains the antidiuretic effect of intravenous hypertonic saline and the diuresis which follows a water load.

Hypovolaemia, however, can overcome the effects of hypo-osmolality and result in antidiuresis. It is necessary to distinguish pituitary diabetes insipidus from the nephrogenic variety (Chapter 8) which does not respond to ADH.

The posterior pituitary and hypothalamus may be damaged by tumour (craniopharyngioma), Hand–Schüller–Christian disease, fracture of the base of the skull and healing tuberculous meningitis. In some cases there is no discoverable cause. Hereditary forms have been described. Both autosomal dominant and X-linked types exist.

Clinical features

The characteristic picture is the sudden onset by day and night of severe polyuria with resultant excessive thirst. Dehydration only develops if fluid intake is limited, voluntarily or during anaesthesia. In the child a common complaint is "enuresis". The urine is very dilute, with a specific gravity of 1.005 or an osmolality of 200 mmol/kg or less. The water deprivation test reveals that the specific gravity and the urine osmolality fail to show the expected increase, while there will be a rapid rise in the plasma osmolality. This must be carefully supervised so that the patient is not allowed to lose more than 5% of his body weight (usually for a period of 6–8 hours). Finally, to distinguish nephrogenic diabetes insipidus 0.4–2 µg of desmopressin is given intramuscularly or intravenously. In pituitary diabetes insipidus this causes immediate abolition of thirst and polyuria with a rise in the urinary specific gravity and osmolality which should be checked every 15 minutes after the injection.

Differential diagnosis

Compulsive water drinking is associated with other signs of psychological disturbance. More common causes of thirst and polyuria are diabetes mellitus and chronic renal failure, both of which should be obvious after simple clinical examination, blood and urine analysis.

Treatment

The most effective preparation for treatment is the intranasal form of desmopressin (DDAVP) which is available in dropper bottles, 100 µg/ml. The dose varies between 10 and 20 µg (0.1–0.2 ml) once or twice daily. If desmopressin is not available, pitressin tannate in oil may be used. In most cases 2–5 units intramuscularly gives an adequate effect for 24–72 hours.

THE THYROID GLAND

Disorders of the thyroid gland are, with the exception of diabetes mellitus, the most common endocrine problems of childhood. The advent of immunoassay techniques has been followed by a vast increase in our knowledge of the physiology and disturbances of thyroid function.

HYPOTHYROIDISM

A classification of the causes of hypothyroidism is shown in Table 12.1. It is designed upon an aetiological basis which will permit the clinician to approach diagnosis and treatment using modern methods. Of the various causes of hypothyroidism in

TABLE 12.1 A classification of hypothyroidism in childhood

Dysgenesis of the thyroid gland

Congenital athyreosis ⎱
Maldescent   ⎰ ⟨ Congenital – cretinism
Maldevelopment   ⎰   Acquired – juvenile myxoedema

Deficiency of iodine (endemic cretinism)

Inborn enzyme defects
   Intrathyroid (familial non-endemic goitrous cretinism)
      Failure of thyroid trapping of iodide
      Failure of organic binding of iodine
      Failure of coupling of iodotyrosines
      Failure of deiodination of iodotyrosines
      Production of abnormal thyroprotein
      Other defects to be defined
   Extrathyroid
      ?Defect in peripheral utilisation of thyroxine

Ingestion of goitrogens (accidental or therapeutic)
   Antenatal (iodine, thiouracil etc. in pregnancy)
   Postnatal

Primary thyroid disease, e.g. autoimmune thyroiditis, carcinoma, etc.

Pituitary hypothyroidism

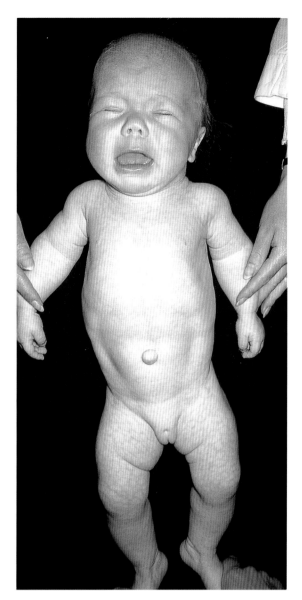

FIGURE 12.2 Sporadic cretin aged 4 months. Note coarse features, large myxoedematous tongue and umbilical hernia.

childhood only endemic iodine deficiency, congenital hypothyroidism and autoimmune thyroiditis will be described in this chapter.

Endemic iodine deficiency

In areas of the world where iodine deficiency is found, up to 8% of the population may have deficient thyroid hormone production, TSH hypersecretion and increased iodine trapping with goitre and a raised plasma $T_3 : T_4$ ratio. Iodination of salt supplies can effectively reduce the prevalence of this condition.

Congenital hypothyroidism

The causes of thyroid dysgenesis in which thyroid tissue may be absent (aplastic), deficient (hypoplastic) or abnormally sited (ectopic) are unknown but affect about 1 in 4000 of all newborns and more commonly affect female infants. Dyshormonogenesis (inborn errors of thyroid hormone biosynthesis) accounts for about 10% of all cases of congenital hypothyroidism, i.e. 1 in 40 000. These autosomal recessively inherited disorders may present with goitre.

Clinical features

The diagnosis of severe cretinism should not be difficult. Indeed, the manifestations are present within a few days of birth. The presenting symptoms are feeding difficulties, noisy respiration and constipation. The undue prolongation of "physiological jaundice" should always arouse the suspicion of hypothyroidism. The appearance of the infant is typical. The facial features are coarse with often a wrinkled forehead and low hairline. The hair may be dry and scanty. The large myxoedematous tongue protrudes from the mouth and interferes with feeding and breathing (Fig. 12.2). The cry has a characteristic hoarseness. The neck appears short because of the presence of myxoedematous pads of fat above the clavicles. The skin, especially over the face and extremities, feels dry, thick and cold. An umbilical

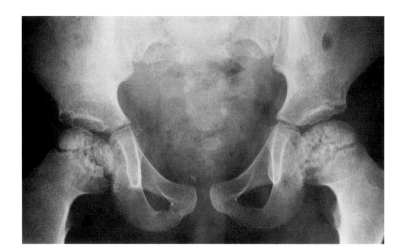

FIGURE 12.3 Epiphyseal dysgenesis in femoral heads. Note stippling and fragmented appearance.

hernia is common. The hands and fingers are broad and stumpy. The hypothyroid (cretinous) infant is frequently apathetic and uninterested in his surroundings. As time goes by, psychomotor retardation becomes obvious and partially irreversible.

Milder degrees of cretinism produce much less striking features. None the less, the marked delay in diagnosis so commonly encountered is unnecessary and it results often in avoidable intellectual impairment. The possibility of hypothyroidism should be considered in every infant or child in whom growth is retarded. Normal linear growth completely excludes hypothyroidism. Most cases of congenital hypothyroidism are detected by detection of increased TSH concentrations in Guthrie card blood spots. Many show no clinical features but some do. It is important not to be lulled into thinking that all cases will be detected by neonatal screening.

In the undetected or untreated child the body proportions remain infantile with long trunk and short legs. A tendency to stand with exaggerated lumbar lordosis and slightly flexed hips and knees is common. The anterior fontanelle is late in closing. The deciduous teeth are slow in erupting and radiographs may show defects in the enamel. The face and hands are frequently mildly myxoedematous and the cerebral activities are slow and sluggish. The mandible is often underdeveloped and the nasolabial configuration may be obviously that of a much younger child. The deep tendon reflexes are sometimes exaggerated with slow relaxation and there may be mild ataxia. In some cases of juvenile myxoedema, however, the only clinical indication of hypothyroidism is dwarfism with infantile proportions. In such cases sexual maturation is delayed (as in all hypothyroid children) so that the condition may be regarded as a "thyrogenic infantilism".

Diagnosis

Linear growth

Short stature is one of the only two invariable findings in hypothyroidism. The ratio of the upper to lower (U/L) skeletal segment is also abnormal (infantile) in hypothyroid children. The lower segment is the distance from the top of the symphysis pubis to the ground; the upper segment is obtained by subtracting the lower segment from the total height. The mean body U/L ratio is about 1.7 at birth, 1.3 at 3 years and 1.0 after 7 years of age. Hypothyroid children have an unduly long upper segment because of their short legs.

Skeletal maturation

Delayed ossification to a more severe degree than the retardation in linear growth is the other constant finding in hypothyroidism. The assessment of bone age is based on radiographs of various epiphyseal areas, chosen according to the child's age, and their comparison with an ossification chart showing the normal ages at which the different centres should ossify (Fig. 12.1). Thus fetal hypothyroidism can be presumed in the full-term baby if the upper tibial or lower femoral epiphyses, which normally ossify at 36 fetal weeks, are absent or if they show epiphyseal dysgenesis. This appearance of dysgenesis of the epiphyses is pathognomonic of hypothyroidism. It may be florid at one area and absent at another, so that radiographs should always be taken of several areas of the skeleton. In some cases dysgenesis only appears after thyroid treatment has been started, but then only in those ossification centres which should have appeared in the normal child before that age. The presence of dysgenesis indicates that the hypothyroid state existed before the affected centre would be normally due to ossify and it permits an assessment of the age, fetal or postnatal, at which the hypothyroidism developed. The characteristic X-ray appearance is of a misshapen epiphysis with irregular or fluffy margins and a fragmented or stippled substance (Fig. 12.3). In the great majority of cases of hypothyroidism measurements of the linear height, the upper and lower segments, and a few well chosen radiographs will establish or exclude the diagnosis of hypothyroidism beyond doubt. They will also determine the age of onset of the hypothyroid state.

Biochemical tests

A particularly sensitive biochemical test for hypothyroidsim lies in measurement of the serum thyroid-stimulating hormone (TSH). The TSH level (normal range = <0.5–4 mU/l) is markedly raised (above 50 mU/l) in primary hypothyroidism, whereas it will be normal in pituitary hypothyroidism. The test can be made even more sensitive by giving thyrotrophin-releasing hormone (TRH) intravenously in a dose of 200 µg. In the normal subject this results in a rise of TSH level from about l to 10 mU/l at 20 minutes. In hypothyroidism there will be a greatly exaggerated rise of an already raised TSH level. The use of this technique may result in a diagnosis of hypothyroidism being established in a few undersized children in whom the standard evidence of hypothyroidism is otherwise lacking, but the diagnosis of hypothyroidism in paediatric practice can be reached with a very high degree of accuracy from a single blood specimen by demonstrating a low total serum T_4 and a high TSH.

Radioactive iodine tests

These are never necessary to establish the diagnosis of hypothyroidism, but they can be used to provide information about the pathogenesis. For the detection and location of thyroid activity in non-goitrous cretins ^{123}I or ^{99m}Tc can be safely given followed by scanning of the neck for radioactivity.

Neonatal screening for congenital hypothyroidism

As irreversible brain damage is a common sequel to a delayed clinical diagnosis of congenital hypothyroidism, which in fact has a higher incidence than phenylketonuria, and as the early results in children who have been detected by screening tests are encouraging, the need for universal screening is now widely accepted. Newborn thyroid screening has been highly successful in improving the prognosis for mental development in hypothyroid neonates. The incidence of congenital hypothyroidism in Europe has been reported to be in the region of 1 in 3600. Screening is usually carried out between the 5th and 14th days

of life. In Europe and Britain the favoured technique is by radioimmunoassay of TSH levels on dried filter paper blood spots obtained by heel stab. It involves an extremely low recall rate for repeat tests but is unable to detect the rare case of secondary (pituitary) hypothyroidism. This disadvantage does not apply to measurement of T_4 levels followed by TSH assay which is confined to specimens with low T_4 values. This method is favoured by many American centres. While both methods are highly reliable it is essential that infants with results in the hypothyroid range have confirmatory tests which should include clinical assessment, TSH assay, quantitative measurements of T_4 and T_3, and assessment of bone maturation by X-ray of the knee. Infants are also missed through newborn thyroid screening programmes because of human error in the infrastructure of the screening programmes. Treatment should be started as early as possible.

Treatment

The drug of choice for the treatment of hypothyroidism is L-thyroxine sodium. In infants a daily dose of 10 µg/kg up to a maximum of 50 µg daily should be given. By 5 years of age the dose should reach 100 µg daily and by 12 years the adult dose of between 100 and 200 µg daily, guided by clinical response, growth assessment and measurements of plasma T_4 and TSH. In the early days of treatment the hypothyroid child frequently shows a disturbed mental performance, unaccustomed restlessness and temporary loss of weight. These manifestations do not indicate overdosage. They are temporary, and parents should be warned to expect them and assured that soon their child will be much better than ever before. The maintenance dose level is that which permits linear growth to proceed at a normal rate and does not leave the bone age retarded. The best guide to adequacy of therapy is periodic measurement of circulating levels of T_4 and TSH. The serum T_4 should be adjusted to the upper normal range. Serum TSH levels may be normal or elevated in adequately treated children. It is undesirable to permit the bone age to advance beyond the chronological age. Treatment must be regularly continued for the duration of the patient's life.

Prognosis

The somatic response to adequate treatment is invariably good but in some cases a disappointing retardation of intellect persists. The principal factors determining outcome are the age at which treatment is started and the amount of functioning thyroid tissue.

Autoimmune thyroiditis (Hashimoto thyroiditis)

Aetiology

Autoimmune thyroid disease is the only primary disease of the thyroid gland which causes hypothyroidism in childhood with any frequency. It is one of the best examples of a strictly organ-specific autoimmunity and the immunological phenomena are usually confined to the thyroid gland. The classic antibodies associated with the thyroid autoimmune state are antithyroglobulin and antimicrosomal antibodies. There is evidence of a familial transmission of thyroid autoimmunity and it more commonly affects girls. The factors which initiate the disease are unknown.

Pathology

The outstanding feature is infiltration of the thyroid by lymphocytes, plasma cells and reticular cells. Hyperplasia of the epithelial cells is commonly seen. In more advanced cases the epithelial cells show degenerative changes and there may be extensive fibrosis with final destruction of the gland.

Clinical features

In most children the only sign is a goitre. It rarely has the firm, rubbery consistency so typical of the adult form of the disease. In fact, almost any goitre in a child may be due to autoimmune thyroiditis and requires specific diagnostic tests for its confirmation or exclusion. It may be smooth in consistency, feel granular and bosselated or become lobulated. Presentation is usually with a euthyroid goitre but in up to 10%, particularly in adolescence, there may be signs of thyrotoxicosis. Only a minority of affected children go on to develop hypothyroidism but it is important to search for signs of this state in every case as the onset is insidious and may be missed.

Diagnosis

In some cases there is a sequential failure of T_4 production followed later by a failure of T_3 production. This explains the case of the euthyroid child with a low T_4 level but a normal T_3 level. In such cases the serum TSH level is almost certain to be elevated.

Treatment

Thyroxine should be prescribed whether or not the child is hypothyroid to suppress the excess secretion of pituitary TSH and diminish the size of the goitre.

These children should be kept under prolonged medical supervision because some later develop other autoimmune diseases such as myasthenia gravis or pernicious anaemia.

HYPERTHYROIDISM

In contrast to hypothyroidism, which is common, thyrotoxicosis is rare in childhood. It usually takes the form of Graves disease with diffuse thyroid hyperplasia and exophthalmos. An uncommon type of hyperthyroidism is encountered in the newborn infant born to a previously thyrotoxic mother.

Graves disease

Aetiology

Graves disease is the most prominent of the autoimmune thyroid diseases. It is believed to be caused at least in part by TSH-receptor antibiotics that have the capacity to stimulate thyroid follicular cell and AMP and produce thyrotoxicosis. Children with Graves disease also have significant circulatory levels of antithyroglobulin and antimicrosomal antibodies and a few children have detectable levels of thyroid growth-stimulating immunoglobulin.

Pathology

The thyroid follicles are hyperplastic and the gland is excessively vascular. Mitotic figures are common in the acinar cells and lymphocytic infiltration may be marked. The alveoli are almost devoid of colloid.

Clinical features

The disease is more common in girls and rare before the age of 7 years. The parents may bring their child for medical advice with a variety of symptoms, such as irritability, fidgetiness, deterioration in school performance, loss of weight in spite of good appetite, excessive sweating, palpitations or nervousness. The child looks thin, and often startled because of her stare and wide palpebral fissures. There may be obvious exophthalmos (Fig. 12.4). Her skin will be flushed, warm and moist. A fine tremor of the outstretched hands is common. The abnormal cardiovascular signs in the child include sinus tachycardia, raised systolic blood pressure and a large pulse pressure. The thyroid gland is visibly enlarged and feels soft. A bruit may be audible over the gland. Emotional lability is frequently very obvious. The upper/lower segment ratio is usually low. Menstruation may be delayed in untreated girls.

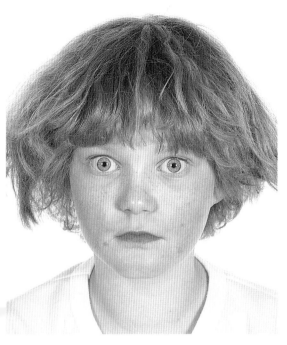

FIGURE 12.4 Thyrotoxicosis showing exophthalmos and goitre.

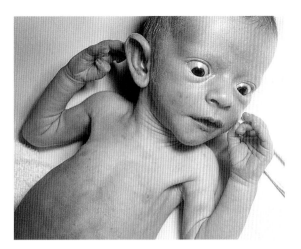

FIGURE 12.5 Neonatal thyrotoxicosis.

Diagnosis

This is usually obvious on simple clinical observation. The most reliable biochemical feature is an elevated serum T_3 level because T_3 levels in Graves disease are often increased to a greater extent than are T_4 levels.

Treatment

A trial of medical treatment should always be made with the objective of rendering the patient euthyroid for 2 years before drug therapy is withdrawn. Suitable drugs and doses are carbimazole 10 mg thrice daily or methylthiouracil 75 mg thrice daily; after 4 weeks or thereabouts the doses can often be reduced to 10–20 mg or 50 mg respectively, daily, according to the clinical state of the child and the T_4 and T_3 levels. At the start of antithyroid treatment the sympathetic overstimulation can be controlled with propranolol 2 mg/kg/day in two or three divided doses. In about 50% of cases we advise partial thyroidectomy. The results in children have been gratifying and complications are uncommon. It must be remembered that all the antithyroid drugs can cause toxic effects, e.g. rashes, agranulocytosis, aplastic anaemia. On the other hand, postoperative hypothyroidism is rare and can, if necessary, be readily corrected with thyroxine. In children there is only rarely a need to use radio-iodine in treatment. It has a place in the rare patient whose thyrotoxicosis relapses following partial thyroidectomy.

Transient neonatal thyrotoxicosis

There have been a considerable number of instances in which women who have or have had thyrotoxicosis have given birth to infants with the unmistakable signs of hyperthyroidism in the neonatal period. The infants have been restless, agitated, excessively hungry and they have exhibited warm, moist flushed skin, tachycardia (190–220 per minute), tachypnoea, exophthalmos and goitre (Fig. 12.5). The diagnosis has been made antenatally because of fetal tachycardia. Some mothers have been previously treated by partial thyroidectomy; others have received thyroid blocking drugs during pregnancy. When the mother is thyrotoxic up to the time of delivery the hyperthyroid state is present in the infant from birth, while if the mother has been rendered euthyroid by drugs the neonatal thyrotoxicosis does not develop for some days because the thyroid gland is suppressed *in utero* and during the infant's first days of life.

There is good evidence that neonatal Graves disease is caused by the transfer of maternal thyroid-stimulating (IgG) immunoglobulins across the placenta from mother to fetus. The presence of such immunoglobulins in mother and infant at the same time has been demonstrated both by mouse bioassay techniques and the radioreceptor assay method. The thyroid-stimulating immunoglobulins disappear from the infant's blood after about 3 months, so that the disorder is a temporary one. Diagnosis in the neonate is confirmed by demonstrating increased levels of total and free T_4 and T_3 and suppressed levels of TSH.

The degree of thyrotoxicosis can be alarmingly severe and prompt treatment of the newborn infant is essential. Treatment can be started with potassium iodide 2–5 mg thrice daily and propranolol 2 mg/kg/day in three divided doses. If the signs of hyperthyroidism are not brought rapidly under control carbimazole should also be given, 2.5 mg four times daily. It is only necessary to continue antithyroid medication for 6–8 weeks. Supportive treatment with digoxin and diuretics may be required if congestive heart failure is present.

Simple and sporadic goitre

It is not uncommon to see children, usually girls, with simple goitres. The goitres vary in size but they are usually diffuse and non-nodular. In adult life some become nodular and thyrotoxicosis or malignant changes are not unknown.

Although these children are clinically euthyroid the serum free thyroxine levels may be slightly subnormal indicating diminished hormone production which results in an increased output of TSH by the pituitary, with resultant goitre.

The causes of sporadic goitre are many. In each case a careful history must be taken with special attention to diet, possible ingestion of drugs, and familial incidence of thyroid disorders or consanguinity in the parents. Most cases are probably due to iodine deficiency as shown by a low level of plasma inorganic iodine. In some parts of the world other factors contribute. Thus, in Tasmania simple goitre has been attributed to a goitrogen in milk derived from weeds in the pastures on which the cows graze. Furthermore, certain foods such as swedes and turnips contain a goitrogen ("goitrin") which may be liberated by the action of enzymes in the intestine. Some cases of sporadic goitre, often familial, are due to partial deficiencies of the same intrathyroid enzymes already described under the causes of hypothyroidism where the deficiency is of more severe degree. Others can be traced to the ingestion of goitrogenic drugs such as iodine, PAS, sulphonamides and cobalt.

Treatment

Simple goitre is best treated with thyroxine in doses just short of those causing toxic effects. It may have to be continued for life. In cases which develop around the time of puberty, however, spontaneous recovery may occur. Goitrogenic drugs should obviously be withdrawn. The addition of potassium iodide to table salt would prevent most simple goitres. It has frequently been advised in the United Kingdom but so far not implemented.

THE PARATHYROID GLANDS

Primary disorders of the parathyroid glands are exceedingly rare in paediatric practice. Much has been learned about the molecular structure and physiological activities of parathyroid hormone in recent years and immunoassay is not practicable. It is hardly possible to consider the actions of parathyroid hormone without consideration of calcitonin. This substance, similar in molecular weight to parathyroid hormone and also a polypeptide, arises, not from the parathyroids as first believed, but from the parafollicular or "C" cells of the thyroid gland. It also is subject to immunoassay. It inhibits the resorption of bone and acts as a physiological antagonist to parathyroid hormone, causing hypocalcaemia. The only primary disorder of calcitonin production yet recognised is in medullary carcinoma of the thyroid in which a state of "hyperthyrocalcitoninism" exists. In some instances the medullary carcinoma occurs as part of a multiple endocrine neoplasia (MEN) due to a specific gene defect.

HYPOPARATHYROIDISM

Aetiology

Hypoparathyroidism may occur as a permanent or temporary state after thyroid surgery or after the removal of parathyroid tumours, but most of the cases reported in children have been of the "idiopathic" variety. A rare syndrome, probably genetic in origin, is hypoparathyroidism which develops in childhood and is associated later with hypoadrenocorticism, and sometimes with steatorrhoeas, pernicious anaemia, diabetes mellitus or elevated sweat electrolytes; moniliasis frequently precedes the endocrine manifestations. Apart from transient neonatal tetany in artificially fed infants which might be regarded as due to temporary hypoparathyroidism, a state of true hypoparathyroidism arises in the infants of 50% of mothers who are suffering from hyperparathyroidism. Spontaneous recovery is usual in these cases. Permanent hypoparathyroidism may, however, present in the neonatal period when it would appear to be inherited as a sex-linked recessive trait and always to affect males. The exceedingly rare association of congenital absence of the parathyroids with aplasia of the thymus (3–4 pharyngeal pouch syndrome) resulting in tetany, failure to thrive, lymphopenia, diarrhoea and immunological paralysis is discussed in Chapter 14 on immunological disorders.

Clinical features

The diagnosis of hypoparathyroidism is not difficult when a child presents with chronic tetany. The symptoms include paraesthesiae ("pins and needles") muscle cramps and carpopedal spasm. Chvostek and Trousseau signs may be elicited. More often the outstanding feature is the presence of recurrent convulsions when an erroneous diagnosis of epilepsy may easily be made. Some affected children have also een mentally retarded and intracerebral calcification may occur. Useful diagnostic clues are delay in the second dentition and defective enamel, ectodermal dysplasia and deformed nails, loss of hair, and moniliasis in the mouth or nails. Cataract develops later in 50% of cases. The characteristic biochemical changes are a low serum calcium (below 2.25 mmol/l; 9 mg/100 ml) and raised serum phosphate (above 2.25 mmol/l; 7 mg/100 ml) in the absence of rickets, renal disease and steatorrhoea.

"Pseudo-hypoparathyroidism" gives rise to a very similar clinical picture but it appears not to respond to parathyroid hormone, possibly because of a failure of the renal tubules to respond so that there is an abnormal reabsorption of phosphate. Characteristic clinical signs include a stocky figure with dwarfism and a rounded face; brachydactyly with shortening of the metacarpals and metatarsals of the first, fourth and fifth fingers and toes; subcutaneous bone formation; mental backwardness and obesity. However, the hypocalcaemia responds to vitamin D.

Treatment

The immediate treatment for tetany is an intravenous injection of 10% calcium gluconate, 10–20 ml, repeated every few hours as necessary. Parathormone may also be given intravenously or intramuscularly, 50–200 units every 12 hours, to raise the serum calcium. For long-term treatment alfacalcidol (1α-hydroxyvitamin D_3; 1α-OHD$_3$), has replaced calcifidrol. It is easier to maintain normocalcaemia and due to the short half-life of 1α-OHD$_3$ any episode of hypercalcaemia during treatment can be quickly corrected by temporary withdrawal of medication.

HYPERPARATHYROIDISM

Aetiology

Adenoma and hyperplasia of the parathyroid glands have both been found, the former being more common.

Clinical features

In some cases bone pains and muscular weakness are the first symptoms. More often nephrocalcinosis and nephrolithiasis result in thirst and polyuria. Peptic ulceration is unduly frequent in these patients. Anorexia, vomiting and severe constipation are common and attributable to the hypercalcaemia. The bone changes of osteitis fibrosa generalisata are found. These include osteoporosis with patches of osteosclerosis. This produces a characteristic granular mottling or discrete rounded translucent areas in radiographs of

the skull. Similar appearances are commonly found in the clavicles and iliac bones. Pathognomonic changes are frequently seen in the terminal phalanges of the hands where there is subperiosteal resorption of bone with a crenellated appearance, best seen with a hand lens. The lamina dura, a dense line of alveolar bone surrounding the roots of the teeth, disappears. A giant-cell tumour (osteoclastoma) may appear as a multilocular cyst on radiographs of the mandible or long bones. Occasionally the presenting sign is a pathological fracture at the site of such a tumour.

The most common biochemical features are a raised serum calcium level (over 2.75 mmol/l; 11 mg/100 ml) and lowered serum phosphate (below 1 mmol/l; 3 mg/100 ml). These values fluctuate and several estimations in the fasting patient at intervals may be required before the diagnosis is confirmed. The plasma alkaline phosphatase is frequently but not invariably raised. There is an increased urinary output of calcium (over 10 mmol/24 hours; 400 mg/24 hours on an ordinary diet). This observation should be followed by estimating the 24-hour calcium output on a low-calcium diet (120 mg/day); an output in excess of 4.5 mmol/24 hours (180 mg/24 hours) is abnormal. A useful diagnostic test is to give cortisone, 50–100 mg daily for 10 days. Hypercalcaemia from other causes will fall on this drug, but hypercalcaemia due to primary hyperparathyroidism is unaffected. When the kidneys have been severely damaged by nephrocalcinosis a high serum phosphate level may simulate secondary hyperparathyroidism. In children, however, renal osteodystrophy includes the changes of rickets which are rare in primary hyperparathyroidism. Furthermore, hypocalciuria is the rule in renal failure, but hypercalciuria usually persists in primary hyperparathyroidism even when there is severe renal damage.

Treatment

The parathyroid tumour or hyperplastic glands should be removed surgically. Transient post-operative tetany is common and best treated with frequent intravenous doses of calcium gluconate. The results of operation are excellent provided the diagnosis has preceded irreversible damage to the kidneys.

THE ADRENAL GLANDS

STEROID SYNTHESIS IN THE ADRENAL CORTEX

The physiological chemistry of the adrenal cortex is exceedingly complicated. It follows that the disturbances which may arise in this system are also

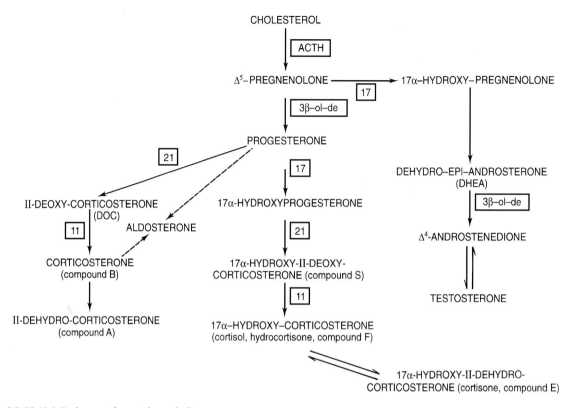

FIGURE 12.6 Pathways of steroid metabolism.

complicated, requiring highly sophisticated laboratory tests for their elucidation. The more important metabolic steps are shown in Fig. 12.6. The three main groups of hormones synthesised by the adrenal cortex are the mineralocorticoids, glucocorticoids and sex steroids.

The function of the chromaffin cells of the adrenal medulla is to secrete the catecholamines, dopamine, noradrenaline and adrenaline. Similar cells are present in the organ of Zuckerkandl and in other organs. They are the site of origin of phaeochromocytoma. There are also sympathetic ganglion cells in the adrenal medulla and their precursors can be the site of origin of neuroblastoma. These cells can also produce dopamine and noradrenaline which may be found in excess in some cases of neuroblastoma.

CONGENITAL ADRENAL HYPERPLASIA

In the most common variants of this disorder there is overproduction of adrenal androgens which results in virilisation of the female (female pseudohermaphroditism) and in macrogenitosomia praecox in the male. The cause is a deficiency of one or other of the enzymes necessary for synthesis of the adreno-

cortical hormones. These defects are transmitted a autosomal recessive traits, being manifest only i homozygotes.

Pathogenesis

Deficiencies, variable in degree from case to case, c several adrenocortical enzymes have now bee defined. The most common involves 21-hydroxylase This results in a diminished production of cortiso and by means of the feedback mechanism, in a increased output of pituitary corticotrophin (ACTH The consequences are adrenocrotical hyperplasia an increased production of 17α-hydroxyprogesterone From this is manufactured an excess of 17 oxosteroids with androgenic properties which caus masculinisation. The urine contains a marked exces of 17-oxosteroids and of pregnanetriol c pregnanetriolone which are derived from 17α hydroxyprogesterone. If the deficiency of 21-hydrox ylase is almost complete, acute adrenal insufficienc with excessive loss of salt in the urine will rapidl develop – "salt-losing syndrome". Less commonl there is a deficiency of 11-hydroxylase. This result in the excessive production of compound S and c 11-deoxycorticosterone (DOC) which is a poter mineralocorticoid with salt-retaining properties an cause of hypertension. Salt-losing crises do not occur. In addition to an increased urinary excretion of 17-oxosteroids large amounts of tetra-hydro-S (THS) derived from compound S are excreted. In a few of these patients the excess manufacture of etiocholanolone causes periodic attacks of fever. Another enzyme defect involves 3β-hydroxysteroid dehydrogenase. This results in deficient production of cortisol and other hormones with salt loss and functional adrenal failure. Pregnanetriol output in the urine is greatly decreased but there is an excessive excretion of 17-oxosteroids, Δ⁵-pregnenolone and dehydroepiandrosterone (DHEA). Affected females show virilisation as in the other enzyme defects, but males show incomplete masculinisation with bifid scrotum and undescended testes. This may be explained by the fact that 3β-hydroxysteroid dehydrogenase is also necessary for the formation of Δ⁴-androstenedione. On the other hand, a defect in the activity of 17-hydroxylase results in impaired formation of cortisol and in the excessive production of DOC and corticosterone. The salt-retaining properties of corticosterone prevent the salt-losing syndrome but result in hypertension. However, failure to produce 17α-hydroxypregnenolone and 17α-hydroxyprogesterone prevents the formation of dehydroepiandrosterone (DHEA) and Δ⁴-androstenedione. Biosynthesis of androgens (or oestrogens) in the adrenals or gonads would, therefore, be negligible so that genetic males with 17-hydroxylase deficiency have abnormal external genitalia with cryptorchidism and hypospadias. They may indeed be misdiagnosed as cases of the testicular feminisation syndrome. Steroid studies of the urine show greatly elevated levels of tetra-hydro-DOC and DOC, but the urinary androgen levels are extremely low and the ratio of pregnanediol to pregnanetriol is excessively high. Blood studies may reveal hypokalaemia and hypoglycaemia. When 18-oxidase, which is necessary for the synthesis of aldosterone, is absent, the genitalia remain normal in both males and females. The clinical presentation is as a salt-losing crisis in the neonatal period. There will be an increased urinary output of corticosterone, but normal levels of pregnanetriol and 17-oxosteroids. Aldosterone, however, will be absent. Another very rare defect can occur early in the biosynthetic pathway preventing the conversion of cholesterol to Δ⁵-pregnenolone. The result is the accumulation of cholesterol and its esters in the adrenal cortex – congenital lipoid adrenal hyperplasia. The enzyme affected is possibly 20,22-desmolase. All affected infants of either genetic sex have female external genitalia because there is, of course, deficient production of androgens, oestrogens, cortisol and aldosterone. The few reported cases have been salt-losers, with an olive-green, bloated appearance, and all have ended fatally.

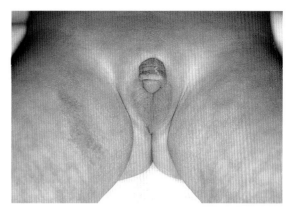

X X

Adrenal

Androgens +

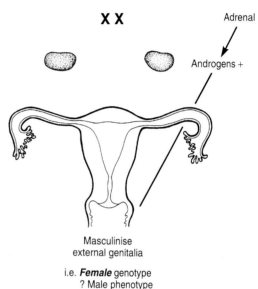

Masculinise
external genitalia

i.e. **Female** genotype
? Male phenotype

FIGURE 12.7 Masculinisation of female genitalia due to congenital adrenal hyperplasia.

Clinical features

Male infants with either 21- or 11-hydroxylase deficiency appear normal at birth apart from rather marked pigmentation of the scrotum. After a short time virilisation is revealed by enlargement of the penis, growth of pubic hair, excessive muscular development and advanced skeletal maturation. These effects are due to the virilising and protein-anabolic action of the excess androgens. The testes, however, remain small and atrophic. The increased stature ultimately gives way to dwarfism due to premature fusion of the epiphyses. In female infants the excessive androgenic effects upon the fetus produce more striking and unwelcome changes. In mild cases there is marked clitoral enlargement (Fig. 12.7). At the other end of the scale there is a penile urethra and fused labia which simulate a scrotum so that the infant can readily be mistaken for a cryptorchid male. Rectal examination will help elucidate the situation as the relatively large uterus can be palpated. Pubic hair of male distribution may also appear soon after birth. However, such female pseudohermaphrodites always possess a uterus, tubes, ovaries and a vagina which usually opens into the urethra. The most common appearance is a large clitoris (phallus) with an opening in the perineum, the urogenital sinus, which is a common outlet for both urethra and vagina. Without treatment such a girl becomes progressively masculinised with excessive muscularity and advanced bone age.

When a 21-hydroxylase defect is complete, an acute adrenal crisis occurs during the neonatal period with vomiting, diarrhoea, severe dehydration and oligaemic shock. The correct diagnosis is easy enough in the virilised female infant but in the male an erroneous diagnosis of pyloric stenosis, gastroenteritis or septicaemia is easily made. The clue to the correct diagnosis is the presence of abundant urinary chlorides in these "salt-losers" in contrast to the diminished urinary chlorides usually found in other types of dehydration. The serum sodium and chloride levels are reduced, and the serum potassium level is high with corresponding ECG changes. In 11-hydroxylase deficiency salt loss does not occur but the characteristic diagnostic feature is hypertension which disappears with treatment. In all types of adrenal hyperplasia excessive skin pigmentation is common.

As stated above the rare cases of 3β-hydroxysteroid dehydrogenase deficiency have all been salt-losers, and most have ended fatally. In the female a degree of virilisation is seen, but the male is always incompletely masculinised with cryptorchidism, hypospadias and scrotolabial folds. Genetic sexing by chromosome analysis is essential to determine the sex in these patients, and, indeed, should be performed in every instance where an infant's sex is difficult to determine. Most cases of 17-hydroxylase deficiency have been diagnosed in females after puberty with amenorrhoea, absence of secondary sex characteristics, hypertension, hypokalaemia and osteoporosis. In males the differential diagnosis is from the androgen insensitivity testicular feminisation syndrome.

Diagnosis

In the cases of 21-hydroxylase deficiency precise diagnosis can be confirmed by the demonstration of a high urinary excretion of 17-oxosteroids (in relation to the patient's age) and of pregnanetriol, whereas the output of 17-hydroxycorticosteroids or 17-oxogenic steroids is not significantly abnormal. However, for rapid and early diagnosis measurements of the plasma 17-hydroxyprogesterone (17-OHP) will reveal a high concentration as a result of the block in steroidogenesis. This should be delayed for 24 hours after birth to eliminate the placental influence on the plasma 17-OHP level. It is important also to recognise that plasma 17-OHP levels may be elevated in ill and preterm infants, and in infants with hyponatraemia from other causes, although rarely to the high values seen in 21-hydroxylase deficiency. The biochemical differentiation of 11-hydroxylase deficiency is essentially based upon the finding of excessive amounts of THS in the urine. The diagnosis of 3β-hydroxysteroid dehydrogenase deficiency rests upon the demonstration of excess dehydroepiandrosterone (DHEA) and other Δ^5 steroids in the urine. The output of pregnanetriol is greatly decreased. In 17-hydroxylase deficiency there are markedly raised urinary levels of DOC and tetrahydro-DOC, whereas androgens are extremely low.

Differential diagnosis

The severely virilised female can best be separated from the hypospadiac male by nuclear sexing methods. Macrogenitosomia praecox in boys with adrenal hyperplasia can be distinguished from true pubertas praecox due to hypothalmic or "constitutional" causes by the fact that in the latter the testes show enlargement and biopsy will confirm spermatogenesis. The masculinising ovarian arrhenoblastoma does not occur before puberty.

An important differentiation in the older child is between congenital adrenal hyperplasia and tumour, adenoma or carcinoma, of the adrenal cortex. Adrenal hyperplasia is pituitary dependent which can be demonstrated by the dexamethasone suppression test. Administration of this drug will markedly suppress the urinary output of 17-oxosteroids. Adrenal tumours remain unaffected in their hormonal activity by dexamethasone. Indeed, in these cases the output of 17-oxosteroids frequently reaches very high levels (above 104 µmol/24 hours; 30 mg/24 hours). The tumour may be outlined by ultrasonography or computed tomography (CT scan).

The female fetus can be severely masculinised when various synthetic progestogens have been given to the pregnant women in the first 12 weeks of pregnancy to prevent abortion. In these cases the urinary output of 17-oxosteroids and pregnanetriol is not increased.

An extremely rare adrenal cortical enzyme defect is of 18-oxidase, required for the synthesis of aldosterone. Severe salt loss results in anorexia, vomiting and severe dehydration during the neonatal period. As cortisol production is normal there is no adrenocortical hyperplasia, nor virilisation due to excess androgens. This rare defect should not be confused with salt-losing cases of congenital adrenal hyperplasia. The urine will show aldosterone to be absent while corticosterone and tetrahydrocortisol are increased. The output of 17-oxosteroids will be normal.

Treatment

Low-dose glucocorticoid replacement therapy is employed to treat all children with congenital adrenal hyperplasia. Hydrocortisone is administered to children in a range of 10–20 mg/m²/day divided equally into two doses. Patients are monitored by measuring serum 17-OHP precursor levels. In children and young adolescents growth velocity and bone age are followed over time to ensure that they are receiving the proper dose. In the salt-wasting forms of congenital adrenal hyperplasia mineralocorticoid replacement is also necessary. The synthetic mineralocorticoid 9α-fluorohydrocortisone (fludrocortisone acetate) in a dose of 0.05–0.2 mg daily orally is suggested with careful monitoring of blood pressure as excess dosage can cause hypertension.

With suppressive therapy, children with adrenal hypertension usually do well. They should always carry a card or identity disc stating the fact that they are on steroid therapy. Any infection, injury or surgical operation must be covered with intramuscular or intravenous hydrocortisone hemisuccinate 100 mg followed by reduced doses at 6-hourly intervals for the next few days.

A difficult problem can be posed by the virilised girl who has remained undiagnosed and has been reared as a "boy" for 3 or more years. Girls reared as boys have obvious sexual and psychological problems, but it would now appear that in late cases of congenital virilising adrenal hyperplasia a change of sex is not so hazardous psychologically as we used to fear, provided the child and her parents receive expert psychiatric and social advice. In most virilised females who have been treated with suppressive glucocorticoids from an early age it is both possible and important to correct the external genitalia, thus permitting a normal sexual life later on. Indeed, some such patients have now been successfully delivered of live babies in adult life. Most would agree that operation should be performed in the first 4 years of life, although not in early infancy. When only the clitoris is enlarged, it often diminishes in size after some years of suppressive therapy. It may, however, require surgical treatment, and an operation has been devised which preserves the glans that may be important for normal sexual experience in adult life (see below).

Surgical treatment has two aims: first of all, to return the appearance of the perineum to that of the female state and secondly, to establish an adequate vaginal cavity with an opening to the perineum. Clitoroplasty is performed by isolating the neurovascular bundles to the glans and removing the corpora of the clitoris from their origins on the pubic rami, then replacing the glans over the pubis. Opening of the vaginal cavity is performed by turning a flap of skin from the perineum into the posterior wall of the existing "proximal vagina" with adjustment of the position of the labio-scrotal folds. These are approximated anteriorly and extended backwards alongside the vaginal opening. Later in childhood, the vaginal size has to be assessed and some girls require further vaginoplasty.

CUSHING SYNDROME

This disease, in contrast to the adrenogenital syndrome, is very rare in childhood. It is much more common in girls than boys.

Aetiology

The clinical manifestations are due to the excess production of cortisol and other hormones by an overactive adrenal cortex. A pituitary basophil adenoma as originally described by Cushing is, in the child, an extreme rarity, although in those cases due to bilateral adrenal hyperplasia there may be some primary hypothalamic or pituitary disturbances which has interfered with the ACTH secretory or release mechanisms. However, in the young child Cushing syndrome is more often due to an adrenal cortical carcinoma than to an adenoma or to adrenal hyperplasia. In the adult, adrenal hyperplasia and Cushing syndrome can result from malignant tumours of the lung, thymus, pancreas, etc. which apparently secrete an adrenocorticotrophic hormone, but this has not been reported in children. It should not be forgotten, however, that all the features of Cushing syndrome can be produced when ACTH or the corticosteroids are given in pharmacological doses in diseases such as nephrosis, juvenile chronic arthritis, rheumatic fever, inflammatory bowel disease and leukaemia.

Clinical features

The clinical features of Cushing syndrome result from the secretion of adrenal hormones and are dominated by the effects of cortisol. Those due to an increased production of glucocorticoids include buffalo-type obesity, moon face, purple striae over abdomen, flanks and thighs, easy bruising, muscle wasting and weakness, osteoporosis, latent diabetes mellitus and polycythaemia (Fig. 12.8). Increased output of mineralocorticosteroids and aldosterone accounts for the hypertension and common hypokalaemic alkalosis. Excessive secretion of androgens may cause hirsutism, acne, baldness and clitoral enlargement. These patients are, in addition, highly susceptible to infection.

Diagnosis

The urinary output of free cortisol and of 17-hydroxycorticosteroids or 17-oxogenic steroids is

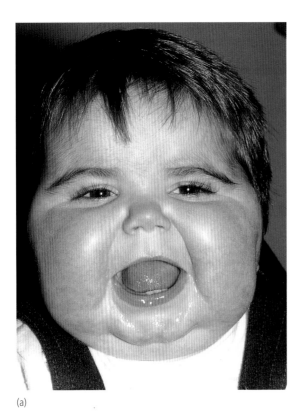

(a)

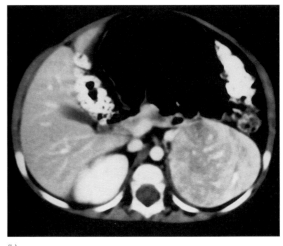

(b)

FIGURE 12.8 (a) Cushing syndrome. (b) CT scan showing a large well encapsulated tumour with calcification of the left suprarenal gland. The liver is normal as is the right kidney. The left kidney cannot be seen because it is displaced by the tumour.

elevated and there may be a raised output of 17-oxosteroids. Plasma cortisol levels are now commonly estimated in routine laboratories. Both the morning and evening levels are raised in Cushing syndrome, especially when the cause is an adrenal tumour and the normal diurnal rhythm disappears. The dexamethasone suppression test is very useful. In cases due to adrenal hyperplasia there is likely to be a 50% reduction in the urinary output of 17-hydroxycorticosteroids. Complete absence of adrenocortical suppression by dexamethasone is strongly suggestive of a tumour. Hypokalaemic alkalosis is commonly found and a glucose tolerance test may give a diabetic curve. The sella turcica should always be X-rayed to exclude a pituitary tumour. X-rays of the spine will reveal the degree of osteoporosis. The site of an adrenal tumour can best be demonstrated by computed tomography (CT scan) which can distinguish adrenal carcinoma from adenoma or bilateral hyperplasia.

Treatment

A tumour of the adrenal should, of course, be excised when this is possible. In most cases of adrenal hyperplasia a satisfactory result can only be obtained by total bilateral adrenalectomy followed by replacement therapy (as in Addison disease). Unfortunately, it appears that this treatment may be followed by the

subsequent appearance of pituitary tumours and severe hyperpigmentation (Nelson syndrome). The prognosis of Cushing syndrome when the cause is tumour will depend upon its nature, extent and removability.

ADDISON DISEASE

This is an exceedingly rare disease in paediatric practice but some cases are probably missed. Correct diagnosis is important because effective treatment is now available.

Aetiology

In some cases there is adrenocortical atrophy of the type common in adults. Such patients show a high incidence of specific type antibodies to adrenal, thyroid and stomach tissues, and relatives may suffer from thyroid disorders or pernicious anaemia. Addison disease is rarely due to tuberculosis of the adrenal glands in Britain nowadays. It is occasionally familial with considerable variation in the age of onset of symptoms. In several reports of congenital adrenal hypoplasia an X-linked mode of inheritance has been demonstrated. This has occasionally been associated with mental retardation and in a few patients it has been accompanied by X-linked glycerol kinase deficiency. There is some support for the suggestion that familial Addison disease of childhood may represent a milder form of the same genetic disorder responsible for congenital adrenal hypoplasia.

Clinical features

In the older child the manifestations closely resemble those seen in the adult – extreme asthenia, cachexia, hypotension and microcardia. Pigmentation of skin and mucous membranes tends to be less marked in children. Dangerous adrenal crises may occur, often precipitated by infections. Hypoglycaemic convulsions may first bring the child to the physician.

In the congenital form of the disease acute adrenal failure may develop with alarming rapidity during the neonatal period. Vomiting, diarrhoea and extreme dehydration can lead easily to an erroneous diagnosis such as pyloric stenosis, high intestinal obstruction or gastoenteritis. The pointer to adrenal insufficiency is the presence of abundant chlorides in the urine.

Diagnosis

During a crisis characteristic blood chemical changes are found. These include low serum chloride and sodium, elevated serum potassium (with changes in the ECG) and hypoglycaemia. The serum sodium : potassium ratio which is normally 30 : 1 falls below 20 : 1. In the absence of a crisis the blood chemistry may not be grossly abnormal and more refined tests are necessary. The simplest of these rests upon the inability of the kidneys in this disease to respond to a water load with a normal diuresis. After an overnight fast the child is given water in a dose of 20 ml/kg to be drunk within 45 minutes. The urine is collected for the next 5 hours. If less than 80% of the water load is excreted there is impaired diuresis. The test can be repeated on the following day, the child having been given 100 mg cortisone by mouth 4 hours before the start of the test. In Addison disease a normal diuresis will then occur.

One of the adrenal stimulation tests is the most reliable method of establishing the diagnosis of chronic hypoadrenocorticism. The best is the intramuscular tetracosactrin test. The plasma cortisol level is estimated before an injection of Synacthen (Ciba) (25 µg), and preferably at 30 minutes and 1½ hours after the dose. In the normal subject the plasma cortisol level will rise more than 193 nmol/l (7 µg/100 ml) above the resting value, the final level being usually about 497 nmol/l (18 µg/100 ml). This response will be absent in Addison disease.

Treatment

The adrenal crisis should be treated along the lines described for salt-losers in the adrenogenital syndrome. This includes intravenous 5% dextrose in physiological saline; hydrocortisone hemisuccinate 100 mg preferably intravenously followed by 50 mg 6-hourly; deoxycorticosterone pivalate 1–2 mg intramuscularly twice daily; and aldosterone 200–500 µg intravenously in frequent doses as determined by repeated ECGs and serum potassium estimations.

Maintenance treatment must take into account the severity of the condition and the patient's age. It must aim at adequate growth, well-being and energy, a normal heart size, normal ECG, normal blood chemistry and blood pressure. Oral cortisone is given thrice daily in individual doses of 5–10 mg. Extra salt (2–5 g/day) is included in the diet. In severe cases it is desirable to give a mineralcorticosteroid such as fludrocortisone 50–200 µg/day by mouth.

The prognosis in older children should be good, although they are susceptible to periodic adrenal crises when they acquire intercurrent infections. Adrenal failure in the neonatal period, however, can prove a most difficult problem and death may occur in spite of the most energetic measures.

PHAEOCHROMOCYTOMA

This is very rare in childhood. The tumour may arise in the adrenal medulla (phaeochromocytoma) or from chromaffin cells elsewhere such as the organ of Zuckerkandl (paraganglioma). In children both adrenals may be simultaneously affected. In some cases the tumour is locally malignant. There is also an association in the adult with thyroid medullary carcinoma and multiple true neuromata.

Clinical features

In some cases hypertension occurs in paroxysms which coincide with the liberation of the catecholamines by the tumour. These cause headaches, palpitations and epigastric pain. Sweating may be profuse and the child becomes prostrated. Frequently he has a characteristically "startled" expression with wide palpebral fissures and dilated pupils. More often, however, the hypertension becomes chronic and produces retinal changes (papilloedema and exudates), cardiomegaly and proteinuria. There may be hyperglycaemia and glycosuria. The intravenous pyelogram is usually normal unless the tumour itself is obstructing the ureter. Whenever recurrent or chronic hypertension is documented in the paediatric patient phaeochromacytoma should be considered in the diagnosis.

Diagnosis

In every case it is essential to prove the diagnosis by demonstrating an excessive urinary excretion of

VMA (3-methoxy-4-hydroxymandelic acid) over 25 μmol/24 hours; 5 mg/24 hours). The site of the tumour can often be defined by intravenous pyelography, computed tomography or ultrasonography. The use of pharmacological agents such as phentolamine (Rogitine) and histamine to aid in diagnosis of phaeochromocytoma should be reserved for some cases in which repeated measurements of catecholamines and their metabolites are normal and suspicion of phaeochromacytoma is high. Metaiodobenzyl guanidine (MLBG) is selectively taken up by this tumour and is useful in identifying the tumour and metastases.

Treatment

The tumour should be removed surgically whenever this is practicable. Chronic hypertension can be controlled while the operation is being arranged with phenoxybenzamine (Dibenyline) 10 mg twice or thrice daily; it must be withdrawn 48 hours before operation. During the operation hypertension must be carefully controlled with intravenous phentolamine. After the tumour has been removed there is a danger of profound hypotension. This must be prevented by the continuous infusion of noradrenaline (Levophed), 8 mg in 1000 ml 5% dextrose in water, for 4–36 hours until the blood pressure remains spontaneously at a safe level. In bilateral adrenal tumours total adrenalectomy should be followed by substitution therapy. Several days after removal of the phaeochromocytoma the 24-hour urinary excretion of catecholamines should be measured to be certain that the functioning tumour has been removed.

THE GONADS

Disturbances of function of the sex glands are rarely evident before puberty. The paediatrician must, however, be familiar with these problems as his patients will reach adult life in good health only if he correctly diagnoses and treats the ailments of childhood. The most common practical problem in this field is the undescended testis (cryptorchidism), although this does not inevitably lead to hypogonadism.

HYPOGONADISM

Failure of the testicular function leads to the state of eunuchoidism. This may be due to such causes as testicular agenesis, mumps orchitis, bilateral cryptorchidism, prolonged malnutrition and castration. A specific variety of male hypogonadism is found in the Klinefelter syndrome in which the buccal smear is chromatin positive (as in the normal female). Chromosome analysis reveals a sex chromosome configuration such as XXY or XXXY. In some cases there has been mosaicism, e.g. XXY/XY. In the female, primary hypogonadism is much less common. The classical example is Turner syndrome (gonadal dysgenesis) in which the buccal smear is chromatin negative and there is only one female sex chromosome (XO). Female hypogonadism will, of course, result from bilateral oöphorectomy. Secondary hypogonadism can result in both sexes from selective failure in the production of pituitary gonadotrophins (hypogonadotrophic hypogonadism).

Clinical features

With the exception of cryptorchidism the features of hypogonadism in the male only become manifest after the time of normal puberty. Growth continues for an abnormally long period because of delay in fusion of the epiphyses. Fat distribution is excessive and in the usual female sites, hips, thighs, breasts. The voice is high-pitched and "infantile". The penis is small and sexual hair is scanty. The degree of eunuchoidism varies in cases of Klinefelter syndrome according to the amount of androgen production but testicular biopsy always shows hyalinisation in the cells of the seminiferous tubules and adenomatous clumping of the Leydig cells. In Klinefelter syndrome there is an extra X chromosome present, i.e. the patient has 47 chromosomes, there being one Y chromosome and two X chromosomes. On some occasions there may be further additional X chromosomes and also mosaicism may occur. The features of Klinefelter syndrome are:

1 Tall male with small and usually undescended insensitive testes.
2 Gynaecomastia.
3 Recession of temporal hair.
4 Scanty body and facial hair.
5 Lack of libido.
6 Mental retardation (up to 50% of patients).
7 High urinary gonadotrophin levels.

The patient may have presented because of undescended testes. Although orchidopexy can be performed, it does not influence the behaviour of the individual.

Turner syndrome occurs in about 1% of conceptuses but only results in 1 in 2000 live births. Nineteen out of 20 abort spontaneously. Approximately 50% of affected infants have a 45 X karyotype, up to 20% have an isochromosome X and up to 40% have mosaicism, usually 45X/46XX. Occasionally the mosaicism is 45X/46XY.

The condition can be diagnosed by standard chromosome techniques following chorionic villus sampling, amniocentesis or cordocentesis. It is suspected in fetuses with cystic hygromata especially when there is coexisting

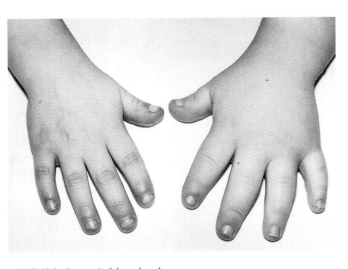

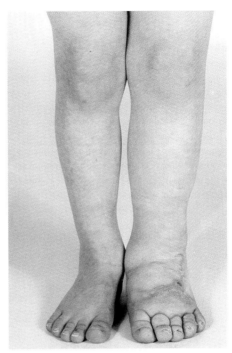

FIGURE 12.9 Congenital lymphoedema.

hydrops fetalis. The cystic hygroma occurs because the communication between the jugular vein and the embryonic lymphatic reservoir fails to develop, resulting in lymphatic stasis and dilatation of lymphatic channels. Many such fetuses die *in utero* but occasionally the cystic hygromas can be seen by ultrasound prenatally and have disappeared by the time of birth. The features of Turner syndrome are: webbed neck; increased carrying angle; sexual infantilism; low birthweight; long gestation; lymphoedema; redundant skin in infancy; coarctation of the aorta plus or minus other cardiac anomalies; valgus knees; digital anomalies; deafness and short stature. In these girls the ovaries are usually replaced with fibrous streaks and there is gonadal dysgenesis together with absence of secondary sexual characteristics. Menstruation does not occur and the uterus remains small and infantile. There is an excessive urinary output of gonadotrophins after the age at which puberty should have occurred. In some cases congenital lymphoedema of the extremities is associated with severe cardiac or renal anomalies (Bonnevie–Ullrich syndrome) (Fig. 12.9).

One form of pituitary hypogonadism is Fröhlich syndrome which can be caused by a tumour such as craniopharyngioma, encephalitis or trauma. This is, in fact, an excessively rare condition. The principal features are gross obesity combined with sexual infantilism. Ossification is delayed. It must not be confused with simple obesity which is very common. A variant of Fröhlich syndrome, transmitted as an autosomal recessive trait, is the Laurence–Moon–Biedl syndrome which is characterised by obesity, genital hypoplasia, polydactyly or syndactyly, retinitis pigmentosa and severe mental retardation.

Idiopathic pituitary hypogonadism has been called hypogonadotrophic hypogonadism. In males the characteristic findings are those of eunuchoidism; in the female there is primary amenorrhoea. This condition not infrequently is associated with growth hormone deficiency. The diagnosis can be confirmed by demonstrating that an intravenous dose of LHRH fails to provoke a rise in the plasma levels of LH or FSH. In "idiopathic" cases there is some evidence to suggest that there is primarily a failure in the synthesis of LHRH by the hypothalamus.

Treatment

Primary hypogonadism in the male may be treated with oxymetholone, 2.5 mg/day. The diagnosis must first be approved by testicular biopsy because these drugs can damage the healthy testis. Turner syndrome is treated with oestrogens, possibly also progestogens, given cyclically. The use of human growth hormone, together with oxandrolone, improves growth rate and will probably allow near normal adult stature. Ovum donation at least offers Turner patients a chance of fertility. It is now possible to restore menstruation and induce ovulation in females with hypogonadotrophic hypogonadism by pulsatile administration of LHRH with a portable pump.

In the presence of a mosaic 45X/46XY the gonads should be removed because of the risk of a gonadal blastoma arising in the streak ovary in association with the Y chromosome. Surgery may also be necessary for orthopaedic complications or to remove the neck webbing. The renal tract is abnormal in up to

50% of Turner patients and early ultrasound diagnosis and long-term management to prevent recurrent urinary tract infections are important. Chronic otitis media is more common and unless carefully managed may lead to deafness. Up to 30% have a risk of hypothyroidism due to antibody formation and those with an isochromosome X have a high risk of Graves disease and Hashimoto thyroiditis. It is not, of course, possible to make these patients fertile. Recently it has been shown that therapy with hGH alone and in combination with oxandrolone can result in a sustained increase in growth rate and a significant improvement in adult height for most prepubertal girls with Turner syndrome.

PRECOCIOUS PUBERTY

If a boy develops secondary sexual characteristics before the age of 9 years or a girl before the age of 8 years the child is considered to have sexual precocity.

Aetiology

There are many causes of precocious puberty. They can be classified into central precocious puberty or peripheral precocious puberty and variations of normal pubertal development. A very rare cause of pubertas praecox in boys is the interstitial (Leydig) cell tumour of the testis. Teratoma is equally rare and may also cause sexual precocity. Germinal cell tumours such as seminoma do not produce androgens. In girls isosexual precocity may be due to a granulosa cell tumour of the ovary; it is usually benign. A teratoma may produce similar effects.

Clinical features

Behavioural changes occur and many exhibit aggressive behaviour. In both sexes the result of hyperactivity of the gonads is isosexual pubertas praecox. In boys the penis and testes enlarge and sexual hair appears at an unduly early age. In girls the genitalia enlarge, menstruation and ovulation occur and sexual hair develops. Bone age is advanced. In boys there is an excess output of urinary 17-oxosteroids. In girls oestrogens reach and may surpass adult female levels.

Differential diagnosis

Sexual precocity may have various causes such as hypothalamic lesions in both sexes and adrenogenital syndrome in boys, although in the latter spermatogenesis does not take place and the testes remain small. It is important to appreciate, however, that the most common type of precocious puberty is "constitutional", 90% in girls, 50% in boys. Here there is no discoverable lesion and future adult development is normal. Interstitial cell tumours of the testis and granulosa cell tumours of the ovary are invariably palpable.

Treatment

Treatment must obviously be directed at the underlying cause such as tumour of testis, ovary or hypothalamus. This is likely to involve surgery, and chemotherapy for malignant neoplasms. When no treatable cause is found, medical therapy is required.

Management of the much more common "constitutional" precocious puberty requires a sensitive understanding of the anxieties and behavioural problems which the child and her family will experience, combined with drug therapy to inhibit the secondary sexual characteristics, skeletal maturation and growth velocity. Medroxyprogesterone in 5 mg daily oral doses will inhibit gonadotrophins but is more effective in girls than boys. The current treatment of choice for central precocious puberty is to administer long-acting gonadotrophin-releasing hormone agonists (GnRH-A). GnRH-A are ineffective in children with peripheral precocious puberty therefore a number of other agents (testolactone) have been used with some success.

INTERSEX

Birth of an infant with genitalia deviant from the normal male or female pattern is a course of major concern for the family. The problem must be handled promptly, honestly and expeditiously. Undue haste or ill-informed decision making is in the long term more deleterious than an explanation of the difficulty and the necessity for consultation with experts before assigning a gender to the infant. Terminology has been confusing and the terms used in this section are defined.

- Ambiguous genitalia and intersex are terms used by different clinicians to identify an infant or child having sexual characteristics intermediate between those of a typical male and a typical female.
- Hermaphrodite: used to describe an individual with parts belonging to both male and female reproductive systems.
- Genotype: the genetic "sex" of an individual as defined by chromosomal analysis, i.e. normally XX or XY.
- Phenotype: the physical appearance and structural make-up of an individual which is determined on clinical examination.
- Sexual differentiation. The fetus for the first 6 weeks inhibits a common appearance whether the chromosome complement be male (XY) or female (XX). Thereafter the "common stem" fetus

progressively differentiates into male or female phenotype (Fig. 12.10). Sexual differentiation in the human female is largely "passive" and the basic development as with many other species is for the embryo to start developing towards femininity. The presence of XX chromosome

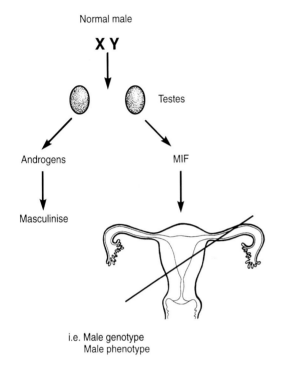

i.e. Male genotype
Male phenotype

FIGURE 12.10(a) Differentiation of male phenotype.

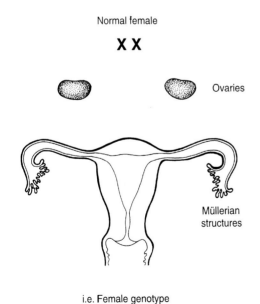

i.e. Female genotype
Female phenotype

FIGURE 12.10(b) Differentiation of female phenotype.

make-up allows this development to proceed with the pubic tubercle, pubic ridges and pubic folds developing into the clitoris, labia minora and labia majora and the urogenital sinus invaginates to meet the fused Müllerian ducts. The lower two-thirds of vagina comes from the urogenital sinus and the proximal one-third from the fused Müllerian ducts which also form the uterus and fallopian tubes. In the male fetus the initial development of Müllerian ducts occurs before the presence of the Y chromosome determines that the primitive gonads become testes. From the testes androgens and Müllerian inhibiting substance (MIS) are subsequently secreted and have two main actions. Androgens cause the pubic tubercle to enlarge to the penis. Active growth of the perineal tissues results in the closure of the urethra and fusion of the two halves of the scrotum. Internally, MIS from the developing testes results in resorption of Müllerian development and the Wolffian ducts develop to form the epididymis, vas and seminal vesicles.

Arrest of either of these lines of development may occur resulting in ambiguous genitalia at birth. The other cause of intersex is overstimulation and overgrowth of the perineal tissues (see adrenal hyperplasia).

Hermaphroditism, uncommon in man, is usually found on investigation of an infant or child who has presented with ambiguous genitalia. Paradoxically the genotype is more often female but the phenotype, although not fully developed, is more often male. The chromosome pattern may show mosaicisms with XY/XX but numerous variations in genotype have been defined. Gonadal make-up is also variable with ovarian and testicular tissue being present in one or both sides or both may be present in one or both gonads. Gonadectomy is usually desirable to prevent cancer developing in the abnormal testis, the rate being as high as 30%. Treatment is to give the child an acceptable phenotype although they will be infertile.

Anorchia

Rarely development of the testes may fail at an early age in an XY genotype individual. This may give rise to poor genital development or external female phenotype. Internally the Müllerian duct development is hypoplastic. These individuals are reared as females.

Androgen insensitivity syndrome (testicular feminisation)

This condition has been called male pseudo-hermaphroditism as the genotype is male but the

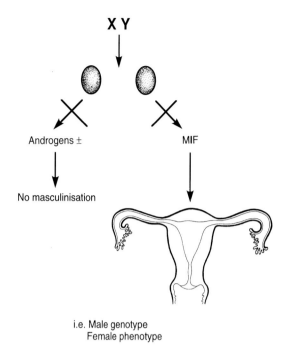

i.e. Male genotype
Female phenotype

FIGURE 12.11 Androgen insensitivity syndrome (testicular feminisation syndrome).

phenotype is female. In this condition the genetic composition is XY and in consequence the primitive gonads develop into testes (Fig. 12.11). The secondary masculinising effects from the testicular hormones do not develop (the complete syndrome) or only partially develop (the incomplete syndrome) with the infant at birth appearing to be a normal female, or in the incomplete expression of the disorder the infant may have an enlarged clitoris or even more masculinisation of the perineal area with the appearance suggestive of an infant with hypospadias and undescended testes. The cause may be either testicular failure or end-organ insensitivity to the androgen stimulus. In addition to the external failure of masculinisation the reduction in or absence of Müllerian inhibiting factor results in persistence of the Müllerian structures and development of unusually hypoplastic fallopian tubes, uterus and proximal vagina.

Presentation of testicular feminisation syndrome can occur at different ages:

1 Neonatal period: ambiguous genitalia, e.g. clitorial enlargement.
2 Infancy: girls with bilateral inguinal herniae.
3 Adolescence: primary amenorrhoea.
4 Adult: lack of pubic and axillary hair or with a pelvic mass (tumour of testes).

The male to female sex incidence for inguinal herniae is 10 : 1. The infant or older girl who has bilateral inguinal herniae has a 2% chance of having testicu-

lar feminisation. Inspection of the gonad at the time of hernia repair can quickly eliminate this diagnosis. If the gonad is not in the hernial sac it can be brought into vision by pulling on the round ligament and bringing the fimbriated end of the tube and gonad into view. If the diagnosis is confirmed by chromosome studies there needs to be a lengthy explanation to, and discussion with, the parents. The child will require bilateral orchidectomy and the optimal age for this remains in doubt. It should be performed before puberty. Usually the girls are very feminine in shape and behaviour and fully accept their reared sex. A major problem is the infertility which is inevitable. In some girls the existing vaginal cavity is adequate but in other vaginoplasty will be required so that normal sexual relationships may be achieved although fertility is excluded. In adolescence, hormone replacement therapy is given.

General management

Intersex problems require a thorough investigation to achieve a diagnosis. Not all features are necessarily found in each individual patient but most important is a thorough clinical examination including rectal examination. Schedule of assessment includes:

1 Clinical examination.
2 Plasma urea and electrolytes.
3 24-hour specimen of urine (for 17-ketosteroid estimation).
4 Chromosomal sex determination.
5 Ultrasound assessment of urinary tract and genital tract.
6 Invasive radiological procedures.
7 Endoscopy.
8 Laparotomy plus biopsy.

XX Males

This rare disorder may present with the stigmata of Klinefelter syndrome including small testes with hypoplastic genitalia prior to puberty, gynaecomastia and infertility. Skeletal proportions and intelligence are normal. The explanation of testis induction in XX males may be that there is reciprocal translocation between the short arms of the X and Y chromosomes leading to transfer of testis-determining genes from the Y onto the short arm of the X.

XYY Syndrome

This chromosomal anomaly is found in 1 in 1000 males. The karyotype is associated with increased growth in early to mid-childhood with about one-third on the 90th centile for height. Intelligence is not significantly different from their chromosomally normal siblings. There is a tendency towards compulive behaviour which may lead to socially deviant behaviour but in the presence of a stable family background this seldom leads to trouble. The initial reports of males with 49 XYY came from institutions or mentally ill criminals which led to the association of the chromosomal anomaly with deviant behaviour. Prospective studies have shown that given a reasonable family upbringing the affected individuals cannot be identified within the normal population except by routine chromosomal screening.

THE PANCREAS

The most common endocrine disorders involving the pancreas in paediatric practice are found in diabetes mellitus and in the babies of diabetic mothers.

DIABETES MELLITUS

Aetiology

There are two types of this disease. Type 1 or insulin-dependent diabetes mellitus (IDDM; juvenile-onset diabetes); and type 2 or non-insulin dependent diabetes mellitus (NIDDM). Type 2 is very uncommon during childhood and the subsequent discussion will be confined to IDDM. Insulin is produced by the β-cells of the pancreas and consists of A and B polypeptide chains linked by disulphide bridges. The pathogenesis of IDDM is by no means well understood although it is clear that both genetic and environmental factors are involved.

There is an association between IDDM and the HLA histocompatibility complex. The first to be recognised was with the B locus and the antigens B8 and B15. However, it is now known that this association is secondary, the primary association being with the D locus. The increase in prevalence of B8 is due to linkage disequilibrium with DR3, and of Bl5 with DR4 in probands with the disease. An increase in prevalence of the heterozygote DR3, DR4 has been noted in Caucasians and is associated with the highest known risk in relatives for IDDM, which suggests that possession of both antigens confers a greater genetic predisposition to IDDM than does possession of either gene alone. There is, however, evidence of further association between IDDM and the Kidd blood-group locus which is, of course, not HLA-linked.

It has further been demonstrated that several different types of islet-cell antibodies can be identified in the blood of IDDM sufferers, sometimes as long as a year before the onset of symptoms. Although these and some other immunological abnormalities (e.g. lymphocytic infiltration of the islets) have not been shown to be the direct cause of damage to the islet cells the phenomenon can be described as "autoimmune".

Lastly, there is some sero-epidemiological evidence that Coxsackie B viruses and particularly B4 may be causally related to IDDM, possibly by triggering the development of clinically overt diabetes in the already predisposed child.

In Caucasians a family history of IDDM is obtainable in at least 20% of cases. The prevalence of the disease appears to be increasing in Britain, doubling roughly every decade, and at age 10 years is now 1.3 per 1000.

Pathology

There has been great variation in the reported findings depending upon the duration of the IDDM before death. In patients who die within the first year or two of onset the striking features are a marked reduction in the islets and the numbers of β-cells, also lymphocytic infiltration of the islets. Deficiency of insulin results in many metabolic upsets. The conversion of glucose to glycogen is diminished, hence the hyperglycaemia and glycosuria. The muscles are unable to utilise glucose as a source of energy. The glucose is excreted in the urine with water and sodium, hence the polyuria and thirst. Protein synthesis is impaired resulting in loss of weight, muscle weakness and slowing of growth. An important effect is a decrease of lipogenesis from carbohydrate and an increased breakdown of fat from which energy is derived. When the production of ketone bodies exceeds their utilisation they accumulate in the blood and spill over into the urine; this leads to the state of ketoacidosis which results in coma.

Terminology

This has been defined in recent years as follows:

- Potential diabetes: individuals with a normal glucose tolerance test (GTT) but a known risk of developing diabetes in later life, e.g. one identical twin already affected, history of the disease on both sides of the family, women who have given birth to babies weighing over 4.5 kg.
- Latent diabetes: individuals with a normal GTT but who have shown an abnormal GTT during infections, pregnancy or when stressed with corticosteroids.
- Chemical (asymptomatic) diabetes: individuals with an abnormal GTT but without symptoms.
- Clinical diabetes: individuals with the clinical features described below.

The term "pre-diabetes" should be reserved for that period of a person's life before the diagnosis of diabetes was made. It cannot properly be used until the diagnosis has been made, save in the case of an identical twin, the other twin already suffering from diabetes mellitus. There is a less than 50% chance of the second twin getting IDDM.

Clinical features

Diabetes mellitus is potentially a much more acute disease in the child than in the adult. The onset is marked by polyuria, excessive thirst and rapid loss of weight. In the untreated case the urine is loaded with sugar and acetone. The plasma CO_2 will be reduced due to metabolic acidosis. At this stage there will develop anorexia, abdominal pain and frequent vomiting. Finally, in a state of profound dehydration, sunken eyes, dry tongue, and scaphoid abdomen, the child lapses into the coma which precedes death. Respiration is rapid, sighing and pauseless. The blood pH is reduced. The serum sodium and chloride levels are also reduced. Haemoconcentration masks the severe losses of intracellular potassium in diabetic coma, but after the dehydration has been corrected there is marked hypokalaemia and the ECG shows characteristic abnormalities.

Diagnosis

This is not difficult in the child because by the time medical advice is sought there is marked glycosuria and ketonuria. The blood sugar level is rarely below 11.1 mmol/l (200 mg/100 ml) and frequently much higher. A fasting blood sugar level over 6.66 mmol/l (120 mg/100 ml) is diagnostic of diabetes mellitus. It is rarely necessary to carry out a glucose tolerance test (after 1.75 g glucose per kg body weight). Haemoglobin A_1C has been used as a diagnostic tool indicating metabolic control in diabetes over the preceding 2–3 months. High values in the treated patient indicate poor control.

Differential diagnosis

One of the authors has seen a child in diabetic coma who had been treated for "enuresis" during the preceding 6 weeks. This can only happen when a physician commits the unforgivable sin of diagnosing "enuresis" without having tested the urine. Diabetes insipidus is extremely rare. The urine will not show the presence of glucose or acetone. Renal glycosuria is not associated with symptoms and the diagnosis is readily confirmed by a glucose tolerance test.

Course and prognosis

Without treatment, death in coma is inevitable within a few months or less. On the other hand, with adequate treatment and supervision the diabetic child is able to live a normal life, to attend an ordinary school, and to engage in all normal physical pursuits, although there is evidence that even when control of the disease is adequate by present standards there is often a degree of growth retardation. The long-term prognosis must be guarded because over 60% of all diabetic children will develop serious complications in early middle age. These include diabetic retinopathy, cataract, renal glomerulosclerosis, coronary artery disease, peripheral vascular disease and various types of neuropathy. It is becoming clearer that these long-term microvascular complications can be reduced or delayed by very good control and stabilisation of the blood glucose levels, although these objectives are not always easy to obtain. The diabetic child with irresponsible or mentally impoverished parents is in a most unenviable position.

Insulins

There have been major changes in the insulin preparations in Britain following the introduction in 198_ of the U100 strength (100 units/ml) and the gradual withdrawal of the 40 and 80 units/ml strengths. All the U100 insulins are highly purified. Those most commonly used in paediatric practice are shown in Table 12.2. Human insulins differ from porcine or bovine insulins in having threonine in place of alanine as the C terminal amino acid of the B chain. They may be produced by enzymatic action to replace the alanine or porcine insulin by threonine, and such insulins are designated by the British Pharmacopoeia as human "emp" (enzymatically modified porcine). They may also be processed by production of separate A and B chains by recombinant DNA technology using *E. coli* fermentation, followed by chemical combination of the chains to produce biosynthetic human insulin. This is designated human "crb" (chain recombinant bacterial). There is no evidence that human insulin has significant advantages over the highly purified beef or pork insulins. It is customary to classify the insulin preparations into short-, medium- and long-acting, but it must be stressed that the duration of action of any preparation may vary from one patient to another so that the choice of dose and preparation is to some extent a matter of trial and error. It is doubtful if there is ever need to use long-acting insulins in children.

Treatment

For newly diagnosed patients and their families, the initial phase of stabilisation is best accomplished in an inpatient setting. Indeed, by the time of diagnosis the patient is only too often in a state of ketoacidosis and dehydration requiring emergency treatment. The diagnosis of diabetic ketoacidosis is seldom difficult. In these circumstances vomiting is often severe.

TABLE 12.2 Some U100 highly purified beef, pork and human insulins

	ANIMAL SOURCE	PEAK ACTIVITY (h)	DURATION (h)
Short-acting insulins			
Neutral soluble insulins			
Actrapid MC	Pork	2–5	6–8
Human Actrapid	Human emp	2–5	6–8
Velosulin	Pork	2–5	6–8
Humulin S	Human crb	2–5	6–8
Hypurin neutral	Beef	2–5	6–8
Neusulin	Beef	2–5	6–8
Quicksol	Beef	2–5	6–8
Intermediate-acting insulins			
Isophane insulins			
Humulin I	Human crb	6–12	12–24
Insulatard	Pork	6–12	12–24
Hypurin Isophane	Beef	6–12	12–24
Neuphane	Beef	6–12	12–24
Monophane	Beef	6–12	12–24
Biphasic (mixed) insulins			
Rapitard MC	Beef and pork	3–8	16–22
Initard	Pork	3–8	16–22
Mixtard	Pork	3–8	16–22
Insulin zinc suspensions			
Amorphous (Semilente) → Semitard MC	Pork	5–10	12–16
Mixed → Monotard MC	Pork	6–14	16–22
Human Monotard	Human emp	6–14	16–22
Long-acting insulins			
Hypurin Protamine zinc	Beef	10–20	20–36
Insulin zinc suspensions			
Hypurin Lente	Beef	6–14	18–30
Lentard MC ⎱ Mixed	Beef and pork	6–14	18–30
Neulente ⎰ Lente	Beef	6–14	18–30
Ultratard MC (Crystalline Ultralente)	Beef	10–24	20–36

and the first requirement is physiological saline given by continuous intravenous infusion after taking blood for glucose estimation and following aspiration of the gastric contents with gastric lavage. Rapid infusions of fluid for vascular volume re-expansion, cardiovascular resuscitation, or establishment of urine flow should be near isotonic in composition. Following this phase of therapy the flow rate for the intravenous saline must be determined on clinical grounds, but as a general guide, 500 ml can be infused in 2–3 hours, and in 30 minutes for those over 6 years of age. Subsequently these rates are reduced to one-third. When the plasma glucose level has fallen to below 16.7 mmol/l (300 mg/100 ml), the intravenous fluid can be changed to 5% glucose in half-strength physiological saline. Even severe degrees of acidosis are rapidly correctable with the above fluid regimen plus insulin; and sodium bicarbonate, if it is used at all, is probably best reserved for patients with a blood pH level below 7.1, when 10 mmol/litre can be added to the infusion fluid. The aim is to raise the pH to 7.1 rather than to normal and a second infusion is rarely needed. The plasma potassium level and ECG should be carefully monitored, and the hypokalaemia

which follows rehydration should be corrected by adding potassium chloride to the infusion fluid in a concentration of 20–30 mmol/litre.

The treatment of diabetic ketoacidosis always requires a soluble form of insulin (e.g. Actrapid). There are two methods of initiating insulin administration, both giving good results in experienced hands. This is best administered in frequent small doses intramuscularly or by slow intravenous infusion. The former method consists of the intramuscular injection of 0.25 units soluble insulin per kg body weight within an hour of starting the intravenous infusion. This is followed by hourly intramuscular injections of 0.1 unit/kg until the blood glucose has fallen below 11.1 mmol/l (200 mg/100 ml). It should be noted that insulin dosage is based entirely upon body weight, irrespective of the blood glucose level. The alternative method is by continuous low-dose intravenous infusion of insulin, for which a constant-infusion pump is essential. To begin with, an intravenous dose of insulin, 0.5 units per year of age, is given. An insulin solution is then constituted with physiological saline to give 30 units in 30 ml. This is then infused at a rate of 2.5 ml/hour for children under 8 years and 5 ml/hour for children of 8 years or older, until the blood glucose has fallen below 11.1 mmol/l (200 mg/100 ml). At this point with either method the insulin administration is changed to the subcutaneous route according to future blood and urine tests. However, during the acute illness the blood glucose and electrolytes, and the ECG, must be monitored every 2 hours, and the urine tested as available. The development of cerebral oedema in patients with diabetic ketoacidosis is the most worrying complication. Once present, cerebral oedema can only be supportively treated with non-specific measures of neurointensive care.

The diet considered appropriate for the diabetic has undergone considerable revision over the years. It is no longer considered desirable to restrict carbohydrates whereas, in an attempt to reduce the risk of arterial disease, fat intake should not be allowed to exceed 35% of the calories consumed. This can be achieved by eating fish and chicken in preference to beef, lamb and pork, by grilling rather than frying and by using yoghurt instead of cream. However, the type of carbohydrate consumed is also important. According to the British Diabetic Association, 50% of the total energy intake should be from carbohydrate. Most should be in the form of polysaccharides (i.e. starch), and foods rich in fibre should be encouraged, e.g. Weetabix, Shredded Wheat, All-Bran and wholemeal bread as well as vegetables, pulses, beans and fruit. Rapidly absorbed mono- and disaccharides should be excluded from the diet. It is convenient if the carbohydrates are presented in 10 g portions because in time the parents and child are able to judge these with considerable accuracy and the necessary early weighing then becomes superfluous. The protein intake should constitute about 15% of the total calorie content of the diet. Saccharin or Aspartame are acceptable as a sweetener, but there is little to recommend the use of sorbitol, fructose or the diabetic specialty foods. The diabetic child's diet should always be planned by the physician in consultation with the dietitian and it is essential that the parents fully understand it before their child leaves the hospital. In the past some physicians recommended the so-called "free" diet for the diabetic child because it was easier for the parents and less likely to result in hypoglycaemic attacks. As it does result in higher blood glucose levels with larger fluctuations we do not recommend its general use, although it may be appropriate for some families.

Consideration must now be given to a suitable regimen for long-term insulin administration. For good control of the blood glucose level throughout the 24 hours, twice daily injections are almost unavoidable. A mixture of short- and medium-acting insulins in equal doses (e.g. Velosulin and Insulatard, or Actrapid and Monotard) may be given 30–45 minutes before breakfast and before the evening meal, with two-thirds of the total daily dose in the morning and one-third in the evening. This regimen can then be modified in accordance with the blood and/or urine tests. In families where there are difficulties in measuring two different types of insulin one of the biphasic insulin mixtures (e.g. Mixtard) may be used, although this lacks the flexibility which can respond to changes in diet or physical activities. Until satisfactory control of the diabetes has been achieved blood and/or urine should be tested before breakfast, lunch, the evening meal and bedtime. Later on twice-daily testing may suffice. The home monitoring may be based either on urine testing (with Diabur Test 5000 strips) or blood glucose measurements using reagent strips (e.g. Glucostix, BM Test-Glycemie) with or without a reflectance meter. An acceptable degree of control can be achieved with either method, but only if sufficient time and effort are given to educating the parents and child in their use and then only if they are sufficiently motivated and intelligent to keep good records of the results. Most children prefer home glucose monitoring and some combine the two methods. Older children should, of course, be taught to inject their own insulin and monitor their own blood or urine tests. In recent years, in adults, the continuous subcutaneous infusion of a short-acting insulin by means of infusion pump has been employed in an effort to achieve optimal diabetic control. This is clearly a method which makes considerable demands on the patient and parents, as well as upon the time which the hospital staff must devote to their education. Despite these reservations it would appear that the insulin pump system is practicable for older children and that it can achieve near physiological control of the blood glucose. Also there are several pen devices available to deliver insulin subcutaneously for older children.

The diabetic child is best supervised at a special clinic where physician, dietitian and social worker are available to continue education and motivation of the child and parents in this life-long disease, and where they learn from other parents and hear of other diabetic children's accomplishments. In all other respects the child should be encouraged to live a normal and unrestricted life. Pancreatic transplantation, although offering the hope of a cure, leaves the patient with a lifetime of immunosuppressions and is currently unwarranted as a therapy for children.

NEONATAL DIABETES MELLITUS

Rarely gross dehydration can occur in light for dates newborn infants as a result of transient neonatal diabetes mellitus. There is severe hyperglycaemia and glycosuria. Usually the infant is very responsive to quite small doses (2–4 units) of insulin. There is spontaneous recovery during the first 3–4 months of life but many develop diabetes again in later life.

INFANTS OF DIABETIC MOTHERS

It has long been known that a high perinatal morbidity and mortality is found in the offspring of diabetic mothers (but not of diabetic fathers). These babies have such a characteristic appearance that they might well be related. Indeed, the appearance of such an infant has frequently led to the diagnosis (later confirmed) of a potential state of diabetes in the mother. The infants of diabetic mothers have an unduly high weight and length for their gestational age. They are obese, covered with vernix caseosa, round-faced and plethoric. They lie on their backs with legs abducted and flexed and with their hands alongside their heads, a posture commonly adopted by the premature infant. They frequently tremble on being stimulated by noise. They show an undue susceptibility to develop the respiratory distress syndrome and to have cyanotic attacks. They are frequently premature by dates, often because birth is by Caesarean section because of the known tendency toward intrauterine death after the 36th week. Hypoglycaemia is more consistently found 2–3 hours after birth than in normal infants, but it is usually corrected spontaneously in 4–6 hours. The most constant necropsy finding is hypertrophy of the islets of Langerhans, mainly due to hyperplasia of the β-cells. These facts correlate with the tendency to early postnatal hypoglycaemia. It has been shown that diabetic mothers' babies have an abnormally high plasma insulin-like activity after a glucose load, and it seems likely that their characteristic obesity is due to their own excess production of endogenous insulin, stimulated by the maternal hyperglycaemia. In known diabetic pregnancies, good diabetic control prevents all of these complications and allows a normally grown, normoglycaemic infant to be delivered spontaneously at term.

HYPOGLYCAEMIA OF INFANCY AND CHILDHOOD

There is no critical level of blood glucose below which symptoms will occur. The normal range is 4.4–6.7 mmol/l (80–120 mg/100 ml). Children can tolerate levels of 2.8 mmol/l (50 mg/100 ml) without symptoms, and newborn infants even lower levels. However, in the newborn hypoglycaemia is defined as a blood glucose concentration of less than 2.5 mmol/l (45 mg/l00 ml) whether the infant is term or preterm.

Hypoglycaemia from an overdose of insulin in the diabetic child is a complication which may result from the attempt to achieve good control of the blood sugar levels throughout the 24 hours. Some physicians recommend that before the diabetic child leaves hospital after stabilisation he should be allowed to experience a hypoglycaemic attack so that his parents may observe it and learn how to deal with this emergency. This is, however, an unpleasant experience for all concerned. The occurrence of hypoglycaemia in the infant of a diabetic mother is also caused by an (endogenous) excess of insulin. A rare but dangerous form of persistent, severe non-ketotic hypoglycaemia in the newborn or very young infant is due to nesidioblastosis (β-cell hyperplasia of the pancreas). The pancreas can be shown by special staining and immunohistochemical studies to be diffusely abnormal, with widespread infiltration of the acinar tissue, by both individual and groups of insulin-containing cells, and also of cells secreting glucagon, somatostatin and pancreatic polypeptide. There is failure to form discrete islets of Langerhans and an abnormal quantification of the individual cell types. The diagnostic criteria for this type of hyperinsulinism are:

1 inappropriately high plasma insulin concentrations for the low blood glucose values;
2 a glucose infusion rate > 15 mg/kg/min to maintain the blood glucose > 2 mmol/l (36 mg/100 ml);
3 low blood ketone bodies during hypoglycaemia;
4 glycaemic response to intramuscular glucagon despite hypoglycaemia.

The hypoglycaemia is exceedingly difficult to control and the affected infants are at great risk of brain damage and subsequent mental retardation. In older children a very rare cause of hypoglycaemic attacks is an islet-cell tumour of the pancreas. This can be a difficult diagnosis but the plasma insulin will be inappropriately high during a hypoglycaemic period, and intramuscular glucagon (100 μg/kg) will produce a further inappropriate increase in the plasma insulin level. A rare cause of hypoglycaemia in the young infant is leucine sensitivity. The attacks follow feeds or meals which are rich in leucine. The term ketotic hypoglycaemia is given to attacks sometimes seen in older infants or children, more often in males. It is by far the most common cause of hypoglycaemia outside of the transient hypoglycaemic neonatal disorders. The attacks are provoked by fasting and most often occur in the early morning, associated with ketonuria. This is often described as the "Sunday morning fit" which occurs when family members sleep in and the child misses breakfast. The diagnosis can be confirmed by putting the child on a high-carbohydrate diet for 5 days followed by a ketogenic diet when ketonuria and then hypoglycaemia will develop.

Hypoglycaemia is also a feature of a variety of metabolic disorders such as coeliac disease, galactosaemia, von Gierke disease, hepatic disorders, growth-hormone deficiency and adrenocortical failure where it only infrequently causes characteristic clinical manifestations.

Clinical features

In older children the early symptoms are sweating, pallor, irritability or irrational behaviour, and tachycardia. Later there are more severe neurological manifestations such as tremors, paralysis, convulsions and coma. In the newborn or young infant hypoglycaemia may cause floppiness, reluctance to suck, jitteriness, apnoeic attacks, convulsions or sudden circulatory collapse. Since the symptoms and signs of hypoglycaemia are non-specific, it is essential to document that they are truly caused by hypoglycaemia and that the correction of the hypoglycaemia results in disappearance of the symptoms.

Treatment

Mild insulin-induced hypoglycaemic attacks in the diabetic child can be corrected with a few lumps of sugar or a glucose drink. In severe attacks, or if there is loss of consciousness, 1 mg of glucagon should be injected intramuscularly followed by an intravenous injection of 20–40 ml of 50% dextrose. It is important to ensure that the plasma glucose concentration remains above 50 mg/dl to prevent the sequelae of hypoglycaemia, mental starvation and neurological damage.

In nesidioblastosis the infant should be given a continuous 10% dextrose infusion, and intravenous diazoxide 5–20 mg/kg/day in three 8-hourly doses, but subtotal (85%) resection of the pancreas should proceed with a minimum of delay. Recent work has indicated that alloxan may have a place in management. If hypoglycaemia still persists a total pancreatectomy will be essential after which the infant will have to be treated as an insulin-dependent diabetic. An islet-cell adenoma should be excised, although it is sometimes difficult to find.

In leucine sensitivity there may be a place for diazoxide, 5 mg/kg/day, in association with a low-protein, high-carbohydrate diet. Ketotic hypoglycaemic attacks can be abolished by a diet low in fat with frequent high-carbohydrate, high-protein meals. The condition of ketotic hypoglycaemia usually resolves spontaneously by 8–10 years of age.

13

Haematological Disorders

HAEMOPOIESIS

Within a few days of embryonic implantation "blood islands" develop in the human yolk sac. Cells from these islands develop into vascular endothelium and primitive blood cells. These pluripotent stem cells known as progenitor or CFU-GEMM (colony forming unit, granulocyte-erythroid/megakaryocyte-macrophage) cells produce red cells, white cells except lymphocytes and platelets (Fig. 13.1) Most haemopoiesis in the fetus takes place from progenitor cells seeded to the liver. Bone marrow haemopoiesis is present from about 10 weeks' gestation and by term has taken over almost all of the fetal haemopoietic function. Control of erythropoiesis in the fetus is through hepatic erythropoietin mediated by fetal tissue oxygen concentration. There is a switch to renal erythropoietin a few weeks after birth.

All of the white cell series and platelets are identifiable in fetal blood by about 14 weeks' gestation and the granulocyte series is controlled by the hormone GSF and platelets by thrombopoietin.

Modern haematology embraces many complicated techniques which have added greatly to our understanding of the nature of some of the less common disorders, e.g. haemolytic anaemias, haemoglobinopathies, megaloblastic anaemias, etc. None the less, the blood disorders commonly encountered in paediatric practice can most often be dealt with by the use of relatively simple standard techniques.

THE NORMAL BLOOD PICTURE IN INFANCY

Considerable variations in normal values during the early days of life have been recorded by different workers. There are several reasons for this. Blood samples obtained by venepuncture in early infancy have lower values for haemoglobin and red cell counts than those obtained by heel prick and individual infants show a wide variation in values. In routine clinical practice only fairly large departures from normal ranges are likely to prove significant.

Haemoglobin

The Hb concentration in blood from the umbilical cord is high with a mean of 17 g/dl (17 g/100 ml). Values up to 20 g/dl may be recorded. A venous sample of the infant's blood some hours after birth may reveal an even higher Hb level with a mean of 19 g/dl, and a skin-prick sample is likely to be still higher with a mean of 21 g/dl. This rise in Hb values just after birth is probably due to haemoconcentration due to diminution in the plasma volume, in addition to the infusion of red cells which may occur when late clamping of the umbilical cord is practised.

The oxygen-carrying capacity of the blood is related to the total circulating red cell mass (RCM) which can vary in normal infants between 30 and 50 ml/kg depending on whether the cord is clamped early or late. Haemoglobin concentration and haematocrit can correlate poorly with the RCM especially in preterm infants. The RCM can vary between 12 and 24 ml/kg in infants with a haematocrit of 0.3 (30%) due to compensatory reductions of plasma volume.

The Hb value falls to 10–11 g/dl by the age of 8–12 weeks but rises again to between 11 and 13 g/dl between the ages of 6 months and a year. Thereafter, the Hb level increases to 11.5–15 g/dl by the age of 10–12 years, and reaches normal adult values (men = 13.5–18 g/dl; women = 11.5–16.5 g/dl) by the age of

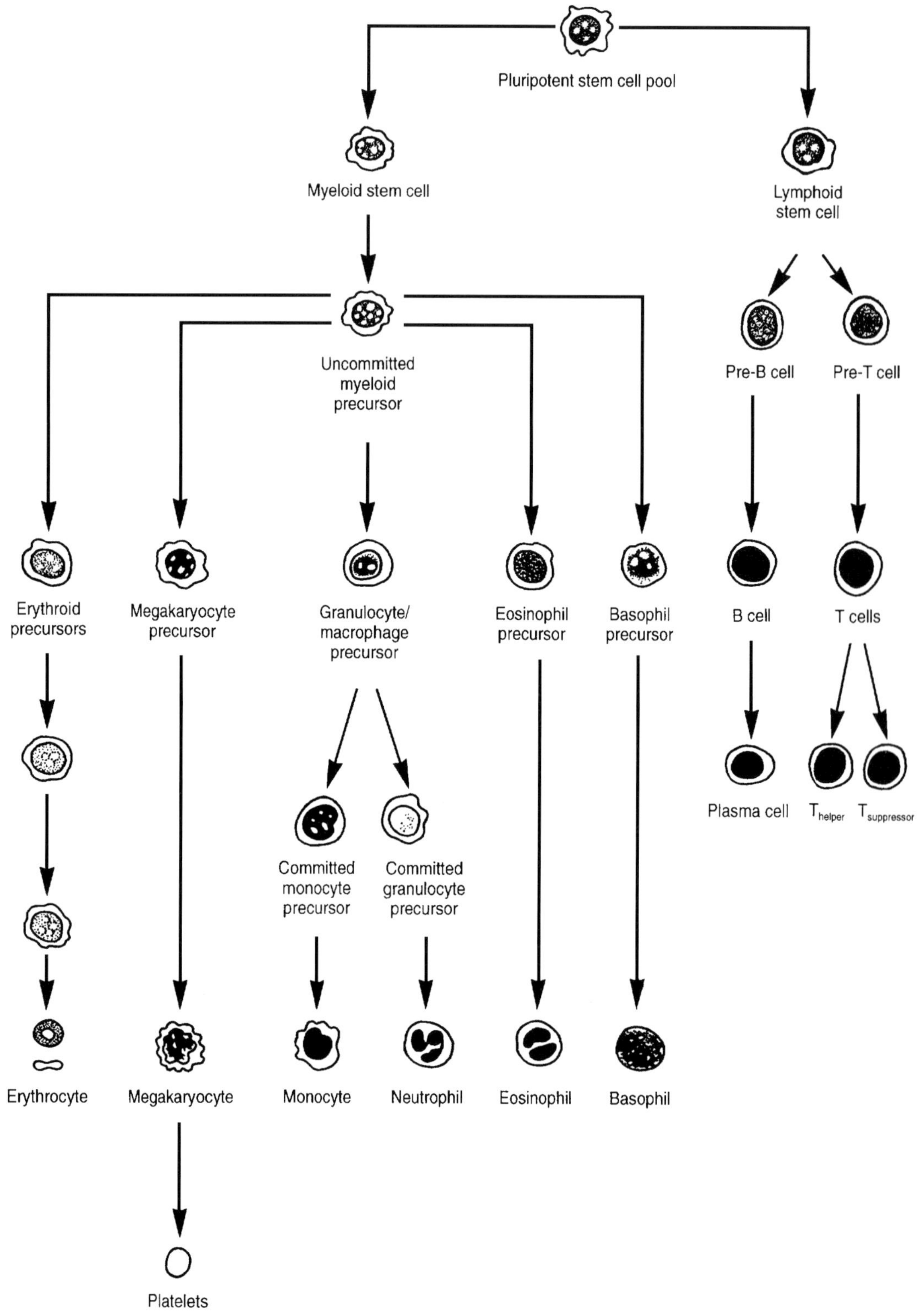

FIGURE 13.1 Haemopoiesis in the embryo and fetus.

15 years. The explanation for the fall in Hb level during the early weeks of life is that, although erythropoiesis continues at a high level found in the fetus for about 3 days after birth, an abrupt decline in erythropoiesis then occurs and the marrow erythroid count falls from 40 000 to 6000 per mm³. This is reflected in a fall in the reticulocyte count from 3 or 4% just after birth to under 1% one week later.

At birth 50–65% of the Hb is of the fetal type (Hb-F) which resists denaturation with alkalis. It has a slightly different electorphoretic mobility and a quite different oxygen dissociation curve from adult type haemoglobin (Hb-A). After birth Hb-F is slowly replaced by Hb-A so that after a year of age only small amounts of Hb-F are still present. In certain diseases, such as thalassaemia and sickle-cell anaemia, Hb-F is produced in excessive quantity. The value to the fetus of Hb-F appears to be that of a greater affinity for oxygen at low tensions than Hb-A and an ability to release CO_2 more readily.

Since the discovery in 1949 of the first abnormal haemoglobin molecule (Hb-S) a great deal of information has accumulated about the molecular structure of haemoglobin. Over 100 variant forms of human haemoglobin have now been recognised. Some of these are associated with serious disease in various parts of the world.

Red cells

The red cell count at birth varies between 5.5 and 7.5 million per mm³. The count falls to about 5–5.5 millions after 2 weeks and thereafter runs parallel to the Hb level. Scanty eosinophilic normoblasts are found in the peripheral blood at birth. Erythrocytes at birth have a larger diameter (about 8.4 μm) than in the adult. The mean adult value of 7.2 μm is reached after 1 year.

White cells

The total white cell count at birth is about 18 000 per mm³. The adult value of 6000–7000 per mm³ is not reached for 7–10 years. At birth about 60% of the white cells are polymorphonuclear (11 000 per mm³) and 30% are lymphocytes (5400 per mm³). During the ensuing 2 weeks the polymorphonuclear count falls to within the normal adult range (3500–4500 per mm³) where they remain during the rest of childhood. On the other hand, the lymphocytes, predominantly of the large type in infancy, rise rapidly to about 9500 per mm³ at 2 weeks and only slowly fall during the next 12 years to the adult level of about 1500–2000 per mm³. It is important to remember the comparatively high lymphocyte count

in normal children if mistaken diagnoses such as glandular fever or leukaemia are to be avoided. The monocyte ratio in children tends to be somewhat higher than in adults. Eosinophils and basophils show no special characteristics.

IRON DEFICIENCY OR NUTRITIONAL ANAEMIA OF INFANCY

This is the only deficiency disease seen commonly among infants and children in the UK at the present time. The highest incidence of anaemia is found in the lower socio-economic groups.

Aetiology

Several factors, singly or in combination, can result in this deficiency state. Unduly prolonged milk feeding (human or cows') or feeding whole cows' milk in early infancy results in iron deficiency. This is perhaps the most commonly found factor. Another important factor is the influence of birthweight. It is well known that preterm infants and others of low birthweight (such as twins or triplets) are particularly likely to develop iron deficiency anaemia. Infants, whatever their maturity, have a body iron content of about 75 mg/kg fat-free body weight. The bulk of the infant's iron endowment (66–75%) is represented by haemoglobin iron. One gram of haemoglobin contains 3.4 mg of iron. Complications of pregnancy or the perinatal period that result in blood loss will compromise the infant's iron endowment. The smaller infant grows more rapidly in proportion to his birthweight than the larger with a corresponding need for a larger increase in his red cells and haemoglobin. As the amount of iron absorbed is very low during the first 4 months of life the small infant more rapidly exhausts his storage iron (in liver and spleen) and develops overt signs of iron deficiency. Unless extreme, the presence of maternal iron deficiency does not appear to compromise the iron endowment of the fetus. Infections, to which the iron deficient infant is prone, further aggravate the anaemia. Finally, the possibility of chronic blood loss from, e.g. oesophagitis, a Meckel diverticulum or hookworm infestation, or of iron malabsorption must always be considered in cases of iron deficiency anaemia. Occult gastrointestinal bleeding can occur in infants who have been started on whole cows' milk early in life.

Clinical features

A mild degree of nutritional anaemia probably affects over 25% of infants during their first year. The onset is rarely before the fifth month of life. When the anaemia is severe there is obvious pallor of skin and mucous membranes. *Splenomegaly* may be present and there may be cardiomegaly and a haemic systolic murmur. The anaemia is microcytic and hypochromic. Serum iron is markedly reduced (normal mean = 18 mmol/l; 100 mg/100 ml), and the saturation of the iron binding protein of the serum is reduced from 30% to 10% or less. The serum ferritin concentration is reduced (less than 10 µg/ml). Bone marrow shows normoblastic hyperplasia and an absence of stainable iron.

Prevention

In the term infant, iron deficiency is best prevented by the avoidance of whole cows' milk as a drink until 12 months and by the introduction of mixed feeding with foods rich in iron at the age of 4 months. In the preterm infant iron should be given orally from the age of 4 weeks. The term infant should receive 1 mg of iron/kg/day and the preterm infant 3 mg/kg/day.

Treatment

In most cases the anaemia can be rapidly corrected with oral iron. Among the ferrous salts such as sulphate, fumarate, succinate, glutamate, gluconate and lactate the sulphate salt is considered to be the salt of choice. The dose of iron in an average child is 2–3 mg of elemental iron per kg administered three times daily between meals. The therapeutic response to iron therapy may be verified by any one of the following methods. A reticulocytosis may be noted 2–3 days after the start of therapy with a peak rise at 7–10 days. The haemoglobin may be rechecked after 2–4 weeks. Once normal haematological values have been attained iron should be continued for an additional 1–2 months to reconstitute depleted iron stores. Intramuscular administration of iron is indicated only if it is not possible to achieve compliance with the use of oral iron or under the unusual circumstances in which iron malabsorption occurs.

THE MEGOBLASTIC ANAEMIAS (FOLATE DEFICIENCY, VITAMIN B$_{12}$ DEFICIENCY)

Folate deficiency

True megoblastic erythropoiesis is rare in paediatric practice. The most common cause is malabsorption of folic acid in the older child with inadequately treated coeliac disease. However, folate deficiency may also be caused by inadequate intake, increased requirements, disorders of folate metabolism (congenital and acquired) and increased excretion. The symptoms of folate deficiency anaemia are similar to vitamin B$_{12}$ deficiency except that neuropathy is not a feature of folate deficiency. Also the peripheral blood and bone marrow changes in folate deficiency are indentical to those found in vitamin B$_{12}$ deficiency.

Hypersegmentation of the neutrophils in the peripheral blood is the single most useful laboratory aid to early diagnosis. The serum folate assay is a sensitive, reliable guide to the presence of folate deficiency and remains the best way of confirming early folate deficiency. Successful treatment of patients with folate deficiency involves correction of the folate deficiency as well as amelioration of the underlying disorder and improvement of the diet to increase folate intake. It is usual to treat folate deficient patients with 1–5 mg folic acid orally daily.

Vitamin B$_{12}$ deficiency

Vitamin B$_{12}$ deficiency in children is exceedingly rare. If it occurs it is caused either by a specific malabsorption of vitamin B$_{12}$ or as part of a generalised malabsorption syndrome. After resection of the terminal ileum there is a risk of a megaloblastic anaemia developing 2–3 years later once the liver stores are depleted. Those most vulnerable are children who lose terminal ileum as a result of tumour (lymphoma), necrotising enterocolitis, Crohn disease or trauma. Most cases of vitamin B$_{12}$ deficiency occur during the first 2 years of life and others manifest later in childhood until puberty.

The clinical signs and symptoms of vitamin B$_{12}$ deficiency are related primarily to the anaemia but can also be complicated by subacute combined degeneration of the spinal cord. Glossitis with papillary atrophy may also be seen.

The haematological findings are indistinguishable from those of folic acid deficiency. The peripheral blood and bone marrow findings can be identical but the serum vitamin B$_{12}$ level is low. A Schilling test may be necessary to diagnose vitamin B$_{12}$ malabsorption.

Most patients with vitamin B$_{12}$ deficiency require treatment throughout life. Vitamin B$_{12}$ therapy results in reticulocytosis that peaks in 6–8 days and falls gradually to normal by 12th day. Bone marrow returns completely from megaloblastic to normoblastic in 72 hours.

THE HAEMOLYTIC ANAEMIAS

The causes of haemolytic anaemia, which may be defined as one in which the life span of the red cells is shortened can be summarised as follows:

- Defects within the red blood cell
  Chemical and structural consequences
  Congenital spherocytosis
  Thalassaemia
  The haemoglobinopathies

  Enzymatic
  G-6-P dehydrogenase deficiency
  Pyruvate kinase deficiency

  Undetermined
  Paroxysmal nocturnal haemoglobinuria (not seen in children)

- Mechanisms extrinsic to the red blood cell
  Infections

  Chemical drugs and physical agents

  Red cell antibodies
  Idiopathic
  Symptomatic – secondary

  Undetermined
  With or without systemic disease

Haemolytic anaemias due to blood group incompatibility between mother and child and G-6-P dehydrogenase deficiency are considered in Chapter 1. It should also be pointed out that the common and classical manifestations of increased haemolysis such as acholuric jaundice, excess urobilinogenuria, reticulocytosis and hyperplasia of the bone marrow need not always be present. Indeed, even anaemia may be absent in mild cases because of the capability of the bone marrow to compensate for increased red cell destruction. On the other hand, the increased folic acid requirements in the presence of haemolysis are well documented and may require supplements of folic acid.

Hereditary spherocytosis (congenital haemolytic jaundice)

Aetiology

Hereditary spherocytosis is one of the most common inherited haemolytic anaemias encountered in paediatrics. This disease is transmitted as a Mendelian dominant trait but in 25% of the cases neither parent appears to be affected. This is most likely the result of spontaneous mutation. At present it seems likely that the physiologically important abnormality is an inherent instability of the red cell membrane. It is certain that the major part of the haemolysis of the abnormal red cells takes place in the spleen.

Clinical features

The disease is quite variable in its severity. However, most affected children will, at some time, manifest one or more of the cardinal features of the disease: anaemia, jaundice and splenomegaly. It can cause haemolytic icterus in the neonatal period and kernicterus has been described. It is, however, rare for the disease to appear in infancy. More commonly it presents during later childhood with pallor and lassitude, less often with jaundice and highly coloured urine. Children may present with an acute abdomen from splenic infarcts. They have a fever, a leucocytosis and a tender enlarged spleen, which can rupture, as well as anaemia and jaundice. It may remain symptomless until adult life when biliary colic due to gallstones is not uncommon. Acute haemolytic crises with severe anaemia and icterus require emergency treatment but they are, in fact, uncommon. Splenomegaly is usually present whatever the degree of haemolysis in hereditary spherocytosis. The red cells are unable to sustain a normal biconcave shape because of their metabolic defect. They are spheroidal with a smaller diameter than normal. It is usually easy to differentiate microspherocytes in well stained blood films. They appear unduly dark in colour and small in diameter than normal biconcave erythrocytes. A significant reticulocytosis is usually found. High figures may be reached during a crisis but the absence of a reticulocytosis does not exclude the diagnosis. The serum unconjugated bilirubin level is increased and there is excess urobilinogen in the urine. Increased osmotic fragility of the red cells is an important diagnostic feature. The test is much more reliable when performed on a quantitative basis but is not pathognomonic of hereditary spherocytosis, being sometimes abnormal in acquired haemolytic anaemia, and infrequently it may be normal in the neonatal period. In hereditary spherocytosis the Coombs' test is negative and the marrow shows normoblastic hyperplasia. Rarely, an aplastic crisis can occur with hypoplasia of the bone marrow resulting in anaemia, leucopenia and thrombocytopenia. Routine ultrasound of the gall bladder should be done to determine whether biliary pigment stones have developed. These should be removed at the time of splenectomy.

Treatment

Splenectomy results in a return to normal health although it does not alter the metabolic defect in the red cells. It should always be advised in the child with hereditary spherocytosis since even mild disease interferes with growth and well-being. Splenectomy renders the child more susceptible to severe bacterial infections and there is good evidence that the risk is greatest in infancy. This can be reduced by immunisation with pneumococcal vaccine, since 50% of post-splenectomy sepsis is due to *Streptococcus pneumoniae*. In addition the child should receive life long oral prophylactic penicillin. If the child has not

TABLE 13.1 Globin chains of normal haemoglobins

Adult	
Hb-A	$\alpha_2 + \beta_2$
Hb-A$_2$	$\alpha_2 + \delta_2$
Fetal	
Hb-F	$\alpha_2 + \gamma_2$
H-Bart's	γ_4
Hb-H	β_4

been previously immunised against *Haemophilus influenzae* it would be worthwhile giving Hib vaccine. In our opinion splenectomy should be postponed until the child is about 5 years old. There is no evidence that further delay is useful, and it may be harmful, since the risk of cholelithiasis increases in children after the age of 10 years. Control of the anaemia can meantime be achieved by blood transfusion. Rarely, in the neonatal period a rising serum bilirubin level may necessitate an exchange transfusion to eliminate the risk of kernicterus.

The thalassaemias

Aetiology

Normal adult and fetal haemoglobin contains four globin chains (Table 13.1). The thalassaemia syndromes are a heterogeneous group of disorders of haemoglobin (Hb) synthesis resulting from a genetically determined reduced rate of production of one or more of the four globin chains of haemoglobin – α (alpha), β (beta), δ (delta) and γ (gamma). This results in an excess of the partner chains which continue to be synthesised at a normal rate. The alpha-chain types are carried on chromosome 16 and the beta, delta and gamma on chromosome 11. Each type of thalassaemia can exist in a heterozygous or a homozygous state. The most common is beta-thalassaemia (Cooley's anaemia) which involves suppression of beta-chain formation. In homozygotes there is a severe anaemia with a high level of Hb-F (α_2, γ_2), some Hb-A$_2$ (α_2, δ_2) and a complete absence of, or greatly reduced (normal) Hb-A (α_2, β_2). Heterozygotes on the other hand suffer from only mild anaemia with reasonable levels of Hb-A, somewhat raised Hb-A$_2$, but Hb-F levels rarely in excess of 3%. Children of the mating of two such heterozygotes have a 1 in 4 chance of suffering from the homozygous state for beta-thalassaemia. They will not present clinically, however, until later infancy when the effects of beta-chain suppression develop because Hb-A formation fails to take over from the production of Hb-F in the normal way. The other main type of thalassaemia involves suppression of alpha-chain production and as alpha chains are

shared by Hb-A, Hb-A$_2$ and Hb-F it is to be expected that alpha-thalassaemia would become clinically manifest in fetal life.

Tetramers of gamma chains may be produced (Hb-Bart's) which result in a clinical picture very similar to that in hydrops fetalis with stillbirth or early neonatal death. In haemoglobin H disease, on the other hand, tetramers of gamma chains (Hb-H) are present in excess and there is considerable clinical variability: from a picture indistinguishable from Cooley's anaemia to an absence of specific signs. Heterozygotes for alpha-thalassaemia cannot be detected with certainty. The thalassaemias are uncommon in persons of British stock but they are commonly seen in children of Mediterranean origin as well as in South-east Asia where they constitute a major and distressing public health problem. The clinical account which follows refers only to the most common variety of beta-thalassaemia in the homozygous state (beta-thalassaemia major – Cooley's anaemia).

Clinical features

This condition is characterised by a chronic haemolytic anaemia which becomes manifest later in infancy but not in the newborn. Pallor is constant and icterus not uncommon. Splenomegaly increases throughout childhood. Hepatomegaly is also present largely due to extramedullary erythropoiesis. Pathognomonic skeletal changes can be demonstrated radiographically. Membranous bones of the skull are thickened and lateral views of the skull show the "hair on end" appearance (Fig. 13.2). The facies has a mongoloid appearance due to thickening of the facial bones. The hands may become broadened and thickened due to changes in the metacarpals and phalanges. These bone changes are due to the hyperplasia of the bone marrow. Blood examination shows a severe hypochromic anaemia with marked anisocytosis and poikilocytosis. Many microcytic red cells lie side by side with large (12–18 μm), bizarrely shaped cells. In some of the latter cells an abnormal central mass of haemoglobin gives them the appearance of "target cells" (Fig. 13.3). Reticulocytosis is marked and Howell–Jolly bodies may be numerous. Serum unconjugated bilirubin concentration is increased. There is increased serum iron while the iron-binding capacity is fully saturated and lower than in normal children. The haemoglobin pattern in beta-thalassaemia major consists mainly of Hb-F, which may amount to 90% of the total and of Hb-A$_2$; Hb-A is totally absent or greatly reduced. Most children affected by beta-thalassaemia major can be kept in reasonable health if they are maintained on a high blood transfusion regimen which prevents the Hb level from falling 11 g/dl. Other laboratory abnormalities commonly found in homozygous beta-thala-

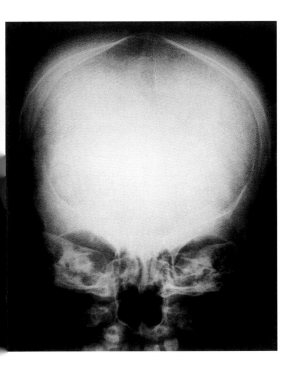

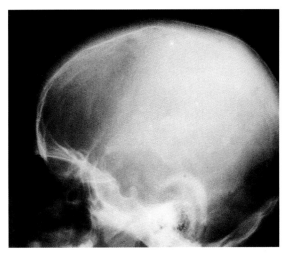

FIGURE 13.2 X-ray of skull of a child with homozygous beta-thalassaemia showing "hair-on-end" appearance associated with chronic marrow hyperplasia.

...saemia are mostly due to complications of transfusional haemosiderosis. However, even with the best available treatment, growth failure becomes apparent before puberty. In boys there is usually a complete or partial failure of pubertal growth and sexual maturation. In girls the failure tends to be less severe with irregular or scanty menstrual periods. However, secondary amenorrhoea may develop from iron overload. Ultimately, death occurs in most patients in adolescence or early adult life due to cardiac failure from iron overload. Other effects may include endocrine, hepatic or renal failure and overt diabetes mellitus.

Treatment

The prognosis in beta-thalassaemia has improved in recent years and could improve still further if the best available management were to be everywhere pursued. This has been well described under three major categories: choice of transfusion scheme; hypersplenism and splenectomy; iron chelation therapy. The objective of the transfusion scheme should be never to allow the Hb value to drop below 11 g/dl and to raise it to 14 or 15 g/dl by a programme of routine red cell transfusions every 3–4 weeks. This regimen will reduce the stimulus to unlimited bone marrow expansion and so prevent such undesirable manifestations as cardiomegaly, stunting of growth and the disfiguring, "Cooley's facies". This regimen has become standard therapy for beta-thalassaemia major. On the other hand, the

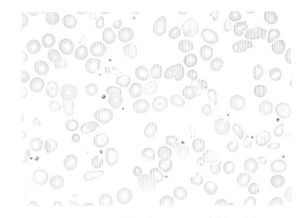

FIGURE 13.3 Peripheral blood smear of a child with homozygous beta-thalassaemia showing a target cell.

degree of hypersplenism has not always been appreciated and it may be marked even in the absence of thrombocytopenia or leucopenia. Its presence greatly increases the blood requirements. The rate of splenic enlargement is variable even in well transfused patients and the massive size of the spleen may lead to abdominal discomfort. Often the transfusion requirement increases as the spleen enlarges. Eventually most patients undergo splenectomy which usually leads to improved physical well-being and a reduction in the transfusion requirement. Splenectomy should be delayed if possible until the child is 4 or 5 years of age. Splenectomised children should receive life-long oral penicillin prophylaxis and polyvalent pneumococcal and Hib vaccine. Desferrioxamine is the only effective agent available for chronic iron chelation. The age at which chelation should be initiated is controversial. Most patients must accrue approximately 3–4 g of iron reflected by a serum ferritin of greater than 500 ng/ml before subcutaneous desferrioxamine leads to significant iron excretion. Desferrioxamine can be administered subcutaneously (25–40 mg/kg/day) with a small infusion pump or it may be given by intravenous infusion (60–75 mg/g/h) either intermittently at the time of transfusion to supplement regular subcutaneous infusions or regularly as an alternative form of therapy. There is also general agreement that ascorbic acid 100–200 mg daily by mouth enhances the effectiveness of desferrioxamine therapy. Most patients older than 3 years appear to reach negative iron balance as calculated from urinary iron excretion. A programme of home chelation therapy has been instituted in several centres. The patients or their parents are trained to administer the drug subcutaneously as an overnight infusion. The child's school life is therefore not affected by the therapy. There is, however, an alternative form of treatment for selected patients with the very severe form of beta-thalassaemia. Bone marrow transplantation can potentially provide a "cure" for thalassaemia; however, risks are too high at this stage to be acceptable and gene therapy is not yet possible.

Prevention

The only rational approach to thalassaemia on a world scale must lie in programmes developed towards prevention. These have been based on the prospective detection of heterozygotes followed by genetic counselling. Prenatal diagnosis of the homozygous fetus can be reached by means of fetoscopy and fetal blood sampling. However, this is not practicable before 18 weeks' gestation which leaves little time for consideration of termination of pregnancy. More recently the technique of transcervical biopsy of chorionic villi during the first trimester of pregnancy promises great potential for fetal diagnosis. The trophoblast tissue so obtained is subjected to restriction endonuclease analysis of fetal DNA. However, while sickle-cell anaemia can be diagnosed in all cases by this highly sophisticated technique, in beta-thalassaemia blood is required from a previous thalassaemic or normal child or from lateral relatives of the parents to achieve fetal diagnosis in 60–80% of cases. Nevertheless, the progress being made in the prenatal diagnosis of thalassaemia suggests that it will not be long before direct gene analysis will become possible both for the detection of carriers and for prenatal diagnosis.

Sickle-cell disease

Aetiology

This disease is almost confined to the black African races. Homozygotes suffer from *sickle-cell anaemia* in which all of their haemoglobin is of the Hb-S variety (homozygous SS disease). The abnormality in Hb-S lies in the beta-peptide chains, the alpha chains being normal. The aberration in the beta chains is due to the substitution of valine for glutamic acid in the no. 6 position. Heterozygotes reveal the *sickle-cell trait* (AS) and their haemoglobin is composed of about 60% Hb-A and 40% Hb-S. The trait is found in about 7–9% of American black people but it is much more prevalent in some African tribes. It provides increased resistance to malignant tertian malaria. Hb-S has a distinctive electrophoretic pattern which is due to its abnormal molecular structure. This type of haemoglobin forms crescent-shaped crystals under reduced oxygen tension, and it is this property which is responsible for the sickled shape of the erythrocytes in people who possess the gene. Haemolysis in sickle-cell anaemia appears to be due mainly to impaction of the sickled cells in the capillaries, especially in organs where the oxygen tension is low. Capillary obstruction leads to infarcts in various organs, e.g spleen, intestine, bones, kidneys, heart, lungs and brain.

Clinical features

The sickle-cell trait (AS) is symptomless unless it is associated with another haemoglobinopathy or with thalassaemia (see below). Sickle-cell anaemia (SS often presents during the first year with pallor listlessness and mild jaundice. The onset of symptom is, however, delayed for 6 months or longer until the Hb-F of the infant has been replaced by Hb-S. In some cases there are recurrent haemolytic crises with acute symptoms such as severe abdominal pain and rigidity, pain in the loins, limb pains, localised paralyses, convulsions or meningism. Symmetrical painful swellings of the fingers and feet (hand-and-foot syndrome) may develop due to infarction in the small bones as the sickle cells stick together and occlude small blood vessels. X-rays show severe bone destruction and periosteal reaction. They may also reveal radial striations in the skull. Chronic haemolytic anaemia interferes with growth and nutrition so that the child is often stunted in later years. Splenomegaly may be marked, but sometimes disappears in late childhood. Cholelithiasis may develop as in other haemolytic anaemias. In adults the large joints may become swollen and painful with serious crippling. The peripheral blood shows a normochromic anaemia, reticulocytosis and polymorphonuclear leucocytosis. In addition there is an increase in th

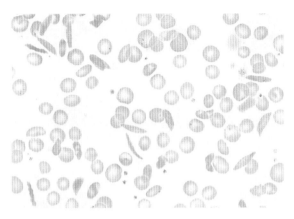

FIGURE 13.4 Peripheral blood smear of a child with sickle-cell disease showing sickled red cells.

serum unconjugated bilirubin and a decrease in red cell osmotic fragility. In a crisis excess urobilino-genuria is marked. Sickled cells may be seen in ordinary blood films. They can always be produced by preparing a fresh drop of blood under a cover-slip which is sealed off from oxygen with Vaseline. After 1–24 hours at room temperature sickled forms will be seen (Fig. 13.4). The diagnosis can be confirmed by demonstration of the characteristic mobility of Hb-S on starch gel electrophoresis. Children affected with sickle-cell anaemia also have some Hb-F in their circulation.

Treatment

There is no cure for sickle-cell disease but blood transfusions are frequently required for anaemia. Because of the high incidence of serious bacterial infections in patients with sickle-cell anaemia, the index of suspicion for infection should be high. Antibiotic choice should include agents effective against pneumococcus, *Haemophilus influenzae*, salmonella and *Staphylococcus aureus*. Antibiotics should be discontinued or modified when culture reports are available. In vaso-occlusive crises, rest in bed and relief of pain are essential. Dehydration and acidosis should be quickly corrected. With careful supervision and the use of blood transfusion many children with sickle-cell anaemia (SS) reach adult life. Splenectomy is indicated when there is evidence of hypersplenism. Folate deficiency is particularly common in sickle-cell disease and 5 mg of folic acid should be given daily. Death can occur suddenly from cardiac failure, renal failure or cerebral infarction and patients of black African extraction should always be tested for sickling before anaesthesia. Sickle-cell testing is an important consideration in any child from geographical areas where sickle-cell disease is prevalent before any elective surgery is carried out.

Post-operative preparation may require blood transfusion, and hypoxia and acidosis should be avoided during the operation. Prevention is to be approached along the same lines as those already described for thalassaemia, but progress on a world scale is likely to be painfully slow.

Other haemoglobinopathies

It has already been noted that there are three *normal haemoglobins* each of two identical pairs of globin polypeptide chains with an iron-containing haem group inserted into each chain. In the healthy adult 98% of the Hb-A is composed of two alpha and two beta chains ($\alpha_2\beta_2$). About 2% of adult Hb is Hb-A composed of two alpha and two delta chains ($\alpha_2\delta_2$). Fetal Hb or Hb-F is composed of two alpha and two gamma chains ($\alpha_2\gamma_2$). However, over 100 abnormal haemoglobins have now been recognised in which the aberration generally consists of a single amino-acid substitution in one pair of the peptide chains due to gene mutation. That is to say, they are determined by alleles of the genes for normal Hb-A, Hb-A_2 or Hb-F. The different haemoglobins carry different electrical charges, so causing them to move at different speeds in an electrical field and they can usually best be identified by electrophoresis. The different haemoglobinopathies vary widely in their effects, from no apparent effect on health to a fatal disease (e.g. Hb-S). The homozygote for the gene will, of course, always be much more severely affected than the heterozygote, as in sickle-cell disease.

The homozygote for Hb-C presents with manifestations similar to those in sickle-cell disease but sickling and bone changes do not occur. The heterozygote is usually symptomless but blood films show target cells and there is increased osmotic resistance. The homozygote for Hb-E, on the other hand, suffers only from a mild normochromic anaemia with numerous target cells and increase in osmotic resistance, while the heterozygote is asymptomatic. Haemoglobin M disease is very different in that it causes methaemoglobinaemia.

Having now considered thalassaemia and a few of the haemoglobinopathies in both the homozygous and heterozygous forms, it remains to point out that some anaemic children are found to have inherited the genes for two abnormal haemoglobins, one from each heterozygous parent, or more commonly for beta-thalassaemia and one abnormal haemoglobin. They are, in fact, mixed or double heterozygotes. Thus there has been described beta-thalassaemia with haemoglobin S (or C, D or E) as well as S/C, S/D combinations, etc. The effects produced by these states depend upon the peptide chains involved. Thus, if both abnormal genes affect the same type of chain the effects are much more severe than if they affect different chains, i.e. the mixed heterozygous state is more crippling than the double heterozygous state. For example, in both S/C disease and Hb-S/beta-thalassaemia the beta chains are involved. This means that no Hb-A can be formed because no normal beta chains can be produced, a state called "interaction" and the resulting clinical manifestations are very similar in severity to the homozygous S/S state (sickle-cell anaemia). On the other hand, when both an alpha- and a beta-chain abnormality are inherited (e.g. as in alpha-thalassaemia with beta-chain haemoglobins S,C or E) the effect is usually no more severe than when only one of the abnormalities is present because no "interaction" has taken place. Some of these abnormal haemoglobin states can only be accurately identified by family studies, employing sophisticated techniques. The matter is of practical importance because of the differences in prognosis.

Autoimmune haemolytic anaemia

Aetiology

This is not a common problem in paediatric practice but it may present as an acute emergency. There are two major classes of antibodies against red cells that produce haemolysis in man: IgG and IgM. The IgM antibody is generally restricted to the clinical entity of cold haemagglutinin disease because it has a particular affinity for its red cell antigen in the cold ($0-10°C$). IgM-induced immune haemolytic anaemia is most commonly associated with an underlying mycoplasma infection or cytomegalovirus, mumps and infectious mononucleosis infections.

The IgG antibody usually has its maximal activity at $37°C$ and, thus, this entity has been termed warm antibody-induced haemolytic anaemia. IgG-induced immune haemolytic anaemia may occur without an apparent underlying disease (idiopathic disease); however, it may also occur with bacterial and viral infections or may be drug induced.

Clinical features

In some children the disease has an alarmingly acute onset (Lederer anaemia) with fever, backache, limb pains, abdominal pain, vomiting and diarrhoea. Haemoglobinuria and oliguria may be present. Pallor develops rapidly and icterus is common. Frequently, the pallor, listlessness and mild icterus develop more insidiously. Splenomegaly is common. The urine may be dark in colour due to the presence of excess urobilinogen. The anaemia is usually orthochromic but it can be either normocytic or macrocytic. Reticulocytosis is often marked and there may be many erythroblasts in the peripheral blood. Spherocytosis with an increased fragility of the red cells may simulate congenital spherocytosis. However, in acquired haemolytic anaemia the Coombs' test is positive and serum unconjugated bilirubin concentration is increased. Autoagglutination may be marked at room temperature. A polymorphonuclear leucocytosis is usual and myelocytes may be numerous. Occasionally a thrombocytopenia and purpura can develop. Both haemolytic and aplastic crises may occur. A false positive serological test for syphilis is a recognised phenomenon.

Treatment

In many patients with IgG- or IgM-induced immune haemolytic anaemia no therapeutic intervention is necessary, since the haemolysis may be mild. However, in some children with significant anaemia complete recovery follows emergency blood transfusion. In less acute cases the haemolytic process continues after transfusion. Corticosteroids are of great value in these circumstances and frequently abolish the need for further transfusions. Oral prednisolone 2 mg/kg/day should be given until the haemolysis is brought under control. Thereafter, the dosage is progressively reduced to achieve the smallest maintenance dose compatible with a reasonable haemoglobin value (10–12 g/dl). When long-term steroid therapy proves necessary a careful watch must be kept for undesirable side effects such as osteoporosis, diabetes mellitus, etc. When haemolysis cannot be controlled with a reasonable dosage of steroid, the question of splenectomy arises. Unfortunately this operation does not always relieve the anaemia. Chromium-labelled red cell kinetic studies are probably unnecessary as they are not a reliable indicator of response to splenectomy. After splenectomy small doses of corticosteroids are usually still required. Another approach has been the use of antimetabolites, such as mercaptopurine, azathioprine or thioguanine to destroy the cells which produce the abnormal autoantibodies. This is potentially dangerous and not recommended for routine use. Plasmapheresis or exchange transfusion has proved beneficial in some patients with autoimmune haemolytic anaemia and has been used as an acute temporary measure in patients with profound haemolysis until other therapeutic measures are effected. Also intravenous gammaglobulin may also be effective in some cases of autoimmune haemolytic anaemia caused by IgG antibodies.

APLASTIC AND HYPOPLASTIC ANAEMIA

This group of anaemias is poorly understood and clearly contains a considerable number of quite separate diseases which present clinically in somewhat similar ways. The defect in erythropoiesis may affect all elements of the marrow or only one, such as the erythropoietic tissue. There may be virtually no formation at all of the precursors or red cells, leucocytes or platelets. Fortunately, these conditions are not common, but those to be considered here occur sufficiently frequently in paediatric practice to merit the attention of all who have to handle sick children.

Congenital hypoplastic anaemia (Blackfan–Diamond anaemia)

Aetiology

This disease presents in early infancy as an apparent aplasia of the red cells. Granulocytes and platelets are unaffected. In most cases the bone marrow shows a gross deficiency or erythroblasts but shows normal maturation of myeloid and megakaryocyte cells. The incidence is the same in boys as in girls but the disease tends to be milder in its effects on boys. Its occurrence in siblings has been reported in several families and family studies have suggested an autosomal recessive mode of inheritance.

Clinical features

The presenting feature is pallor, which becomes apparent in the early weeks or months of life. Irritability becomes obvious only when the anaemia is severe in degree. Physical examination is usually unrevealing. There are no haemorrhagic manifestations. Hepatic or splenic enlargement is unusual but may develop as a consequence of cardiac failure. Haemic systolic murmurs are common. The anaemia, often severe, is normocytic and normochronic. Reticulocytes are absent or scanty. White blood cells and platelets show no abnormalities.

Course and prognosis

This is greatly influenced by treatment. Repeated blood transfusions lead to haemosiderosis which causes a typical muddy bronze skin pigmentation. Cirrhosis of the liver ultimately develops with failure of sexual maturation. Portal hypertension and hypersplenism occasionally develop. The long bones often show marked growth-arrest lines. Osteoporosis and delayed bone age are common. Affected children are frequently dwarfed but mental development proceeds normally. The prognosis is not good in the long term; on the other hand, spontaneous remissions have frequently been reported, even after puberty and several hundred transfusions.

Treatment

Repeated transfusions of packed red cells, always after careful cross-matching, are frequently required over periods of many years. In some cases there is a marrow response to prednisolone in an initial dose of 2 mg/kg/day in four divided doses, but only if treatment is started before 3 months of age. The dosage should thereafter be reduced to the smallest which will maintain a reasonable haemoglobin level and normal reticulocyte count and is given on alternate days. Continuous steroid therapy is likely to be necessary, with side effects such as retardation of growth. In these children bone marrow transplantation may be considered. When repeated transfusions are necessary the development of haemosiderosis can be delayed with the iron chelating agent desferrioxamine. Chelation of iron with subcutaneous desferrioxamine should be given 1 or 2 years after the patient is placed on a chronic transfusion programme and iron stores are shown to be elevated. A great increase in the urinary output of iron can be demonstrated with this treatment, particularly if steps are taken to ensure that the child is not deficient in ascorbic acid.

Fanconi-type familial aplastic anaemia

Aetiology

This autosomal recessive disorder affects all three elements of the bone marrow (pancytopenia). Chromosomal studies in some cases have revealed an abnormally high number of chromatid breaks, endoreduplications and other minor abnormalities.

Clinical features

Pallor may become obvious in early infancy, but more often the onset is delayed until between the ages of 3 and 10 years. Purpura and ecchymoses are not uncommon and there may be bleeding from mucous membranes. Defects in the radius and/or thumb or accessory thumbs are common. Mild hyperpigmentation, hypogonadism and short stature have frequently been reported, and endocrine studies have revealed growth hormone deficiency, isolated or combined with deficiencies of gonadotrophins and ACTH. Other congenital abnormalities seen less frequently include microcephaly, squints and anomalies of the heart or renal tract. Exaggerated tendon reflexes have been noted. The blood shows a normocytic, normochromic anaemia, leucopenia, granulocytopenia and thrombocytopenia. Reticulocytes are scanty or absent. Leukaemia not infrequently appears in relatives and occasionally in the patient. The diagnosis is readily overlooked in patients who lack the characteristic congenital abnormalities but useful diagnostic pointers are the presence of Hb-F, 1–2 g/dl in the blood and of chromosomal abnormalities in the lymphocytes.

Treatment

Repeated blood transfusions may be necessary in spite of the risks of transfusion haemosiderosis. Death is common during childhood but a sustained remission can sometimes be obtained with a combination of prednisolone 0.4 mg/kg on alternate days and oxymetholone 2–5 mg/kg daily. The latter drug can give rise to hepatoblastoma. Therapy with human growth hormone may cause an increase in growth velocity if a deficiency of GH has been confirmed. Also successful bone marrow transplantation has been reported in 40 patients with Fanconi anaemia.

Acquired hypoplastic anaemia

Aetiology

This is a rare disease in childhood and most cases are "idiopathic". The bone marrow is rarely completely aplastic in such patients. Some cases are secondary to the toxic effects of drugs such as chloramphenicol, phenylethylacetylurea, carbimazole, thiouracil, phenybutazone and gold salts.

Clinical features

The onset may be acute or insidious with increasing pallor, listlessness, malaise, bruises, purpura and sometimes bleeding from mucous membranes. Death is due to haemorrhage into internal organs or to intercurrent infection. The blood shows a normocytic, normochromic anaemia, thrombocytopenia, leucopenia and granulocytopenia. Bone marrow must always be examined by needle biopsy or trephine. Marrow examination is, furthermore, the only way in which hypoplastic anaemia can be distinguished from aleukaemia leukaemia. The prognosis is grave when the marrow examination reveals gross hypoplasia of all the blood forming elements, but in less severe cases there is always hope of a spontaneous or induced remission.

Treatment

Life can be prolonged by repeated transfusions of packed red cells. Platelet transfusions can also help to prolong life. Remissions can sometimes be obtained with a combination of prednisolone and oxymetholone as described for the treatment of Fanconi anaemia. However, the treatment of choice is bone marrow transplantation from histocompatible sibling or family donor. Unfortunately, the small size

of families in Europe and North America restricts this approach to 1 in 3 affected patients. More recently success has been achieved using histocompatible unrelated volunteer donors but this procedure raises many clinical, ethical and logistical problems. Bone marrow transplantation is more likely to be successful if blood transfusions have been irradiated and kept to a minimum to avoid sensitisation to donor transplantation antigens.

Albers–Schönberg disease (osteopetrosis)

Aetiology

This is a genetic disorder of bone, usually autosomal recessive. The cortex and trabeculae of the bones are thickened and the marrow is crowded out. Extramedullary erythropoiesis in the liver and spleen may prevent anaemia for a variable period. It is now recognised that the cause of osteopetrosis is a defect or deficiency of osteoclasts or their precursors which are derived from the pluripotent haemopoietic stem cells. Bone resorption is inhibited.

Clinical features

The disease may present in infancy with progressive loss of vision due to optic atrophy, with cranial nerve palsies or with deafness. In later childhood the mode of presentation is a pathological fracture or increasing pallor. The anaemia is leuco-erythroblastic in type. There is progressive hepatosplenomegaly. The most characteristic diagnostic signs are to be found in radiographs of the skeleton (Fig. 13.5). The bones, including the base of the skull, ribs, vertebrae, scapulae and pelvis show increased density (Fig. 13.6). Typical zones of decreased density can be seen at the metaphyses and running parallel to the borders of scapulae and ilia; these still contain marrow.

Treatment

It is now possible to cure some infants with the severe form of the disease by bone marrow transplantation from a histocompatible sibling. Infants with compatible donors should be transplanted as early as possible to avoid irreversible damage from bone encroachment on cranial nerves.

THE THROMBOCYTOPENIC PURPURAS

Purpura is an extremely common clinical phenomenon in childhood and has many causes. The principal pathogenic factors are capillary defects and thrombocytopenia, sometimes both being present. In

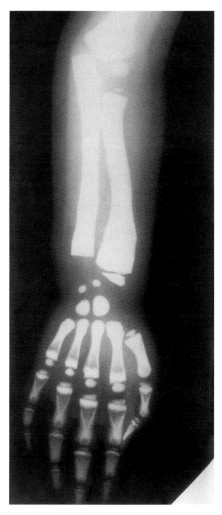

FIGURE 13.5 Osteopetrosis showing zones of increased density at metaphyseal ends of long bones.

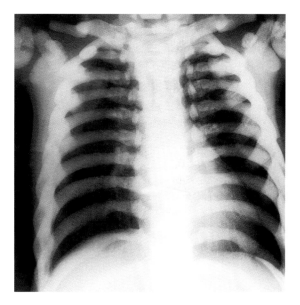

FIGURE 13.6 Osteopetrosis showing increased density in ribs.

most cases the purpura is symptomatic of another disease. It occurs due to decreased capillary resistance or bacterial microemboli in acute infections such as meningococcal (and other) septicaemia, bacterial endocarditis, typhus and typhoid fever, scarlet fever, etc. It may arise in scurvy, uraemia and snake bite. Severe intrapartum hypoxia sometimes causes petechiae, especially over the head, neck and shoulders of the newborn. A similar mechanical effect is sometimes seen in the child who has had a severe and prolonged convulsion and in whooping cough. Symptomatic thrombocytopenic purpura occurs in leukaemia, hypoplastic anaemia and in states of hypersplenism. Fragmentation of platelets as well as red cells, with thrombocytopenia and haemolytic anaemia, may occur in cases of giant haemangioma and after cardiac surgery. Congenital defects in the capillaries are seen in such rare conditions as hereditary haemorrhagic telangiectasia (Osler disease) and cutis hyperelastica (Ehlers–Danlos syndrome). It will be clear, therefore, that purpura reflects a blood disorder in only a minority of cases. None the less, the more important primary diseases in which purpura is a prominent feature are conveniently discussed in this chapter.

Idiopathic thrombocytopenic purpura

Idiopathic thrombocytopenic purpura (ITP) accounts for the majority of cases of childhood thrombocytopenia and has been classified into acute and chronic forms. It is a clinical diagnosis reached by exclusion of other causes of thrombocytopenia.

Clinical features

Most cases in childhood have an acute onset. There has frequently been a recently preceding, non-specific upper respiratory infection or other common childhood illness and immunisations have been associated. The first manifestation may be bleeding from mucous membranes such as epistaxis, bleeding gums or haematuria. Generalised purpura and/or ecchymoses are characteristic and often profuse. The spleen may be palpable but never becomes very large. Life may be endangered in severe cases by blood loss or by subarachnoid haemorrhage. The differentiating characteristic of this acute form is the spontaneous and permanent recovery within 6 months of onset.

Chronic cases are also seen in which crops of purpura and ecchymoses persist beyond 6 months and occur more frequently in girls. Children who have the chronic form of idiopathic thrombocytopenic purpura may present at any age, although children over 10 years of age are a greater risk than those in the younger age group.

The blood shows a diminished platelet count. Spontaneous bleeding can occur when the count falls below 25 000 per mm³. The bleeding time is prolonged and clot retraction is defective but the clotting time is normal. The Hess capillary resistance test is positive during the active phases. A post-haemorrhagic anaemia and leucocytosis may be present. Bone marrow examination must always be carried out to exclude other blood disorders. Megakaryocytes will be found in normal or increased numbers and although hyperplasia may appear as a response to haemorrhage the other elements in the marrow will be normal in ITP.

Treatment

Unfortunately the clinician cannot predict whether a given child will have the more common acute self-limiting form, develop a chronic course, or be in the 1% of children who have their course complicated by a sudden spontaneous life-threatening gastrointestinal or central nervous system haemorrhage. However, in most children the acute attack of thrombocytopenic purpura undergoes spontaneous remission and does not again appear. There is rarely any need for a quick decision about some form of specific treatment. When bleeding is severe and persistent, blood transfusion combined with steroid therapy is usually successful in initiating a remission. This may be permanent or temporary. Platelet transfusions should be used only when life-threatening bleeding episodes occurs, since they achieve only a transient haemostatic response. Intravenous administration of very large doses of human immunoglobulins also can lead to a rapid but usually transient rise in platelet count.

Elective splenectomy is followed by permanent return of the platelets to normal levels in only about 80% of cases. For this reason we have been reluctant to recommend it unless the disease is persistent or there are repeated acute attacks. For the relatively rare cases of chronic thrombocytopenia in which splenectomy has failed, a trial of immunosuppressive therapy with azathioprine and cyclophosphamide has been advocated.

Congenital thrombocytopenic purpura

It is well recognised that the infant of a mother who is suffering from idiopathic thrombocytopenic purpura or thrombocytopenia secondary to systemic lupus erythematosus may be born with severe thrombocytopenia. The infant usually exhibits generalised purpura, and during the first few days of life there is a risk of severe haemorrhage into organs such as the brain, adrenals or pericardium. The pathogenesis has been shown to be the transplacental passage of antibodies which are directed against antigens common to all platelets (Chapter l). If the infant's platelet count falls below 10 000 per mm³, prednisolone 2 mg/kg/day should be prescribed for 2–3 weeks with later reduction of the dosage. This type of congenital thrombocytopenia has to be differentiated from neonatal, also immune thrombocytopenia in which there is fetomaternal incompatibility for a platelet antigen absent in the mother and expressed on the fetal platelet membranes. This antigen induces the maternal production of an antibody which crosses the placental barrier and destroys the fetal platelets. The situation is analogous to Rh or ABO incompatibility, but there are as yet no reliable tests to predict the birth of an affected baby during pregnancy. In contrast to Rh sensitisation, first-born infants may be affected and the risk of recurrence in future pregnancies is high. The diagnosis can be confirmed by the demonstration of antiplatelet antibodies in the maternal serum reacting with paternal platelets. These tests, together with a normal maternal platelet count and the exclusion of other known causes of neonatal thrombocytopenia (e.g. neonatal infection, disseminated intravascular coagulation, drug-induced or autoimmune thrombocytopenia) often establish the diagnosis of neonatal alloimmune thrombocytopenia. The best form of treatment is probably transfusion of platelets lacking the offending antigen, i.e. only the mother's platelets, which can be obtained by platelet-pheresis. Exchange transfusion, steroids and intravenous immunoglobulins have also been used but the more effective treatment remains the transfusion of compatible platelets.

Wiskott–Aldrich syndrome

This is a rare X-linked recessive disorder affecting only males. It is characterised by the triad of severe thrombocytopenia, eczema and repeated infections with all classes of micro-organisms. The majority of children die from overwhelming infection at an early age. Those who survive may develop reticuloendothelial malignancies such as lymphoma and myeloid leukaemia. The usual mode of presentation is during infancy with typical atopic eczema which may later be superseded by asthma. The bleeding tendency results in purpura or oozing from mucous membranes. Infections such as otitis media, pneumonia, septicaemia, meningitis and virus diseases constitute the major threat to life. Recent studies have revealed a broad immunological deficiency in this disease involving both humoral and cellular responses, in spite of the fact that the total serum immunoglobulin levels are normal and that the lymphocytes respond normally to *in vitro* stimulation with phytohaemagglutinin. On the other hand, delayed hypersensitivity responses are absent when tested with various skin test antigens (PPD, *Candida*, mumps, etc.) and dinitrochlorobenzene (DNCB) sensitisation. The serum IgM levels are reduced because of defective responses to polysaccharide antigens such as blood group antigens, *E. coli* antigens, pneumococcus polysaccharide, etc.

Treatment

Apart from blood and platelet transfusions little could be done for children with this disease until recently. However, complete correction of all the problems can now be achieved by bone marrow transplantation, when a histocompatible sibling is available, and after marrow ablation with busulphan and immunosuppression with cyclophosphamide.

Henoch-Schönlein purpura

See Chapter 15 on Connective Tissue Disorders.

BLOOD CLOTTING DEFECTS

The mechanism of blood clotting is extremely complex and modern tests used to define the various congenital and acquired defects in this mechanism are only for the expert haematologist. The paediatrician must, however, have sufficient knowledge of the clinical types of clotting deficiency to use rationally the help which the haematologist has to offer.

Mechanism of blood clotting

Only a brief description will be given. The basis of our present knowledge was laid down initially by Morawitz as follows:

Prothombin + Calcium ions + Thromboplastin → Thrombin
(Factor II)   (Factor IV)   (Factor III)

Thrombin + Fibrinogen (soluble) → Fibrin (insoluble)
(Factor I)

There are also anti-clotting factors normally present in blood. The most important is probably heparin which has an anti-thrombin activity. Another is an enzyme (plasmin) which has a fibrinolytic activity; it exists in precursor form as plasminogen which is "activated" under certain circumstances, e.g. tissue damage.

However, many other factors are now known to be required for normal clotting. The formation of active thromboplastin in blood requires the presence of anti-haemophilic globulin (AHG: Factor VIII). Christmas factor (plasma thromboplastin component: PT Factor IX), and plasma thromboplastin antecedent (PTA: Factor X) in addition to platelet factor. The tissues also produce their own thromboplastin. The conversion of prothrombin to thrombin also requires additional factors, namely, pro-accelerin (Factor V: labile factor), and proconvertin (Factor VII: stable factor). Two other factors necessary for the formation of thromboplastin are Stuart–Prower factor (Factor X) and Hageman factor (Factor XII).

It is clear that congenital deficiency of any of these factors could result in abnormalities of haemostasis. A considerable number have been described but haemophilia and Christmas disease are the major problems.

Haemophilia A

Aetiology

Deficiency of anti-haemophilic globulin is inherited as an X-linked recessive trait affecting males. Affected females are extremely rare.

Clinical features

It is rare for haemophilia to become manifest during the first year of life. The outstanding feature is bleeding. This may take the form of prolonged oozing from a minor injury such as a cut lip or finger, from an erupting tooth, after the loss of a decidious tooth or from the nose. There may be dangerous and persistent bleeding from circumcision or tonsillectomy if haemophilia has not been discovered. A common event is severe haemarthrosis, especially in a knee joint after quite minor strain. A blow may result in a massive haematoma on any part of the body. A deeply situated haematoma may threaten life by pressure on vital structures such as the trachea or a large artery. In some children who are severely affected repeated haemarthroses may lead to fibrous ankylosis and crippling. Bleeding from gastrointestinal or renal tracts is not rare. Cases vary considerably in severity but run true to type within each individual family. There is a fairly high mutation rate, and the absence of a family history of "bleeders" does not exclude the diagnosis.

Diagnosis

Haemophilia A and B cannot be differentiated on clinical grounds. The classical coagulation abnormality in haemophilia is a prolonged clotting time. While this is certainly to be found in most cases, it may become normal between attacks of bleeding, and in mild cases it may never be possible to demonstrate a delay in clotting. Furthermore, this simple and time-honoured test cannot distinguish true haemophilia from some of the other clotting factor deficiencies. It is, indeed, no longer acceptable as the sole basis of diagnosis which must rest upon more refined tests. The most valuable of these is the *thromboplastin generation test*. This test reveals the inefficient formation of thromboplastin, due in haemophilia to lack of AHG, which factor is found in normal plasma treated with aluminium hydroxide but which is absent from normal serum. There is, therefore, a demonstrable defect in clotting when the test is performed with the patient's alumina-plasma, normal serum, platelets and calcium chloride. Clotting proceeds normally, however, when normal alumina-plasma is used along with the patient's serum. The one-stage "prothrombin time" test gives a normal test in haemophilia. It is possible by the use of these two tests to separate out the various deficiencies of clotting factors which have not been defined. In haemophilia the prothrombin consumption test, the kaolin cephalin clotting time and the partial thromboplastin time are also normal.

Differential diagnosis

Haemophilia may obviously be simulated clinically by a deficiency of any one of the clotting factors described above. None of these is as common as haemophilia, but the minor differences in clinical behaviour which they exhibit do not allow a firm diagnosis to be based upon anything less than a detailed laboratory investigation. Misdiagnosis of haemophilia A as haemophilia B or vice versa can be disastrous.

Treatment

The objective is to correct the clotting defect as soon as possible after bleeding has started, or to prevent bleeding in the case of dental extraction or surgery. This is achieved by the intravenous administration of one of the concentrated preparations of Factor VIII. Fresh frozen plasma is no longer used for the treatment of haemophilia. In the United Kingdom cryoprecipitate has been widely used. This preparation, which contains Factor VIII and fibrinogen, is manufactured by allowing frozen plasma to thaw at 4–80°C when it comes out of the ice as a "sludge". It is, however, tedious to prepare for use, its Factor VIII content varies from one batch to another and the need to store it in a deep freezer is inconvenient. Cryoprecipitate is prepared in plastic bags, one of which is equivalent to 250 ml of fresh frozen plasma. A suitable dosage which will raise the plasma Factor VIII level to at least 20% of normal is two "bags" per 10 kg body weight. A more accurate and satisfactory control of the clotting defect can be obtained with freeze-dried human Factor VIII concentrates.

These concentrates usually contain 180–220 units per vial. The dose in units of Factor VIII can be calculated from the formula:

$$\frac{\text{Patient's wt in kg} \times \text{required rise in Factor VIII}}{K}$$

where K is a constant for a given type of material, being 1.5 for human Factor VIII concentrates and 1.0 for animal AHG. The latter is antigenic and mainly indicated for emergency treatment of patients who have developed a high titre of Factor VIII antibodies. To control early haemarthrosis or other bleeding, an *in vivo* level of 20% Factor VIII activity is generally adequate but major surgery or dental extractions require that the Factor VIII activity be raised to over 40% and kept there until healing is complete. This necessitates injections of the concentrate several times daily. However, in the case of simple dental extraction, after the Factor VIII level has been raised with concentrate, bleeding can be prevented with tranexamic acid 0.15 mg/kg given intravenously and followed by oral administration of 30 mg 6-hourly until gum healing is complete. Topical thrombin may also be used to dry the socket and some dentists like to apply dental splints. It should be noted that haemophiliacs must never be given intramuscular injections but immunisations can be given by subcutaneous or intradermal injections.

In a small percentage of haemophiliacs antibodies to Factor VIII ultimately appear and make treatment very difficult. The dose of human Factor VIII will have to be greatly increased, or animal AHG may be used with its attendant risk such as allergic reactions or thrombocytopenia. It is also possible to lower a high AHG antibody level by plasmaphaeresis, exchanging 4–6 litres of the patient's plasma with plasma protein fraction or fresh frozen plasma. This should be immediately followed by an appropriate dose of Factor VIII concentrate.

In addition to the problem of an antibody response to human Factor VIII there is a risk of transmitting infection from the human donors. Hepatitis and AIDS occurred in many patients who received multiple blood transfusions and blood products derived from pooled plasma. Clinically obvious symptomatic acute hepatitis occurs with very low frequency and is caused by the non-A, non-B hepatitis viruses. In the United Kingdom approximately 30% of haemophiliacs are HIV positive. It is recommended that all haemophiliacs should be vaccinated against hepatitis B. Clinical trials of artificial Factor VIII and virally inactivated fresh frozen plasma are currently underway. In the UK there is mandatory screening of blood donated by syphilis, hepatitis B and C and HIV. There remains a theoretical risk that donations may contain viruses to which the donor has not seroconverted or other viruses which are not screened for.

Long-term management involves education of the child and his parents in a way of life which makes minor injuries less likely to be sustained. It is now common practice in the case of a child with good parents and good veins to teach the technique of intravenous administration of Factor VIII concentrate in the home. Attendance at an ordinary school is often possible through the cooperation of the teaching staff and the boy's friends. A useful adult life is usually attainable, especially in mildly affected cases. One of the most difficult tasks is to convince the parents of the need for regular expert conservative dental care. The removal of a carious and neglected permanent tooth in an adult haemophiliac involves the medical staff in a major effort and the patient in a most unpleasant experience. The fact that crippling deformities can now be prevented is worthy of emphasis. Every child with a clotting deficiency should be issued with a Haemophilia Card (stating blood group) and the parents advised to contact the Haemophiliac Society.

Haemophilia B (Christmas disease)

Aetiology

Deficiency of Christmas factor is inherited as an X-linked recessive trait. It accounts for about 15% of all "bleeders", being much less common than true haemophilia A.

Clinical features

The disease cannot be distinguished from haemophilia on clinical grounds. It can best be differentiated by means of the thromboplastin generation test. Defective clotting will be found when the test is performed with the patient's serum and normal alumina-plasma, whereas a normal response will be found with the patient's alumina-plasma and normal serum. The one-stage prothrombin time is normal, as in haemophilia A.

Treatment

Several Factor IX concentrates are now available to stop bleeding. The appropriate intravenous dosage can be calculated from the formula on page 368 taking the K constant as 0.7 for Factor IX concentrates. They usually contain 300 units per vial.

Haemophilia C

Aetiology

Deficiency of Factor XI is inherited as an incompletely recessive characteristic, affecting both males and females. Homozygotes bleed severely while heterozygotes bleed only mildly.

Clinical features

The diagnosis of this rare disease can be shown in the thromboplastin generation test which will be normal only when it is performed with both the patient's alumina-plasma and the patient's serum. The one-stage prothrombin time is normal as in haemophilia A and B.

Treatment

Bleeding is easily controlled with intravenous fresh frozen plasma, 15 ml/kg.

Congenital afibrinogenaemia

Aetiology

This severe and rare disease is transmitted as an autosomal recessive characteristic, both sexes being equally affected.

Clinical features

Severe haemorrhagic episodes may first appear in the neonatal period, e.g. in the form of haemorrhage from the umbilical cord. In other respects the clinical picture simulates that of haemophilia A although haemarthrosis is rarely seen. The blood is completely incoagulable and the plasma fibrinogen level is absent or grossly reduced.

Treatment

Bleeding can be temporarily controlled by blood transfusions or by the transfusion of concentrated fibrinogen.

Von Willebrand disease

Aetiology

This bleeding disorder has been recognised with increasing frequency in young children (3–5 years) in recent years. Indeed, the tendency to haemorrhage may lessen in adult life. It is inherited as an autosomal dominant characteristic.

Clinical features

The haemorrhage is of the "capillary" type rather than the "clotting deficiency" type as seen in haemophilia. Common presenting features include epistaxis, prolonged bleeding from cuts or dental extractions and excessive bruising. Gastrointestinal bleeding can occasionally be alarming and menorrhagia may be a problem in the adult.

The diagnosis is based on a prolonged bleeding time, reduced platelet adhesiveness, defective platelet aggregation with ristocetin and Factor VIII assay below 50% of normal.

Treatment

Simple local haemostatic measures such as nasal packing or a pressure bandage usually suffice. If bleeding continues, cryoprecipitate 2 bags/10 kg should be given. Blood transfusion is only rarely required.

Disseminated intravascular coagulation (DIC) consumption coagulopathy

Disseminated intravascular coagulation is an acquired haemostatic defect that occurs when there is *in vivo* activation of the coagulation mechanism resulting in an accelerated rate of conversion of fibrinogen to fibrin. Fibrin may or may not be deposited within blood vessels. It is always caused by some underlying disease process. Infection is the most common cause of disseminated intravascular coagulation. Within this category bacterial septicaemia (Gram-negative bacterial infections) with associated septic shock is the most frequent infectious cause of DIC. Haemolytic uraemic syndrome, meningococcal septicaemia, falciparum malaria, haemolytic transfusion reactions and some snake venoms can induce a consumption coagulopathy. Virus-induced DIC occurs predominantly in immunocompromised patients. Fungal infections are rarely a cause of DIC. Regardless of the underlying primary disease in the majority of patients the main clinical finding is bleeding and only a small number of patients will show thrombosis or thromboembolic episodes.

The laboratory findings in this clinical condition consist of a reduction of Factors II, V, VIII and fibrinogen, thrombocytopenia and secondary activation of the fibrinolytic system with prolongation of the prothrombin time (PT), partial thromboplastin time (APTT) and thrombin time (TCT).

Therefore, the most useful screening tests for the diagnosis of DIC are the platelet count, prothrombin time and the presence of fibrin degradation products. To make a definite diagnosis of DIC the tests available are those that would detect the presence of soluble fibrin complexes and coagulation factor assays for Factor II, V, VIII and fibrinogen.

Treatment

The aim of treatment of DIC is to control bleeding and to eliminate the threat of fibrin deposition. The management objectives include control or removal of the underlying disease, replacement of depleted procoagulants with fresh frozen plasma, cryoprecipitate and platelets and in selected cases medical interruption of the consumptive process with anticoagulants and platelet inhibitor drugs. Also, the use of exchange transfusion in newborns and plasma exchange in older children has been reported to be beneficial in some cases.

THE ACUTE LEUKAEMIAS

In childhood, leukaemia is nearly always of the acute variety. On the basis of morphological classifications they are divided into lymphoblastic (ALL) and non-lymphocytic (ANLL) or myeloblastic (AML) types.

Approximately 80–85% of acute leukaemias in children are lymphoblastic and 15–20% are myeloblastic (non-lymphocyte). The remainder (1–5%) of leukaemias are difficult to characterise as either ALL or AML and are therefore referred to as undifferentiated or unclassified leukaemias (AUL). The exact cause of leukaemia remains unknown although the list of risk factors associated with childhood ALL is substantial.

In 1976, the French–American–British (FAB) collaborative group proposed criteria for classifying ALL into three subtypes based on blast cytology, as seen in Romanowsky's stained bone marrow smears (Fig. 13.7). Assignment to one of these groups, L1, L2 or L3, depended on cell size, nuclear to cytoplasmic ratio, and other factors. Approximately 84% of childhood ALL is L1, 14% is L2 and 1% is L3.

As one learns more about the biology of leukaemic cells it is possible to define groups of patients with characteristic clinical, immunological and genetic properties. In this way, it is becoming increasingly evident that ALL is not one disease but several diseases. Therefore, on the basis of immunological classification ALL may be classified into T-ALL, B-ALL and non-T-, and non-B-ALL, according to the presence or absence of surface characteristics of these two lymphocyte lines on the leukaemic blast cells. About 85% of childhood ALL falls into the non-B-ALL group and in the great majority of such cases the blast cells carry the common ALL (CALL-A) antigen on their surface. This antigen appears to be characteristic of early B lymphoblasts and perhaps about one-third of patients with CALL-A also have immunoglobulin chains in their blast cell cytoplasm enabling further classification as pre-B-cell ALL. It seems that in future the better definition of distinct subtypes of ALL will lead to the design of specific therapies and thus improved survival of all children with ALL.

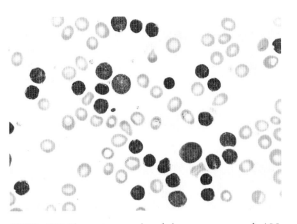

FIGURE 13.7 Photomicrograph of bone marrow of ALL subtype L1 and the blasts shown are typical small dense cells with a very high nuclear cytoplasmic ratio and indistinct nucleoli.

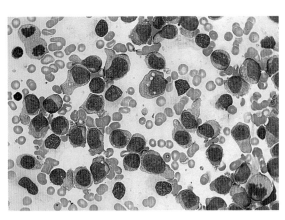

FIGURE 13.8 Photomicrograph of bone marrow of a child with acute myeloid leukaemia showing myeloblasts.

In the UK the annual incidence of ALL is in the region of 26 per million. The peak incidence in children is between the ages of 3 and 5 years. ALL below the age of 15 years is approximately 30% more common in males than females.

On the basis of cytogenetic studies it has been possible to classify childhood ALL into five "cytogenetic groups". Children who have more than 50 chromosomes have the best prognosis (hyperdiploid), those with diploidy (normal number of chromosomes and no structural abnormality) have an intermediate prognosis and those with pseudodiploidy (with 46 chromosomes with structural abnormality) have a poor prognosis. Also specific translocations such as the Philadelphia chromosome (tg;22, t8;14 and others) have a poor prognosis.

Clinical features

The most common symptoms and clinical findings reflect the underlying anaemia, thrombocytopenia and neutropenia that result from the failure of normal haemopoiesis. Therefore, the most common presenting features are rapidly progressive pallor and spontaneous haemorrhagic manifestations such as purpura, epistaxis and bleeding from the gums. These are associated with increasing weakness, breathlessness on exertion, malaise, anorexia and fever. In some cases the onset takes the form of a severe oropharyngeal inflammation and enlargement of the cervical lymph nodes which does not respond to antibiotics. In two-thirds of children with ALL the onset is with bone pains and half of these will have radiological bone changes. Arthralgia, secondary to leukaemic infiltration of joints may be difficult to differentiate from other non-malignant disorders such as juvenile chronic arthritis or osteomyelitis.

Extramedullary leukaemic spread causes lymphadenopathy, hepatomegaly and splenomegaly. In some patients, however, the signs are confined to pallor and haemorrhage of variable severity and distribution. Infrequently jaundice may develop or there may be early evidence of involvement of the central nervous system. Ophthalmoscopy frequently reveals retinal haemorrhages. As the leukaemia progresses severe sepsis often develops, sometimes in the form of necrotic ulceration of skin or mucous membrane. A somewhat characteristic terminal event often associated with extreme neutropenia, is a distressingly painful gangrenous ulceration of the lower rectum, perianal region, vulva and perineum. Alternatively, severe haemorrhage into the brain, or from the bowel, stomach or kidneys may lead rapidly to death.

However, clinicians should be aware of the fact that ALL may mimic a number of non-malignant conditions.

Blood picture and bone marrow findings

In addition to severe anaemia the peripheral blood films will show immature cells. These are most often lymphoblasts, less commonly myeloblasts and other granulocytic precursors, rarely monoblasts or neoplastic megaloblastic erythroid cells. The total white cell count is often raised to between 20 000 and 30 000 per mm³, only rarely to a very high figure. Thrombocytopenia is almost invariably found. Reticulocytes are usually scanty. It is, however, rarely justifiable to base the diagnosis of leukaemia on the peripheral blood picture alone. Bone marrow biopsy will nearly always confirm the diagnosis beyond doubt, the films and sections showing gross leukaemic infiltration by immature or abnormal white cell precursors, diminution in erythropoietic activity and disappearance of megakaryocytes.

The majority of children presenting with ALL will have more than 80% of their marrow cells consisting of lymphoblasts, whereas it is not uncommon to see the presence of only 30–50% blasts in the bone marrow in acute non-lymphocytic leukaemia. The majority of childhood acute leukaemias (85–90%) can be readily separated into lymphoid or myeloid (Fig. 13.8) subtypes on the basis of morphology alone. Thus, although in most cases the diagnosis is apparent from the morphology, the final diagnosis of ALL rests on confirmatory cytochemical staining patterns and in some situations on additional immunological and cytogenetic studies. These studies are of therapeutic significance in lymphatic leukaemias.

Meningeal and testicular leukaemia

Meningeal and testicular leukaemia became a major problem when the duration of life for children with acute leukaemia progressively lengthened as the result of treatment with modern anti-leukaemic drugs. These manifestations commonly develop in patients who are in complete haematological remission and the incidence has exceeded 50% in some series. Not infrequently the meningeal relapse coincides with a systemic relapse. It is probable that a few nests of leukaemic cells are already present when the patient first presents, and as the cytotoxic drugs do not readily cross the blood–brain barrier these neoplastic cells are able to multiply in the largely protected environment of the brain and meninges. The child, who has been in systemic remission for months or even some years, develops headache, vomiting and meningism. A rapid increase in weight due to the increased appetite of hypothalamic damage is not uncommon. There may be neurological signs such as squint, ataxia, or visual disturbance, but more often the only signs are of increased intracranial pressure including papilloedema. Cerebrospinal fluid will show a pleiocytosis due to leukaemic blast cells with increased protein and reduced glucose. The recent introduction of cranial or craniospinal radiation combined with intrathecal methotrexate has drastically reduced the incidence of meningeal relapses.

Testicular

The testes are a major site of extramedullary relapse in boys with ALL. Clinically, overt testicular relapse presents as painless testicular enlargement that is usually unilateral. (In contrast ovarian relapse is rare.)

Treatment

Since the recognition that ALL is a heterogeneous disease and that affected children can be classified into various risk groups it is no longer appropriate for all children to be treated with a "standard therapeutic regimen". Modern protocols now include stratifying patients at the time of diagnosis and tailoring therapy according to the prognostic characteristics of the patient. For these reasons, the best results are only obtainable in special centres with experienced staff, specialised equipment and sufficient turnover of cases to maintain expertise.

Most ALL treatment regimens divide therapy into four main treatment phases: remission induction, CNS treatment, intensification and maintenance. Complete remission is the absence of clinical signs and symptoms of disease and the presence of normal blood count and a normocellular bone marrow with 5% or fewer morphological blast cells. In the UK this arbitrary definition of remission is sufficient to make a diagnosis of a complete remission (CR) in ALL but in cases of AML other marrow cellular elements should return to normal.

The initial aim in the treatment of acute leukaemia is induction of remission. These days most treatment centres are using intensive (consolidation/intensification) chemotherapy schedules once complete remission (CR) has been obtained. In consolidation therapy a further course of treatment using the same drugs and dosage used to achieve CR are given on the assumption that the leukaemia cell mass had already shown some responsiveness. This approach is used mainly in treating AML. Intensification regimens use different drugs from those used during induction in the hope of eliminating resistant leukaemia clones and residual disease in sanctuary sites (e.g. CNS and testes). Drugs used include prednisolone, vincristine, 6-mercaptopurine, methotrexate, cyclophosphamide, cytosine arabinoside, daunorubicin and asparaginase.

Induction for remission for ALL

Although the basic two-drug combination of intravenous vincristine and oral prednisolone can induce remission in approximately 85% of children with ALL, the addition of intramuscular L-asparaginase will improve the remission induction rate to approximately 95%. Furthermore, adding a third drug to prednisolone and vincristine has resulted in improved remission duration. The effectiveness of this combination has been well substantiated by various collaborative groups including the Medical Research Council (MRC), Berlin–Frankfurt–Munster group (BFM) and the USA Children's Cancer Study Group (US CCSG). The addition of CNS prophylactic therapy and maintenance therapy resulted in long-term disease-free survival of approaching 50%.

The agreed UK schedule (UK ALL VIII0) used a three- (prednisolone + vincristine + asparaginase) or four-drug (prednisolone + vincristine + asparaginase + daunorubicin) randomised remission induction regimen and the four-drug combination regimen showed an improved disease-free survival. This improvement may have been due to continuing therapy without interrupting drug induction, a long course of intramuscular asparaginase over 3 weeks, full dose mercaptopurine and co-trimoxazole during CNS prophylaxis, and the use of sustained maximum tolerated doses of mercaptopurine and methotrexate maintenance. Hyperuricaemia due to the release of nucleoprotein from disintegrating nucleated cells poses the threat of uric acid nephropathy and subsequent acute renal failure. Renal damage can be prevented during the period of rapid reduction in blast cells with oral allopurinol, adequate hydration and alkalinisation of urine.

Central nervous system leukaemia

Preventative therapy for ALL

The recognition that central nervous system relapse was a major obstacle to overall treatment success stimulated efforts to prevent central nervous system disease. It was due to the fact that the leukaemic cells in the central nervous system remained protected by the blood–brain barrier from cytotoxic concentrations or systemically administered anti-leukaemic therapy.

There are several different regimens possible but most now favour a combination of cranial irradiation usually combined with intrathecal methotrexate. However, a variety of other methods have been used in an attempt to avoid cranial irradiation. These include triple intrathecal therapy (methotrexate, cytarabine and hydrocortisone) alone; intermediate dose systemic methotrexate (with or without intrathecal methotrexate); intrathecal methotrexate alone; and high-dose systemic methotrexate.

The choice of CNS therapy for relapse is partly dependent upon the initial preventative treatment.

Intensification therapy for ALL

It is now quite clear that intensification chemotherapy is a rational approach to curative treatment for ALL. The factors which are potentially responsible for the failure of treatment of ALL are: inadequate initial reduction in the leukaemic cell load, the development of resistant leukaemic clones and the presence of "sanctuary" sites (e.g. CNS and testes) of resistant disease. Various groups suggest that children with high-risk ALL should have an element of early intensification therapy and thus reduce their risk of relapse.

Maintenance therapy for ALL

Once complete remission has been achieved maintenance chemotherapy is required. Early studies involved the use of vincristine and prednisolone but it was not until the addition of mercaptopurine and methotrexate that any advantage to survival was found. The optimal duration of maintenance chemotherapy has not yet been defined although there is now fairly wide agreement that continuation of this phase of treatment for more than 2–3 years carries no advantage.

Bone marrow transplantation for ALL

It has been suggested that allogeneic bone marrow transplantation should be considered as part of the therapeutic approach for patients who fail to enter a remission with standard aggressive chemotherapy. The preparatory regimen can be used in these circumstances both to achieve a remission and potentially to gain long-term control of the disease. Marrow transplantation which would ordinarily be used in such patients with poor prognosis should be considered earlier in the course of their therapy.

Prognosis for children with ALL

The prognosis for children with ALL has been vastly improved in recent years by the use of several drugs in combination. At present, approximately 60% of children with ALL are in continuous complete remission (CR) for 5 years following their initial diagnosis and the majority are considered cured. Recognition that certain clinical features evident at diagnosis have prognostic value has allowed ALL to be divided into groups with relatively favourable or unfavourable prognosis. Consequently this dramatically altered the therapeutic approach to this disease.

Not all the adverse prognostic features listed in Table 13.2 are of equal weight, and the apparent prognostic significance of many of them has varied widely from one series of patients to another.

TABLE 13.2 Adverse prognostic features in ALL

High peripheral white blood cell (WBC) count
ALL (FAB L2 or L3)
Age < 2 or > 8 years
High Hb
T- or B-ALL
Hepatosplenomegaly
Male gender
Pseudodiploidy
Slowness to remit
Early CNS disease
Black race
Low Ig
Low PAS score

Sequelae of therapy

Learning difficulties, precocious puberty, growth deficiencies due to insufficiency of thyroid and growth hormone and sterility have been reported in children after chemotherapy and whole body irradiation. To avoid the trauma and pain of repeated venepuncture most children receiving chemotherapy, whether for leukaemia or solid tumours, have a central line inserted under general anaesthesia. These lines engender a significant morbidity with rates of infection varying from 10 to 30%.

Despite dramatic improvements in the prospects for a child with acute leukaemia over the past two or three decades there is still a great need to improve therapy, particularly for the high-risk patient.

AGRANULOCYTOSIS

Aetiology

This is, fortunately, extremely uncommon in children. It may, of course, be part of other blood diseases such as hypoplastic anaemia and leukaemia. It may also complicate a severe or fulminating bacterial or virus infection. A few cases are "idiopathic". The majority are due to an idiosyncrasy towards commonly used drugs including thiouracils, troxidone, phenytoin, potassium, perchlorate, carbimazole, phenylbutazone, chloramphenicol and carbutamide.

Clinical features

The onset is usually sudden with fever, severe toxaemia, limb pains, anorexia, vomiting and sore throat. Severe necrotic and membranous lesions may affect the mouth and throat, less commonly the vulva or rectum. Jaundice and purpura are uncommon but do occur. The characteristic haematological finding is severe leucopenia with gross neutropenia. The red cells or platelets are also affected in some cases. The marrow usually shows an isolated but gross deficiency of myeloid precursors.

A chronic cyclical neutropenia has been described in a few children who suffer from recurrent attacks of infection and malaise. They can develop severe infections such as osteitis and septicaemia in their neutropenic spells. It is necessary in these children to institute permanent prophylactic antibiotic therapy.

Prognosis

Acute "idiopathic" or drug-induced cases carry a grave prognosis.

Treatment

The first essential is careful enquiry about possible drugs and their immediate withdrawal. Blood transfusion is indicated only if there is anaemia.

14

Immune Deficiency Disorders

The basic function of the immune system is to protect the human body from diseases caused by microorganisms present in the environment – bacteria, viruses, fungi and parasites. The primary response consists of phagocytosis and the inflammatory response. These functions are carried out primarily by polymorphonuclear leucocytes, macrophages (monocytes) and the complement system. Secondary immune responses consist of two mechanisms, namely antibody production and cell-mediated responses. Lymphocytes which are the main cells controlling the immune response have the ability to recognise "foreign material" and distinguish it from the body's own components. Thus, lymphocytes react to foreign material but not against the body's own tissue. Lymphocytes are of two main types: B cells, which develop in fetal liver and subsequently in bone marrow and T cells which develop in thymus.

It is essential for both B and T cells to recognise the antigen to produce an antibody response. Such antigens are called T-dependent antigens to differentiate them from T-independent antigens which can stimulate B cells directly. T-helper cells (TH) and B cells usually recognise different parts of the antigen and the T cell usually recognises different parts of the antigen and the T cell delivers a signal to the B cell. This process is referred to as T-cell help. The B cells are stimulated to proliferate and differentiate into antibody-forming cells which secrete antibody.

Antibodies are a class of serum proteins which are induced following contact with antigen and can be measured in the serum as immunoglobulin (Ig). Most antibodies are found in the gammaglobulin fraction of serum. Normal immunoglobulin values vary with age and assay method. There are five antibody classes: IgG, IgM, IgA, IgD and IgE. Some of these are further divided into subclasses. The number of subclasses varies between different species, e.g. in man there are four subclasses of IgG: IgG_1, IgG_2, IgG_3 and IgG_4. IgG is the major serum immunoglobulin and constitutes the majority of the secondary response to most antigens. It is transferred across the placenta in humans to provide protection in neonatal life. IgG antibodies are most important in defence against pyogenic organisms. IgA is the major mucosal immunoglobulin, coating mucosal surfaces and protecting against bacterial adhesion and/or viral penetration. Also there are two subclasses of IgA: IgA_1 and IgA_2. IgM is the first immunoglobulin to be produced both during the development of the immune system and during the initial response to viral and Gram-negative bacterial infections. IgM is responsible for the early and transient response to neoantigens. IgE immunoglobulin is the principal anaphylactic antibody in humans. IgE responses are encountered in hypersensitivity reactions in atopic subjects and during allergic states. The function of IgD immunoglobulin is not entirely clear.

Resistance to infection with virulent bacteria is mainly dependent upon antibody-enhanced phagocytosis. Resistance to infection by viruses and fungi seems to be dependent upon the integrity of the cell-mediated aspect of immunity. T-cell lymphocytes are derived from bone marrow and, after maturation in the thymus, have a key role in cell-mediated defences. They help identify and kill intracellular organisms directly and by activation of macrophages and other cellular defence mechanisms.

In children with recurrent or severe infections the possibility of an underlying immunodeficiency should be considered. Immune deficiency disorders reflect impairment in one or both of the major immune responses – the primary immune mechanisms (phagocytosis and the inflammatory response) and/or the

TABLE 14.1 Immune deficiency disorders

Defects of primary immune function
Defects of phagocytosis
   Qualitative (neutrophil dysfunction syndrome)
     Chronic granulomatous disease
     Job syndrome
     Chediak–Higashi syndrome
   Quantitative
     Neutropenia: congenital or acquired
Defects of complement
C3 deficiency, C5 deficiency, chemotaxis inhibition
Defects of secondary immune function
Defects of humoral function (thymic independent, primary B-cell deficiencies)
   Agammaglobulinaemia: congenital, acquired, physiological
Defects of cell-mediated function (thymic-dependent)
   Nezelof syndrome, Di George syndrome
   Immunodeficiency with ataxia telangiectasia
   Immunodeficiency with thrombocytopenia and eczema
   (Wiskott–Aldrich syndrome)
Combined defects of thymic dependent and independent functions
   Severe combined immune deficiency (SCID)
   Adenosine deaminase deficiency (ADA)
   Purine nucleoside phosphorylase deficiency (PNP)
   Paediatric AIDS
   Overwhelming post-splenectomy infection (see Chapter 13)

secondary immune mechanisms (antibody- and cell-mediated responses). A classification of the immune deficiency disorders is shown in Table 14.1.

It is proposed in this chapter to describe only the most clearly defined of these disorders.

DEFECTS OF NEUTROPHIL FUNCTION

Children with primary inherited defects of neutrophil function have recurrent infections, fevers, aphthous ulcers, abscesses (cervical, perianal and hepatic) and otitis media with common pathogens which fail to be eradicated by appropriate antibiotic therapy and cervical drainage. Defects of neutrophil function in such children can involve one or several mechanisms which encourage normal neutrophils to migrate from the circulation to the site of infection and there to recognise, attach to, ingest and destroy the offending bacterium or yeast. These disorders of chemotaxis, opsonisation, phagocytosis, degranulation, lysozyme and acid hydrolase activity and of superoxide/hydrogen peroxide systems all have similar clinical presentations.

Chronic granulomatous disease (CGD)

Chronic granulomatous disease was the first of the neutrophil dysfunction syndromes to be described. Initially this disease was thought to be confined to

males but recently there have been a number of reports of its occurrence in females. It is characterised by recurrent and persistent bacterial infections usually involving the skin, lymph nodes, liver, spleen and lungs but any organ may be involved.

Recurrent infections in these patients are always due to a particular group of organisms especially *Staphylococcus aureus*, *S. typhimurium*, *Aerobacter aerogenes*, *Escherichia coli* and *Serratia marcescens*. The common denominator with these bacteria is that they are all catalase producers. A peculiar feature of the disease is the formation of non-caseating granulomas containing pigmented lipid histocytes. The recurrent infections are due to an intracellular defect of leucocytes which renders them incapable of destroying ingested catalase-producing bacteria. This intracellular defect can be readily detected by the nitroblue tetrazolium (NBT) dye reduction test.

Antibacterial drugs achieve only limited success but some antibiotics, e.g. rifampicin, penetrate CGD neutrophils better than normal neutrophils and may be useful in infection. Infusions of normal granulocytes harvested from the child's parents or volunteers can prove life-saving. More severe cases of CGD may need bone marrow transplantation.

Job syndrome

In Job syndrome red-haired girls are affected by recurrent staphylococcal abscesses but without granulomata. There is a neutrophil mobility defect but other defects probably exist. It is characterised by very high serum IgE levels.

Chediak–Higashi syndrome

This is an autosomal recessive disorder characterised by partial oculocutaneous albinism, frequent bacterial infections with the later development of lymphadenopathy and hepatosplenomegaly and also mental retardation. Chemotaxis is abnormal and the circulating neutrophils contain giant greenish-grey granules related to impaired lysosomal activity and bacterial killing. Most patients die in childhood from infections or a peculiar malignant lymphoma. In addition to prophylactic or prompt treatment of acute infection with antibiotic therapy some of these patients benefit from bone marrow transplantation.

DEFECTS OF COMPLEMENT-DEPENDENT SYSTEM

The complement system includes a group of nine serum proteins which interact with one another in a cascading fashion similar to the blood clotting sequence. Some of the components synthesised during this interaction promote chemotaxis (C5, C6 and C7), phagocytosis (C3) and bacteriolysis (C1–C9).

Specific defects of the complement system that have been described are associated with an undue susceptibility to infection. Deficiencies of C5, C6, C7 and C8 result in undue susceptibility to severe infections with bacteria of the *Neisseria* genus.

DEFECTS OF SECONDARY IMMUNE FUNCTION (PRIMARY B-CELL DEFICIENCIES)

These patients have normal T-cell function; therefore they show normal immune response to most viral, fungal and mycobacterial infections. The clinical manifestations in children with defects of B-cell function are recurrent infections with pyogenic bacteria. More sensitive techniques have shown that gammaglobulin is probably never completely absent and it would, therefore, be preferable to call these conditions hypogammaglobulinaemias rather than agammaglobulinaemias.

There are two types of inherited hypogammaglobulinaemia: the most common X-linked recessive (congenital agammaglobulinaemia – Bruton type) disorder and the sporadic (autosomal recessive) type affecting both males and females. Acquired agammaglobulinaemia, either primary or secondary, affects both males and females. Transient hypogammaglobulinaemia of infancy is characterised by low serum concentrations of gammaglobulin after birth when the maternal gammaglobulin is gradually disappearing and the infant's own synthesis has not yet been established. This conditions differs from the others in that it is transient. The aetiology of this transient hypogammaglobulinaemia is unknown.

Congenital hypogammaglobulinaemia (Bruton type)

Aetiology

This form of the disease is generally inherited as a sex-linked recessive and confined to males. In a few instances inheritance has appeared to be autosomal recessive.

Pathogenesis

In this form of hypogammaglobulinaemia there is a severe deficiency in the ability to synthesise the principal immunoglobulins and the child is immunologically deficient from the time the maternal antibodies

have gone from the circulation which is between 6 months and 1 year. Lymph nodes and other tissues are characteristically lacking in germinal centres and plasma cells. On the other hand, although the lymphoid structures and thymus may be somewhat smaller than normal, the tissues of such patients contain relatively normal numbers of lymphocytes. It is characteristic that the same bacterial pathogen recurrently infects these children.

Clinical features

Most commonly the disease presents in a young male child with repeated severe bacterial infections, e.g. pneumonia, otitis media, sinusitis, furunculosis and pyogenic meningitis. Gram-negative infections tend to be less common with the exception of pyelonephritis. They have a peculiar susceptibility to infection of the lungs by the protozoon *Pneumocystis carinii*. This should be suspected when a child known to be hypogammaglobulinaemic develops progressive dyspnoea with few clinical signs of chest infection. Radiographs show a characteristic symmetrical ground glass opacity spreading outwards from the hilar regions. The protozoa may be found in material obtained by lung puncture, bronchoscopy or by tracheal intubation and suction. Prenatal diagnosis can be made by sex determination of the fetus of known heterozygous parents or by direct fetal blood sampling confirming the absence of mature B cells.

Treatment

Infections should be treated with appropriate antibacterial drugs. Long-term management should be with monthly administration of 200–800 mg/kg intravenous immunoglobulin (IV Ig) which greatly reduces the incidence of severe infections.

DEFECTS OF THYMIC-DEPENDENT (CELL-MEDIATED FUNCTION)

Children who suffer from T-cell deficiencies are more susceptible to serious infections than are children with partial or complete B-cell deficiencies. Unlike the infections seen in B-cell deficiencies, which are primarily bacterial in origin, children with T-cell deficiency disorders manifest viral and fungal infections with onset commonly at about 3 months of age. Opportunistic organisms are difficult to eradicate in these children.

Nezelof syndrome

In this disorder there is faulty development (dysgenesis) of the thymus gland. This form of immunoparalysis is inherited as an autosomal recessive trait. It is characterised by the onset during early infancy of severe and recurrent infections. Diagnosis of the syndrome is made by the finding of normal serum immunoglobulins and impaired cell-mediated immunity. The absence of metabolic and structural abnormalities differentiate it from Di George syndrome. Some patients may respond to fetal thymus transplantation.

Di George syndrome (congenital thymic aplasia)

This rare disease consists of a complete absence of the thymus and of the parathyroids which develop from the third and fourth pharyngeal pouch endoderm. The syndrome is not genetically determined but appears rather to result from some intrauterine accident before the eighth week of gestation. There is commonly an associated anomaly of the aortic arch. Other associated findings include dysplasia of the ears and mouth, hypertelorism and imperforate anus. Affected infants present with neonatal tetany, prolonged hypocalcaemia, increased susceptibility to infections (particularly fungal and viral) and failure to thrive.

Circulating lymphocyte counts and appearances are normal as are the serum immunoglobulins and antibody responses. The thymic shadow is absent from chest X-ray. Delayed-type hypersensitivity is completely absent. The majority of infants die within the first month usually from the cardiovascular defect.

Long-term treatment of the hypoparathyroidism is with oral calcium gluconate and vitamin D, 10 µg/kg/day. Transplants of fetal thymus into these infants result in a rapid reconstitution of T-cell function. Bone marrow transplantation has also been successful.

Immunodeficiency with thrombocytopenia and eczema (Wiskott–Aldrich syndrome)

See Chapter 13.

Immunodeficiency with ataxia telangiectasia

This condition has now been defined as a specific entity transmitted as an autosomal recessive characteristic. A constant feature of all the investigated cases and one which explains the extreme susceptibility to severe sinopulmonary infection is absence or gross reduction in the serum IgA globulin. Some of these children also have IgG_2 subclass deficiency and

approximately 80% have depressed IgE concentration. There may be reduced responsiveness of cultured lymphocytes to phytohaemagglutinin suggesting dysfunction of the thymus-dependent lymphocytes.

The clinical features are diagnostic when fully developed. First to appear is a progressive cerebellar ataxia in the course of the second or third year of life, occasionally even earlier. There may be, in addition, choreo-athetotic movements and a tendency to turn the eyes upwards when focusing. Telangiectases make their appearance between the ages of 3 and 7 years. They are found on the bulbar conjunctiva, malar eminences, ears, antecubital fossae and elsewhere. These children suffer severely from infections of the sinuses and lungs; indeed bronchiectasis is a frequent cause of death. In other cases death has been due to development of malignant tumours particularly of the lymphoid system. There is no specific treatment yet available. Infection should be controlled with suitable antibiotics. Immunological reconstitution with transplants of bone marrow in these infants is still in the experimental stage. Intrauterine diagnosis of this disorder has been accomplished.

Severe combined immunodeficiency (SCID)

This form of immunoparalysis is an autosomal recessive condition in which affected patients usually have no T or B cells.

Pathogenesis

There is absence or gross deficiency in all three immunoglobulins (IgG, IgA and IgM). There is severe hypoplasia of the complete lymphoreticular system. The thymus is rudimentary, virtually devoid of lymphocytes and without Hassall corpuscles – thymic alymphoplasia. These patients lack the capacity to develop delayed-type hypersensitivity reactions such as lymphocyte transformation on stimulation by phytohaemagglutinin or sensitisation to dinitrochlorobenzene (DNCB).

Some infants with severe combined immunodeficiency have shown abnormalities affecting the enzymes adenosine deaminase (ADA) or purine nucleoside phosphorylase (PNP). Adenosine deaminase deficiency (ADA) is almost exclusively associated with defective T- and B-cell immunity whereas PNP deficiency is associated with T-lymphocyte immunodeficiency alone.

Clinical features

This is a very severe form of immunoparalysis and affected infants usually died of severe infection during the first 2 years of life. Infants suffer from persistent lung infection with monilial infection of the oropharynx, oesophagus and skin. Chronic diarrhoea and wasting begins in the early months of life. Pneumonia may be due to CMV, *Pneumocystis carinii* or bacteria. Viruses may be excreted persistently from several sites. All these infections are particularly resistant to treatment. Radiological findings include pulmonary infiltration and absence of a thymic shadow. Patients show a characteristic and severe lymphopenia and occasionally neutropenia is found.

Successful treatment has resulted from bone marrow transplants obtained from donors who are compatible by leucocyte typing at the HLA locus and also by mixed leucocyte culture (MLC). When appropriate marrow is unavailable, enzyme replacement therapy using bovine PEG-ADA can provide sufficient ADA to reduce the risks of overwhelming infections. Recently human gene therapy has been used for correction of adenosine deaminase (ADA) deficiency in patients with ADA-deficient severe combined immunodeficiency (SCID).

Antenatal diagnosis of SCID may be made in some cases by fetal blood sampling through lymphocyte subset identification and functional studies.

Paediatric AIDS (acquired immunodeficiency syndrome)

The acquired immunodeficiency syndrome (AIDS) is a multisystem disease of infants and children caused by the retrovirus of the lentivirus subfamily, human immunodeficiency virus type 1 (HIV-1) and type 2 (HIV-2). Paediatric HIV infection has become one of the major health problems in parts of Africa. The virus may remain latent for prolonged periods. However, at any time, the virus can return to its infectious state; this usually occurs when its host T cell is activated in response to other immunological stimuli such as viral infections.

The predominant mode of transmission of HIV infection to children is vertical. Children contracting HIV-1 via vertical transmission are usually born to HIV-1 infected mothers who became infected via IV drug abuse or exposure to HIV-1 infected sexual partners (drug abuse, bisexual or HIV seropositive). Since sensitive methods for screening the supply of blood and blood products have become available the incidence of HIV infection secondary to blood and blood product transfusion has declined dramatically. Other historical features that should be considered as an indication for HIV testing in a child include a history of sexual abuse. There is ample evidence to suggest that casual contact between infants and children and HIV-1 infected individuals does not lead

to HIV infection. More than half of vertically infected children have symptoms by age 1 year and 78% by age 2 years. Some children infected with HIV remain symptom free for many years. Maternal HIV antibody can be detected on Guthrie card infant blood by a simple screening procedure. Up to 30% of these HIV antibody positive infants may subsequently be found to be infected with the virus.

The disease is characterised by failure to thrive, respiratory infections mainly due to bacterial opportunistic infection or interstitial pneumonitis of undetermined aetiology or from *Pneumocystis carinii*, diarrhoea, chronic candidiasis, lymphadenopathy and hepatosplenomegaly. Some of these children may develop signs of progressive neurological disorder.

The laboratory diagnosis of HIV infection is made by testing serum for HIV-1 specific IgG antibodies by ELISA confirmed by Western blot analysis. Sometimes to clarify the diagnosis more specific tests such as HIV culture or detection of specific HIV DNA after PCR enhancement are necessary. HIV infects lymphocytes and cells of monocyte/macrophage lineage, expressing the surface receptor CD4 both *in vitro* and *in vivo*. As the disease progresses the percentage and absolute number of CD4 positive lymphocytes decreases, thus producing inversion of the CD4 (T4)/CD8 (T8) ratio. Also delayed hypersensitivity skin tests become nonreactive.

The approach to the care of children with AIDS should be comprehensive and co-ordinated as with any chronic disease of childhood. While the advances in therapeutic regimens promise to extend the length and quality of life of these children, the diagnosis of HIV infection carries a grim prognosis. The only drug licensed for use in HIV infection is the antiretroviral agent zidovudine (AZT). The drug's principal mode of action is to block HIV replication by inhibition of the DNA polymerase reverse transcriptase. Because of the danger of transmitting HIV to an uninfected infant via breast feeding, HIV positive mothers in developed countries should not breast feed their babies. Children should be immunised as needed (i.e. BCG, rubella, hepatitis B, tetanus booster, measles, pneumococcal and influenza vaccines).

Overwhelming post-splenectomy infection (OPSI)

The post-splenectomy syndrome of overwhelming sepsis in children is well known. The risk of infection is lower in those who are splenectomised after 5 years of age. Splenectomised children should receive prophylactic antibiotics and polyvalent pneumococcal vaccine.

15

Connective Tissue Disorders

In view of the voluminous information available on the structure and biosynthesis of collagen it has become possible to explain a number of genetic diseases on the basis of molecular defects in collagen biosynthesis. Acquired diseases involving collagen are clearly important in medicine but knowledge of how acquired diseases alter collagen synthesis or metabolism is still fragmentary. At present there are a number of diseases which can not clearly be classed as collagen diseases until they are fully understood. In the following pages only the inflammatory diseases of connective tissue which are of significance to paediatricians (Table 15.1) will be dealt with in order of clinical importance.

TABLE 15.1 Connective tissue diseases in children

Acute rheumatic fever

Juvenile chronic arthritis
  Systemic onset
  Polyarticular onset
  Pauciarticular onset

Viral arthritis

Dermatomyositis-polymyositis

Vasculitic syndromes
  Henoch–Schönlein purpura (anaphylactoid purpura)
  Polyarteritis
  Kawasaki syndrome (MLNS; mucocutaneous lymph node syndrome)

Systemic lupus erythematosus

Scleroderma (PSS; progressive systemic sclerosis)

Ankylosing spondylitis

Psoriatic arthritis

Reiter syndrome

Behçet syndrome

Lyme arthritis

ACUTE RHEUMATIC FEVER

Over the past few decades major changes have occurred in the epidemiology of acute rheumatic fever resulting in a decline of the disease in Europe and the developed countries. Despite these changes acute rheumatic fever remains the leading cause of acquired heart disease in the developing countries of the world. In fact, rheumatic heart disease is the most common cause of cardiovascular death in the first five decades of life in many of these countries and is responsible for very significant morbidity and mortality.

Aetiology

Acute rheumatic fever is perhaps unique among the connective tissue disorders in that there is a clear association between the disease and the Lancefield group A β-haemolytic streptococcus. A high titre of the most commonly measured antistreptolysin-O (ASO) in the blood is so regularly a feature of this disease as to be almost a diagnostic *sine qua non*.

The incidence of acute rheumatic fever and chorea in childhood shows marked variation with age. Acute rheumatic fever is rare below the age of 5 years and even rarer below the age of 3 years. The peak incidence of first attacks is highest between the ages of 10 and 14 years. First attacks of acute rheumatic fever after the age of 30 years are rare but do occur. The sex incidence of acute rheumatic fever shows a slight preponderance of females. In girls approaching puberty there is an inexplicable predominance of chorea.

Clinical manifestation

There are five major clinical features of the clinical complex of acute rheumatic fever, namely: polyarthritis, carditis, erythema marginatum, subcutaneous nodules and chorea. To these may be added a few non-specific clinical features which occur frequently in rheumatic fever. Because they also often occur in numerous other diseases their diagnostic value is limited. The usefulness of these manifestations is in supporting the diagnosis of rheumatic fever when only a single major manifestation is present.

The diagnosis of acute rheumatic fever should be made by using the revised Jones criteria. This requires two major or one major and two minor criteria plus evidence of streptococcal infection by throat swab or streptococcal antibodies (Table 15.2).

Polyarthritis

The polyarthritis of acute rheumatic fever renders the diagnosis easy when it results in the classical swelling, redness, pain and limitation of movement of the large joints and when it flits from joint to joint. In children, however, arthritic manifestations are often mild,

TABLE 15.2 Jones criteria (revised) for guidance in the diagnosis of rheumatic fever

MAJOR MANIFESTATIONS	MINOR MANIFESTATIONS
	Clinical
Carditis	Previous rheumatic fever or rheumatic heart disease
Polyarthritis	Arthralgia
Chorea	Fever
Erythema marginatum	
Subcutaneous nodules	
	Laboratory
	Acute phase reactants
	ESR
	C-reactive protein
	Leucocytosis
	Prolonged P-R interval

Supporting evidence of streptococcal infection
Increased titre of antistreptococcal antibodies
Positive throat cultures for group A streptococcus
Recent scarlet fever

amounting perhaps to pain with only minimal objective evidence of joint involvement. Occasionally the disease presents as an acute arthritis confined, for a few days at least, to one joint such as the hip, when a wrong diagnosis of pyogenic arthritis can easily be made. In some children involvement of the small joints of the hands or feet can make early differentiation from juvenile chronic arthritis impossible. In most cases, however, a few days' observation will allow the situation to become clearer. The spine is unaffected in acute rheumatic fever.

Carditis

In acute rheumatic fever during the acute phase the cardiac disease is more widespread than the mere involvement of the endocardium. Myocarditis is the rule rather than the exception and pericarditis occurs more often than the clinical signs would suggest showing up on the echocardiogram. In mild cases no demonstrable indication of cardiac involvement may be present. A soft systolic murmur may be the first indication of rheumatic carditis but such murmurs are so common in children as to be of limited value in the diagnosis of rheumatic carditis. Therefore the appearance of abnormal signs in the heart of a child known previously to have been healthy is almost certain evidence of rheumatic carditis. A soft mid-diastolic murmur at the apex is of much more significance and usually indicates myocarditis. Tachycardia is an important indication of carditis, especially if the pulse rate is taken when the child is asleep, and there may be little difference between waking and sleeping pulses. Other more objective factors may be of help. On ECG a prolonged P-R interval to more than 0.18 seconds, indicating delayed conduction is of some importance. Pericardial friction rub is a clear indication of severe cardiac involvement. Under the age of 5 years carditis predominates and joint symptoms are mild. It should be noted that severe cardiac crippling is rarely the sequel to a first attack of acute rheumatic fever but that it indicates repeated attacks or continued rheumatic activity. However, in the developing countries a schoolchild may present with gross rheumatic heart disease but no history suggestive of acute rheumatic fever in the past.

Subcutaneous nodules

These are small firm nodules most often found over bony prominences, e.g. occiput, olecranon, humeral condyles, knees, knuckles and malleoli, or in the tendon sheaths on the flexor aspects of the wrists or the dorsum of the foot. They are more readily detected by the blanching of the skin seen when it is stretched by flexion of the joint than by palpation.

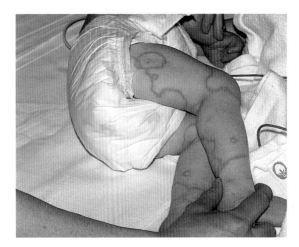

FIGURE 15.1 Erythema marginatum.

They are of great prognostic significance because their presence always indicates active carditis and the likelihood of severe residual damage in the heart.

Erythema marginatum

This typical rash with map-like defined erythematous markings and pale centres of normal skin which changes shape continuously is pathognomonic of rheumatic fever. However, it is lacking in any particular prognostic significance and, in fact, it may persist after all the other signs or rheumatic fever have vanished. It may appear over trunk or limbs (Fig. 15.1).

Rheumatic chorea (Sydenham chorea, St Vitus dance)

This major manifestation of rheumatic fever may occur in association with other manifestations such as polyarthritis and carditis but it frequently appears as a solitary and rather odd phenomenon. It is, in fact, the only major rheumatic manifestation which can affect the same child more than once, and sometimes several times, without the development of any of the other manifestations of acute rheumatic fever. For these reasons and also because the ESR and ASO titre remain normal in uncomplicated chorea, the precise relationship of this disease to rheumatic fever has been the subject of an unresolved controversy. It is more common in girls. The clinical features fall into four main groups:

1 Involuntary purposeless, non-repetitive movements of the limbs, face and trunk, e.g. grimacing, wriggling and writhing. The movements can be brought under voluntary control temporarily. They are aggravated by excitement and they disappear during sleep. The first indication may be that the child begins to drop things or her handwriting suddenly deteriorates or she gets into trouble with her elders for making faces. Sometimes the movements are confined to one side of the body (hemichorea).

2 Hypotonia may result in muscular weakness. It also causes the characteristic posture of the outstretched hands in which the wrist is slightly flexed, whereas there is hyperextension of the metacarpophalangeal joints. Occasionally the child is unable to stand or even to sit up (chorea paralytica).

3 Inco-ordination may be marked or only obvious when the child is asked to pick a coin off the floor.

4 Mental upset is often an early sign. Emotional lability is almost constant. School work usually deteriorates. Infrequently the child becomes confused or even maniacal (chorea insaniens).

As regards the management, rheumatic chorea needs little treatment apart from rest and quiet. Haloperidol has been used with possible benefit. If the involuntary movements are very severe, as the condition shows a relapsing course, treatment with steroids may be tried. Prophylactic chemotherapy is required as for rheumatic fever.

Treatment

The most important single therapeutic measure in rheumatic fever is rest in bed. It is traditional to urge that the child with acute rheumatic fever be kept in bed until all signs of rheumatic activity have ceased. The ESR has proved to be a more precise criterion of activity than the clinical signs. Once the initial acute phase of the illness is over, exercise with tolerance is beneficial rather than the reverse even if the heart is affected. It is therefore suggested that the duration of bed rest should vary according to the severity of rheumatic fever present.

The elimination of any streptococci remaining in the upper respiratory tract should be ensured with high doses of benzylpenicillin. A suitable dosage is 250 000 units given intramuscularly or intravenously 6-hourly for 3 days and then oral phenoxymethylpenicillin 250 mg 6-hourly for a further 10 days. Thereafter the prophylactic regimen takes over.

In acute rheumatic fever two anti-rheumatic drugs are used almost exclusively, salicylates and glucocorticoids. The salicylates abolish fever and joint manifestations rapidly but their value in arresting carditis is doubtful. Acetylsalicylic acid (aspirin) 80–100 mg/kg body weight per day given orally in four equal doses will rapidly abolish fever and joint pains. The optimal duration for salicylate therapy is a matter of personal opinion. Some would continue until all signs of activity have disappeared, others would use salicylate only to alleviate symptoms. Many paediatricians give full doses of salicylates for 6 weeks. Children on salicylates must be carefully watched for signs of overdosage such as overbreathing tinnitus, deafness, nausea and vomiting. Avoidable fatalities have been reported and can be prevented by maintaining blood salicylate concentrations of 25–30 mg/100 ml (2 mmol/l).

Corticosteroids are best reserved for those patients with moderate to severe carditis or when there is congestive cardiac failure; they are certainly very much more potent than salicylates in suppressing acute inflammation. There is no clear evidence that cardiac damage is prevented or minimised by steroids even if used early in the course of the disease.

Our present practice is to rely on salicylates alone in the dosage given above in first attacks of the disease. However, if cardiac signs progress on this regimen and also in all relapses, prednisolone is given in addition. The dosage schedule is 15 mg four times daily for 10 days; 10 mg four times daily for 10 days; 5 mg four times daily for 10 days; and 5 mg twice daily for 10 days. The salicylate is continued for at least 2 weeks thereafter in an effort to diminish the incidence of the "rebound phenomenon" as shown by a rise in the ESR. In both types of regimen it is essential that the cardiac state and the ESR be regularly assessed as the best guides to progress.

Course and prognosis

An average attack of rheumatic fever usually lasts for about 6 weeks. About 50% of patients escape lasting cardiac involvement in their first attack. Repeated attacks tend to mimic each other so that, if there is no carditis in the first attack, it is unlikely that there will be carditis in the second and subsequent attacks. Cardiac involvement is much more likely in children under the age of 12 years and unlikely in adults over the age of 25 years. Prognosis is worse where presystolic or aortic systolic murmurs develop or where there is progressive cardiac enlargement or pericarditis. Persistent subcutaneous nodules are a bad prognostic feature.

Prevention of relapses

It has been established that the prevention of further streptococcal infections reduces the risks of relapse in rheumatic children to very small proportions and drug prophylaxis with phenoxymethylpenicillin 250 mg twice daily has constituted a major advance in the management of this crippling disease. This should be continued until the age of 18 years. Some parents and adolescent patients are of course careless and for them an alternative routine is a monthly intramuscular injection of 1.2 mega units of benzathine penicillin.

JUVENILE CHRONIC ARTHRITIS

The well known clinical picture of chronic polyarthritis with lymphadenopathy, splenomegaly, a rash and pericarditis was first described in Britain by George Frederic Still in 1896. Since then the term "Still disease" had been used to encompass the whole spectrum of rheumatoid arthritis in children. Recently the problem of nomenclature and classification was reviewed and the term juvenile chronic arthritis (JCA) has been accepted. It can present with a variety of clinical manifestations which will distinguish it from the clinical picture of rheumatoid arthritis in adults. We propose to recognise these clinical variations by separating juvenile chronic arthritis into three subtypes:

1 systemic-onset JCA (Still disease);
2 polyarticular-onset JCA; and
3 pauciarticular-onset JCA.

Clinical features

Systemic-onset JCA (Still disease)

The major signs and symptoms of this subtype of juvenile chronic arthritis are systemic. The most common age of onset of the disease is under 5 years but it can occur throughout childhood. Boys are affected as frequently as girls. Characteristic features are high remittent fever, generalised lymphadenopathy (including epitrochlear nodes), splenomegaly, polymorphonuclear leucocytosis and a rash. The rash has an irregular outline and is of coppery red colour. The best time to look for the rash is just after the child has had a hot bath or at the height of the temperature elevation. The fever shows diurnal swings as large as 2 or 3°C which are rarely seen in acute rheumatic fever. Acute pericarditis is not very rare in this form of JCA but endocardial involvement is extremely rare. Joint manifestations are usually present at an early stage although they may initially amount to arthralgia without visible swelling.

When the joints are involved they are frequently large ones, e.g. knees, hips, ankles, elbows and wrists. The cervical spine is another commonly affected site, presenting with pain, limitation of movement and torticollis. Also, peripheral joints may be involved. The surrounding muscle atrophy and increasing limitation of movement and muscle weakness can lead to severe crippling. This subtype of JCA frequently runs a course of remission and relapses.

Polyarticular-onset JCA

This type involves five or more joints but is not accompanied by the severe systemic disturbance such as high fever and rash of systemic-onset type JCA. Girls are much more frequently affected than boys

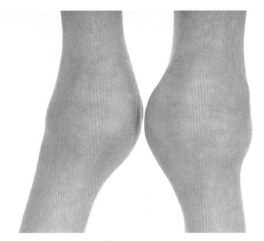

FIGURE 15.2 Juvenile chronic arthritis, pauciarticular type. Swelling of knees.

and although this type of JCA can occur at any age it is more often seen in children over the age of 5 years. The small joints of the hands and fingers may be severely affected.

Children with polyarticular-onset are divided into two groups: those with a negative blood rheumatoid factor present and a small group (10%) with a positive rheumatoid factor. Those with a positive rheumatoid factor are usually over 10 years of age and are more likely to develop destructive joint disease.

Pauciarticular-onset JCA

In this group there is arthritis in one to four joints. Previously, a monoarticular type had been considered as a separate entity but now it is reasonable to include it within the pauciarticular-onset subgroup of JCA. It is essential to remember that children with pauciarticular type do not have symptoms and signs of a systemic or chronic illness. If the pauciarticular-onset type is considered as a single entity, the knee and then the ankle are the most commonly involved joints (Fig. 15.2) but other large and small joints may be involved in this subtype of JCA. While the risk of chronic anterior iridocyclitis exists in all forms of JCA it is particularly common in the pauciarticular-onset type, especially in those with a positive antinuclear antibody (ANA) test. Iridocyclitis is often painless and thus it is important to arrange periodic slit lamp examination for children with pauciarticular-onset JCA.

Course and prognosis of JCA

Rheumatoid arthritis is a chronic systemic disease with a markedly fluctuating but ultimately self-limiting course. In some children remission may occur within a few months or years resulting in little or no deformity; in others the course is more prolonged and in these a greater degree of articular deformity, possibly permanent, is likely.

The overall incidence of chronic iridocyclitis is 10% but in the pauciarticular type it is much higher. A routine slit lamp examination is mandatory in every child with JCA.

Amyloid disease is a rare but potentially fatal complication and progressive enlargement of the liver and spleen and proteinuria are likely warning signs of this. The diagnosis of amyloidosis is confirmed by rectal or renal biopsy.

Treatment of JCA

Rest

It is recommended that a child with JCA should have an adequate period of rest in bed during the night-time and also some rest during the day-time. Complete bed rest is advised only for those children who are severely ill.

Anti-rheumatic drugs

The main aim of treatment in all of the subtypes of JCA is to relieve pain by using a relatively non-toxic drug. Some children with mild symptoms do not require drug treatment, only reassurance, supervision and physiotherapy. Some have intermittent problems that can be solved by the use of simple analgesics taken on demand, while others will require regular treatment with anti-rheumatic drugs. Most doctors caring for children with arthritis realise that treatment with a single anti-rheumatic drug may not help all children and that a combination of anti-rheumatic drugs may be required. The major anti-rheumatic drugs can be divided into first-line, second-line and third-line therapies.

First-line drugs

Non-steroidal anti-inflammatory drugs (NSAIDs) are used initially for the acute flare-up of rheumatic disease and later for long-term maintenance therapy. A 2-week trial is probably adequate to judge the efficacy of any of the NSAIDs. All NSAIDs are acids.

Salicylic acids (aspirin) should be given with caution to children who have a history of chronic asthma, sensitivity reaction to drugs, or other allergies. Children tolerate aspirin well but should be observed closely for evidence of salicylism as mentioned previously (see acute rheumatic fever). Oral aspirin (80–100 mg/kg daily) should be given in four divided doses to maintain plasma salicylate concentrations within the therapeutic range (25–30 mg/100 ml or 2 mmol/l).

Ibuprofen used in children with chronic arthritis is a useful drug and toxicity seems to be low. The daily recommended dosage for children is 20 mg/kg/day. In children weighing less than 30 kg the daily dose should not exceed 500 mg.

Naproxen appears to be extremely well tolerated in children. Recent studies suggest that a daily dosage of 15 mg/kg given in two divided doses produces very little in the way of side effects.

Indomethacin is one of the most popular NSAIDs but should be used cautiously in children. A single dose at night is often helpful in relieving early morning stiffness. The total daily dose should not exceed 2.5 mg/kg.

Full salicylate, ibuprofen or naproxen dosage by day and indomethacin by night is a satisfactory combination.

Tolmetin sodium therapy in JCA is started at 20 mg/kg in three or four divided doses. Dosage higher than 30 mg/kg is not recommended.

Second-line drugs

If a child continues to show evidence of active and progressively destructive joint disease despite an adequate trial of first-line drugs, one should consider using disease-modifying drugs such as gold, penicillamine or hydroxychloroquine.

Patients who respond to gold treatment (*chrysotherapy*) tend also to respond to penicillamine and vice versa. There are no immediate results and maximal effects develop after 4–6 months. The amount of supervision required is the same as with penicillamine, i.e. a full blood count including platelets and urinalysis at least once a month. The current practice is to begin progressively with test doses of sodium aurothiomalate 0.25 mg, 0.5 mg and 0.75 mg/kg intramuscularly at weekly intervals before continuing with 1 mg/kg intramuscularly once a week for 6 months to a maximum of 50 mg/week. If effective, the treatment should not be interrupted but should be continued on an indefinite basis with a reduction in dosage (giving the same amount per injection but less frequently such as every 2, 3 or 4 weeks).

Penicillamine, like gold, has no immediate effect in rheumatoid arthritis and begins to work only after several weeks. The starting dose is 50 mg daily given orally before food, increasing by 50 mg at intervals of not less than 4 weeks. It is recommended that a dose of up to 450 mg daily be given to children under 20 kg body weight and up to 600 mg to the rest, but maintenance doses of less than 375 mg are often adequate.

Because of the risk of retinopathy, *hydroxychloroquine* should only be used when regular ophthalmology review is available. An oral dose of up to a maximum of 6.5 mg/kg daily of hydroxychloroquine will not usually be associated with the development of side effects. If at the end of 6 months there has been no effect, treatment should be stopped.

Third-line drugs

The decision to start a child on corticosteroids should not be taken lightly because of the well known side effects, in particular growth retardation and osteoporosis. However, they should be used in the following situation:

1 Acute systemic involvement.
2 Severe inflammatory joint disease refractory to other drugs.
3 Chronic uveitis unresponsive to local steroid therapy.

Prednisolone can be given orally in doses of 1 mg/kg on alternate days to minimise both adrenal suppression and growth retardation. ACTH has been used instead of oral steroids, as growth retardation is less of a problem, but repeated injections may distress a child.

There is usually little place for *immunosuppressant therapy* in the management of JCA.

Splints, physiotherapy and occupational therapy

Joints may need to be splinted to prevent deformities. Rest splints on wrists, knees and ankles worn at night avoid the development of flexion deformities which, if untreated, may progress to contractures.

A physiotherapist should plan an exercise programme tailored to the child's needs. The purpose of the exercise programme is to maintain joint motion and muscle strength and may be performed in the warm water of the hydrotherapy pool.

The role of the occupational therapist is to keep the child as independent as possible. The occupational therapist will assess any difficulties the child with arthritis may have and will teach the child techniques to make problem activities easier, e.g. by using specially designed cutlery.

Surgery

Most cases of JCA do not require surgery. However, soft tissue release is occasionally required for progressive hip disease that is associated with flexion deformity. Some children may need total hip replacement or knee arthroplasty. Every attempt should be made to delay surgery until growth has ceased.

VIRAL ARTHRITIS

Viral infections commonly cause generalised musculoskeletal complaints. Localised joint symptoms are uncommon and are usually acute and self-limited.

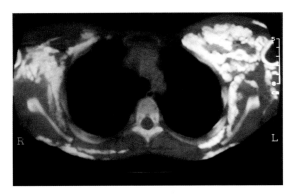
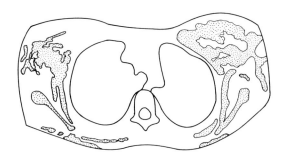

FIGURE 15.3 Dermatomyositis. CT scan of upper thorax showing extensive soft tissue calcification.

Viral infections that may be associated with arthropathy include rubella, both natural and vaccine-induced, mumps, chicken pox, glandular fever, cytomegalovirus, hepatitis B, adenovirus (type 7), influenza and arboviruses. The arthropathy is usually polyarticular transient, non recurring and resolves spontaneously.

Neuro-musculo-skeletal manifestations of malignancy in childhood, e.g. neuroblastoma, Ewing sarcoma, primitive neurectodermal tumours (PNET) may present as a "pseudo-rheumatoid-like diagnosis" and this should be borne in mind as it may result in a considerable delay in diagnosis.

DERMATOMYOSITIS-POLYMYOSITIS

Dermatomyositis-polymyositis is a rare connective tissue disorder in children. Polymyositis is characterised by predominantly proximal muscle weakness but without any evidence of skin involvement. In dermatomyositis the muscle involvement is clinically and histologically indistinguishable from that of polymyositis but there is also a rash involving the face and extremities.

The onset is usually insidious with facial erythema, proximal muscle weakness and fatigue and general constitutional upset but occasionally the onset is acute. It may occur at any age from the second year into adolescence. A heliotrope colour of the eyelids and periorbital skin is quite characteristic of this disorder and periorbital oedema is also common. Calcinosis of the affected areas is common in children and readily demonstrated by X-ray or CT scan (Fig. 15.3).

The diagnosis of dermatomyositis is based mainly on the combination of the clinical features of symmetrical muscle weakness and the typical cutaneous manifestations. It may be confirmed by the finding of an elevation in the serum muscle enzymes (creatine kinase) and/or a muscle biopsy showing inflammatory myositis. The ESR in this condition is unhelpful and may be normal. EMG findings of myopathic/neuropathic pattern are helpful in supporting the diagnosis of inflammatory muscle disease.

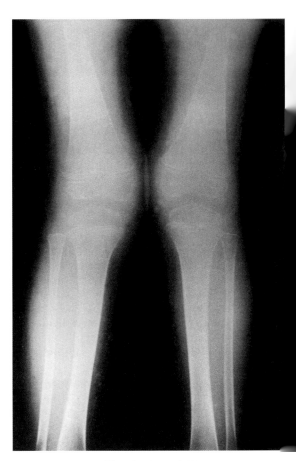

FIGURE 15.4 X-ray of leg showing calcification.

Treatment

Various therapeutic measures have been employed at one time or another but corticosteroids have received considerable attention. A high dosage of steroid such as oral prednisolone is recommended, beginning with 1.5–2 mg/kg/day as a single morning dose rather than in divided doses. Once the acute phase is controlled it is desirable to reduce the dose to an alternate day regimen. A good prognosis is commoner in children than in adults.

VASCULITIC SYNDROMES

Henoch–Schönlein purpura (anaphylactoid purpura)

The disorder known as Henoch–Schönlein purpura is a systemic vasculitis of unknown aetiology involving skin, joints and some viscera. The disease has a wide variety of manifestations but the diagnosis is rarely difficult and based essentially on the rash of characteristic appearance and distribution. In most cases there is a history of a preceding sore throat or respiratory infection. The most prominent symptoms may arise from swollen painful joints, or from areas of angio-oedema elsewhere. In other children the onset is with severe abdominal pain with or without melaena. It is in such cases that a mistaken diagnosis of intussusception has sometimes led to an unnecessary laparotomy. Another mode of presentation in boys is with an acute scrotal swelling which can be mistaken for a torsion of the testis. In the majority of cases the rash is the most striking feature and causes the parents to seek medical advice but it may appear after the abdominal pain. It appears first as small separate urticarial lesions, both visible and palpable. These soon become dusky red or frankly purpuric and they no longer fade on pressure. In the typical case the rash is most profuse over the extensor surfaces of the knees, ankles and dorsum of the feet, arms, elbows and forearms; it is also marked over the legs (Fig. 15.5). The face is completely spared but when the disease appears in an infant, which is quite rare, the face may be markedly involved.

The platelet count and bleeding time are within the normal limits.

Renal involvement is more common than is usually recognised and may occur in 20% of patients. The clinical presentation can vary from microscopic haematuria to a typical acute glomerulonephritis or to a nephrotic syndrome. The renal biopsy findings vary from minimal glomerular changes to proliferative glomerulonephritis and all variations of the latter

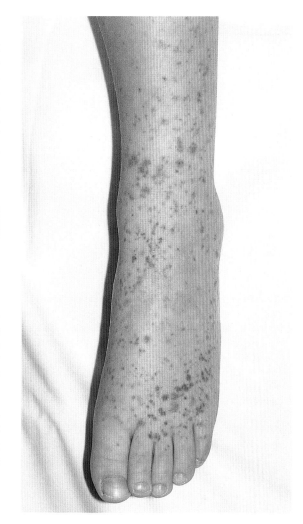

FIGURE 15.5 Henoch–Schönlein purpura. Purpuric rash on dorsum of foot and ankle.

from minor lesions to focal distribution to diffuse involvement with crescent formation may be encountered. While the majority of children with renal involvement make a complete recovery, a few may go on to develop persistent proteinuria, hypertension and deteriorating renal function.

There are no specific laboratory findings to help with the diagnosis of this disease. A raised ASO titre (above 200 units/ml) has been found in approximately a third of cases.

Treatment

There is no specific treatment for Henoch–Schönlein purpura. Bed rest should be encouraged until fresh lesions cease to appear. Penicillin is indicated only if β-haemolytic streptococci are isolated from the throat. (For glomerulonephritis management see p. 220.) Severe abdominal pain may develop at any

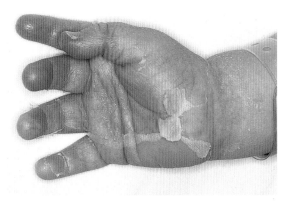

FIGURE 15.6 Kawasaki disease.

TABLE 15.3 Diagnostic guidelines for Kawasaki syndrome
Principal signs
Fever persisting 5 days or more
Polymorphous rash
Bilateral conjunctival congestion
Changes of lips and oral cavity
Reddening of lips
Strawberry tongue
Diffuse hyperaemia or oral and pharyngeal mucosa
Acute non-purulent cervical lymphadenopathy
Changes of peripheral extremities
Reddening of palms and soles
Indurative oedema of hands and feet
Membranous desquamation from fingertips

stage of the illness. It is best relieved with oral pethidine or oral pentazocine both given in the dosage of 1 mg/kg body weight. Corticosteroids and immunosuppressive drugs are of no therapeutic value. A surgical opinion should be sought to ensure no abdominal complications have occurred, e.g. a duodenal intramucosal haematoma causing intestinal obstruction.

Polyarteritis

Polyarteritis may be subdivided into at least five different entities: infantile polyarteritis, polyarteritis of older children, polyarteritis associated with hepatitis-B antigen, cutaneous polyarteritis and Kawasaki syndrome.

Infantile polyarteritis

This affects children under 12 months of age and is very rare. Coronary arteries are the primary site involved. Respiratory symptoms and a morbilliform rash are common and the course tends to be brief. Diagnosis is usually made at post-mortem examination.

Polyarteritis of older children

This resembles the adult form of the disease. Fever is present in almost all cases as are irritability, weight loss and lethargy. Skin rashes of different kinds have been described. Significant arteritis involving the kidneys, heart, CNS and gastrointestinal tract result in clinical manifestations related to these organs. The pathology in children is similar to that in adults with polymorphonuclear infiltration and necrosis occurring mainly in small and medium sized muscular arteries involving all layers of the vessel. It would appear that patients treated with steroids and/or cyclophosphamide have a better prognosis, otherwise prognosis is poor.

Polyarteritis associated with hepatitis-B antigen

No children have as yet been described with this type of polyarteritis.

Cutaneous polyarteritis

This type primarily affects the skin in children and presents with crops of small, painful nodules. Fever and arthralgia are common features. Skin necrosis and ulceration are frequent. Most patients respond to a low dose of steroids.

Kawasaki syndrome (mucocutaneous lymph node syndrome; MLNS)

Kawasaki syndrome is an acute, largely self-limited multisystem disease affecting infants and children which is characterised by prolonged fever, mucosal inflammation, skin changes and cervical lymphadenopathy (Fig 15.6). The disorder is a systemic vasculitis with predilection for the coronary arteries. It was described by Dr Tomasaku Kawasaki in the Japanese literature in 1967 and in the English literature in 1974. It has been subsequently recognised in children of every ethnic group. The aetiology of the disease remains unknown although it is widely believed to be a microbial agent. It is a disease of young children and 80% of cases are younger than 4 years. The peak age of onset is 1 year and the disorder is more common in boys.

The generally accepted diagnostic criteria are outlined in Table 15.3.

A definite diagnosis of Kawasaki syndrome can be made when at least five of the six principal signs are present. However, children with only four of the six principal signs can be diagnosed as Kawasaki syndrome only if coronary artery aneurysms are demonstrated by two-dimensional echocardiography. Illnesses producing similar findings such as streptococcal, staphylococcal and leptospiral infection must be excluded. In the absence of pathognomonic clinical or laboratory signs it is extremely difficult to diagnose mild or incomplete cases. Therefore it is essential sometimes to keep an open mind and occasionally follow a child as a "possible case" with repeated clinical and cardiac evaluations. However, in most cases the diagnostic criteria are clearly indentifiable and a definite diagnosis of Kawasaki syndrome can be made.

Cardiac involvement

Cardiac disease occurs in at least 30% of children with Kawasaki syndrome. In the acute period it may present as myocarditis, pericarditis, valve dysfunction, mitral insufficiency, non-fatal myocardial infarction or sudden death due to coronary thrombosis.

Two-dimensional echocardiography will detect nearly all patients with acute coronary disease and has reduced the need for invasive procedures such as coronary angiography. It should be performed weekly for the first 4 weeks of illness. It has been shown that the peak frequency of coronary dilatation or aneurysms occurs within 4 weeks of onset. In the majority of children coronary aneurysms show regression within 6 months to 2 years. Coronary occlusion with death due to myocardial infarction occurs in fewer than 1% of patients and 85% of deaths occur between days 10 and 40 of illness.

Other less frequent features include arthritis and arthralgia, urethritis, diarrhoea, aseptic meningitis, proteinuria, with sterile pyuria, myocarditis, pericarditis, alopecia, mild jaundice, uveitis and hydrops of the gall bladder with severe upper right quadrant abdominal pain. Blood tests show leucocytosis, a raised ESR and during the second week of illness there may be thrombocytosis.

Treatment

Early initiation of aspirin therapy remains the mainstay of treatment to prevent thrombus formation and ischaemic heart disease. The aspirin should be used in the dosage of 5–10 mg/kg/day until ESR has returned to normal or, if aneurysms have developed, indefinitely. Dipyridamole in a dosage of 3–5 mg/kg/day in three divided doses should be added whenever a patient's platelet count rises above $1000 \times 10^9/l$ or if coronary artery ischaemia is detected. Treatment with IV gammaglobulin (400 mg/kg/day for 4 days) for all children diagnosed within the first 10 days of illness significantly reduces the risk of aneurysms. The mechanism by which this occurs has not been ascertained.

SYSTEMIC LUPUS ERYTHEMATOSUS (SLE)

SLE is a multisystem disease and the literature continually expands our notions of the varied and

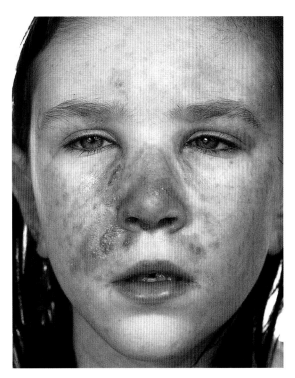

FIGURE 15.7 Typical "butterfly" rash of systemic lupus erythematosus.

seemingly infinite manifestations of this complex disorder. The disease in children is thought to be more severe than in adults and almost invariably results in a fatal outcome. Only a few children develop SLE in the early school years. Most cases occur between 11 and 15 years of age and it is more common in girls.

SLE is a disease of unknown aetiology in which immunological mechanisms play a vital role in the pathogenesis. The hallmark of this disorder is the presence of serum antibodies directed against a wide variety of nuclear, cytoplasmic and serum protein antigens.

Drug-related lupus is clinically identical with idiopathic lupus. In children the most common cause of drug-related lupus is the administration of anticonvulsant drugs. No conclusive criteria exist which will discriminate between idiopathic and drug-related lupus.

Clinical manifestations

In the childhood form of SLE, as in the adult, the clinical symptomatology may be variable and unpredictable with any number of organ systems eventually becoming involved. The disease in childhood is either acute or subacute and rarely chronic. The characteristic erythematous rash with its "butterfly" distribution on the cheeks and bridge of nose is usual in the systemic form of lupus erythematosus in children (Fig. 15.7). In addition, various skin manifestations may occur such as non-specific erythemata, purpura, telangiectasia, urticaria, abnormal pigmentation, Raynaud phenomenon and alopecia. Anaemia in which there may be evidence of haemolysis, thrombocytopenia and leucopenia may occur.

Renal involvement – the so-called lupus glomerulonephritis characterised by red cells, white cells, protein and casts in the urine progressing to significant renal damage associated with uraemia and hypertension – is a characteristic and grave manifestation, being the most commonly identifiable cause of death in SLE.

Joint involvement is not uncommon and varies from mild joint pain to a deforming arthritis closely resembling that of juvenile chronic arthritis.

Heart involvement may occur in this disease in the form of myocarditis, endocarditis and pericarditis. Manifestations of central nervous system involvement include convulsions and mental confusion and various localising manifestations due to focal vascular lesions. Enlargement of the liver and spleen may be found. Lymphadenopathy with generalised lymph gland enlargement is yet another clinical manifestation. There may be a rapidly progressive retinopathy and extensive retinal haemorrhages, exudates and papilloedema.

Laboratory findings

The diagnosis of systemic lupus erythematosus (SLE) is associated with a large assortment of autoantibodies. Presence or absence of particular autoantibodies influences the confidence with which this diagnosis is made. Anti-double-stranded DNA (dsDNA) is now considered the most specific antibody for lupus, while anti-single-stranded DNA (ssDNA) is relatively non-specific and commonly found in many "rheumatic" syndromes. Also, anti-double-stranded DNA is often the harbinger of renal disease, particularly when consistent with evidence of serum complement (C3, C4) consumption. Anaemia is present in most patients but only a fraction of these have a positive Coombs' test. Lymphopenia is possibly one of the most common manifestations of SLE and thrombocytopenia may be seen in some SLE patients.

Treatment

Treatment is directed towards immunosuppression. Prednisolone can be given in high dosage (1–2 mg/kg/day) either alone or in conjunction with azathioprine (2–5 mg/kg/day) or other immunosuppressants. Such treatment is not without significant side effects and therapy should therefore be guided by the severity of the disease which, in its milder form, may be less harmful than the therapy.

Prognosis

The course of SLE in childhood is highly variable an unpredictable. In children under 12 years of age was usually fatal but the increasing use of corticosteroids appears to be improving the outlook.

PROGRESSIVE SYSTEMIC SCLEROSIS OR SCLERODERMA

The term progressive systemic sclerosis is nowaday preferred to that of scleroderma as indicating th important and often lethal nature of the systemi manifestation of this disorder. The disease is excep tionally rare in childhood. Although scleroderma ha been recognised for a considerable time, its aetiolog is still in doubt and its course unpredictable. Therap is of little benefit and the literature yields conflictin views on the prognosis in childhood. Various patche of skin become oedematous and then atrophic an inelastic, becoming adherent to the underlyin tissues. The consequent atrophy and tightening o the skin gives a characteristic appearance of pinche nose and pursed lips. The hands become shiny wit tapered finger ends and restricted movemen producing claw-like deformities which may als affect the feet. Raynaud phenomenon is commor The well known gastrointestinal system involvemen with oesophageal fibrosis and dysphagia is much les common in the childhood form of the disease Pulmonary fibrosis and renal involvement ma occur. Sjögren syndrome (sicca syndrome of dr mouth and eyes) more commonly occurs in SLE bu is not uncommon in this condition. Linear sclero derma is strange condition in which half the body i affected while the other half remains untouched (Fig 15.8).

Although in some children the disease may becom quiescent and even regress, it can equally well becom progressive and rapidly fatal as in adults. An appar ently slowly developing form of scleroderma described largely in adults and called the CREST syndrome, may be found in children. CREST is a acronym for calcinosis, Raynaud phenomenon oesophageal dysfunction, sclerodactyly and telangiec tasia.

Laboratory findings

There are no specific laboratory tests diagnostic o scleroderma. In some cases there may be antinuclea antibodies and even a positive LE cell phenomenon and a positive rheumatoid factor. The ESR i frequently raised and where there is considerabl muscle involvement the transaminases are also increased.

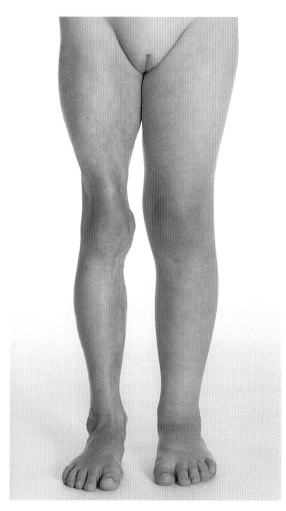

FIGURE 15.8 Scleroderma. Linear scleroderma affecting the right leg.

Treatment

No treatment at the present time is of any certain value. It is important to provide physical and occupational therapeutic measures to attempt to maintain good position and function of the joints and to maintain muscle strength. Corticosteroid therapy has not seemed to alter the progression of the disease. Immunosuppressive agents and penicillamine have been reported to be of benefit to some patients but both these forms of therapy should still be considered to be experimental.

JUVENILE ANKYLOSING SPONDYLITIS (JAS)

Juvenile ankylosing spondylitis is a rare condition in childhood which may present an asymmetrical polyarthritis of hips and knees rather than the classical lumbo-sacral manifestations. Iritis and scleritis may precede the joint involvement and it may take several months or years before a definite diagnosis can be made.

Laboratory findings are not particularly helpful in this disorder as rheumatoid factor and antinuclear antibody tests are normal. The presence of HLA-B27 does not confirm the diagnosis since 10% of normal population has this antigen. However, HLA-B27 positivity will support the diagnosis provided other clinical features of JAS are present. X-ray examination is unhelpful because the typical changes in the sacroiliac joints described in adults are rarely seen in JAS during the childhood years.

The treatment of JAS consists of the use of anti-inflammatory drugs and a physical therapy programme.

PSORIATIC ARTHRITIS

Psoriatic arthritis is rare in childhood. It is more common in girls than in boys. The mean age of onset of arthritis is about 10 years but children of any age can be affected. Asymmetrical polyarthritis, frequently involving the distal interphalangeal joints, is the most frequent pattern. Pauciarticular large joint involvement is seen in some patients, and a minority have sacroiliitis and spondylitis. The major difference between JCA and psoriatic arthritis is the paucity of systemic manifestations. It is interesting that nearly 50% of children with psoriatic arthritis will have either minimal skin disease or no skin involvement at all for several years and therefore are initially diagnosed as cases of JCA. Most children with psoriatic arthritis can be treated satisfactorily with non-steroidal anti-inflammatory drugs but a small group may require slow-acting drugs such as gold therapy.

REITER SYNDROME

Reiter syndrome with the typical triad of urethritis, arthritis and conjunctivitis is rare in childhood. The most common cause of this syndrome in childhood is an infective diarrhoea due to shigella or salmonella or other enteric pathogens. The knee is the most commonly involved joint but ankles and single toes or fingers can be affected. Systemic signs are not prominent although low-grade fever and malaise may be present. Diagnosis of Reiter syndrome is primarily clinical. Rheumatoid factor and antinuclear factor are absent but there is a high association of HLA-B27 in these patients. The prognosis is usually good with gradual amelioration of signs and symptoms.

BEHÇET SYNDROME

This syndrome is rare in children and is characterised by recurrent oral and genital ulceration and eye inflammation. Additonal associated clinical features are arthritis, fever and less commonly there can be involvement of gastrointestinal, cardiovascular and nervous systems. Laboratory findings are not diagnostic. There is no effective treatment although some children may benefit from high-dose corticosteroids.

LYME ARTHRITIS

In 1977 Steer and his colleagues announced the discovery of a new disease called "Lyme arthritis" which they proved was transmitted by the deer tick, *Ixodes dammini*. In 1982 it was discovered that the infectious agent is a spirochaete (*Borrelia burgdorferi*). The clinical syndrome consists of a febrile illness with a characteristic rash, erythema chronicum migrans and cardiac, neurological and articular manifestations. Arthritis may be the initial manifestation of Lyme arthritis. In a series of 25 children with Lyme arthritis recently reported in the United States all patients had a pauciarticular type of joint involvement. The joints predominantly involved were knees, elbows, wrists, ankles and hips, in that order.

Lyme arthritis may also be confused with acute bacterial septic arthritis especially when the synovial fluid leucocyte counts are very high and show a neutrophilic preponderance. It is important that Lyme arthritis should be ruled out in patients with episodic, self-limiting attacks of arthritis even in the absence of the typical rash. All patients in the above series had borrelia-specific antibody which is indicative of Lyme disease and the usual cut-off for diagnosis in the immunfluorescent assay test is 1:256. Therefore, the finding of an elevated titre in association with clinical manifestations is considered diagnostic of Lyme disease. Lyme disease can be treated with high-dose penicillin given intravenously for 10 days during the early course of the disease.

16

Inborn Errors of Metabolism

There has been a remarkable increase in our knowledge of the inborn metabolic errors in recent years, largely brought about by the introduction of new biochemical techniques. The term "inborn errors of metabolism" was first used by Garrod in 1908 when he described albinism, alkaptonuria, cystinuria and pentosuria. Garrod, noting the frequency of consanguineous matings in the pedigrees of his patients, correctly inferred the genetic origin of these disorders. He went further and suggested that they arose through the medium of defective enzyme activities. At the present time there are over 1500 known recessive and X-linked human genetic diseases, all of which can be expected to have an underlying specific inherited metabolic disorder. So far in only about 200 is the precise enzyme defect known, although the chromosomal location of more than 700 of these genes is now known. In this book it would clearly be impracticable to consider the whole subject, which is, indeed, now far beyond the competence of any one individual. An attempt has been made to portray a broad outline of the subject and some of the more common or important diseases in the group receive more detailed considerations. Others are considered in other chapters under the various systems of the body.

GENERAL AETIOLOGICAL CONSIDERATIONS

It is now certain that genes act through the control of complex intracellular biochemical reactions. The concept of "one gene – one enzyme" is useful. It follows, therefore, that an abnormal or defective enzyme activity can be related to an abnormal or mutant gene. Our understanding of the nature of gene activity was greatly furthered by the work of Watson and Crick when they described the structure of the deoxyribonucleic acid (DNA) molecule. A gene is composed of DNA and the structure of the DNA molecule determines the specific function of the gene. This structure consists of two helical chains of phosphate-sugar each coiled round the same axis. The chains are held together by purine and pyrimidine bases which are at right angles to the axis of the molecule. There are four such bases in the DNA molecule – adenine (a purine), thymine (a pyrimidine), guanine (a purine) and cytosine (a pyrimidine). The genetic function is coded, as it were, by the particular sequence of these alternating pairs of purine and pyrimidine bases along the length of the

DNA molecule. The activity of the DNA molecules on the chromosomes transmits information to the molecules of ribonucleic acid (RNA) within the cell nucleus. There are also four nitrogen bases in the RNA molecule – adenine, guanine, cytosine and uracil (instead of thymine as in DNA). RNA or "transfer" molecules then diffuse out into the cytoplasm and pick up individual amino acids which come together to form polypeptide chains and proteins on the ribosomes. The sequence of bases along "messenger" RNA is the code which determines the order of incorporation of amino acids into the particular polypeptide chains. A mutation, therefore, consists of an alteration in the sequence of bases in the DNA molecule and consequently in the messenger RNA molecule. This usually results in the substitution of one amino acid for another in the polypeptide chain. For example, the haemoglobin in sickle-cell anaemia (Hb-S) differs from normal haemoglobin (Hb-A) only in that valine occupies the position in the haemoglobin peptide sequence normally occupied by glutamic acid.

In the case of a defective enzyme system it is also likely that there is formed an enzyme protein which is structurally abnormal. Thus, a single amino-acid substitution at the active centre of the protein could profoundly alter the kinetics of the catalytic process and so result in loss of activity. The same kind of thing could obviously occur in peptides and protein macromolecules other than haemoglobin and enzymes, and the inborn errors of metabolism should now be taken to include all the specific molecular abnormalities which are genetically determined. They can for clinical purposes be divided into four types.

1 Disturbances in structure of protein molecules, e.g. the haemoglobinopathies.
2 Disturbances in synthesis of protein molecules, e.g. haemophilia, Christmas disease, congenital afibrinogenaemia, congenital hypogammaglobulinaemia, and Wilson disease where ceruloplasmin is deficient.
3 Disturbances in function of protein molecules, e.g. enzyme deficiencies like phenylketonuria, galactosaemia, adrenocortical hyperplasia and many others.
4 Disturbances in transport mechanisms, e.g. Hartnup disease, cystinuria, nephrogenic diabetes insipidus, renal glycosuria, de Toni–Fanconi syndrome, vitamin D resistant rickets.

In 1961 the first success was achieved in "breaking the code" which the sequences of base-pairs in the DNA and RNA molecules represent. Each amino acid is specified by a set of three bases out of the possible four nitrogen bases in the DNA and RNA molecules. This is a triplet code which gives $4^3 = 64$ different possibilities, and each base triplet has been called a "codon". Some examples of the code in relation to the RNA molecule are as follows:

Phenylalanine = Uracil/Uracil/Uracil
Methionine = Uracil/Guanine/Uracil
Tryptophan = Uracil/Guanine/Guanine
Leucine = Uracil/Uracil/Adenine

A mutation usually involves the addition or deletion of a single base and as this may occur at random anywhere along the base-pair sequence it follows that many different (alternative) genes (or alleles) may be generated by different mutations in any given gene. For example, in a typical gene with 900 nitrogen bases coding a polypeptide chain of 300 amino acids, as many as 2700 different alleles might arise from different mutations, each causing the replacement of a single base because, of course, each of the 900 bases may be altered to one of three others by different mutational events. Such a great variety of different mutant alleles is not merely theoretical. Over 300 variants of haemoglobin A have now been identified, the great majority differing from normal Hb-A by only a single amino acid substitution, although only a few are associated with overt disease. In the same way an enzyme protein can be altered in many ways by different mutant alleles, although when they result in the loss of enzyme activity they will all have similar metabolic and clinical consequences. In phenylketonuria different degrees of enzyme deficiency have now been recognised which are believed to reflect the effects of different mutations of the same gene, and a similar explanation has been suggested for the fact that some patients with homocystinuria respond to pyridoxine and others do not.

As the triplet code from four bases gives 64 different possibilities it follows that any one of the 20 amino acids must be able to be coded by more than one base triplet or codon. It would appear that of the 64 possible triplet sequences 61 each specify one out of the 20 amino acids, and that most amino acids are coded by two or more different base triplets. The remaining three, sometimes called "nonsense triplets" do not code for any amino acid. They are concerned with chain termination, i.e. they define the point in the synthesis of the polypeptide at which the end of the chain is reached. In the majority of mutations involving a single base change the base triplet (or codon) for one amino acid is replaced by the base triplet for another, resulting in the substitution of one amino acid for another in the polypeptide chain – as in the abnormal haemoglobins. On the other hand, if this single base change were to involve one of the "nonsense triplets" which code for chain termination the result would be the synthesis of a greatly shortened polypeptide chain which would fail to add up to a viable and functional form of protein. The effect could be a complete failure to synthesise the specific enzyme protein or, alternatively, a severe reduction in the rate of its synthesis so that very little is actually present at any one time. In other rare instances complete failure to form the enzyme may arise from a deletion of parts of the DNA sequence of the gene rather than from a single base change.

The basis of many of the inborn errors of metabolism is highly complex and even now not fully worked out. There are, in fact, certain other factors still to be mentioned and which are known to be concerned with the activity of any enzyme. This activity is, of course, determined by the amino-acid sequence of its constituent polypeptide chains which dictate its three-dimensional molecular structure. But the quantity of enzyme which is actually present is also clearly important, and this is the result of the rates at which it is being synthesised in the cells and at which it is being broken down and denatured. Enzyme activity is further influenced by the presence of particular activators, inhibitors, repressors, coenzymes, etc. It will become clear in the accounts of some of the individual inborn errors which follow that these factors may sometimes explain the variations which are now being demonstrated within diseases previously thought to be more or less uniform in their manifestations.

Diagnosis depends both on the clinician having a high index of suspicion and on the appropriate test(s) being carried out. The local laboratory has a key role to play by guiding these investigations so that the most appropriate preliminary "screening" tests are carried out first. Many of the more specialised tests (i.e. specific enzymes) will only be required later to confirm a diagnosis.

such names as atypical PKU, mild PKU, phenylalaninaemia, etc. Recent genetic studies have provided an explanation for this variation. Over 150 different mutations of the phenylalanine hydroxylase gene have been identified.

Pathogenesis

In normal individuals phenylalanine, which is an essential amino acid, is converted in the liver to tyrosine by the activity of phenylalanine hydroxylase. The gene for phenylalanine hydroxylase is located on chromosome 12 and contains 13 exons. A high proportion of affected subjects are compound heterozygotes rather than homozygotes. In affected infants the blood phenylalanine increases to 1815–6050 µmol/l (30–100 mg/100 ml) within 2 or 3 weeks of birth, and after a phenylalanine load the blood level of tyrosine does not rise. The blood phenylalanine is then converted by phenylalanine transaminase to phenylpyruvic acid and other degradation products such as phenyllactic acid, phenylacetic acid and *ortho*-hydroxyphenylacetic acid. The precise chemical cause for the inevitable mental retardation in "classical" PKU is not known but is probably related to the high phenylalanine concentration and to deficiencies of the neurotransmitters noradrenaline, adrenaline and dopamine. The fair hair and blue eyes are due to a deficiency of melanin which is synthesised like the neurotransmitters from tyrosine (Fig. 16.1).

DISORDERS OF AMINO-ACID METABOLISM

Phenylketonuria

Aetiology

"Classical" phenylketonuria (persistent hyperphenylalaninaemia > 240 µmol/l, relative tyrosine deficiency and excretion of an excess of phenyl ketones) is transmitted as an autosomal recessive trait, so that in any family in which the disease has appeared the chances of future children being affected will be 1 in 4. The incidence of the "classical" form of PKU in the United Kingdom is about 1 in 10 000 births. In recent years the development of sensitive screening tests based upon the estimation of blood phenylalanine has shown that hyperphenylalaninaemia is not necessarily associated with the presence of phenylketones in the urine. The terminology relating to these other types of hyperphenylalaninaemia is confused, as is our understanding of their aetiology and has included

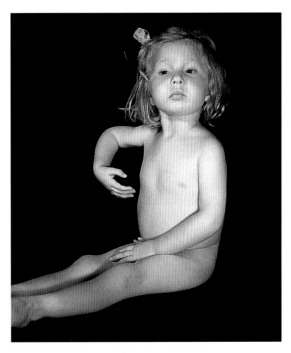

FIGURE 16.1 Untreated phenylketonuria.

The pathogenesis of the other types of hyper-phenylalaninaemia is much less clearly defined. In one group, which may be called "mild" PKU, the blood phenylalanine values remain between 1210 and 1815 µmol/l (20 and 30 mg/100 ml). The urinary ferric chloride test for phenylpyruvic acid is usually weakly positive, but if it is not, phenylketonuria develops if a high-protein diet or a phenylalanine loading dose is given. Enzyme studies on some of these patients have shown complete absence of phenylalanine hydroxylase. In a third group of cases the blood phenylalanine ranges from 302 to 1210 µmol/l (5–20 mg/ml), and phenylpyruvic acid is not excreted in the urine because the level of blood phenylalanine is too low for transamination to occur. In a few such infants enzyme study of liver biopsy material has shown phenylalanine hydroxylase activity of less than half to one-tenth of normal. There are, however, other possible causes of hyper-phenylalaninaemia. Several patients have been described with choking attacks, muscular hypotonia, developmental delay and convulsions, and mild to moderate hyperphenylalaninaemia. Liver phenylalanine hydroxylase activities have been normal and there has been continued clinical deterioration in spite of adequate dietary control. In these patients there is defective synthesis of tetrahydrobiopterin or of biopterin from dihydrobiopterin. As tetrahydrobiopterin is the cofactor for phenylalanine hydroxylase its deficiency prevents the conversion of phenylalanine to tyrosine even though the phenylalanine hydroxylase enzyme is normal. Deficiencies of tetrahydrobiopterin will also interfere with the conversion of tyrosine to dihydroxyphenylalanine (DOPA) and noradrenaline and the conversion of tryptophan to serotonin, as tetrahydrobiopterin is also a cofactor for the enzymes involved. These tetrahydrobiopterin defects are found in about 1% of hyperphenylalaninaemic children and treatment is with tetrahydrobiopterin L-DOPA (dihydroxyphenylalanine) and L-5-hydroxytryptophan and a peripheral decarboxylase inhibitor. There is a blood spot screening test available for total blood biopterin and this should be done in all hyperphenylalaninaemic children. The diagnosis of dihydropteridine reductase deficiency can be made prenatally on amniotic fluid cells and underlying gene defects have been identified. Other instances of hyperphenylalaninaemia may be due to deficiency of phenylalanine transaminase which converts phenylalanine to phenylpyruvic acid and in these patients neither an increased protein intake nor a phenylalanine load would result in phenylketonuria. In this group of patients, not only diagnosis but the question of management raises considerable anxiety. Finally, in some infants there seems to be only a delayed maturation of one or more enzyme systems, especially if they are prematurely born and receiving parenteral nutrition. Such infants, in whom the biochemical findings may mimic permanent hyperphenylalaninaemia, can only be identified when after a lapse of time there is normal restoration of enzyme activity. This emphasises the need for repeated serum phenylalanine estimations during treatment with a low-phenylalanine diet.

Clinical features

Untreated "classical" phenylketonurics have severe learning disorders (IQ 30 or lower). They are frequently blue-eyed, fair-haired and with fair skins. Eczema is often troublesome. Some have convulsions, athetosis and electroencephalographic changes. Many show psychotic features such as abnormal posturings with hands and fingers, repetitive movements such as head-banging or rocking to-and-fro and complete lack of interest in people as distinct from inaminate objects. The tendon reflexes are often accentuated. It should be noted that infants born homozygous for the phenylketonuric trait are not brain-damaged at birth. They only become so after they start to ingest phenylalanine in their milk.

Maternal PKU

As a consequence of defects of phenylalanine and tyrosine metabolism in the mother abnormalities have been reported among a large number of infants of phenylketonuric women. These include mental retardation, microcephaly, congenital heart disease and intrauterine growth retardation. Congenital anomalies are uncommon in the offspring of mothers with phenylalanine concentrations below 600 µmol/l at the time of conception. However, head size, birth-weight and intelligence have been shown to be inversely and linearly associated with maternal phenylalanine concentrations. Phenylalanine concentrations during pregnancy and in the period prior to conception should be maintained between 60 and 250 µmol/l. Effective contraception should be continued until control has been achieved. Biochemical monitoring should be at least twice weekly and careful fetal ultrasound examinations to assess fetal growth and anatomy should be performed. Restriction of maternal dietary phenylalanine with tyrosine supplementation when necessary begun prior to conception controls the blood phenylalanine level and metabolite accumulation in the pregnant mother with PKU just as it does in the child with PKU. Dietary treatment begun after conception seems to be much less effective. It is essential therefore that women with PKU should be appropriately counselled and supported so that their children are conceived under the best possible phenylalanine control.

TABLE 16.1 Nutrient analysis of products for phenylketonuria

	MANUFACTURER	PHENYLALANINE (mg)	N EQUIV IN g OF PROTEIN	CHO (g)	FAT (g)	Kcal	kJ
Infant feeds per 100 ml							
Analog XP	SHS*	0	1.95	8.1	3.5	70	292
Minafen	Cow & Gate	3	1.7	6.5	4.2	69	290
Lofenalac	Mead Johnstone	12.2	2.3	9.2	2.8	68	288
Amino-acid mixtures per 100 g							
XP Albumaid	SHS	<10	33	50	0	320	1350
Albumaid XP Conc	SHS	<25	70	0	0	280	1190
Aminogran Food Supplement	UCB Pharma	0	82	0	0	400	1675
XP Maxamaid	SHS	0	25	51	<0.5	300	1260
XP Maxamum	SHS	0	39	34	<0.5	290	1226
Milupa PKU1	Milupa	0	50	19.3	0	278	1183
Milupa PKU2	Milupa	0	67	7.6	0	298	1265
Milupa PKU3	Milupa	0	68	3.4	0	286	1214
PK Aid 3	SHS	0	82	0	0	330	1400

*SHS, Scientific Hospital Supplies Ltd.

Diagnosis

When it became clear that a low-phenylalanine diet improved the intelligence of patients with PKU the need for early diagnosis, before intellectual impairment had occurred, was recognised. This requirement demands the "screening" of all newborn infants in a community. Those infants found to give a positive result with the screening test require to be submitted to more detailed confirmatory tests.

Screening tests

The presence of phenylpyruvic acid in the urine can be quickly detected by adding a few drops of 5 or 10% aqueous solution of ferric chloride to 5 ml of acidified urine, when a green colour will rapidly develop. Alternatively, a wet napkin can be tested with Phenistix (Ames & Co.) which is pressed between two layers of the napkin to be followed by a similar green colour. This technique was widely adopted as a screening test in the United Kingdom but was soon shown in practice to have real limitations in that many cases (45%) were missed during the neonatal period. The neonatal screening programmes which are now used permit the accurate detection of infants who have raised blood phenylalanine levels from the fifth day of life. Such infants are clearly suspect for PKU and demand confirmatory investigations. As we have already noted, some of these infants will have hyperphenylalaninaemia without phenylketonuria. The most commonly used screening test for raised blood phenylalanine in the United Kingdom at the present time is the Guthrie bacterial inhibition test which has been proved to be extremely reliable. There are, however, several other accurate methods for the detection of hyperphenylalaninaemia such as spectrofluorimetry or one-dimensional chromatography of plasma. Both the Guthrie test and chromatog-

raphy can be modified to "screen" for several other inborn errors such as galactosaemia, tyrosinaemia, homocystinuria, maple syrup urine disease and histidinaemia. The former test is, indeed, being so used now in some areas of the United Kingdom. Blood for the test is obtained from a heel stab between the fourth and 11th day of life, either by hospital staff or the Health Visitor in the baby's home.

Confirmation of the diagnosis of PKU

All infants in whom the Guthrie or other screening test has shown a blood phenylalanine of more than 240 μmol/l (4 mg/100 ml) on two occasions should be further investigated. The urine of an affected infant may be noted to have a mousy smell caused by phenylacetic acid.

Treatment

The accepted dietary treatment of phenylketonuria consists of reducing the intake of phenylalanine to a level which will prevent serious hyperphenylalaninaemia. A low phenylalanine diet cannot fully substitute for the phenylalanine turnover normally exerted by hepatic phenylalanine hydroxylase. As most food proteins contain phenylalanine it is obvious that a low phenylalanine diet must be largely synthetic and consequently expensive. Such a diet is complex and depends on the use of manufactured substitutes for many natural foods (Tables 16.1 and 16.2). There is, however, strong evidence that phenylalanine (Phe) restriction can prevent mental retardation if treatment is started during the first 3 weeks of life. Infant screening programmes now instituted have resulted in the untreated older sufferer from PKU becoming a rarity.

In infancy we prefer to start treatment with a low Phe protein hydrolysate with added tyrosine, tryptophan, carbohydrate, fat, minerals and some vitamins

TABLE 16.2 Low-protein products prescribable for phenylketonuria and other metabolic conditions

BREAD, ROLLS & PIZZAS

Juvela (SHS*)

Low-protein loaf (vacuum packed, sliced & unsliced)	400 g
Low-protein bread rolls (vacuum packed)	5 × 70 g pack

Loprofin (Nutricia)

Low-protein loaf (vacuum packed, sliced & unsliced)	400 g
Low-protein white bread with salt	227 g tin

Rite-Diet (Nutricia)

Low-protein white bread (with added fibre, vacuum packed)	400 g

Ultra (Ultrapharm)

Low-protein & gluten-free white bread (NB the brown bread is *not* suitable)	350 g tin
Ultra PKU bread	6 × 400 g loaves
Ultra PKU pizza base – vacuum packed	5 × 80 g pizzas

FLOUR

Aproten (Ultrapharm)

Low-protein gluten-free bread mix	250 g box
Low-protein gluten-free cake mix	300 g box
Low-protein gluten-free flour	500 g box

Juvela (SHS)

Low-protein mix	450 g box

Loprofin (Nutricia)

Low-protein flour mix	500 g box

Rite-Diet (Nutricia)

Low-protein flour mix	400 g box
Low-protein baking mix	500 g box

Ultra (Ultrapharm)

PKU flour mix	500 g box

Aproten (Ultrapharm)

Crispbread	200 g box
Low protein biscuits	200 g box

dp (Nutricia)

Chocolate chip cookies	170 g box
Butterscotch chip cookies	170 g box

Juvela (SHS)

Gluten-free low protein

orange cookies	175 g box
cinnamon cookies	175 g box
chocolate chip cookies	175 g box

Loprofin (Nutricia)

Cinnamon cookies	100 g box
Chocolate chip cookies	100 g box
Sweet biscuits	150 g box

Cream wafers

vanilla	100 g box
chocolate	100 g box
orange	100 g box
Chocolate cream filled biscuits	125 g box
Crackers	150 g box

Ultra (Ultrapharm)

PKU Savoy biscuits	150 g box
PKU cookies	250 g box
PKU biscuits	250 g box

PASTA & RICE

Aproten Pasta (Ultrapharm)

Anellini (tiny pasta rings)	250 g box
Ditalini (small macaroni)	250 g box
Rigatini (ribbed)	250 g box
Tagliatelli (flat noodles)	250 g box
Spaghetti	500 g box

Loprofin Low Protein Pasta (Nutricia)

Macaroni	250 g box
Spaghetti – short cut	250 g box
Spirals	250 g box

Aglutella (Ultrapharm)

Low-protein rice	500 g box

Organ (Foodwatch Health Products Ltd)

Low-protein pasta	250 g pkt
Low-protein annelini	250 g pkt
Low-protein rigati ribbons	250 g pkt

Promin (Firstplay Dietary Foods Ltd)

Low-protein + gluten-free pasta

shells	250 g pkt
short-cut spaghetti	250 g pkt
macaroni	250 g pkt
spirals	250 g pkt

Low-protein + gluten-free tricolour pasta

spirals	250 g pkt
shells	250 g pkt
alphabets	250 g pkt

The following are only prescribable for phenylketonuria:

Loprofin PKU drink (Nutricia)	200 ml carton
Sno-Pro (SHS)	200 ml carton

Not all of these products will be suitable for your child. Please check with your dietitian if you need any of these foods.

MISCELLANEOUS

Calogen (SHS)	1 & 2 litre bottles
Maxijul Super Soluble (SHS)	560 g or 2.5 kg tin
Duocal Super Soluble (SHS)	400 g tin
Metabolic Mineral Mixture (SHS)	100 g tub
Aminogram Mineral Mixture (Ultrapharm)	250 g tub

Flavour Module System (SHS)

Orange, blackcurrant, pineapple, savoury tomato 100 g tub
(*NB*: only to be used for *unflavoured* Maxamaid and *unflavoured* Maxamum)

Duobar (SHS)

Protein-free energy bar: vanilla and strawberry flavours 100 g bar

Loprofen (Nutricia)

Low-protein egg replacer	250 g tub

Suitable low protein products not available on prescription. These can be bought in large branches of "Boots the Chemist" or some health food shops will stock them:

Rite-Diet (Nutricia)

Tinned low-protein gluten-free spaghetti in tomato sauce	375 g can
Tinned low-protein gluten-free macaroni in mushroom sauce	375 g can
Egg white replacer	75 g tub

(Table 16.1). The bottle fed infant's dietary phenyl-alanine is obtained from measured quantities of proprietary baby milk which should be sufficient to maintain the blood phenylalanine concentration between 182 and 484 µmol/l (3 and 8 mg/100 ml). The baby milk is divided between the day's feeds and given prior to the low Phe feed. The low Phe feed is fed to satiety although care must be taken to ensure that the infant's nutritional needs are met.

Breast fed infants obtain phenylalanine from their mother's milk. Human milk contains less phenylalanine than baby milk formulae so that more mother's milk and less low Phe formula is required to control the infant's blood phenylalanine concentrations. Mothers are encouraged to continue breast feeding on demand but prior to three or four of the breast feeds low Phe formula 15–20 ml/kg (i.e. 60 ml/kg/day) is given. The volumes of low Phe formula given are adjusted to maintain a blood phenylalanine concentration of 120–360 µmol/l (2–6 mg/100 ml).

Mixed feeding should be introduced between 4 and 6 months. Infants who are not breast fed should initially have solids containing negligible amounts of phenylalanine, e.g. strained vegetables and fruit, Aminex low-protein biscuits (Cow & Gate) or manufactured baby foods known to have a very low phenylalanine content. Breast fed infants should be introduced to solids which contain some phenylalanine. Initially 50 mg phenylalanine should be given, e.g. one Farley's rusk or specific quantities of baby foods known to contain 50 mg phenylalanine. Close and relatively frequent monitoring of the blood phenylalanine levels is necessary at this stage to ensure a correct balance between the amounts of phenylalanine received from solid food and the amount received from breast milk.

Between the ages of 9 and 12 months a gradual changeover from low phenylalanine milks to one of the amino-acid mixtures can be given (Table 16.1). This is necessary because of the relatively low protein value of preparations such as Minafen. We have adopted a diet which is easy to prepare and reasonably acceptable to the child. The parents of young children starting solid food are given food tables indicating the weight of individual foodstuffs which contain 50 mg phenylalanine (one phenylalanine exchange). The number of exchanges required will be determined by regular measurements of the child's blood phenylalanine levels. By this means the child's food preferences can best be catered for. Fruit and vegetables (except peas and beans) can be given without restriction. The same applies to the low-protein foods shown in Table 16.2 and which are prescribable under the National Health Service in the UK.

On this diet a child can sit down to a meal which, apart from the lack of meat and other protein, looks very like that of the rest of the family. PKU children can be taken to hotels and holiday camps, and we have experienced no difficulty in arranging for schools to provide the special diet. Indeed, we have been told that sometimes the child's classmates envy them their special diet.

The dietary treatment of phenylketonuria has been considered in some detail because the same principles are applicable in several of the other inborn errors of metabolism which involve the essential amino acids. It will be obvious to the reader that the adequate treatment of the inborn errors of metabolism requires that such patients attend special centres with the necessary dietetic and laboratory facilities. Children with phenylketonuria vary greatly in their tolerance to phenylalanine and the frequency of blood testing will need to be more in some than in others. In general we test blood phenylalanine concentration weekly up to the age of 4 years, every 2 weeks thereafter up to the age of 10 years and thereafter monthly. The parents require constant guidance and support particularly from the dietitian and, indeed, the factors which mostly determine whether a child does well intellectually are the intelligence and sense of responsibility of the parents. It is, of course, important also to perform psychometric tests of a type suitable for age and development periodically throughout childhood. There are as yet no clear guidelines to indicate whether the special diet can be stopped. At the present time we recommend that the diet should be continued for life.

There has been a striking difference in the state of the children who attend a PKU Clinic over the past 30 years. Then, most were retarded. Some did quite well on their special diet, but others remained on the diet for only a short period before it was decided that they were too late for significant improvement. Even although treated individuals may achieve a high academic status there can be subtle global impairment determined by the degree of control in the early years of treatment. Magnetic resonance imaging is revealing abnormal myelin structure in most adolescents and adults with phenylalanine concentrations greater than 400 µmol/l. Overt neurological deterioration is found in some. It is now evident that we must aim for very strict control in earlier life, promote a policy of lifetime treatment and ensure a strict diet pre-conception in women likely to conceive. Effective safe gene therapy may be a reality in the not too distant future.

OTHER DISTURBANCES OF AMINO-ACID METABOLISM

Tyrosinaemia

Hereditary tyrosinaemia type I (hepatorenal tyrosinaemia) is due to a deficiency of the enzyme fumarylacetoacetase. The gene defect is in chromosome 15 (q23–q25). It presents acutely in the newborn infant with failure to thrive, vomiting, diarrhoea, hepatomegaly and bleeding disorder with bruising, haematemesis, melaena and haematuria. Plasma and urinary concentrations of tyrosine and methionine are increased and death from haemorrhage and liver failure is common. Patients with a more chronic form may occur within the same family and have, in addition to liver disease, renal tubular dysfunction, hypophosphataemia and rickets. In later life hepatoma develops in more than half of those surviving the first year and many develop hepatic cirrhosis and episodes of severe acute peripheral neuropathy. Treatment with a low phenylalanine, low tyrosine diet may improve the clinical state and reduce the urinary excretion of succinylacetone and tyrosine. Liver transplantation at an early stage should be considered to avoid hepatocellular carcinomas and the renal tubular problems.

Tyrosinaemia type 2 (oculocutaneous tyrosinaemia) is due to a deficiency of tyrosine aminotransferase. This disorder, like the type 1 defect, is inherited in an autosomal recessive mode. It is characterised by lacrimation, photophobia with tyrosine crystals in the cornea and with associated dendritic keratitis and ulcers. Keratitis also affects the skin and mental retardation is a feature in some affected children. Early treatment with a low phenylalanine/low tyrosine diet offers a good prognosis. The gene defect is on chromosome 16 (q22–q24). The inheritance is autosomal recessive. The primary enzymatic defect is a reduced activity of fumarylacetoacetase. Mental retardation is not a feature of hereditary tyrosinaemia.

Alkaptonuria

Alkaptonuria is due to deficiency of homogentisate oxidase so that homogentisic acid, instead of being converted to maleylacetoacetate, accumulates in the tissues and is excreted in the urine. The urine is noted to turn dark on standing or it can be made to do so immediately by the addition of ammonia or sodium hydroxide. The alkaptonuric is symptomless in childhood but in adult life develops ochronosis. This causes an ochre-like pigmentation of sclerae, ears, nasal cartilages and tendon sheaths, also kyphosis and osteoarthritis of the large joints. The disease is usually inherited as an autosomal recessive. A few families have shown dominant inheritance. There is no specific treatment.

Total albinism

Another disturbance which also arises from defective metabolism of the aromatic amino acids is total albinism. Consanguineous mating has been especially frequently recorded in this autosomal recessive trait. One of the various pathways of tyrosine metabolism is its conversion to 3,4-dihydroxyphenylalanine (DOPA) by the enzyme tyrosinase. This is converted to DOPA quinone which is then converted to melanin. In albinism tyrosinase is lacking. The patients are exceedingly fair-skinned and fair-haired with red pupils and pink or bluish irises. Astigmatism and nystagmus are common. Some are mentally backward. The only available treatment is to protect the eyes and skin from bright sunshine and to correct any refractive errors.

DISORDERS OF BRANCHED-CHAIN AMINO-ACID METABOLISM

Maple syrup urine disease

In maple syrup urine disease (MSUD) so called because the urine from affected infants has an odour (sweet, malty, caramel-like) of maple syrup or burnt sugar, neurological disturbances appear soon after birth, e.g. difficulties with feeding, absence of the Moro reflex, irregular respirations, spasticity and opisthotonus. Pronounced dehydration and metabolic acidosis are not features of acute MSUD in contrast to other disorders of organic acid metabolism. Death occurs within a few months. Early diagnosis and management are essential to prevent permanent brain damage. The ferric chloride test on the urine gives a colour reaction which could be mistaken for phenylpyruvic acid. Urine chromatography will reveal abnormally high concentrations of the branched-chain amino acids valine, leucine and isoleucine and of their corresponding keto and hydroxy acids. The abnormal presence in the urine of the hydroxy acids, which are responsible for the characteristic smell, suggests that the keto acids are reduced by an abnormal pathway, due to deficiency of the branched-chain 2-oxoacetodehydrogenase. The enzyme defect can be demonstrated in leucocytes and patients' cultured skin fibroblasts and it is also possible to detect heterozygous carriers by this technique.

Treatment and prognosis

Very high blood and tissue levels of branched-chain amino acids in the acutely ill newborn will require urgent treatment in the form of haemodialysis, peritoneal dialysis or blood exchange transfusions. Long-term treatment by a life-long diet low in the three branched-chain amino acids has been successful in preventing the manifestations of this disease when diagnosis was made very soon after birth

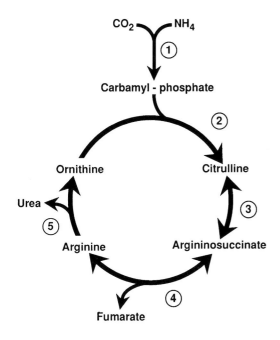

FIGURE 16.2 The ornithine–urea cycle.

① = Carbamyl phosphate synthetase

② = Ornithine transcarbamylase

③ = Argininosuccinate synthetase

④ = Argininosuccinate cleavage system

⑤ = Arginase

the most commonly encountered abnormal organic acidaemias in children. There is at present an ever-increasing number of errors of intermediary metabolism being identified using these techniques and in some effective therapies are available.

Infants with isovaleric, propionic and methylmalonic acidaemias have many symptoms in common. Babies after an initial symptom-free period may present with feeding difficulties, vomiting, lethargy, respiratory distress, hypotonia and generalised hypertonic episodes. Metabolic acidosis, ketonuria, hyperammonaemia, hypocarnitinaemia, neutropenia and thrombocytopenia are almost constant findings. The acute presentation is frequently precipitated by infection or some other form of stress. Treatment includes stopping all protein intake and maintenance with dextrose and bicarbonate to control acidosis. The emergency treatment of organic acidurias consists of removal of toxins by haemodialysis or peritoneal dialysis and/or blood exchange transfusions. In addition glycine in isovaleric, biotin in propionic and vitamin B_{12} in methylmalonic acidaemias should be given in all cases. L-carnitine (125 mg/kg/day) should be given to patients with all three disorders. The long-term treatment involves reducing accumulated toxic products, maintaining normal nutritional status and preventing catabolism. Therefore in these children protein intake is largely restricted. Prenatal diagnosis can be made by enzyme studies in amniotic fluid cells and in uncultured chorionic villi as early as the 12th week of gestation.

Supplementation with an amino-acid mixture lacking the branched-chain amino acids is necessary in a protein restricted diet. The long-term outcome depends on early diagnosis and management. Prenatal diagnosis is possible by enzyme studies on culture amniotic fluid cells and on chorionic villi.

ORGANIC ACIDAEMIAS

There are now described more than 30 inherited conditions characterised by an excessive urinary excretion of acidic metabolites of amino acids, carbohydrates and fats. Infants with otherwise unexplained metabolic acidosis who become acutely ill should have plasma and urine levels of a specific organic acid and its byproducts analysed by gas chromatography and mass spectrometry (GLC-MS) in order to detect conditions such as 3-methylcrotonyl glycinuria, isovaleric acidaemia, glutaric aciduria, propionic acidaemia and methylmalonic acidaemia. Of these, propionic and methylmalonic acidaemias constitute

UREA CYCLE DISORDERS

Only an outline of those biochemical reactions responsible for the breakdown of amino acids leading to the formation of ammonia which is then converted into urea and CO_2 will be presented here (Fig. 16.2). This requires five enzymes (the ornithine–urea cycle). Carbamyl phosphate synthetase converts ammonia and bicarbonate to carbamyl phosphate which then condenses with ornithine under the action of ornithine transcarbamylase to form citrulline. The conversion of citrulline to argininosuccinic acid is catalysed by argininosuccinate synthetase, and argininosuccinic acid is cleaved to form arginine and fumaric acid by argininosuccinate cleavage enzyme (argininosuccinase). The enzyme arginase finally converts arginine into urea and ornithine. This synthetic process takes place in the liver and at least some of the enzymes have also been demonstrated in brain tissue, red cells and fibroblast cultures. Defects in the activity of several of these enzymes have been associated with inborn errors of metabolism in each of which mental retardation is a prominent feature due either to the toxic effects of ammonia accumulation or to the toxic effects of urea-cycle intermediates in the brain. The mechanisms leading to the toxicity of ammonia are not fully understood. The clinical manifestations of urea-cycle disorders are mainly abnormalities secondary to hyperammonaemia and protein intolerance. A rapid diagnosis and institution of diet is essential for a good prognosis.

Hyperammonaemia

Hyperammonaemia can be due to deficiency of ornithine transcarbamylase which is inherited as an X-linked trait affecting males with variable expression in the female, and in which increased amounts of orotic acid are found in the urine; or of carbamyl phosphate synthetase. Signs usually develop in infancy with failure to thrive, vomiting, floppiness, increasing developmental delay and episodic lethargy. A positive association between the clinical features and protein intake is a valuable diagnostic clue and episodes of coma with convulsive twitchings have been provoked by a high protein intake. The fasting plasma ammonia level is usually greatly elevated, e.g. 205–704 µmol/l (350–1200 µg/100 ml) as against the normal range of <35 µmol/l (<60 µg/100 ml). Diagnosis is confirmed by assay of the urea-cycle enzymes in liver biopsy material. In suspected cases the institution of a high-carbohydrate, protein-free diet often produces a dramatic improvement after a few days. Plasma amino acids and urinary orotate levels when measured in hyperammonaemic, non-acidotic infants provide positive identification of the specific enzyme deficiency. Long-term treatment is with a low-protein diet but the condition shows a variable clinical expression in age of onset and severity of symptoms. Even with early institution of a low-protein diet and prompt treatment of metabolic crises, prognosis for normal development is guarded.

Argininaemia

Argininaemia presents in childhood with hyperammonaemia, vomiting and retarded development with spastic quadriplegia, convulsions and hepatomegaly. Plasma and CSF arginine concentrations are grossly elevated and the urine contains excessive quantities of cystine, lysine, ornithine, arginine and citrulline. Arginase deficiency can be demonstrated in erythrocytes.

Citrullinaemia

Citrullinaemia arises from a deficiency of argininosuccinate synthetase and produces a clinical picture similar to that seen in hyperammonaemia, i.e. mental retardation, episodic vomiting and coma with convulsions. The disorder is transmitted as an autosomal recessive trait. Raised levels of citrulline are found in the plasma, urine and cerebrospinal fluid and the plasma ammonia level rises sharply following protein-rich diet and during intercurrent viral and other illnesses, particularly if calorie intake is reduced so that the child becomes catabolic. Defective enzyme activity can be demonstrated in liver and skin fibroblasts. Prenatal diagnosis is possible by demonstrating enzyme deficiency in cultured amniotic cells. A low protein diet and arginine supplement is worth a trial.

Argininosuccinic aciduria

Argininosuccinic aciduria is due to a deficiency of the argininosuccinate cleavage enzyme. There is a severe often fatal neonatal form and a late onset form in which there is severe mental retardation. Convulsive seizures, EEG abnormalities and ataxia may be present. In some children the hair is short and brittle (trichorrhexis nodosa). Argininosuccinic acid is normally present in very low concentrations in body fluids but in this disease high concentrations are found in the urine and cerebrospinal fluid. Deficiency of the enzyme may be demonstrated in liver, fibroblasts or erythrocytes. This disease is inherited as an autosomal recessive. The only treatment available is a restricted protein intake as the plasma ammonia level may be intermittently elevated. Prenatal diagnosis is possible either by demonstrating enzyme deficiency in cultured amniotic fluid cells or the presence of large amounts of argininosuccinic acid in amniotic fluid.

Ornithinaemia

Ornithinaemia can occur in association with homocitrullinaemia when there is deficiency of ornithine decarboxylase. There is mental retardation, ataxia and hyperammonaemia. There is a second type in which there is no hyperammonaemia or homocitrullinaemia but mental retardation, hepatic and renal disease and a generalised aminoaciduria are major features associated with a defect in hepatic ornithine keto-acid transaminase. A third type presents usually with a visual defect and bizarre changes in the optic fundi due to gyrate atrophy of the choroid and retinae associated with a defect in ornithine amino transferase. Low-ornithine diets may help.

In urea-cycle disorders with hyperammonaemia the blood ammonia can be reduced with haemodialysis. Maintenance therapy with sodium benzoate, phenyl acetate or phenylbutyrate may reduce persistent hyperammonaemia and can be given IV in acute episodes.

HISTIDINAEMIA

Histidinaemia is due to a deficiency of histidase which normally catalyses the conversion of histidine to urocanic acid. The urine contains considerable quantities of imidazolepyruvic, imidazoleacetic and imidazolelactic acids. The first of these substances reacts positively with ferric chloride solution and could lead to an erroneous diagnosis of phenylketonuria. There has always been doubt as to whether the biochemical abnormality relates to any clinical manifestations. However, prospective studies of untreated siblings with histidinaemia ascertained through probands and early detected but untreated children have indicated that the prevalence of impaired intellectual or speech development, convulsions, behavioural or learning disorders is not greater than in the non-histidinaemic population. Routine screening for early diagnosis is, therefore, probably not justifiable.

DISORDERS OF THE SULPHUR-CONTAINING AMINO ACIDS

Homocystinuria

Homocystinuria is the most common defect of the sulphur-containing amino acids. Inheritance is as an autosomal recessive, and the defect is in cystathionine β-synthetase. This enzyme catalyses the condensation of homocysteine (derived from methionine) with serine to form cystathionine. The result of this enzyme block in homocystinuria is accumulation of homocysteine in blood and tissues, and its excretion in the urine in its oxidised form, homocystine. There will also be raised blood levels of methionine. Cystathionine levels in the brain are grossly reduced. Usually the four systems involved are the eye, the skeleton, the central nervous system and the vascular system. The fully developed clinical picture includes mental retardation, seizures, malar flush, fair hair, downward dislocation of the lens, livido reticularis and thromboembolic episodes in both arteries and veins. Skeletal changes have been common, e.g. genu valgum, pes cavus, arachnodactyly, irregular epiphyses, vertebral changes, osteoporosis and pectus carinatum or excavatum. The fully developed picture resembles that of Marfan syndrome (Marfanoid habitus of the body) but in the latter there is no mental retardation, no osteoporosis, no thrombotic tendency, the dislocation of the lens is upwards and inheritance is dominant. Some children with homocystinuria exhibit a characteristic shuffling or "Charlie Chaplin" gait; others have shown severe

fatty change in the liver with little disturbance of liver function tests. Epileptic seizures may also occur. On the other hand, a considerable number of patients have a normal level of intelligence and not all cases are associated with the progressive deterioration described above.

The diagnosis can be made early in infancy during screening programmes, and before clinical abnormalities have become manifest. A simple screening test when the diagnosis is suspected in the older patient is the nitroprusside/cyanide test which does not, however, discriminate between an excess of cystine or homocystine in the urine. A positive reaction is an indication for chromatographic examination of blood and urine for increased concentrations of homocystine or methionine. When treatment is started in the neonatal period with a diet low in methionine, plus cystine supplements, normal development may be expected. Suitable amino-acid mixtures with added cystine are now commercially available from Scientific Hospital Supplies Ltd.* Monitoring of treatment requires that the blood methionine be kept below 67 μmol/l (1 mg/100 ml) and that there should be very low levels of homocystine in the blood and urine; it is also important to watch the blood cystine level. There are two distinct types of homocystinuria in that some cases respond completely to treatment with pyridoxine 150–450 mg/day alone. The treatment is more successful when the diagnosis is made early. Prenatal diagnosis can be made by enzymatic assay in cultured amniotic cells and chorionic villi.

It should be noted that Scientific Hospital Supplies Ltd manufacture a range of protein substitutes for a variety of inherited metabolic disorders including phenylketonuria, maple syrup urine disease, tyrosinaemia, homocystinuria, hyperlysinaemia, urea-cycle disorders and organic acidurias.

GALACTOSAEMIA

Aetiology

Classical galactosaemia (transferase deficiency) is another example of autosomal recessive inheritance and it results from the combination in one individual of two recessive genes.

Pathogenesis

Galactose is ingested as lactose in milk which undergoes splitting in the intestine into its component

---

*Scientific Hospital Supplies Group UK Ltd, 100 Wavertree Boulevard, Wavertree Technology Park, Liverpool L7 9PT, UK.

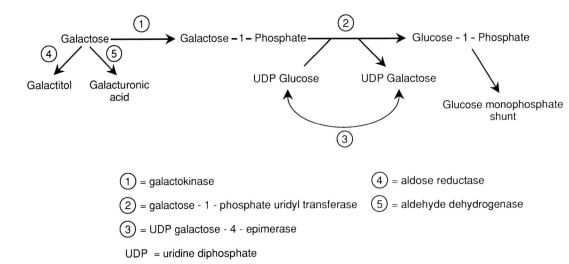

(1) = galactokinase   (4) = aldose reductase

(2) = galactose - 1 - phosphate uridyl transferase   (5) = aldehyde dehydrogenase

(3) = UDP galactose - 4 - epimerase

UDP = uridine diphosphate

FIGURE 16.3 Enzyme steps in galactose metabolism in erythrocytes.

monosaccharides glucose and galactose. Milk and its products is virtually the sole source of dietary galactose in man. Galactose is then converted to glucose or energy in a series of enzyme steps (Fig. 16.3). Although the liver is the main site of this conversion, the demonstration of a similar series of enzyme reactions in red cells and the excess accumulation of galactose-l-phosphate in the erythrocytes from galactosaemic patients made it likely that the defect lay in the activity of galactose-l-phosphate uridyltransferase and in the inability to convert galactose-1-phosphate to glucose-1-phosphate (step 2 in Fig. 16.3). The accumulation in the erythrocytes of galactose-1-phosphate, believed to be the major toxic substance in galactosaemia is evidence that hexokinase activity is normal. In fact, galactosaemic red cells have been confirmed to be defective in Gal-1-P uridyltransferase and a similar deficiency has been demonstrated in liver tissue from affected patients. Gal-1-P uridyltransferase is absent in all tissues and the enzyme deficiency persists throughout life.

Clinical features

Two main clinical types occur. The more severe develops its clinical features within 2 weeks of birth, after milk feeding has been started, with vomiting, disinclination to feed, diarrhoea, loss of weight, dehydration, hypoglycaemia, hepatocellular damage and renal tubular damage. The liver is enlarged with a firm, smooth edge and there may be jaundice. Splenomegaly is common. Cataracts may be seen with a slit-lamp. Finally the infant becomes severely marasmic with hepatic cirrhosis, ascites and hypoprothrombinaemia. Obvious signs and symptoms are later to appear in the less severe type although a

history suggesting some early intolerance of milk ma be obtained. The child may present with menta retardation, bilateral cataracts and cirrhosis of th liver. The explanation for the less severe cases ma be the existence of an alternative pathway for galac tose metabolism in the liver. All the abnormalities i this disease save the mental retardation may regres rapidly on a galactose-free diet. It is, therefore, c prime importance that the diagnosis be made befor irreversible brain damage has occurred. Undiagnose cases may succumb to Gram-negative sepsis.

Diagnosis

The first clue to the disease may be the finding of reducing substance in the urine. Proteinuria may als be present. However, although the Benedict test : positive, tests based on the enzyme glucose oxidas (Clinistix) will be negative. Clinistix measures urin glucose specifically and instead a method for measur ing total reducing substances (Clinitest) must be usec Chromatography will then confirm that the reducin substance is galactose. There is, also, marke aminoaciduria due to renal tubular damage Galactitol can be detected in blood and urine an may be a major factor in the toxic damage to th developing infant tissues. A valuable method c diagnosis, which can be used for umbilical-cor blood testing in the infant born into a known galac tosaemic family and before milk feeds have startec is the demonstration of the absence of galactose-1 phosphate uridyltransferase activity in the red cell An alternative test for use in the newborn is based o the excess accumulation of galactose-1-phosphate i the erythrocytes in this disease. Heterozygous carrie of the gene can be detected by quantitative estimatio of Gal-1-P uridyltransferase activity in erythrocytes. It is possible to "screen" for galactosaemia during the neonatal period by a modified Guthrie test or chromatography of heel-stab blood and to start treatment before clinical features have appeared. Prenatal diagnosis by amniotic fluid cell enzyme assay is possible. In some commoner gene defects prenatal diagnosis and heterozygote testing can be performed using gene probes for the defects on chromosome 9 (p13).

Treatment

The infant should be placed on a diet that is milk free and free from all products made with milk. When previously affected siblings are known to exist the diagnosis can and should be confirmed before the infant receives his first milk feed. Suitable milk substitutes which are almost free from lactose are Galactomin 17 (Cow & Gate) and Nutramigen and Pregestimil (Bristol-Myers) or any of the proprietary soya-based baby milks, e.g. Formula S (Cow & Gate), Prosobee (Bristol-Myers) and Wysoy (Wyeth). Supplementary vitamins and minerals must be given if Galactomin 17 is used. Dietary restriction should be fairly strict during the first 2 years and probably there should be some life-long restriction of milk and milk products intake. Unfortunately, galactosaemic children tend to fall below the average in mental development in spite of dietary treatment, although they remain within the educable range and have good physical health. They may also exhibit psychological disturbances, a phenomenon previously noted in phenylketonuric children also maintained on rigid dietary control. Now it is clear that the current methods of treatment, even if strictly followed, may not ameliorate the long-term sequelae which occur regardless of when treatment was commenced. As adolescents, many develop educational difficulties, memory loss and abnormal neurological findings including ataxia, inco-ordination and brisk reflexes. Young women develop ovarian cysts and poor ovarian function with subfertility. Therefore a guarded prognosis should be given to parents of newly diagnosed cases. Maternal restriction of galactose is usually recommended to prevent prenatal damage in pregnancies known to be at risk of producing a galactosaemic infant. However, it is not established that this is effective.

Galactokinase deficiency

While the term "galactosaemia" has become established to denote the serious disease described above, an elevated blood galactose level may also result from a deficiency of the enzyme galactokinase by which galactose is phosphorylated to galactose-1-phosphate

(Fig. 16.3). Galactokinase deficiency is also an autosomal recessive disorder associated with galactosuria, but the only significant pathology is the development of cataracts which may be nuclear or zonular and is due to accumulation in the lens of galactitol. Liver, renal and brain damage do not occur. The dietary treatment as for galactosaemia prevents the development of cataracts and should be started as early in infancy as possible.

Epimerase deficiency

Deficiency of epimerase enzyme may produce a clinical picture similar to that of the transferase defect or may be asymptomatic. Those affected also, if symptomatic, respond to milk-free diets.

HEREDITARY FRUCTOSE INTOLERANCE

Aetiology

This disease causes severe metabolic disturbances and it is inherited as an autosomal recessive trait. It must be clearly distinguished from benign frustosuria which is due to a deficiency of fructokinase and which produces no clinical disease.

Pathogenesis

The metabolic pathways of fructose are complicated. The primary enzymatic defect is in fructose-1-phosphate aldolase which in the liver and intestine splits fructose-l-phosphate into two trioses, glyceraldehyde and dihydroxyacetone phosphate. This defect results in the accumulation of fructose-1-phosphate which inhibits fructokinase and leads to high blood levels of fructose after its ingestion in the diet. The mechanisms which produce gastrointestinal symptoms and hypoglucosaemia in affected infants are not yet fully understood but the intracellular accumulation of fructose-1-phosphate probably prevents the conversion of liver glycogen to glucose.

Clinical features

Symptoms only appear when fructose is introduced into the diet as sucrose in milk feeds, as sorbitol or as fruit juices. The condition tends to be more severe the earlier the exposure to fructose. They vary in severity, partly according to the amounts of fructose ingested, and the wholly breast fed infant remains symptomless. Common features are failure to thrive, severe marasmus, anorexia, vomiting, diarrhoea and hepatomegaly.

Hypoglucosaemia may cause convulsions or losses of consciousness. Liver damage may result in jaundice, and liver function tests give abnormal results. Albuminuria, fructosuria and excess aminoaciduria may be present. Hyperfructosaemia and hypoglucosaemia develop following upon the ingestion of fructose or sucrose (glucose + fructose). Death ensues in undiagnosed infants. In milder cases in older children gastrointestinal symptoms predominate, and in some a profound distaste of anything sweet develops spontaneously as a protective mechanism.

Diagnosis

The diagnosis is usually suspected because of its clinical presentation, by a dietary history and by a favourable response to removal of fructose from the diet. An oral fructose tolerance test (1 g/kg up to a maximum of 50 g) results in a marked and prolonged fall in the true blood glucose level and a fall in the inorganic phosphorus. There will also be raised blood levels of fructose, free fatty acids and lactic acid. Fructosuria may be detected.

Treatment

Early diagnosis is important. The treatment consists simply in the life-long removal of all fructose-containing foods from the diet and of sucrose from the milk feeds. Sorbitol, a fructose polymer, must not be used as a sweetening agent.

HYPOPHOSPHATASIA

Aetiology

This disease is transmitted as an autosomal recessive characteristic and the heterozygous carrier state can usually be detected. Heterozygotes may have low serum alkaline phosphatase concentrations, high urinary excretion of phosphoethanolamine, or both, without bone disease.

Pathogenesis

In some inborn errors of metabolism the absence of an enzyme activity is deduced indirectly from the demonstration that a metabolic pathway has gone wrong. In hypophosphatasia the enzyme which is defective (alkaline phosphatase) can be directly measured. Further evidence of the nature of hypophosphatasia was the demonstration by chromatography of an abnormal metabolite – phosphoethanolamine – in the plasma and urine of affected patients. Phosphoethanolamine seems to be a naturally occurring physiological substrate of alkaline phosphatase.

The consequence of this enzyme deficiency is a failure of mineralisation of the skeleton, both membranous and cartilaginous. Long bones at the metaphyses show a wide irregular zone of proliferative cartilage with disorganised maturation of the cells and no evidence of calcification of the intercellular matrix. Osteoid tissue is deposited on the cartilaginous intercellular substance and on the outside of the shafts, and as it is almost completely uncalcified, fractures readily occur. There is, however, no shortage of osteoblasts which are the normal source of alkaline phosphatase in bone.

Clinical features

Three clinical types of hypophosphatasia have been described: infantile, childhood and adult. In the infantile type the disease becomes obvious within a few weeks of birth. In one case, where a previous sibling had been affected, the diagnosis was established radiologically before birth. Many of the signs resemble those seen in rickets, e.g. enlarged epiphyses, "beading" of the ribs, kyphoscoliosis, bowing of the long bones which sometimes show spontaneous fractures, failure to thrive and hypocalcaemia. However, as the membranous bones are also affected the skull may be so poorly mineralised that it feels like a balloon filled with water. The anterior fontanelle and sutures may be wide and tense, but subsequently there may be premature fusion with microcephaly. In the childhood type the presenting sign may be premature loss of the deciduous teeth, increased susceptibility to infection and somatic retardation. Radiographs show an abnormal patchy calcification at the metaphyses producing an ill-defined margin distal to which there is a zone of poorly calcified osteoid. The epiphyseal lines are irregularly widened. There may also be periosteal elevation due to deposition of osteoid. The adult form may present with spontaneous fractures and radiolucent bones in the skeleton.

Diagnosis

The diagnosis should be based on a very low level of serum alkaline phosphatase for the patient's age. Biopsy of tissues normally rich in alkaline phosphatase, such as bone, will also show a greatly reduced enzyme content. The histological picture is generally indistinguishable from that of true rickets.

An inconstant but serious finding is hypercalcaemia. It may lead to renal failure. Abnormal quantities of phosphoethanolamine may be demonstrated in the urine and plasma of patients. Prenatal diagnosis of severe hypophosphatasia may be made by ultrasound evaluation of fetal skeletal calcification and reduced alkaline phosphatase activity in amniotic fluid or cells obtained from this fluid.

Treatment

Cases which are diagnosed in early infancy do not survive long. Treatment of children with hypophosphatasia with vitamin D has not been successful. At present there is no effective treatment for this condition.

DISORDERS OF PURINE AND PYRIMIDINE METABOLISM

Inherited disorders of purine and pyrimidine metabolism are rare disorders. In addition to gout and the previously described ADA and PNP deficiencies (see Chapter 14) there remains to be described two rare inherited disorders.

Hereditary orotic aciduria is an autosomal recessive condition in which there is failure to thrive, hypochromic anaemia with megaloblasts in the bone marrow, and increased urinary excretion of orotic acid. The underlying enzyme defect may involve one or both of the enzymes concerned in the synthesis of uridine monophosphate, orotate phosphoribosyltransferase and orotidylate decarboxylase. Treatment with uridine, 1 g/day, results in correction of the anaemia and impaired growth. Prenatal diagnosis of this disorder has never been performed although theoretically this is possible.

The Lesch–Nyhan syndrome is an X-linked recessive disorder in which male infants are generally normal at birth. It is characterised by central nervous system disorders of various types and excessive quantities of uric acid in blood, tissue and urine. The disorder is caused by deficiencies of the enzyme hypoxanthine-guanine phosphoribosyltransferase. Affected boys can be severely mentally retarded and have choreo-athetosis, spasticity and distressing compulsive self-mutilation, or they may present with gouty arthritis and pain from ureteric colic caused by urates. A definitive diagnosis of the Lesch–Nyhan syndrome can be made by demonstrating the absence of hypoxanthine-guanine phosphoribosyltransferase in the erythrocytes. Allopurinol and probenecid will reduce the hyperuricaemia but will not correct or help the neurological problems. Prenatal diagnosis can be made by the culture of cells obtained by amniocentesis.

CONGENITAL METHAEMOGLOBINAEMIA

Aetiology

The most common form of congenital methaemoglobinaemia is inherited as an autosomal recessive trait and it is due to the absence of a normal intra-erythrocytic enzyme activity. A rare type, inherited as an autosomal dominant, has a quite different aetiology in that it is due to the formation of an abnormal haemoglobin (haemoglobin M) with a defective globulin component.

Pathogenesis

In normal haemoglobin the iron of the four haem groups is in the reduced or ferrous state. In methaemoglobin the iron is in the oxidised or ferric state and it is incapable of combining with oxygen. In normal erythrocytes methaemoglobin is constantly being formed and in normal blood a small amount is always present. It is, however, continuously being reduced back to haemoglobin by a complex series of enzyme steps. In congenital methaemoglobinaemia there is an intra-erythrocytic defect in one of these enzyme reactions. The other form of congenital methaemoglobinaemia belongs to the haemoglobinopathies and haemoglobin M can be differentiated from normal haemoglobin by electrophoretic techniques.

Clinical picture

The primary sign is a dusky slate-grey type of cyanosis which is present from birth. It is free from respiratory or cardiac symptoms and clubbing of the fingers and toes does not develop. Some patients develop compensatory polycythaemia and some have been severely mentally retarded.

Diagnosis

The presence of excess methaemoglobin in the blood should be demonstrated by spectrophotometry.

It is important to distinguish the congenital and permanent form of methaemoglobinaemia from the temporary but dangerous acquired form, which may follow the entry into the body of certain poisons such as aniline dyes, nitrites, acetanilide and potassium chlorate. Outbreaks of acquired methaemoglobinaemia have occurred in newborn nurseries when new napkins marked by aniline dyes have been used before laundering and cases have occurred in children drinking well-water containing nitrites. Therefore assays of methaemoglobin reductase and detection of Hb-M are essential to confirm the specific diagnosis.

It is also important to remember that cyanotic children without heart murmurs may have methaemoglobinaemia. We have seen the mistaken diagnosis of congenital heart disease made in two such cases and, in fact, one child was unnecessarily submitted to cardiac catheterisation.

Treatment

Methaemoglobinaemia due to the deficiency of enzyme methaemoglobin reductase may respond to ascorbic acid 200–500 mg/day or methylene blue 5 mg/kg/day, given orally or intravenously. These drugs do not, however, have any beneficial effect in haemoglobin M disease.

GLYCOGEN STORAGE DISORDERS

Glycogen is a complex high molecular weight polysaccharide composed of numerous glucosyl units linked together in the form of many branches. It is mainly found in the liver and muscle. The glucosyl units are mainly linked together through carbon atoms 1 and 4 but at the branch points the bonds are between C1 and C6. Multiple enzymes are involved in the synthesis (glycogenesis) and breakdown (glycogenolysis) of glycogen. There are still several gaps and uncertainties which make classification of the metabolic errors of glycogen metabolism difficult. In practical paediatric practice, however, a somewhat oversimplified concept of these physiological steps will prove sufficient for the clinician's purpose. In health, human liver glycogen content varies from 0 to 5%, while muscle glycogen is rarely as high as 1%. Hepatic glycogen functions as a reserve of glucose and is utilised during fasting to maintain normoglycaemia.

Glycogenesis

Glucose reacts with ATP under the catalytic activity of hexokinase to form glucose-6-phosphate and ADP. Glucose-6-phosphate is then converted to glucose-1-phosphate by phosphoglucomutase. The next step is the conversion of glucose-1-phosphate to glucosyl units in 1,4 linkage. While this can be achieved *in vitro* by phosphorylase, it is possible that *in vivo* it proceeds independently of phosphorylase and by means of two other steps involving UDP-glucose pyrophosphorylase and UDPG glycogen-transglucosylase. This could explain the observation of several workers that the activation of phosphorylase *in vivo* always leads to glycogen breakdown and never to glycogen synthesis. When a chain of the growing glycogen molecule reaches a critical level a branch point is established by transfer of the 1,4 linkage to a 1,6 linkage, this being mediated by amylo (1,4–1,6)-transglucosidase (brancher enzyme).

Glycogenolysis

Glycogen can be converted back to glucose-1-phosphate by the enzymes phosphorylase, which breaks the 1,4 linkage, and amylo-1,6-glucosidase (debrancher enzyme) which breaks the 1,6 linkage. Glucose-1-phosphate is then converted to glucose-6-phosphate, a reversible reaction, by phosphogluco-mutase. Finally, glucose-6-phosphate can be converted to free available glucose by glucose-6-phosphatase. This enzyme is found only in the liver and kidneys. Glycogen in the muscles cannot be converted to free glucose but only to pyruvate and lactate via the Embden–Meyerhof glycolytic pathway.

At least nine types of glycogenosis can now be delineated and this number is likely to increase as further enzyme deficiencies are detected by modern biochemical techniques. The investigation of such cases nowadays can only be considered complete when the chemical structure of the deposited glycogen has been determined and when the various enzymes mentioned above have been assayed. Some types have so far only been described in adults and we shall describe here only those types of glycogen storage disease which, not infrequently, can provide diagnostic difficulties for the paediatrician.

Glycogen storage disease of liver and kidneys (von Gierke disease; glucose-6-phosphatase deficiency type I)

Aetiology

This was the first of the glycogenoses to be recognised. It is inherited as an autosomal recessive disorder in which consanguinity is a common feature. The heterozygous, and apparently healthy, carriers of the gene can be detected by the lowered glucose-6-phosphatase level in the intestinal mucosa.

Pathogenesis

The absence of glucose-6-phosphatase activity has been proved in this form of the disease. This enzyme normally liberates free glucose from glucose-6-phosphate in the liver.

Clinical features

Gross enlargement of the liver is the most constant feature and it is often recognised in early infancy. It

he severe form it may present in the neonatal period
vith profound hypoglycaemia and acidosis. Growth
s stunted and the protuberant abdomen is often
ssociated with an exaggerated lumbar lordosis. Genu
algum (knock knees) is common. There may be an
xcess deposition of fat, and xanthomatous deposits
re commonly found on the knees, elbows and
uttocks. Indeed, affected infants are often fat with a
haracteristically round face (doll-like) (Fig. 16.4).
here is no splenomegaly and there are no signs of
irrhosis. Gout and uric acid nephropathy may
evelop and there are reports of hepatic adenomata
ormation. The presence of fever may lead to an
rroneous diagnosis of sepsis.

iochemical findings

cetonuria is common in the fasting state.
Iypoglycaemia may be so severe as to precipitate
onvulsions and even lead to mental impairment.
Iyperlipaemia and hypercholesterolaemia are
narked and may even interfere with accurate
neasurement of plasma electrolytes. Episodes of
evere metabolic acidosis develop in some cases.
lasma pyruvate and lactate concentrations are
ncreased and the phosphate may be reduced. Renal
lamage from glycogenosis can cause glycosuria and
minoaciduria.

iagnosis

Iepatomegaly with the combination of hypogly-
aemia, hyperlacticacidaemia and hyperuricaemia is
irtually diagnostic of type I glycogenosis. Further
vidence of von Gierke disease may be obtained from
variety of tests.

The glucose tolerance test (after 1.5 g glucose/kg)
shows an abnormally high increase in blood sugar
and a delayed fall.
There is a marked resistance to the hyperglycaemic
response to adrenaline (0.3–0.5 ml subcutaneously) or glucagon (1 mg intravenously). In
normal subjects these agents cause glycogen breakdown to glucose-1-phosphate, its subsequent
conversion to glucose-6-phosphate, and liberation
of free glucose therefrom by the action of glucose-
6-phosphatase. The last step is, of course, deficient
in this disease. The adrenaline or glucagon is given
after an 8-hour fast and immediately after removal
of a specimen of blood for estimation of the true
glucose level. Thereafter the blood glucose concentrations are measured every 10 minutes for 1 hour.
In healthy individuals the values increase 40–60%
above the fasting value. In von Gierke's disease a
"flat" curve is obtained.
Another indirect measurement of glucose-6-
phosphatase activity can be obtained after an

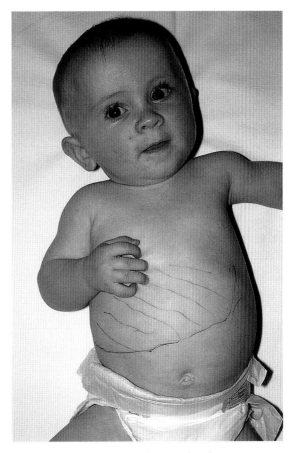

FIGURE 16.4 Four-month infant with glycogen storage
disease. Note rounded facies and gross hepatomegaly.

intravenous dose of galactose 1 g/kg, or fructose
0.5 g/kg. Blood glucose concentrations at 10-
minute intervals are compared with the pre-injec-
tion value. In healthy persons galactose and
fructose are converted via glucose-6-phosphate to
free glucose, but this metabolic pathway is blocked
in von Gierke disease.

Conclusive proof of the diagnosis, however, can
only be obtained from a liver biopsy. The findings in
this type of glycogenosis will be:

1 A liver glycogen content over 5% of wet weight.
2 Glycogen of normal chemical structure.
3 Absent or very low glucose-6-phosphatase activity.

Treatment

Although the enzyme failure cannot be corrected,
considerable benefit can accrue from a diet in which
a high intake of carbohydrate is given in frequent
feeds throughout the 24 hours. Where hypoglycaemia occurs in the early hours of the morning
overnight continuous intragastric feeding can
produce remarkable clinical benefit. Use of slowly

digested carbohydrate such as cornflour can help to maintain blood glucose concentration. Episodes of severe metabolic acidosis, often precipitated by inter-current infections, can endanger life. They must be promptly treated with intravenous glucose and sodium bicarbonate under careful biochemical control. Diazoxide may be of help in infants with intractable hypoglycaemia. Portacaval anastomosis which acts by diverting glucose from the liver to the tissues may be of help. If these children can be tided over the dangerous early years their health often improves greatly during adolescence. Prenatal diagnosis is not possible.

Glycogen storage disease of the heart (cardiomegalia glycogenica; idiopathic generalised glycogenosis; Pompe disease type II)

Aetiology

Once again autosomal recessive inheritance is involved and consanguinity has been reported.

Pathogenesis

The disease may involve the central nervous system and skeletal muscles as well as the myocardium. It has been shown that the primary defect is of the lysosomal enzyme acid α-1,4-glucosidase (acid maltase). In biopsy specimens spontaneous glycogenolysis is rapid and the glycogen does not show the abnormal stability which is a characteristic finding in the other types of glycogenosis.

Clinical features

The infant becomes ill in the early weeks of life with anorexia, vomiting, dyspnoea and failure to thrive. The heart is enlarged, tachycardia is present, and a systolic murmur is commonly heard. Oedema may also develop. The ECG shows a shortened P-R inter-val, inverted T waves and depression of the S-T segments. When skeletal muscles are severely involved the degree of hypotonia may simulate Werdnig–Hoffmann disease. In some infants macroglossia has been so marked as to arouse the suspicion of cretinism. On the other hand, hepatomegaly is not prominent until cardiac failure is advanced. Glucose tolerance, adrenaline and glucagon responses are all normal. The diagnosis may be estab-lished by muscle biopsy and the demonstration of increased glycogen content. There will also be low acid maltase activity in the leucocytes. An electromyo-gram reveals a primary disorder of the muscles.

Treatment

Death is inevitable, usually during the first year. Digoxin and antibiotics, when respiratory infection supervenes, can only have a temporary effect. No specific treatment is available for this disorder.

Glycogen storage disease of liver and muscle (limit dextrinosis; debrancher enzyme deficiency type III)

Aetiology

It is probable that this form of glycogen storage disease is also inherited as an autosomal recessive. It cannot be differentiated reliably from von Gierke disease by clinical examination alone.

Pathogenesis

The debrancher enzyme (amylo-1,6-glucosidase) is absent from liver, skeletal and cardiac muscle. Glycogen deposition in the heart and skeletal muscles does not occur in von Gierke disease.

Clinical features

Hepatomegaly is marked but hypoglycaemic problems are less troublesome and there is less interference with growth. It is common to find the same plump appear-ance and round face as in von Gierke disease (Fig. 16.4). In some cases, the involvement of skeletal muscles gives rise to weakness and hypotonia.

Diagnosis

Acetonuria may appear during fasting and there is a diminished hyperglycaemic response to adrenaline or glucagon. However, de-esterification of glucose-6-phosphate to glucose can proceed normally and there is, therefore, a normal hyperglycaemic response to intravenous galactose or fructose. The serum lactate level is not often raised, but there is a raised blood lipid content. The liver glycogen content is increased and it is abnormal in structure with short external chains and an increased number of 1,6 branch points. Activity of liver amylo-1,6-glucosidase is not detectable. It is also possible to demonstrate an elevated erythrocyte glycogen of the limit dextrin type and the enzyme deficiency can also be demonstrated in erythrocytes and leucocytes. Direct assay of the enzyme in liver and muscle tissue is confirmatory.

Treatment

Frequent feedings with a high-carbohydrate, high-protein diet and overnight nasogastric feedings can be very beneficial. Cardiac involvement is rarely clinically demonstrable but strenuous exercise should probably be avoided. No specific treatment is available for this disorder.

Familial cirrhosis of the liver with abnormal glycogen (amylopectinosis; brancher enzyme deficiency type IV)

This appears to be an excessively rare disease in which amylo-(1,4–1,6)-transglucosidase deficiency results in deposition of an abnormal glycogen with a molecular structure resembling the amylopectins of plants. This substance is toxic so that the patient presents with cirrhosis of the liver, splenomegaly and jaundice. Liver function tests yield grossly abnormal results and death is preceded by the development of ascites and deep jaundice. This diagnosis should be considered in all cases of familial hepatic cirrhosis. Deficiency of the branching enzyme can be demonstrated in liver and leucocytes. Patients usually succumb to the complications of cirrhosis.

Glycogenosis type V (myophosphorylase deficiency, McArdle disease)

Children with myophosphorylase deficiency are asymptomatic at rest but muscle cramps occur with moderate exercise. These symptoms are usually absent or slight during the first decade. A diagnosis is made on the basis of history and the absence of elevation of lactate after exercise. No specific treatment is available. In the absence of severe exercise the patients remain asymptomatic.

Glycogen storage disease due to liver phosphorylase deficiency (type VI)

In this form of glycogenosis the clinical picture simulates that described in von Gierke disease and in limit dextrinosis, although the characteristic rounded facial appearance is absent. The striking feature is hepatomegaly. Growth retardation is slight. Clinically these children have a very mild disease. Ketoacidosis is absent. Hypoglycaemia is mild and inconstant. The serum lactate level is not usually raised but there may be elevation of the serum uric acid. The blood glucose level rises after intravenous galactose. There is usually a moderate rise in the blood lipids and the red cell glycogen is elevated. Phosphorylase activity is demonstrably low in liver tissue and in the leucocytes. There is no specific therapy for this disorder.

INBORN ERRORS OF LIPID METABOLISM (THE LIPIDOSES)

This group includes Gaucher disease, Niemann–Pick disease, Tay–Sachs disease and probably also metachromatic leucodystrophy and Krabbe leucodystrophy. The chemical pathways of lipid metabolism are at present imperfectly understood. Here it will only be stated that in the lipidoses there is an abnormal intracellular deposition of sphingolipids, often widely spread throughout many organs and tissues as in Gaucher and Niemann–Pick diseases.

Gaucher disease

Aetiology

In Gaucher disease a glucocerebroside (glucosylceramide) is deposited in the tissues. The glycolipids which go to form glucocerebroside are derived from senescent leucocytes and erythrocytes. They are normally broken down by a series of enzymes, one of which is glucocerebrosidase. In the type 1 form of the disease the spleen has only about 15% of normal enzyme activity whereas in the type 2 acute form glucocerebrosidase is completely absent from the spleen and other organs (including the brain).

Clinical features

This disease appears to occur in three forms, type 1 adult, chronic, non-neuropathic form, type 2 infantile, acute, neuropathic form, and type 3 juvenile subacute neuropathic form. All are inherited as autosomal recessive traits but the condition runs true to form in any single family. Gaucher type 1 disease is particularly common in Jewish families.

The type 1 chronic form is the most common. It presents at any age from a few months to late adulthood with gross splenomegaly. Hepatic enlargement may also be marked. There is also a progressive anaemia, and leucopenia and thrombocytopenia due to hypersplenism develop early in its course. Bone involvement may give rise to limb pains. Radiographs reveal a characteristic flaring outwards of the metaphyseal ends of the long bones with thinning of the cortex. This is most marked at the lower ends of the femora which have an Erlenmeyer flask appearance. These features develop in childhood or early adult life. In older patients especially, the face, neck, hands and legs may show a characteristic brownish pigmentation, and the conjunctiva may show a wedge-shaped area of thickening with its base to the cornea (pinguecula). The serum cholesterol level is normal. The diagnosis can be confirmed by finding the lipid-filled cells which have a typical fibrillary appearance of the cytoplasm. These should be sought in material obtained by needle puncture of the bone marrow, spleen or lymph nodes. The disease runs a slow course but death is inevitable if untreated.

The type 2 infantile acute form is a rare phenomenon confined to infancy. In addition to hepatosplenomegaly there is evidence of severe cerebral involvement which is rarely seen in the chronic form. There may be hypertonia, catatonia, trismus, ipisthotonus, dysphagia, strabismus and respiratory difficulties. Death occurs by the age of 3 years.

The type 3 juvenile subacute form shares some characteristics of types 1 and 2. Neurological features may appear early in addition to hepatosplenomegaly but the time course of progression is slower. Spasticity, ataxia, ocular palsies, mental retardation and seizures are later features. Ultimate proof of diagnosis would require tissue or white blood cell β-glucosidase assay, or liver or spleen glucocerebroside determination. Prenatal diagnosis is possible using cultured amniocytes.

Treatment

Treatment is now available with synthetic enzyme and bone marrow transplantation. Results of such treatments are being evaluated.

Niemann–Pick disease

Aetiology

Sphingomyelin, a component of myelin and other cell membranes, accumulates within cells throughout the central nervous system and other tissues. Sphingomyelin is normally catabolised by the action of sphingomyelinase but in Niemann–Pick disease this enzyme activity is only about 7% of normal.

Clinical features

This disease also consists of a group of disorders characterised by hepatosplenomegaly and accumulation of sphingomyelin (ceramide phosphorylcholine) in organs and tissues. Three clinical forms have been identified. In type A (acute neuropathic), which is the commonest, there is hepatosplenomegaly by 6 months of age and there are severe feeding difficulties related to central nervous system involvement. It is inherited in an autosomal recessive fashion and is more common in infants of the Jewish race. The infant's abdomen becomes greatly protuberant due to massive hepatosplenomegaly. Skin pigmentation is common and severe wasting is invariable. Deterioration in cerebral functions appears early and progresses to a state of severe incapacity with generalised muscular weakness and wasting. Pulmonary involvement is commonly found. Anaemia of severe degree is an early sign but

thrombocytopenia develops late, in contrast to its earl appearance in Gaucher disease. In some affected infant ophthalmoscopy reveals a cherry-red spot at the macul resembling the retinal appearance in Tay–Sachs diseas and corneal opacities may be found.

Definitive proof of diagnosis would depend o demonstration of increased sphingomyelin levels i tissue specimens (usually liver or spleen) and/o identification of a specific sphingomyelinas deficiency in white blood cells, fibroblasts or viscera specimens.

In type B (chronic non-neuropathic) there is slightly later onset and no evidence of central nervou system impairment. Pulmonary infiltration ca predispose to recurrent respiratory infections. In typ C (chronic neuropathic) there is gradual onse usually after the age of 18 months, of neurologica impairment manifest as ataxia, loss of speech wit dysarthria and convulsions. Most die before the ag of 15 years.

Prenatal diagnosis on cultured amniocytes is onl possible for types A and B.

Treatment

None is available at present.

Tay–Sachs disease

Aetiology

An abnormal accumulation of Gm_2 ganglioside i confined to the brain resulting in progressive cortica failure and death by 2½–5 years of age. These ar complex lipids and their catabolism involves a succes sion of enzymes of which hexosaminidase is lackin in Tay–Sachs disease. There are two hexosaminidase in the body, A and B. In classical Tay–Sachs diseas (type I) only hexosaminidase A is lacking whereas i the non-Jewish form (type II, Sandhoff disease) which is clinically indistinguishable, both A and B ar absent. There are also extremely rare adult an juvenile forms which have their onset after the age o 1 year and in which hexosaminidase A activity i from 10 to 12% of normal. All types are inherited a autosomal recessive and consanguinity is not uncom monly found.

Clinical features

In this disease because the deposition of lipid i confined to the central nervous system the feature are neurological in character. They appear betwee the ages of 4 and 6 months as delay in psychomoto development, irritability, hyperacusis for sudde noises, spasticity, generalised weakness and muscl wasting. An outstanding feature is progressive loss o vision leading to complete blindness. The deep reflexes are exaggerated, at least to begin with, and the plantar responses are extensor. Ophthalmoscopy reveals primary optic atrophy and the diagnostic macular cherry-red spot on each side, surrounded by a greyish-white halo appearance. Convulsions may occur. Ultimately there are dysphagia, dementia, blindness and a tendency to repeated respiratory infections due to accumulation of mucus. Diagnosis can be confirmed by enzyme estimations on leucocytes or in skin fibroblasts growing in tissue culture. Rectal biopsy may also prove confirmative. Death usually occurs before the age of 3 years.

Treatment

None is available. Heterozygote screening in Ashkenazi Jewish populations, where a carrier rate of 1 in 27 is found, with appropriate genetic counselling can reduce the disease incidence.

Generalised gangliosidosis

Aetiology

The enzyme defect has been defined in this disease which has previously been described by such names as the late infantile amaurotic family idiocy of Bielschowsky–Jansky, pseudo-Hurler and the juvenile form of Spielmeyer–Vogt. However, some cases of the last-mentioned have probably been cases of Batten disease in which the cerebromacular degeneration is related to a lipid called ceroidlipofuscin, an unrelated disorder. There are, in fact, two biochemically distinct forms of the disease under consideration – juvenile Gm$_1$ gangliosidosis (type II) and generalised gangliosidosis (type I). In the latter, three acid β-galactosidases (A, B and C) are absent, whereas in type II only B and C are absent. The effect of the enzyme deficiency in type 1 is the accumulation in the brain, viscera and bones of Gm$_1$ ganglioside. In type II Gm$_1$ accumulates only in the neurones.

Clinical features

In generalised Gm$_1$ gangliosidosis (type I) neurological manifestations – hyperacusis, muscle weakness, inco-ordination, convulsions, loss of speech, mental retardation – develop during infancy and progress inexorably. Splenomegaly and hepatomegaly develop and in due time facial and skeletal changes resembling those of gargoylism become more obvious. Eye changes include macular degeneration, cherry-red spot, nystagmus and blindness. The full clinical picture is rarely present before the age of 18 months. Diagnosis can be based upon enzyme assays in leucocytes, and rectal biopsy will also reveal characteristic changes. Death occurs before the age of 5 years.

In the juvenile form (type II) the viscera are not involved and the bones only to a slight degree. Slowly progressive neurological deterioration is the principal feature. Diagnosis is suggested by mucopolysaccharidosis-type dysmorphism (with normal urinary mucopolysaccharides), eye changes, multi-vacuolated foam cells in the bone marrow and vacuolisation of lymphocytes in peripheral blood smear.

Treatment

None is available.

THE MUCOPOLYSACCHARIDOSES

This group of disorders, classified into six types, is characterised by the widespread intracellular deposition of complex substances called mucopolysaccharides (MPS) or sulphated glycosaminoglycans. They present primarily as disorders of the reticulo-endothelial system or as progressive disorders with visceral and skeletal manifestations. The mucopolysaccharides which appear in the urine show variations between the different clinical types and this is of help in differential diagnosis. All types of this disorder are inherited in an autosomal recessive fashion with the one exception of Hunter syndrome (MPS type II) in which transmission is as a sex-linked recessive. The aetiology appears to be a fault in the degradation of the mucopolysaccharides to their constituent sugars, this being related to a deficiency of one of several lysosomal enzymes, each of which normally breaks a specific bond in the mucopolysaccharide molecule. Specific enzyme deficiencies have now been identified. In Hurler syndrome (MPS type I-H) the missing enzyme activity is α-L-iduronidase and in Scheie syndrome (MPS type I-S) the same enzyme is absent in spite of marked clinical differences. This suggests that Hurler and Scheie syndromes represent different mutations of the same gene with resulting but different alterations in the composition of the enzyme protein. In Hunter syndrome the missing enzyme is iduronate sulphatase. The Sanfilippo syndrome, however, appears in biochemical terms to be four diseases: Sanfilippo A, due to deficiency of heparan sulphatase; Sanfilippo B, related to N-acetyl-α-glucosaminidase; Sanfilippo C, related to α-glucosaminide-N-acetyl-transferase; and Sanfilippo D, related to N-acetyl-α-D-glucosaminide-6-sulphatase. There are two forms of Morquio disease, types A and B which comprise MPS type IV. Morquio A is related to galactosamine-6-sulphate sulphatase and Morquio B to β-galactosidase. In the Maroteaux–Lamy syndrome (MPS type VI) the enzyme deficiency is of arylsulphatase B. A few cases of "atypical" Hurler syndrome have been described in which β-glucuronidase was the missing factor and this can be

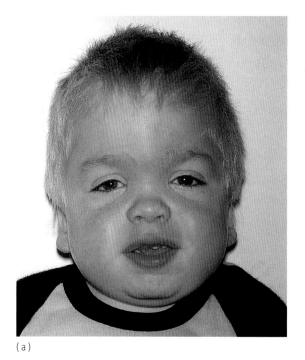

(a)

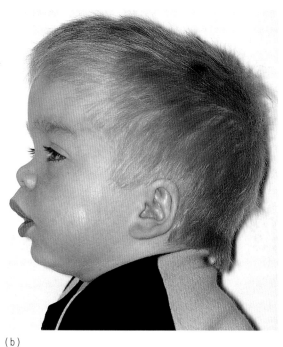

(b)

FIGURE 16.5a,b,c Hurler syndrome.

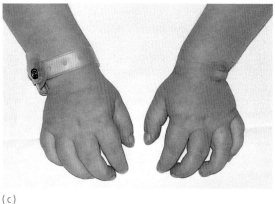

(c)

called MPS type VII or Sly syndrome. The number of disorders which may present with a Hurler-like phenotype and the complexities of establishing a specific diagnosis require a combined clinical and laboratory approach.

Mucopolysaccharidosis type I: Hurler syndrome

This type of mucopolysaccharidosis is associated with excessive amounts of dermatan sulphate and heparan sulphate in the urine in a ratio of about 2:1. There is deficiency of α-L-iduronidase. The superficial appearances in a typical case of "gargoylism" allow immediate diagnosis (Fig. 16.5). The head is large and scaphocephalic. The eyes are set wide apart and there are heavy supraorbital ridges and eyebrows. The nose is broad with a flattened bridge and the lips are thick. The skin is dry and coarse. The corneae usually show a marked spotty type of opacity or cloudiness. The neck is short, there is a lumbodorsal kyphosis and the protuberant abdomen often has an umbilical hernia. The spleen and liver are considerably enlarged. The hands tend to be broader than they are long. There is characteristic limitation of extension (but not of flexion) in many joints, most marked in the fingers. The fourth and fifth fingers may be short and curved towards the thumb. Genu valgum and coxa valga are common. There are also very characteristic radiological changes in the bones. The skull shows an elongated sella turcica, widened suture lines and an unduly large fontanelle. The long bones and phalanges are broader and shorter than normal and they are often bizarre in shape. The ribs too are excessively thick. The pelvis is distorted with abnormal acetabula. The vertebral bodies have an abnormal shape with concave anterior and posterior margins and there is often a hook-like projection from the anterior border of the first or second lumbar vertebra which tends to be displaced backwards. Bone age is usually delayed. Affected children are severely mentally retarded. They show diminished physical activity. This is partly due to excessive breathlessness on exertion when the heart is involved. Cardiomegaly, precordial systolic and diastolic murmurs, and electrocardiographic evidence of left ventricular hypertrophy are commonly found. Death takes place before adult life from congestive cardiac failure or intercurrent respiratory infection.

While the child with this disorder somewhat resembles a cretin, there are very obvious clinical differences, e.g. corneal opacity, hepatosplenomegaly, limitation of extension of the interphalangeal joints, and characteristic radiological findings in the skeleton. The precise diagnosis should be based on demonstration of the specific enzyme deficiency in leucocytes or cultured fibroblasts.

Mucopolysaccharidosis type II: Hunter syndrome

This form of mucopolysaccharidosis is X-linked. It differs from Hurler syndrome in usually being less severe, but there is a severe form which results in death by the age of 15 years and a milder variety with survival to middle age. Clouding of the cornea does not occur but deafness is common. The urine contains large amounts of dermatan sulphate and heparan sulphate in approximately equal quantities. It reacts well with alcian blue to produce a metachromatic effect. The enzyme defect can be demonstrated in the lymphocytes. By 12 months of age radiographs show a mild but complete pattern of dysostosis multiplex.

Mucopolysaccharidosis type III: Sanfilippo syndrome

In this variety heparan sulphate is excreted in the urine almost exclusively. Mental deficiency is severe and there may be hyperactivity and destructive behaviour. Visceral and corneal involvement is relatively mild and the only skeletal signs may be biconvexity of the vertebral bodies and some degree of claw hand. There may also be a very thick calvarium. The enzyme deficiency can be demonstrated in cultured fibroblasts.

Mucopolysaccharidosis type IV: Morquio syndrome

This is probably the disease first described by Morquio in Montevideo in 1929. The urine contains large amounts of keratan sulphate, a mucopolysaccharide which is unrelated to dermatan or heparan sulphate. Mental deficiency is not a usual finding and the face and skull are only slightly affected. The neck is short, there is marked dorsal kyphosis and the sternum protrudes. The arms are relatively long for the degree of dwarfism and may extend to the knees. There is, however, no limitation of flexion of the fingers. Genu valgum with enlarged knee joints and flat feet are present. There is a waddling gait. Radiographs may reveal platybasia, fusion of cervical vertebrae and flattening of the vertebral bodies. The metaphyses of the long bones may be irregular and the epiphyses are misshapen and fragmented. Mild degrees of corneal opacity may appear at a late stage of the disorder.

Mucopolysaccharidosis type I-S (previously type V): Scheie syndrome

The outstanding features are stiff joints, aortic regurgitation and clouding of the cornea (most dense peripherally). The facies shows the characteristics of gargoylism to a lesser extent than in Hurler syndrome, intellect is but mildly impaired and survival to adulthood is common. The urine shows the same distribution of mucopolysaccharides as in Hurler syndrome.

Mucopolysaccharidosis type VI: Maroteaux–Lamy syndrome

The principal features are severe corneal and skeletal changes as in Hurler syndrome and valvular heart disease, but mental deficiency does not occur. Hepatosplenomegaly is usually of mild degree. The urine contains dermatan sulphate almost exclusively. Leucocytes or cultured fibroblasts can be tested for enzyme activity.

Treatment

In all types of MPS the parents must be given genetic counselling and prenatal diagnosis is also possible. Encouraging results in Hurler syndrome are being obtained with bone marrow transplantation when an appropriate well matched donor is available.

MITOCHONDRIAL DEFECTS

Energy, in the form of ATP, is generated by oxidative phosphorylation of breakdown products of metabolic fuels such as glucose, fatty acids, ketone bodies and organic and amino acids in the mitochondria. This breakdown of nutrient fuels (oxidation) generates reduced factors – NADH and reduced flavoproteins. These must be re-oxidised for re-utilisation in this process by the respiratory chain. The mitochondrial respiratory chain is a series of five complexes situated within the inner mitochondrial membrane. There are also two small mobile electron carriers ubiquinone and cytochrome c involved in the process. Energy substrates cross the double phospholipid mitochondrial membrane usually with a specific carrier (L-carnitine). The proton pumps of the respiratory chain components produce an electrochemical or proton gradient across the inner membrane and this charge is subsequently discharged by complex V (ATP synthase) and the energy thus released is used to drive ATP synthesis.

Clinical presentation

The first of the mitochondrial respiratory chain diseases were described in relation to disorders of muscle and this resulted in the term mitochondrial myopathies. It is now known that other tissues, particularly the brain may be involved. Respiratory chain defects may produce isolated myopathy, eye movement disorder (ophthalmoplegia) with or without myopathy and occasionally with CNS dysfunction such as ataxia, multisystem disease, fatal lactic acidosis of infancy, and single organ dysfunction such as cardiomyopathy. The encephalopathies contain a number of recognisable syndromes such as the Kearns–Sayer syndrome characterised by progressive external ophthalmoplegia, pigmentary retinopathy and heart block, myoclonus epilepsy with ragged red fibres (MERRF) where in addition to myoclonic seizures there is weakness, ataxia, deafness and dementia. Myopathy, encephalopathy, lactic acidosis and stroke-like episodes (MELAS) is characterised by the recurrence of stroke-like episodes with onset usually before the age of 15 years. Cortical blindness and hemianopia usually accompany the stroke-like episodes which may be preceded by a migraine-like headache, nausea and vomiting. Dementia frequently ensues. Another syndrome known as NARP is comprised of neurogenic weakness, ataxia and retinitis pigmentosa. Unlike the other syndromes described there are no morphological changes in skeletal muscle and the mtDNA defect affects ATP synthesis. Leigh syndrome of subacute necrotising encephalomyopathy presents with vomiting, failure to thrive, developmental delay, muscular hypotonia and

respiratory problems. There may also be ophthalmoplegia, optic atrophy, nystagmus and dystonia. The disorder usually presents at around the age of 6 months but may be present from birth or may not appear until the late teens. In Leigh encephalopathy like many of the mitochondrial syndromes, it is difficult to pinpoint a single biochemical abnormality. There are defects of the respiratory chain, pyruvate dehydrogenase complex and biotinidase variably present in this syndrome. Lactate and pyruvate concentrations are frequently elevated in blood and CSF and MRI scans show characteristic low density areas within the basal ganglia or less commonly the cerebellum. There is occasionally an autosomal recessive pattern of inheritance in Leigh syndrome which suggests that it may be caused by a nuclear gene rather than a mitochondrial defect. However, in some patients mutations have been found in mtDNA. There are some patients who do not fit into these clinical patterns of disease and many have been shown to have multiple defects of respiratory chain complexes due to mtDNA disorder.

Leber hereditary optic neuropathy (LHON) is one of the commonest inherited causes of blindness in young men due to a disorder of mtDNA. Some men with the disorder have an encephalopathy with deafness and dystonia and a few develop cardiac conduction defects. There is some evidence that a gene on the X chromosome may be linked with this disorder.

There are various syndromes with non-neuromuscular presentation which involve the gastrointestinal tract with anorexia and vomiting and occasionally hepatic failure, yet others have cardiomyopathy with different degrees of heart block, renal disease with generalised aminoaciduria and haematological disorders affecting bone marrow function. In Pearson syndrome which presents at birth or early infancy there is refractory sideroblastic anaemia, thrombocytopenia, neutropenia, metabolic acidosis, pancreatic insufficiency and hepatic dysfunction. Renal tubular disorder, diarrhoea, steatorrhea and skin lesions with eventual liver failure have been described. Deletions of mtDNA have been identified.

Many of the respiratory chain disorders may present in the very young but there are three specific syndromes affecting the infant. The first is fatal infantile lactic acidosis. Infants present with hypotonia, vomiting and ventilatory failure and die often before the age of 6 months. A generalised aminoaciduria (de Toni–Fanconi–Debré syndrome), grossly increased plasma lactate concentrations, hypoglycaemia, liver dysfunction, convulsions and increased plasma calcium have been reported. The second clinical presentation is benign infantile lactic acidosis which may present with failure to thrive, respiratory failure and hypotonia with increased plasma lactate concentrations but the condition gradually remits and by

12–18 months these infants are often normal. There is a cytochrome oxidase defect which appears to improve with age and may be related to a switch from a fetal to an adult form of complex IV. The third syndrome is the mtDNA depletion syndrome in which the infant is weak, hypotonic and has respiratory difficulties together with renal tubular disorder and convulsions. The condition is usually fatal before the age of 1 year.

Treatment

Children with respiratory chain defects have been treated with vitamin C (4 g/day), vitamin K (menadione 50 mg/day) and ubiquinone (100 mg/day) in the hope that these vitamins may act as artificial electron acceptors. Some improvement in electron transfer have been suggested by NMR studies in these patients but there is some doubt as to the overall clinical benefit. Other treatments have included thiamine, biotin, L-carnitine, riboflavin and dichloracetate. As the mitochondrial respiratory chain generates free radicals, scavengers such as vitamin E might be of some clinical benefit. Unfortunately most of these conditions are progressive and result in significant disability and/or death. Considerable support of the families involved is required during the care of these infants and genetic counselling with prenatal diagnosis is available for some of these conditions.

PEROXISOMAL DISORDERS

Peroxisomes are present in every body cell except the mature erythrocyte and are particularly abundant in tissues active in lipid metabolism. They do not contain DNA and are therefore under the control of nuclear genes. A number of clinical and biochemical disorders have now been ascribed to disorders of peroxisomal metabolic functions. These functions may be catabolic and include β-oxidation of fatty acids, oxidation of ethanol and hydrogen peroxide based cellular respiration and the breakdown of purine. The anabolic functions of the peroxisomes include plasmalogen, cholesterol, and bile acid synthesis.

Table 16.3 gives a tentative classification of the peroxisomal disorders. In the group I disorders there is a reduction or absence of functional peroxisomes. Zellweger syndrome is a lethal disease presenting with severe hypotonia, typical craniofacial abnormality with a high domed forehead, severe developmental delay with neuro sensory defects and progressive oculomotor dysfunction. These neurological abnormalites may be related to the neuronal migration disorders found in the brain at post mortem. There is also progressive liver dysfunction with chondrodys-

TABLE 16.3 Classification of peroxisomal disorders

Peroxisome deficiency disorders
    Zellweger (cerebrohepatorenal) syndrome
    Neonatal adrenoleucodystrophy
    Infantile Refsum disease
    Hyperpipecolic acidaemia

Disorders with loss of multiple peroxisomal functions and peroxisome structure in fibroblasts
    Rhizomelic chondrodysplasia punctata
    "Zellweger-like" syndrome

Disorders with an impairment of only one peroxisomal function and normal peroxisomal structure
    Disorders of peroxisomal β-oxidation
        Adrenoleucodystrophy (X-linked) and variants
        Acyl-CoA oxidase deficiency
        Bi(multi)-functional protein deficiency
        Peroxisomal thiolase deficiency

    Other disorders
        Acyl-CoA: dihydroxyacetone phosphate acyltransferase (DHAP-AT) deficiency
        Primary hyperoxaluria type I
        Acatalasaemia
        Glutaryl oxidase deficiency

plasia calcificans of the patellae and the acetabulum. In neonatal adrenoleucodystrophy there is progressive demyelination of the cerebral hemispheres, cerebellum and brain stem with neuronal migration disturbances and perivascular lymphocytic infiltration. There is also adrenal atrophy. In infantile Refsum disease (IRD) there is developmental delay, retinitis pigmentosa, failure to thrive and hypocholesterolaemia. In the group II disorders, rhizomelic chondrodysplasia punctata (RCDP) is an autosomal recessive disorder characterised by short stature, a typical facial appearance, joint contractures and X-ray changes showing stippling of the epiphyses in infancy and severe symmetrical epiphyseal and extraepiphyseal calcifications in later life. Only two patients have been described as having the Zellweger-like syndrome which is clinically indistinguishable from the classical Zellweger but shows abundant peroxisomes in the liver. In the third group of disorders with impairment of a single peroxisome function and with a normal peroxisome structure adrenoleucodystrophy, an X-linked recessively inherited disorder, usually affects males between the ages of 4 and 10 years.

Initially there may be attention deficit noticed in school followed by convulsions, visual disturbance with the later manifestations of paralysis and death. This phenotype known as childhood adrenoleucodystrophy (ALD) has been treated with long-chain polyunsaturated fatty acids but there is some doubt as to the overall benefit of this form of therapy.

About 25% of ALD cases present in adulthood with paraparesis whilst a few may exhibit adrenocortical insufficiency without neurological involvement. Twenty per cent of female heterozygotes develop mild or moderate progressive paraparesis after the age of 40 years.

Pseudoneonatal ALD presents with early convulsions, muscular hypotonia, hearing loss and visual impairment due to retinopathy. *Bifunctional protein deficiency disorder* has occurred in only one patient with hypotonia and macrocephaly at birth and a single patient with *pseudo-Zellweger syndrome* had marked facial dysmorphia, muscle weakness and hypotonia at birth. The liver contained abundant microsomes but the enzyme defect was subsequently identified. The other disorders are also rare apart from primary hyperoxaluria type I in which autosomal recessive disorder of glyoxylate metabolism there is recurrent calcium oxalate nephrolithiasis and nephrocalcinosis presenting during the first decade. There are a few, however, who present with an acute neonatal form of the disorder and early death.

Treatment

Apart from the attempt to treat X-linked ALD with fat restriction and supplementation with glycerol trioleate and glycerol trierucate which has been shown to improve peripheral nerve function but not as yet to effect long-term benefit, there are recent reports that bone marrow transplantation may be effective in mildly affected childhood ALD patients. In more advanced X-linked ALD, bone marrow transplantation worsened the clinical picture. It is hoped that gene therapy might improve the outlook for this condition. Treatment with pyridoxine may be effective in a small number of patients with primary hyperoxaluria type I. Haemodialysis may be required during end-stage renal failure in this disease and surgical removal of oxalate stones may be required. Eventually combined liver and kidney transplant becomes necessary for survival.

INHERITED DISORDERS OF INTERMEDIARY METABOLISM

Every newborn infant with unexplained neurological deterioration, ketosis, metabolic acidosis or hypoglycaemia should be suspected of having an inherited metabolic error of intermediary metabolism (Table 16.4). A high index of suspicion and rapid diagnosis can prevent death and severe neurological damage in a significant number of affected infants and will ensure adequate prenatal diagnosis in subsequent pregnancies. The newborn has a limited repertoire of responses to severe illness whether caused by overwhelming infections or metabolic defects. Most inborn errors of intermediary metabolism fall into two categories namely "intoxications" and "energy deficiencies". *Intoxications* are secondary to an accumulation of toxic compounds such as branched-chain keto acids in maple syrup urine disease, most organic acidurias, urea-cycle defects, galactosaemia,

TABLE 16.4 Hypoglycaemia

Energy deficiencies (usually with ketonaemia)
    Ketotic hypoglycaemia
    Tyrosinaemia
    Maple syrup urine disease
    Glycogen storage diseases
    Galactosaemia
    Fructosaemia
    Reye syndrome
    Poisoning – alcohol and aspirin
    Jamaican vomiting sickness

Hyperinsulinism (no ketones)
    Insulinoma or nesidioblastosis
    Leucine sensitivity
    Poisoning – insulin

TABLE 16.5 Initial investigations to help categorise metabolic disorders

Urine
    Smell
    Acetone
    Reducing substances
    Keto-acids (dinitrophenylhydrazine test)
    Sulphites (Sulfitest, Merck)
    pH

Blood
    Blood cell count
    Electrolytes (look for anion gap)
    Calcium
    Glucose
    Blood gases (pH P_{CO_2}, HCO_3, P_{O_2})
    Ammonia
    Lactic acid and pyruvic acid
    3-Hydroxybutyrate, acetoacetate
    Uric acid

Store at −20°C
    Urine (as much as possible)
    Heparinised plasma, 2–5 ml
    Do not freeze whole blood!
    CSF, 0.5–1.0 ml

Miscellaneous
    EEG
    Bacteriological samples
    Chest X-ray
    Lumbar puncture
    Cardiac echography
    Cerebral ultrasound

fructosaemia and tyrosinaemia. The clinical features (vomiting, lethargy, coma, liver failure, acidosis, ketosis, hyperammonaemia) are common to most of these conditions. Treatment has to be aimed initially at removal of the toxic metabolites by peritoneal or haemodialysis, exchange transfusion and special diets. *Energy deficiencies* are due in part at least to a deficiency of energy production or defect in utilisation. Defects of gluconeogenesis, congenital lactic acidaemias (pyruvate carboxylase and dehydrogenase deficiencies), fatty acid oxidation defects, disorders of mitochondrial respiratory chain and disorder of peroxisomal metabolism belong to this group. Clinical features common to this group include severe hypotonia, cardiomyopathy, failure to thrive, circulatory collapse, sudden infant death and hyperlacticacidaemia. There may also be congenital malformations such as absent corpus callosum and cerebral malformations with congenital lactic acidaemia and facial and bone anomalies with peroxisomal defects. There can be overlapping of the clinical features between the toxic and energy deficient disorders where there is accumulation of toxic compounds in addition to a deficiency of energy production. A third category of clinical presentation is *hypoglycaemia with liver dysfunction*. Convulsions and hepatomegaly with ketosis and lactic acidosis are the usual presenting features. The main diseases in that group are the glycogen storage diseases.

Table 16.5 gives a list of initial investigations which can help categorise the metabolic disorder. More specialised investigations such as amino and organic acid analyses can then be arranged.

If the child dies it is important to have obtained urine, plasma, white blood cell DNA, fibroblast culture, and muscle and liver biopsies stored deep frozen. Subsequent analyses may help determine the nature of the metabolic defect and allow a diagnostic and proper genetic counselling to be given to the family.

CONCLUSION

Although individual inherited metabolic diseases are rare and this book contains only a limited review of some of the disorders, collectively they form a major grouping of disorders causing significant mortality and an overwhelming burden of morbidity for families and the community.

17

Trauma

Trauma is the commonest cause of death in childhood. In the post-neonatal period to the age of 1 year, only 3% of deaths are due to injury or poisoning, whereas in the 1–4 years group it is 26%, from 5 to 9 years it is 35% and from 10 to 14 years the rate in boys has risen to 44%. Many other children who survive injuries go through life handicapped and often have severe physical and deep psychological scars. It is important that children are brought up in an environment in which it is safe and healthy for them to play and grow whilst allowing them to gain enough experience in living. Many injuries can be prevented and it is the realisation of the dangers in the home and on the roads that has encouraged people through bitter experience to introduce legislation to prevent these hazards. Some examples are:

1 Seat belt legislation and campaigns to educate the public about road safety codes.
2 Bicycle helmets introduced to minimise head and neck injuries.
3 Childproof caps for containers of dangerous medicines and bottles containing dangerous solvents, e.g. bleach.
4 Smoke alarms in homes.
5 Legislation against the use of materials which are flammable in the household, especially for clothing such as pyjamas, nightgowns and shell suits.
6 Protection from open fires and campaigns on the safe use of fireworks.
7 Many modern appliances in the home and garden have locks and devices to cut electrical circuits if tampered with by children.
8 Vigilance and awareness especially at certain times of year when bonfires and fireworks may be particular hazards.
9 The introduction of new toys using mercury/alkaline batteries has introduced a new hazard of severe burns and perforation of the oesophagus when these are accidentally swallowed.

The infant's mobility between the ages of 1 and 2 brings with it many falls and accidents. From the ages of 2 to 5, the child's world continues to expand rapidly and the danger of accidents increases. More time is spent out of doors playing with other children, exploring and investigating their environment. A different set of dangers arises as the child begins school.

Children who suffer a minor injury, e.g. a cut or an abrasion, are readily frightened and struggle if restrained and have to be continually reassured preferably by their parents. Cuts and lacerations are only too common and frequently the parents are more apprehensive than the child. It is preferable to achieve skin closure with a Steristrip rather than suturing wounds in nervous children when practical. Administration of a general anaesthetic for wound suturing may be necessary. Children are subject to the same forms of trauma as are adults, and the principles of treatment are similar. There are certain types of injury which are particularly common in childhood and merit description.

BATTERED BABY SYNDROME OR NON-ACCIDENTAL INJURY IN INFANTS AND CHILDREN

Caffey in 1956 published an article entitled "Some traumatic lesions in growing bones other than fractures and dislocations" in which he stated this to be the least well known and the most abused subject in the entire field of paediatrics and radiology. Since that time, more people have come to realise that

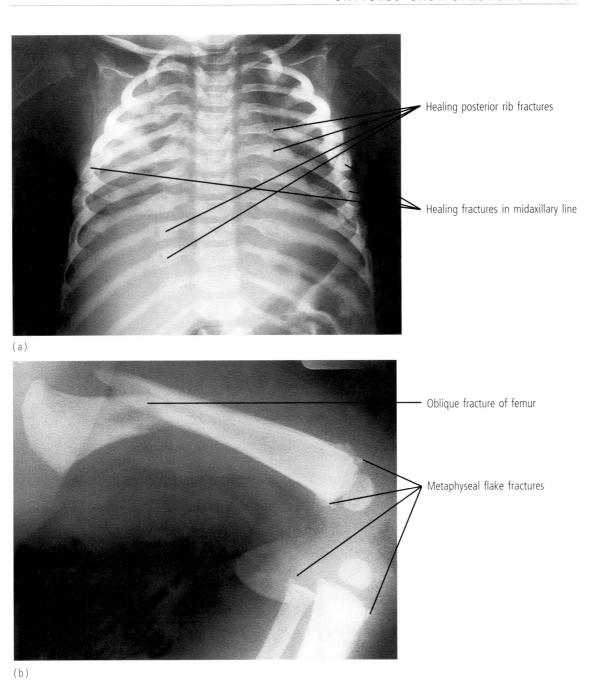

Healing posterior rib fractures

Healing fractures in midaxillary line

(a)

Oblique fracture of femur

Metaphyseal flake fractures

(b)

FIGURE 17.1 Non-accidental injury (NAI). (a) A post-mortem X-ray of the chest showing numerous fractures of varying age posteriorly and laterally. There is also a healing fracture of the right clavicle. The infant also had retinal haemorrhages and subdural collections and had a total of over 30 fractures. (b) X-ray of left femur and knee demonstrating metaphyseal flake fractures at the lower end of the femur and upper ends of the tibia and fibula. These appearances are diagnostic of NAI. There is also a fracture of the upper part of the femur.

many children are injured non-accidentally and awareness of this condition has increased. An injury in a child which does not fit in with the explanation given should be suspect. Subdural and retinal haemorrhages produced by severe shaking, metaphyseal fractures of the long bones and displacement of the epiphysis may occur with twisting of the arms and legs. An infant may be brought to hospital because of swelling of a limb or with a history of screaming when the limb is touched, or because of failure to move the limb. A history of trauma is usually unobtainable. Examination may reveal evidence of old bruising suggestive of previous child abuse. The typical lesion seen on X-ray is a small metaphyseal fracture which can easily be overlooked. Early recognition is of great importance since it may well prevent more serious injuries in these children. A full skeletal survey should be carried out in order to detect other injuries which have occurred in the past (Fig. 17.1). Some infants and children present with head injuries, others with burns or scalds. Injury to internal organs can result from blows to the chest or abdomen. The first concern of the doctor is the safety of the child.

If there is suspicion of deliberate injury the child should be admitted to hospital. The accusation that parents or others have injured a small child is a very serious one which may lead to prosecution. Social work and legal enquiries should be initiated only by senior members of the hospital staff and the situation requires delicate but firm handling.

SPIKE INJURIES

Children quite frequently impale themselves on spike railings and penetrating wounds are sustained to the buttocks, perineum and less commonly to the chest or abdomen. Where there is injury to the chest and abdomen, urgent surgical intervention may be necessary even though the child appears well at the time. Such wounds should be carefully examined. Penicillin and tetanus toxoid are administered and the wound fully explored under general anaesthetic. The outer portion of the wound is usually excised and the depth explored thoroughly to remove any foreign material which may have been introduced. Examination of the underlying viscera should be undertaken for signs of trauma where body cavities have been penetrated.

FOREIGN BODIES IN THE SOFT TISSUES

It is not uncommon for foreign bodies such as grit, stones, and splinters of wood to become embedded in a child's tissues through very small wounds of entry. If not removed these may present at a later date as an inflammatory lesion or even a growing mass. When removed, the foreign material is found in the centre of a fibrotic lesion.

MAJOR TRAUMA IN CHILDHOOD

Road traffic accidents are the most common cause of death in childhood. With the introduction of car seat belts, the pattern of trauma in childhood has changed significantly. In the past many children would have been killed outright. Now with restraints in the car, children are admitted to hospital alive but sometimes with severe visceral injuries. It is important that these are identified early and treated accordingly. When there is notification of a major accident, the resuscitation team should be available in the Accident and Emergency Department to receive the injured victims. When many children are involved in an accident, e.g. a bus outing, the Major Accident Policy of the hospital has to be activated and help sought from all the relevant departments. Triage in the Accident and Emergency Department is performed by senior medical staff, and the injured are directed to the various parts of the hospital which have been identified for dealing with major accidents. The child requiring resuscitation is admitted to the intensive care unit, where, after assessment of the injury the A, B, C system is followed, as below.

Airway (A)

This involves dealing with any respiratory difficulties that the child might have. The commonest cause of respiratory obstruction is the presence of vomit or foreign material in the pharynx. Suction of the oropharynx with endotracheal intubation and ventilation to prevent hypoxic brain damage may be required. It is important to establish whether there is any chest injury such as fractured ribs producing a flail chest, or a tension pneumothorax which requires urgent insertion of a chest drain.

Blood pressure (B)

A major haemorrhage may be overt or cryptogenic such as major haemorrhage into the chest or into the abdomen from a ruptured spleen or liver. It is important to establish early venous access. Large volumes of colloid may have to be given as a matter of urgency to correct hypovolaemia and shock until blood becomes available. An adequate blood volume has to be established and maintained to allow adequate perfusion of tissues. Heart rate, blood pressure, the gradient between skin and core temperatures, urine output and skin capillary refilling are clinical indicators which must be serially assessed. Attempts should be made to control on-going haemorrhage. Fractured limbs should be stabilised by splinting. Compound fractures should be covered with a sterile dressing and splinted until definitive treatment is given. Sites where fractures are overlooked include the faciomaxillary region, the cervical region, and the pelvis where soft tissue injuries such as ruptured bladder or bowel can occur.

Conscious state (C)

Lowering of the conscious state may be due to a direct injury of the head and/or hypotension. Measurement of the state of consciousness according to the modified Glasgow Coma Scale (Table 17.1) should be made. Additional factors which may alter the conscious state such as pneumothorax or severe bleeding should be identified and treated. CT scan or MRI will allow the identification of intracranial bleeding and help determine the need for burr holes to decompress the cranium. Other injuries which may be easily missed are spinal injuries which may cause paraplegia.

Where there is an open injury prevention or control of infection is important and antibiotic therapy may be indicated. Patients are monitored for their heart rate, respiratory rate and TcO_2 saturation and the child should be constantly observed for signs of deterioration of, or loss of consciousness, the presence of poor capillary return indicating poor peripheral circulation, neck veins which may be empty suggesting hypovolaemia, or full suggesting pneumothorax or cardiac tamponade. Insertion of a large bore central line for monitoring venous pressure and for IV therapy is advantageous in all severely injured patients. Fluids which may be required include whole blood, Haemaccel, plasma, albumin, nutrient fluids and electrolytes.

NEONATAL INJURIES

Neonatal head injuries can be difficult to differentiate from hypoxic cerebral damage or other prenatal brain insult especially in the preterm infant. Superficial injuries from forceps or ventouse extraction may produce abrasions, petechia or haemorrhages often after a difficult labour. Loss of an area of skin on the scalp due to congenital aplasia of the scalp may be mistaken for an injury. Caput succedaneum consists of oedematous swelling often associated with ecchymoses over the presenting part of the baby. It is most commonly seen over the parietal region in vertex deliveries, but may occur over any presenting part. In breech presentations, the scrotum, labia or buttocks may be severely oedematous and markedly discoloured and bruised. The swelling subsides within days, but bruising may take some time to disappear. In cephalhaematoma haemorrhage occurs between the periosteum and the skull, usually in the parietal region. The haematoma is limited to the area of the affected bone by attachment of the periosteum at the suture lines. It usually appears on the second day of birth and may persist for several weeks, but almost invariably it disappears without any intervention. Later calcification at the edge of lifted periosteum may give the impression of a ring of bone with a central depression and the condition can be mistaken for a depressed fracture when noticed at a later date. Aspiration is never indicated and may indeed cause infection of the haematoma with serious complications. Bruising and ecchymoses from birth trauma are not uncommon and require no treatment. Abrasions and lacerations may be caused by slipping of obstetric forceps and scalpel lacerations during an emergency Caesarean section. These should be treated in the conventional manner and leave very little scarring because of the good healing qualities of neonatal tissues. The presence of areas of fat necrosis in a newborn baby may be due to intrauterine pressure and very often disappears spontaneously within a year of birth. Rarely an expanding skull fracture can occur when the underlying dura is torn and becomes interposed between the edges of the fracture, thus preventing healing. Brain tissue may herniate through this gap. Treatment is surgical repair of the dural defect.

Neonatal subdural haemorrhages may result from tears of the straight cerebral vein (vein of Galen) during a difficult vaginal delivery or rarely from an underlying bleeding disorder. Expanding subdural collections of fluid may develop 10 days or more after the acute bleed and may cause raised intracranial pressure and be mistaken for a brain tumour. If the collection reaccumulates after an initial trial of repeated aspiration neurosurgical drainage or excision may be required.

Nerves

Forcible manipulation or traction on the arm during the delivery may damage the brachial plexus. In *Erb–Duchenne paralysis* the fifth and sixth cervical nerves or the roots are damaged, causing paralysis of the abductors and lateral rotators of the shoulder and flexor of the elbow. The arm lies at the side of the trunk in a position of internal rotation with the forearm pronated and with fingers and wrist flexed (waiter's tip position). The differential diagnosis is from a fracture of the clavicle or humerus and from neonatal osteitis (Fig. 17.2). If there is no permanent damage to the plexus, recovery is usually complete within 3 months. Subluxation of the head of the radius may be associated with Erb palsy and leads to limitation of flexion and external rotation at the elbow. Lower brachial plexus injuries involving C8 and T1 produce the condition known as Klumpke paralysis. The clinical features are wrist drop, flaccid paralysis of the hand with absence of the grasp reflex and sometimes local swelling and redness. A splint is applied which extends the wrist at the same time keeping the hand flat. Complete recovery is rare. A phrenic nerve injury which involves C3, C4 and C5

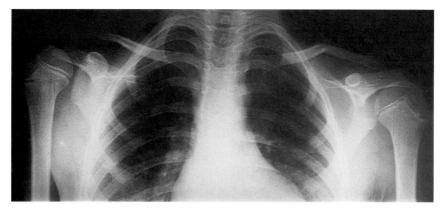

FIGURE 17.2 X-ray of fracture of clavicle with callus formation.

may cause diaphragmatic palsy and respiratory difficulty and be associated with Erb palsy. Other nerve injuries at the time of forceps delivery include a facial palsy with a characteristic drooped angle of the mouth on the side of the palsy.

Fractures

Skull and limb fractures occurring during labour and delivery are now infrequent and may present as a swelling over the bone. Fractures of the limbs and the clavicle may be detected by an absent Moro reflex in the affected quadrant. The site of the fracture may be missed initially and detected later as a swelling due to callus formation (Fig. 17.2). The bones should be carefully palpated for signs of tenderness or swelling. Healing is more rapid with complete remodelling in early infancy.

Visceral injuries

Subcapsular haematoma of the liver is a rare injury nowadays and occurs in babies who are asphyxiated at birth and particularly after assisted breech extraction. Congestion predisposes to the formation of the subcapsular haematoma. Should the capsule rupture, extensive intraperitoneal bleeding occurs. There is usually a symptom-free period of from 1 to 7 days, and abdominal distension may be delayed for several hours after the capsule has ruptured. An erect abdominal X-ray will show small bowel floating on the blood which has collected in the pelvis. The baby is anaemic and jaundiced. Staining of the abdominal wall, particularly around the umbilicus, may be noted and if a processus vaginalis is patent, that side of the scrotum becomes distended and stained by the blood. Treatment involves restoring and maintaining the circulating blood volume and giving IV vitamin K.

Haemorrhage usually arrests spontaneously but suture of the liver may be necessary in rare cases.

Adrenal haemorrhage may be unilateral or bilateral but is very rarely so severe as to cause serious complications from hypovolaemia or adrenal failure. This condition should be kept in mind at operation for haemoperitoneum. Adrenal haemorrhage may be subcapsular and trickle down to surround the kidney, impeding its function, and can be detected on ultrasound examination of the abdomen. Minor bleeding may escape clinical detection and may present in later life with suprarenal calcification (Fig. 17.3). This can be mistaken for a neuroblastoma.

Pneumothorax

Pneumothorax in the newborn may be spontaneous or induced. Too rapid expansion of one portion of the lung during attempts at resuscitation may lead to overdistension and rupture of alveoli and pneumothorax. In a typical pneumothorax with lung collapse, there is severe dyspnoea, cyanosis, mediastinal shift easily confirmed by cold light transillumination and X-ray. Insertion of a cannula through the fifth and sixth intercostal space in the mid-axillary line and attaching it to an underwater drain or Heimlich valve may be life saving. After the airleak ceases the cannula can be removed.

Gangrene

Neonatal gangrene of a terminal phalanx or a toe is an uncommon occurrence. It is usually caused by snaring of a digit with a loose loop of thread in the finger of a glove. If the hands and feet must be covered, mittens, i.e. without separate fingers, are worn and should be turned inside out before use and any free loops of thread divided (Fig. 17.4).

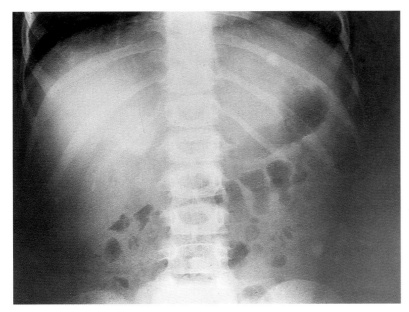

FIGURE 17.3 X-ray of calcified adrenal.

Cold injury of the newborn

The infant is susceptible to cold injury, as heat loss is more marked because of the proportionally greater surface area to body mass. The hypothermic infant may be admitted with abdominal distension and vomiting and on X-ray examination there is widespread dilatation of the bowel. The skin appears and feels cold, and temperature taken with a low registering thermometer will reveal the hypothermia. Rewarming in an incubator reverses the condition but it is important to maintain normoglycaemia with IV infusion of 10% dextrose.

Sclerema is a rare complication in sick newborn infants and may occur after operations. Chilling of the body surface alone does not cause the syndrome, but dehydration and infection contribute. The infant becomes progressively stiff and active treatment of the primary cause is necessary to reverse the sinister sign.

INJURIES IN INFANTS AND CHILDREN

Head injuries

These are the commonest injuries in infants and young children. The injury is often nothing more than a simple contusion but when it results from a fall from a height, a blow from a swing or a golf club, or as a result of a road traffic accident, it can be lethal. The infant's skull is relatively elastic and its resilience cushions and protects the brain. This alters

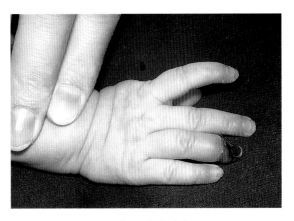

FIGURE 17.4 Gangrene of terminal phalanx.

with growth and in older children the consequences of head injury resemble those in adults. The outcome is exceptionally difficult to predict in the young child since it has been recognised that trivial head injuries cannot be regarded lightly and, conversely, signs suggestive of grave intracranial haemorrhage can be followed by spontaneous recovery.

Most children with head injuries make an uncomplicated recovery. A few lives are saved by painstaking management or operative intervention. It is well known that apparently trivial injuries can be followed by intracranial haemorrhage, meningitis, or fits, and these complications may develop rapidly with little warning. Close observation using the Glasgow Coma Chart is best achieved be admitting the patient to a hospital ward for at least 24 hours following the injury where there has been a loss of consciousness.

TABLE 17.1 Paediatric Glasgow coma score

		> 1 year	<1 year	
Eye opening	4	Spontaneously	Spontaneously	
	3	To verbal command	To shout	
	2	To pain	To pain	
	1	No response	No response	
Best motor response	5	Obeys commands		
	4	Localises pain	Localises pain	
	3	Flexion to pain	Flexion to pain	
	2	Extension to pain	Extension to pain	
	1	No response	No response	
		>5 years	2–5 years	0–2 years
Best verbal response	5	Oriented and converses	Appropriate words and phrases	Smiles and cries appropriately
	4	Disoriented and converses	Inappropriate words	Cries
	3	Inappropriate words	Cries	Inappropriate crying
	2	Incomprehensible sounds	Grunting	Grunting
	1	No response	No response	No response
		Normal aggregate score:		
		<6 months	12	
		6–12 months	12	
		1–2 years	13	
		2–5 years	14	
		>5 years	14	

From Simpson DA, Reilly PL. Paediatric coma scale. *Lancet* 1982; **ii**: 450. See also Reilly PL *et al. Child's Nervous System* 1988; **4**: 30–33. Modified GCS (Glasgow).

Other indications for admission to hospital after a head injury include excessive vomiting, dizziness, or a fit. The early assessment of head injury in young children is important, as most blows to the head produce nothing worse than a transient interruption of activity occasionally with vomiting and frequently tears. With a more severe injury, rapid assessment of the level of consciousness and airway patency is the essential first step. Immediate treatment of hypoxia takes precedence over further examination (Fig. 17.5). Once the airway is cleared and adequate ventilation is established, detailed evaluation is undertaken. Haemorrhage with oligaemic shock is the next priority for treatment. Bleeding is commonly due to cuts but concealed haemorrhage may result from injuries to the trunk or limbs. A significant amount of blood can be lost into the tissues.

If the child is unconscious at the time of examination, a cerebral contusion is probable and this can result in prolonged coma. Concussion which is often witnessed by those at the scene is rarely seen by the time the child arrives at the doctor as the child recovers consciousness within a few moments of injury. The next priority is recording a baseline by which further progress can be judged. It is often difficult if

not impossible to discover the duration of a post-traumatic amnesia to indicate the likely extent of injury to the brain in young children. The time and circumstances of the injury are noted, together with the time of examination. Assessment of the depth of coma on the Glasgow Coma Scale should be commenced and recorded. A record of the vital signs (respiration and pulse rates, temperature and blood pressure) ranks next in importance to the level of consciousness record.

Further neurological examination focuses on a search for paralysis or meningism. The motor activity of the cranial nerves is tested and the relative size of the pupils and their response to light is noted. Power of all four limbs is assessed and if seizures occur a note is made of the limbs involved. Tendon reflexes may be informative. Meningeal irritation which provokes neck stiffness and limitation of straight leg raising can develop soon after an injury associated with intracranial haemorrhage. Meningeal irritation arising some days later suggests complications of infective meningitis. The portal of entry in this case is usually secondary to a compound fracture. An occult compound fracture can occur with an apparently closed intracranial injury. Fractures

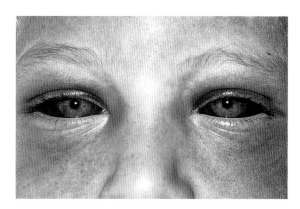

FIGURE 17.5 Traumatic asphyxia.

through the base of the skull allow cerebrospinal fluid or blood to escape from the nose or the ears. Paradoxically not all overt compound fractures provide spontaneous decompression of the brain. Most of these fractures will be found on inspection, palpation or probing of the scalp wounds during toilet in preparation for suture. In general, open head injuries with wounds that expose the brain either kill quickly or heal well.

The search for trauma is completed by examining the body and limbs for bruising and fractures of the limbs, pelvis and spine and for visceral injuries within the thorax or abdomen.

Indiscriminate X-rays of every child who has had a bump on the head is useless and costly. Plain X-rays cannot reveal injuries to the brain and no treatment is specifically required for a simple fissure fracture of the skull. On the other hand, the absence of a fracture does not guarantee that an infant or child will not develop a subdural or extradural haemorrhage. The need for operative intervention in a closed head injury is *never* determined by the radiographic findings. Statistically, the presence of a skull fracture on X-ray increases the chance of finding intracranial bleeding in the child with impaired consciousness or neurological signs. X-ray of the skull is helpful in indicating the likely site of bleeding but CT scan is more informative for selected patients. Rarely, radiographic examination is indicated in the child with a compound fracture of the skull and in the child with a depressed fracture.

In the unconscious child it is essential that a CT scan is carried out in order to determine whether there is intracranial haemorrhage which might require an emergency craniotomy (Fig. 17.6). Only a very small proportion of children who injure their heads need decompression of the brain to overcome the effects of acute intracranial haemorrhage and cerebral oedema, but when it is indicated it must be performed immediately if life is to be saved and brain tissue preserved.

Acute subdural haemorrhage

This is a feature of most fatal closed head injuries. The brain is often severely damaged and progressive intracranial compression develops very shortly after injury. If there is a lucid interval it will be relatively short. Operative decompression is undertaken when signs of progressive increase in intracranial pressure are detected.

Extradural haemorrhage

This diagnosis is usually suggested when there has been a distinct lucid interval after injury followed by rapidly deepening coma. The patient is often restless and the scalp becomes oedematous at the site of injury. Fixed dilatation of the pupil on the side of the bleeding is common and there may be muscular weakness or seizure of the limbs on the opposite side of the body. Decompression is indicated as soon as the condition is recognised.

General care of the patients

Maintaining the airway

A clear airway is needed for adequate respiration. This can often be obtained by nursing a comatose child almost prone with the face turned to one side and removing secretions or vomit by repeated suction. Endotracheal intubation is often safer.

Hypoxia

This is usually the result of airway obstruction or of convulsions. Oxygenation must be restored and then the metabolic acidaemia due to the hypoxia can be treated if severe or persistent.

Cerebral oedema

Cerebral oedema is often due to hypoxia rather than due to brain contusion. It can be treated by intravenous administration of mannitol. Hyperventilating the patient to reduce the $P\text{CO}_2$ and reduce the venous congestion in the brain might speed the resolution of the cerebral oedema.

Pyrexia

Lethal hyperpyrexia can develop at an alarming speed and the body temperature must be reduced to normal by tepid sponging the skin and using a fan. Additional cooling can be obtained by packing crushed ice around the patient but is rarely necessary.

Sedation

The use of opiates or similar drugs is absolutely contraindicated. Restlessness may be due to hypoxia, thirst or a full bladder and appropriate treatment may eliminate the restlessness. If necessary, paracetamol may be given to relieve pain.

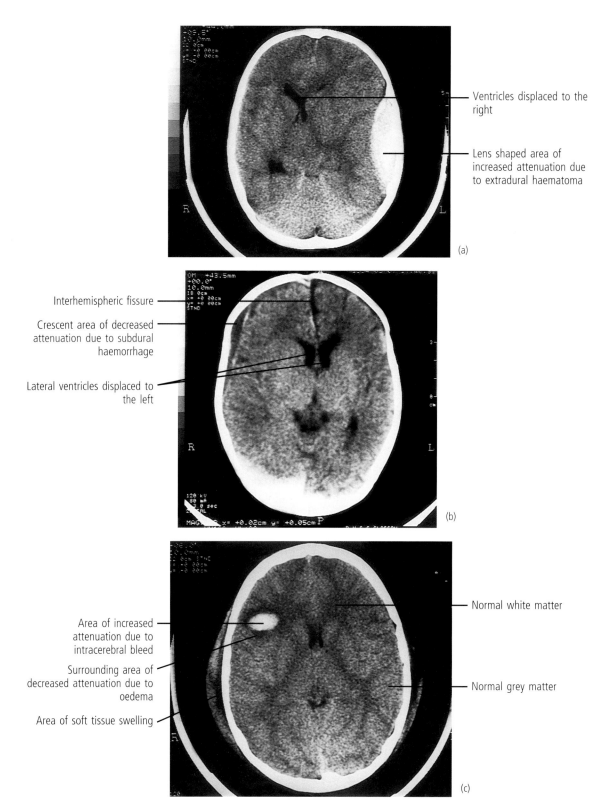

Ventricles displaced to the right

Lens shaped area of increased attenuation due to extradural haematoma

(a)

Interhemispheric fissure

Crescent area of decreased attenuation due to subdural haemorrhage

Lateral ventricles displaced to the left

(b)

Normal white matter

Area of increased attenuation due to intracerebral bleed

Surrounding area of decreased attenuation due to oedema

Area of soft tissue swelling

Normal grey matter

(c)

FIGURE 17.6 (a) Epidural haematoma. Unenhanced axial CT scan showing a lens-shaped haematoma in the left parietal region with displacement of the midline structures of the brain to the right. (b) Subdural haematoma. Unenhanced axial CT scan showing a crescent-shaped low attenuation area over the right frontal and parietal region with shift of the midline to the left. This appearance resulted from an acute injury 3 weeks earlier. (c) Intracerebral haemorrhage. Unenhanced axial CT scan showing an intracerebral haematoma in the right fronto-parietal region.

Infection

Where there is an overt or an occult compound fracture of the cranium antibiotics are administered to counter the risk of infection. Infective meningitis is best prevented by prescribing a 7-day course of a third generation cephalosporin. Lumbar puncture in a head injury is only indicated to resolve any suspicion of infective meningitis.

Fluid balance and feeding

Fluid intake should be restricted when there is evidence of cerebral oedema. An intravenous infusion of mannitol will allow time for scanning or transfer to an appropriate centre.

Instructions to nurses

Much of the minute to minute observation and care of patients with head injuries falls to the nurses who must know when to summon medical aid. The specific instructions for when to call for help are as follows:

1 If the airway is compromised or if the breathing becomes rapid or irregular.
2 If coma gets deeper.
3 If pyrexia exceeds 38.5°C.
4 If seizures occur.
5 If the pulse rate falls below 60/min or rises to over 140/min.
6 If urine output drops.

The nurse will endeavour to keep the patient's airway clear and will attend to pressure areas as the injuries allow. In addition, a record of progress will be maintained half-hourly or more frequently in an unstable patient during the first 12 hours, and hourly thereafter if coma persists. This will include all the parameters recorded in the Glasgow Coma Chart.

Sequelae of head injuries

Most children recover and have no long-term sequelae but a few become nervous and irritable, may suffer nightmares, and have a change of personality for some months. Headaches, epilepsy and permanent injuries to the cranial nerves are fortunately rare in children.

Subacute and chronic subdural haematoma

This complication does not demand immediate operation but any collection of subdural fluid which fails to reabsorb or increases in size will require evacuation.

Injuries to the chest

Non-penetrating injuries

These vary from simple contusions of the chest wall to gross damage to the lung, thoracic duct, heart and the

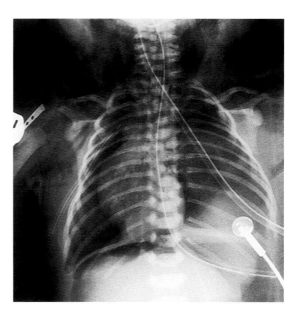

FIGURE 17.7 Surgical emphysema.

aorta. Localised contusion which resolves in 2–3 weeks is the most common visceral injury. Children with flexible thoracic cages may have severe visceral injuries without fracture, but ribs can be broken by crushing or direct blows. Such injuries can be complicated by subcutaneous surgical emphysema where the child may "blow up" like a "Michelin man" and on palpation one can detect crepitus beneath the skin (Fig. 17.7).

Pneumothorax, haemothorax or chylothorax

Sudden compression of the thorax can produce traumatic asphyxia. The mechanism by which this occurs is a retrograde pressure wave moving up to superior vena cava and valveless great veins to cause interstitial haemorrhage in the skin of the head, neck and shoulders. Subconjunctival haemorrhage and submucous petechiae as well as a purple skin suffusion may be evident. This skin suffusion must be differentiated from cyanosis which may result from additional intrathoracic damage. Post-traumatic flail chest is rarely seen in childhood.

Management of closed chest injuries

X-ray examination of the chest is mandatory as soon as the shock state is treated. This often demonstrates any contusion of the lungs or presence of pneumo-haemothorax which can be evacuated by an intercostal underwater sealed chest drain. Any contusion or collapse of lung tissue requires prophylaxis with antibiotics to prevent secondary infection. If there is respiratory insufficiency, oxygen is usually administered via a face mask and simple analgesia is given to relieve pain associated with the contusion. Opiates carry the risk of respiratory depression which can lead to retention of CO_2 and narcosis. It is of note that severe injury to the chest with fractured ribs is often accompanied by trauma to other parts of the body notably the diaphragm, liver, spleen, kidney (haematuria) fractures of the spine, long bones and other abdominal viscera.

Penetrating wounds of the chest

These uncommon childhood injuries may follow impalment by a spike when falling off a fence or falling out of a tree. Life is threatened as soon as the pleural cavity is opened, survival may be complicated by a haemothorax or an empyema. Wounds of the heart or great vessels are usually rapidly fatal, but prompt resuscitation and surgery may achieve a successful outcome.

Fracture of the ribs

Broken ribs are usually due to a crush injury or fall. They usually heal without any problems within 2–3 weeks. Early analgesia is necessary but pain soon disappears. Liver damage with right-side injury or splenic damage with left should be excluded.

Fractures of the sternum

This rare entity if isolated requires no treatment.

Zip-fastener injuries

The prepuce may be caught firmly in the zip and it may be impossible to free the foreskin even under a general anaesthesia. This injury may be numbered among the rare indications for circumcision.

Closed abdominal trauma

Such injuries occur in road accidents after a blow to the abdominal wall. Contusion of the abdominal wall may simulate visceral damage, but only too often serious visceral damage is slow and insidious in manifesting itself. There may be damage to the mesentery, intramural haematoma, or perforation of the gut, most commonly affecting a proximal jejunal loop. As in the adult, there may be contusion of the liver, spleen or contusion or rupture of the kidney but rarely the pancreas. On rarer occasions rupture of the urinary or gall bladder is found. In the presence of leakage of blood, urine or bile, signs of peritonitis may develop. The prognosis is excellent after laparotomy and repair of the damage.

Fractures

General considerations

In children, healing of fractured bones is rapid and they do not suffer the consequence of stiff joints requiring physiotherapy or the added complication of deep vein thrombosis found in adults. A birth fracture is firmly united in 3 weeks, but as the child ages the speed of repair diminishes. If a fracture unites with angulation of fragments, the resulting deformity usually corrects in an infant within a few months and the older child within a year or two. Not only is angulation corrected, but if shortening results then the rate of growth of the fractured limb increases beyond its fellow until the limbs once more are equal in length.

A good blood supply of a growing bone results in extensive haemorrhage at the site of a fracture, and may result in considerable blood loss, especially when the pelvis or femur is fractured. If the periosteum remains intact, a closed haematoma results and decalcification and absorption of the bone ends proceeds concurrently with the deposition of new bone and callus formation. Parents should be warned about a hard visible palpable swelling at the site of the fracture which will disappear with remoulding. When there is a tear of the periosteum blood extravasates into the adjacent tissues.

Except in the bones of the skull and the clavicles which develop in membrane, primary and secondary centres of ossification appear in regular sequence. The radiologist or surgeon called upon to interpret the X-ray film of a suspected fracture must be familiar with the times of their appearance and of their fusion. Two centres of ossification are not uncommon in children and their appearance on an X-ray may be mistaken for a fracture. The incomplete or greenstick fracture is common in childhood and may be found in three forms:

1 A hairline crack in the cortex resulting from torsional strain and presenting with slight local pain and tenderness. This may be overlooked on the immediate X-ray, and only after several days once there is a new bone formation present is the diagnosis obvious. This fracture may be accompanied by a slight pyrexia which suggests an inflammatory cause for the local pain and tenderness.

2 The compression fracture in which the X-ray film shows a horizontal line of compressed cortex. Deformity is absent and local pain and tenderness subside quickly with rest and immobilisation in a plaster splint.

3 The common and typical greenstick fracture in which the cortex has broken through on one side and is only bent or incompletely broken at the opposite side. Deformity, local pain and tender-

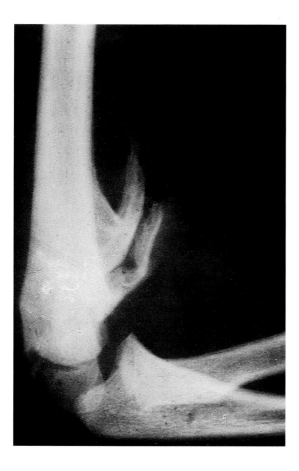

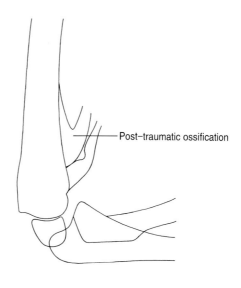

FIGURE 17.8 Post-traumatic ossification.

ness are present, but there is no abnormal mobility or crepitus, the periosteum frequently remaining intact. Where the force of an injury has been applied at the end of a long bone there may result not a fracture but a separation of the epiphyses. In minor degrees of this injury displacement is negligible and exact diagnosis is only evident on X-ray. In more severe forms the epiphyses may displace a triangular fragment of the metaphases.

Complications of fractures

Non-union

Non-union in children is extremely rare. Delayed union is far commoner because of the inability of the child to keep still which results in inadequate immobilisation. This however, merely increases the amount of callus formation and never results in non-union. Re-fracturing a site in a child may result in prolonged non-union or a fibrous union.

Localised traumatic ossification

Where a muscle has been torn from its attachment a mass of bone may form within the muscle, restricting its movement and limiting the range of movement of the joint (Fig. 17.8).

Interference with the circulation

This is not a common complication of fractures in childhood but may follow injuries in the region of the elbow and the forearm. The results of unrelieved arterial or venous obstruction are disastrous for the child. The mechanism of obstruction and the resulting changes in the tissues are varied. Inspection of the limb in all fractures is essential to make sure that the circulation of the limb is intact. If plaster of Paris is applied too tightly it may cause vascular compromise.

The branchial artery may be occluded by pressure of bony fragments as a direct result of an accident. This may produce pallor of the limb and absence of the radial pulse. The vessel may be in spasm due to bruising or partial occlusion by a bony fragment. Treatment of this clinical situation is immediate exploration of the fracture site. If not relieved the long-term results may be disastrous, varying from losing the limb to severe ischaemia which affects not only the forearm muscles but also the median and ulnar nerves.

The clinical picture of venous obstruction develops much more slowly than that of arterial obstruction. The pulse usually remains palpable but there are persisting signs of cyanosis of the hand and increasing pain. The presence of tissue oedema, coupled with slow and continuous haemorrhage under a deep fascia, may result in this clinical picture. Prophylactic elevation of the limb and removal of any tight plasters may be indicated to relieve the venous obstruction.

Nerve injury

Primary nerve injury as a complication of fractures in childhood is uncommon. The bruising of the radial and ulnar nerves may occur in supracondylar fractures of the humerus and of the perineal nerve in fractures of the upper end of the fibula. Recovery is usually rapid.

Damage to the growth area of a long bone

Separation of any epiphysis in a child is rarely accompanied by damage to the neighbouring growth area. A crush injury, however, may cause damage to this area, resulting in very severe intractable deformity.

Pathological fractures

Spontaneous and pathological fractures are not uncommon in childhood and are met in:

1 General affections of the skeleton such as osteogenesis imperfecta.
2 Neoplastic disease.
3 Generalised decalcification of bone.
4 Paralysed limbs or following prolonged recumbancy with immobilisation, there is decalcification of bones of the affected limbs.
5 Pseudoarthrosis is also rare, with persistent non-union of the clavicle. Similar appearances may occur in other bones in association with neurofibromatosis. The radiographic appearance is of bone sclerosis and expansion of the bone ends at the site of non-union. Improvement in appearance can be obtained by excision of the defect and the excessive bone with bone grafting and internal fixation.
6 Hyperaemic decalcification may result from a local focus of chronic bone infection and occurs quite early in acute haematogenous osteitis.

Treatment

First aid treatment of fractures

As in the adult, the joint above and below the fracture must be immobilised before the child is moved from the scene of the accident. This is especially so in the unconscious child who may have a severe head injury and other injuries to the chest and abdomen. In the upper limb, the arm is held to the side of the body or supported by a sling and thus immobilised. In the leg it is best to immobilise in a splint, but if no splint is available, bandaging one limb to the other would be sufficient for transport.

The speed of repair of a child's bone calls for the early correction of deformity as callus develops rapidly within a few days. By manipulation under anaesthesia, accurate alignment of the fragments becomes possible. Repeated manipulations in children cannot be too strongly condemned. With each attempt fresh haemorrhage occurs followed by an increased swelling and not only is reduction increasingly difficult, but there is a real danger of producing heterotopic ossification. The capacity for the restoration of normal structure is so great in children that it is often wiser to be content with less than complete correction in the knowledge that nature will in due course make good the shortcomings of the surgeon. Where traction is employed it should be remembered that the ratio of the muscle power to body weight is high in the child. A relatively greater weight is thus required in the child to overcome muscle spasm and reduce shortening. Skeletal traction should seldom be employed as the child's bone will be cut through readily by fixation wires with consequent risk of damage to the epiphyses. Skin traction correctly applied will carry all the weight required. Where external splintage is called for, plaster of Paris offers the simplest and most effective method. In children, the need for open operations on fractures is very limited. Condylar fractures at the elbow which will not respond to manipulation calls for open replacement to avoid disturbance of the carrying angle. Fractures of the olecranon and the patella with wide separation of the fragments may require replacement and suture. There is also some justification for operation in fractures or fracture dislocation of both bones of the forearm when there is rotation of the fragments.

Dislocation of traumatic origin

The joint of a growing child is normally more flexible and is possessed of a greater range of movement than that of the adult. Actual dislocation is less common in children although minor sprains with or without an effusion of fluid in the joint can occur. Reduction of a dislocation under general anaesthesia is usually obtained without difficulty, and restoration of normal function is almost invariable. Physiotherapy is rarely necessary.

Injuries of the spine

The spine of a child is normally much more flexible than that of an adult, and consequently fractures of the spine are uncommon but may be missed when they do occur. Usually, injuries are in association with other more extensive injuries in the body. Although intrathecal fracture is rare, haemorrhage s less uncommon and may cause pressure on the cord with resulting paralysis which may be temporary or permanent. As in an adult at the scene of injury, a child should not be lifted from the scene of the accident until some form of immobilisation of the neck is achieved, in order to avoid a cervical cord injury as a result of flexion of the child's spine. The diagnosis and treatment of injuries to the cord are along the same lines as those adopted in the adult.

Cervical spine

Fractures and dislocations of the cervical spine are uncommon in childhood and may cause transection of the cord. This is rare. Subluxation of the cervical spine can occur but complete dislocation is rare. Head traction relieves pain and spasm and allows the facets to reset. Delay in recognition of cervical cord damage with consequent paraplegia may occur.

Dorsal spine

Compression fracture may occur in an injury as a result of falling from a height or a car accident. Usually there is no permanent disability and after a period of bed rest recovery is complete.

Lumbar spine

Fractures below the first lumbar spine are rare in children. Fractures of transverse processes or pedicles are rare but may follow a torsion injury. Bed rest is all that is necessary and complete recovery is the rule.

Shoulder and upper limb

The clavicle

The clavicle forms the only bony connection between the shoulder girdle and the trunk. It is one of the most commonly fractured bones in the body. The clavicle is liable to break when force is applied to the outstretched hand, elbow or shoulder. Injuries to the clavicle may result from birth trauma. In infancy, fractures of the clavicle may present with a pseudoparalysis and pain when the arm is moved. It must be differentiated from Erb palsy, osteitis of the clavicle, scapula or upper humerus. At times, children present with a swelling due to massive callus over the clavicle after the initial injury may have been missed. This usually disappears in a few months – no treatment is necessary. In children, reduction of a fractured clavicle is rarely necessary under the age of years. The use of a figure of eight bandage or simple support in a sling may help relieve discomfort.

The scapula

Most fractures of the scapula are due to direct violence. Even if there is marked displacement treatment is conservative. Bed rest or a simple sling is the only treatment necessary. Winging of the scapula as the arm is held forward is normally the result of paralysis of muscles around the scapula as in poliomyelitis or after damaging the long thoracic nerve of Bell following thoracotomy, e.g. after the repair of an oesophageal atresia. Winging may also be due to a benign exostosis on the deep surface of the scapula which can be removed surgically, or as a result of a condition known as fibromatosis.

Injuries at the shoulder joint

Dislocation of the shoulder is rare in childhood. Fractures of the surgical neck and upper third of the humerus are not uncommon (Fig. 17.9). Anterior, posterior, and rotational displacement may accompany both adduction and abduction types of injury. Lateral as well as antero-posterior X-ray films are essential in all cases. Impaction of the fracture is common and 10–20 degrees of angulation is permissible without attempting correction. Moulding of the fracture takes place in 6 months to a year and what initially might appear unsatisfactory is usually passed

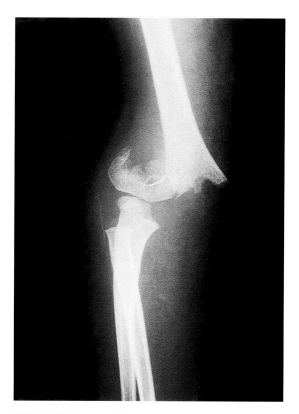

FIGURE 17.9 Fracture of humerus.

as normal at the end of that period. If the fracture is not impacted it may be aligned by a hanging plaster cast as in the adult. Reduction by open operation should be avoided especially if the child is a girl in whom the presence of an unsightly scar may be resented later in life.

Injuries about the elbow

The elbow joint is very vulnerable in the child and there is a wide range of degree of fracture displacement. Because of the lack of ossification in the epiphyses around the joint, experience is required to interpret the exact nature of the fractures on X-rays. Failure to correct displacement may result in deformity and loss of function in the joint.

Supracondylar and intercondylar fracture

There are two forms of these fractures, extension type (99%) and flexion type (1%). The extension type of fracture is caused by a fall on the outstretched hand. The fracture line runs transversely across the shaft immediately above the condyles and from below upwards and backwards. The deformity is threefold, the lower fragment being displaced backwards, tilted to the medial or lateral side, and rotated relative to the long axis of the humerus. Reduction is an emergency and effected as soon as possible after the injury. The patient is admitted to hospital and detained for 24 hours after reduction to observe the peripheral circulation. Should there be any sign of circulatory impairment, treatment which involves exploration of the branchial artery should be instituted immediately. Failure to do so invites Volkmann paralysis. Reduction should be performed by an experienced surgeon. Traction is applied to the distal fragment with the elbow flexed to overcome the upward and backward displacement; the lateral or medial displacement is then corrected. Confirmation of reduction by X-ray is essential. Medial angulation must not be accepted since this will result in cubitus varus. Minor displacement is of little importance in the presence of correct alignment. Mobilisation is by a plaster cast from shoulder to wrist with as much elbow flexion as possible. The radial pulse must not be obliterated by overzealous flexion. The plaster is usually removed in 3 weeks and replaced by a triangular sling. Active movements of the elbow are encouraged and the sling is removed in a further 2 weeks. On no account should massage or passive movement be permitted. Open reduction of this fracture is seldom necessary. However, this is necessary when the fracture is compound and when there is gross deformity of the fracture.

Flexion type occurs with a fall on the flexed forearm or on the elbow. The line of fracture runs upwards and forwards, the displacement is usually slight and there is no rotational deformity. The fracture is reduced and immobilised in extension fo[r] 10 days. The elbow is then brought to a 90 degree[e] angle and immobilised for a further 10 days in [a] dorsal plaster slab.

Fracture of the lateral condyle

Fracture of the lateral condyle may vary from a[n] incomplete fracture or a flake injury, to a complet[e] separation of the condyle. Displacement in the incom[-]plete fracture is minimal and may only be shown a[s] a thin flake of bone on an X-ray. This may appea[r] following a severe jerk of the elbow. In older childre[n] the injury results from a fall on the outstretched han[d] causing the radial ligament to tear away. Treatmen[t] consists of a few weeks rest in a plaster slab with th[e] elbow in flexion followed by active use. A complet[e] fracture of the lateral condyle is more serious a[nd] permanent disability may result if treatment is inade[-]quate. When displacement is gross and the fractur[e] surface faces outwards open reduction and fixatio[n] with screws is the method of choice. Complication[s] of this injury may result in an ulnarneuritis or eve[n] osteoarthritis of the joint later in life.

Fracture of the medial condyle

Although a fracture of the medial condyle is rare i[n] children, fracture of the epicondyle is not uncommo[n]. The flexor muscles tear off their attachment follow[-]ing a severe strain. In the uncomplicated cas[e] immobilisation of the elbow in flexion for 3 weeks i[n] a plaster slab is all that is needed. The ulnar nerve i[s] vulnerable because of its anatomical position an[d] may be injured.

Fracture of the olecranon

This is uncommon and results from a fall on the poin[t] of the elbow. It may produce a simple crack or [a] complete fracture with considerable separation of th[e] fragments. Minor injury requires only symptomati[c] treatment with a sling. Open reduction may be nece[s]-sary with internal fixation of the fragments whe[n] there is a wide separation in an extensive fracture.

Pulled elbow

This is a descriptive term for the injury at the uppe[r] end of the radius in an arm subjected to sudde[n] traction, i.e. snatching the arm to save a falling chil[d]. There is a subluxation of the radial head downward[s] through the annular ligament. This causes discomfo[rt] and the arm hangs by the side unused. There is n[o] gross deformity and the ability to allow full flexio[n] and extension adequately excludes more sever[e] injury. Supination is limited and attempts to produc[e] this cause pain. The diagnosis of a pulled elbow is [a] clinical one. Radiographs are usually normal an[d] diagnosis rests upon the above physical finding[s] together with the history of a traction injury. Th[e] condition wears off rapidly if a simple manipulatio[n] into full supination is carried out during which it is usual to feel a "click" as the radial head is reduced. In the minority in which a satisfactory outcome is not readily obtained, the child can be given a broad arm sling to rest the arm and spontaneous resolution will occur in 1–3 days.

Fracture of the neck of the radius

This is a comparatively rare type of fracture due to a fall on the outstretched hand with the forearm in supination. Manipulative reduction should be attempted but even if not completely successful, open reduction should seldom be undertaken. Excision of the head of the radius may ultimately be necessary.

Dislocation of the elbow joint

Posterior dislocation of the forearm bones behind the humerus is a common injury of childhood and is usually the result of a fall upon the outstretched hand. The loss of mobility and derangement of the normal relations of the olecranon and condyles enable the injury to be differentiated from a supracondylar fracture. The diagnosis is confirmed by X-ray. Reduction by traction is usually easy but in children a general anaesthetic is needed. The joint is rested at 90 degrees in a dorsal slab for 3 weeks. Active exercise is encouraged thereafter.

Injuries of the forearm

Fractures of the forearm occur in the following order of frequency: distal third, 75%; middle third, 20%; proximal, 5%. Fractures of the upper third of the ulna is an uncommon injury in children and results from a fall on the outstretched hand with the forearm in pronation. When a fracture with angulation occurs in a single bone of the forearm, the X-ray must include both the elbow and wrist joints, lest dislocation is overlooked. In children it is possible to reduce both fracture and dislocation by fully supinating the forearm. The limb is immobilised in this position for 6 weeks.

Fractures of the middle third of both bones of the forearm

Though violence is indirect, the bones frequently break at the same level. The line of fracture is usually oblique, commonly the fracture is of a greenstick type, either of both bones or of one only, the other being complete. Reduction of the displacement without rendering the fracture complete is not easy and deformity will usually recur within the cast. Immobilisation is by means of a padded plaster cast from axilla to the metacarpophalangeal joints, with a plaster strap across the palm. The elbow is held in the 90 degree position. In general, full supination is used for fractures in the upper third, mid-pronation for fractures of the middle third and full pronation

for fractures of the lower third and immobilisation is maintained for about 6 weeks.

Fractures of the lower third of the forearm

These are of three common types:

1 Incomplete compression fracture of the lower third of the radius (buckle fracture). Local tenderness is the only sign of injury to the bone and an X-ray shows the transverse line of compressed cortex. Symptomatic treatment only is needed. A dorsal plaster slab from elbow to metacarpophalangeal joint immobilises the wrist and relieves pain which settles in 10 days.

2 Separation of the lower radial epiphysis. In the majority of injuries, the epiphysis carries with it a wedge of dorsum of the metaphysis and the injury is more accurately described as a fracture. This clinical picture resembles that of the Collé fracture which is much less common in children. The typical dinner-fork deformity is present, the epiphysis being displaced and rotated dorsally. Correction of the deformity is usually obtained without difficulty. The method of reduction is similar to that employed in the treatment of Collé fracture. It is wiser to place the wrist in a position of slight flexion before applying the plaster, as there is a greater risk in children of the epiphysis slipping back when the swelling has subsided.

3 Fractures of both bones about 2–5 cm above the epiphysis may be complete or incomplete and the common deformity is a backward displacement of the lower fragments. Reduction is usually easily achieved but the deformity is very liable to recur. This can be prevented by immobilising the forearm in full pronation.

The wrist and hand

Sprained wrist and fracture or dislocation of one of the carpal bones are extremely rare in young children, but from the age of 10–12 years fracture of the scaphoid is not infrequent. Any child at this stage who is supposed to have a sprained wrist should be subjected to a careful X-ray examination. As in the adult, the line of fracture is easily missed unless oblique views of the wrist with the hand in radial deviation are taken. Fracture of the scaphoid tubercle is the more usual type of injury in children, but fracture of the waist of the scaphoid may occur. The former unites quickly whereas the latter requires prolonged immobilisation as in the adult. Ligamentous injuries of the carpus require 2 weeks of complete immobilisation.

Fractures of the metacarpals and phalanges follow the same pattern as in adults. Flexion fractures of the neck of the metacarpal bone of the index or little finger are not uncommon. Correction of the deformity can be effected by direct pressure on the head through the flexed proximal phalanx. The fingers are strapped over a rolled bandage in the palm for 2 weeks. In the common oblique fracture of the shaft of the metacarpal there is rarely any displacement and the application of a dorsal plaster of Paris slab for 3 weeks is all that is necessary. Local splinting of fingers is difficult in children because of their size. It is quite justifiable to include adjacent fingers as natural splints. Fractures of the metacarpals and the phalanges unite rapidly and immobilisation beyond 3 weeks is rarely required.

Open injuries of the hand are extremely common in children but fortunately most are of a minor nature which include abrasions and superficial skin wounds that require only first aid treatment. This is aimed at cleaning the wound and preventing infection. A sterile dressing is applied and the hand bandaged in the position of function. Examination of an injured hand is important in order to assess whether deeper damage has occurred to tendons or nerves. The posture of the hand results from a balance of the muscles controlling the fingers, both agonists and antagonists, and when this is impaired due to division of the tendons or paralysis of the nerves, there is an obvious deviation from the normal position. Damage to a flexor tendon results in greater extension whereas an extensor tendon cut will result in the finger being pulled into greater flexion. Immediate repair of divided tendons and nerves is important and should be done by a surgeon experienced in this work.

If the fingertip is crushed but the bone is not denuded the wound is gently but thoroughly cleansed. Damaged tissue is approximated and a firm dressing applied. Fractures of the distal phalanx require no further treatment. If the nail is partially avulsed it is trimmed off proximally, leaving the distal part as a splint. If the tip of the finger is partially amputated it is stitched back on as the regenerative ability of the tissues of the child are indeed remarkable.

The pelvis

Fracture of the pelvis occurs in children as a consequence of falls, crushing injuries or by direct trauma in road traffic accidents (Fig. 17.10). Of itself, fracture of the pelvis is not serious although considerable blood loss into the tissues may occur. Bed rest with analgesia until the patient becomes comfortable is the only treatment necessary. Fractures of the pelvis do become very important when other soft tissues are damaged, in particular when the urethra suffers either partial damage as it passes through the pelvic floor or in more severe injury complete disruption of the urethra may occur. Extravasation of urine will occur

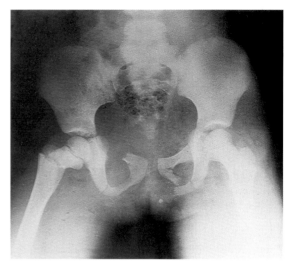

FIGURE 17.10 Fracture of pelvis.

if early recognition and treatment is not instituted. Passage of a catheter along the urethra to the bladder if possible and if not then exposure of the bladder and passage of a catheter, with control from above and below should be performed and urinary drainage continued for 10–14 days.

The hip and lower limb

All fractures in children except those in certain pathological bone disorders unite without difficulty provided the bone ends can be kept close together. Rigid fixation is not required unless one fragment is intra-articular when good position is impossible to maintain without operation and internal fixation. Open reduction plays some part in the wider displaced fractures of the upper third of the femur, but plating is not often advisable. Skeletal traction should not be used in children and repeated manipulation aimed at achieving anatomical reduction should be avoided. A plaster of Paris splint should be used only if:

1 It makes the child more comfortable.
2 It prevents the fracture from displacing.

If a plaster cast is used a layer of cotton wool must separate it from the skin and instructions given for the child to be seen immediately if pain or discolouration of the limb ensues.

Femur

Fractures of the femoral neck follow major violence (Fig. 17.11). They are treated by reduction and internal fixation. Fractures of the shaft are either transverse and caused by major violence or oblique caused

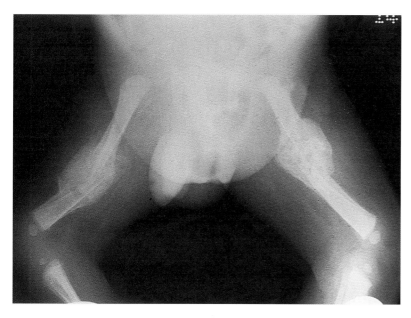

FIGURE 17.11 Bilateral femoral fracture with extensive callus formation.

by twisting injury which might be apparently trivial. Skin traction and a Thomas splint is preferred. The splint is fixed at the foot of the bed and the end of the bed raised on an elevator to avoid discomfort from pressure by the splint in the groin. These fractures heal readily and 1 week of splintage per year of age to a maximum of 6 weeks is sufficient to mobilisation. Foot movement is encouraged throughout this period and a close watch is kept for evidence of pressure on the lateral peroneal nerve in the region of the neck of the fibula. After the period of immobilisation an X-ray is taken and if the fracture is clinically and radiologically firmly united the splint is removed and knee movement commenced.

Fractures around the knee

The cruciate ligaments are firmly attached to the head of the tibia and their function is to prevent excessive gliding of the tibia on the femur. After a severe injury the entire articular facet of the tibia can be pulled out of the tibial head by these ligaments. There is always a severe haemarthrosis. The fragment avulsed is often bigger than it appears on a radiograph. The fragment needs to be replaced under general anaesthesia during which procedure the femoral condyles thrust the displaced fragment of bone downwards into its proper position. A plaster cylinder is applied to the leg for 4 weeks.

Fractures of tibia and fibula

As in the femur, transverse fractures indicate severe direct violence and oblique fractures are due to twists. The latter are more common and may be overlooked unless radiographs in two planes are studied. Manipulation of transverse fractures is aimed at getting end-to-end apposition and angulations are corrected as a plaster of Paris cast is applied. It is important to immobilise the knee with 25 degrees of flexion and the ankle at right angles in order that quick recovery of muscle power and joint movement will occur after union of the fracture and removal of the plaster.

Fractures of the bones of the foot

The more severe types of fracture of os calcis are rare but cracks may occur and are not uncommon. Diagnosis is made on an X-ray film. A below-knee walking plaster cast is applied, extending to the base of the phalanges and weight bearing is allowed. The plaster is removed after 3 weeks.

Fracture of the talus, although uncommon, may occur in association with severe crushing injuries, the bone being driven upwards between tibia and fibula. Avascular necrosis may result if the blood supply is damaged. Regeneration is slow and prolonged freedom from weight bearing is essential. Fracture of other small bones of the foot is uncommon. Union occurs readily if the foot is immobilised in a plaster cast for 4 weeks.

Fracture of the metatarsal bones and phalanges

Fractures of the base of the fifth metatarsal are not uncommon and require no treatment beyond rest for 2 weeks. Alternatively, a light walking plaster may be applied for the same period. Care must be taken not to mistake the common presence of an accessory bone, the vesalianum, for a fracture. A badly crushed foot is moulded back to its normal contours, held in a padded plaster cast and elevated on pillows. The metatarsals eventually remould themselves and function is excellent. Broken phalanges are splinted or bound to an adjacent toe.

Burns and scalds

It is usual to describe lesions due to dry heat as burns, and those from moist heat as scalds. There is, however, no essential difference except that in scalds the lesions are usually more superficial and dermal necrosis is less common. In infants and young children, scalds are more common than burns and are usually caused by hot water, soup, tea or coffee (Fig. 17.12). Burns are sustained by clothes catching fire or the child clutching the bar of an electric fire (Figs 17.13 and 17.14). Exploding fireworks can cause deep burns of the hands, face and body. More recently, deep socket burns of the lips and tongue may be caused by plugs of television sets placed in the mouth. Apparently there can be a discharge from the condenser in some sets for at least an hour after the set is switched off. Most domestic burns and scalds are preventable and in many homes the elementary precautions against accidents are

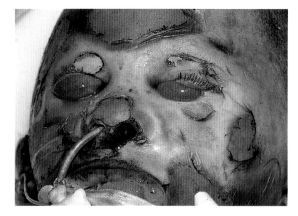
FIGURE 17.13 Burn.

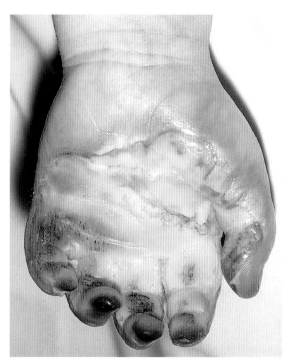
FIGURE 17.14 Electrical burn of hand.

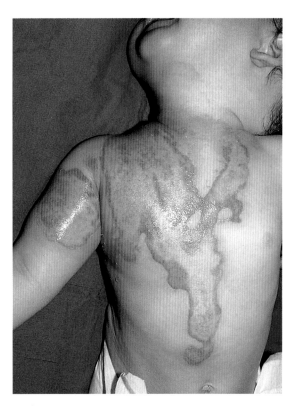
FIGURE 17.12 Scald.

neglected. Inhalation of hot air in a house fire damages the epithelial lining of the upper airway including the Eustachian tubes. Open fires should be adequately protected by fireguards. The common fabrics used for children's clothing should be flame resistant. Materials can now be rendered relatively flame resistant by chemical processes.

The diverse mechanism of scalds presents a serious problem to all parents and it is a duty of the family doctor to point out hazards which exist in the home. The main agents responsible for scalds in the home are:

1 Pulling cups, jugs and teapots off the table.
2 Knocking pans and kettles off the hob or kitchen stove.
3 Falling into a bath of hot water.
4 Collision with another child or adult carrying a utensil full of hot fluid.

Clinical features

The severity of burn in a young child can be difficult to assess as there is a striking lack of anxiety after the initial fright has passed and the child appears to suffer little pain. Primary shock is uncommon and there is usually a marked contrast between the child and the frightened parents.

Secondary (oligaemic) shock soon develops due to loss of fluid both externally and into the tissues unless haemoconcentration is prevented. In spite of copious oral fluids the patient may shiver and complain of cold. The pulse rate increases and the extremities feel cold. Restlessness sets in and the colour of the patient becomes poor with a tinge of cyanosis. Vomiting may begin and there may be alternating periods of drowsiness and restlessness. Only then is there a marked fall in blood pressure and a drop in urine output by the oligaemic and hypoxic kidneys. A haematocrit obtained at this stage will indicate haemoconcentration. Loss of consciousness may follow quickly unless the oligaemia is rapidly corrected by the administration of intravenous fluids. If a scald involves the chin, neck, chest, lips and mouth, the oropharynx should be examined for evidence of damage. Children may attempt to drink from the spout of a kettle and hot water or steam may be inhaled or swallowed, causing oedema of the glottis and severe respiratory difficulty. Lung damage may follow inhalation of noxious gases and smoke, particularly in situations such as house fires, and there can be serious and difficult management problems. Blood carboxyhaemoglobin measurements can give an indication of the severity of the problem and response to treatment.

Treatment

Most small superficial lesions heal well irrespective of the method of local management. The best first aid measure is immediate chilling of the injured part in cold water. This supports the acute inflammatory reaction if performed in time, and usually relieves pain in a dramatic fashion. Most scalds affect small areas and are managed at home. If the burn is more than trivial the patient would benefit from hospitalisation. Admission is desirable where the burn is extensive or deep or where the domestic circumstances are poor. Burnt clothing is often sterile and can be bandaged in place to form a good first aid dressing. Freshly laundered domestic linen can also be

used with safety. If the patient is far from hospital and the burn extensive, an intravenous infusion is given and continued during transport to combat oligaemic shock. The principles and priorities in the treatment of burns can be summarised as follows:

1 The child is weighed.
2 Pain relief (Omnopon 0.3 mg/kg) is given.
3 Extent and depth of burn are assessed. If over 10% intravenous fluids are given.
4 Fluid replacement is commenced.
5 Local care of burn/scald is performed.
6 Long-term management.

Pain

Relief of pain is important in the management of the infant or child who has had a hot thermal injury as failure to do so will increase the shock suffered by the patient. To give adequate but safe medication, it is necessary to know the patient's weight which should be obtained as soon as possible after admission. A usual medication would be 0.3 mg/kg intramuscular Omnopon.

Assessment

Initially, the extent rather than the depth of injury determines the threat to life caused by loss of fluid from the circulation. Discounting erythema, burns involving more than 10% surface of a child will provoke significant circulatory embarrassment. Treatment should be instituted before shock develops.

The rule of 9s used for adults is used as a basis for initial assessment, although it should be remembered that in the infant, the head and neck is double and the lower limbs are half the area of an adult. The palm of the hand is approximately 1%. Accurate assessment and recording is achieved by mapping out the affected areas on body charts (Fig. 17.15).

Fluid replacement

Oligaemic shock in the extensively burnt patient can be prevented by adequate and early intravenous infusion. The circulating volume must be replaced rapidly at first to keep pace with losses. In the first 8 hours after injury the amount needed will be about half the quota for the first 24 hours. The volume required to replace loss is Wt × % area in the first 8 hours after injury, i.e. not 8 hours after admission. A similar volume is given in the next 16 hours and again in the next 24 hours with the addition of the patient's normal daily fluid requirements. Half of the burn replacement fluid is given as colloid and the remainder as crystalloid fluids.

This forecast must be modified according to the response of the patient, who is reviewed at least hourly during the first 8 hours of treatment. No fluid for infusion is clinically superior to reconstituted dried human plasma; plasma/saline mixtures and

RECORD CHART FOR **BURNS and SCALDS**	Surname _____	Hosp No _____
	Other Names _____	D of B _____
	Address _____	Sex _____
	_____	Clinic Ward _____

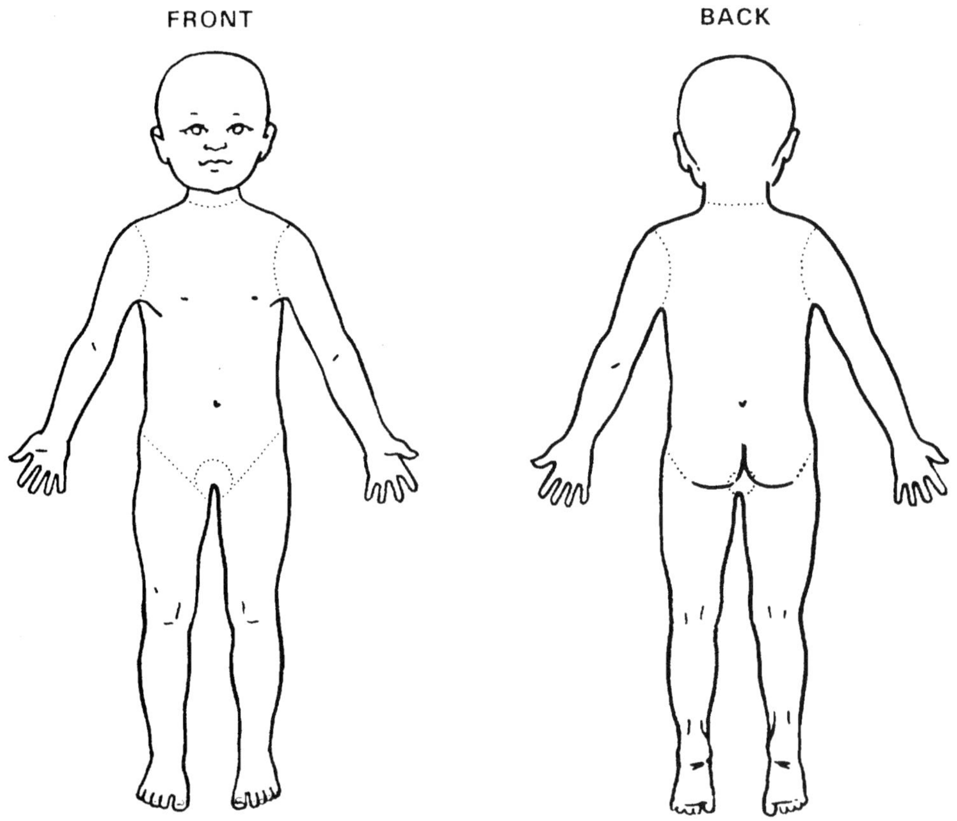

FRONT   BACK

DATE | MARK CHART AS FOLLOWS :— | Superficial Skin Injury
(Excluding Erythema) | ///// |
| | Deep or full thickness Skin Injury | ##### |

APPROXIMATE % AREA OF SKIN IN RELATION TO AGE
(Enter estimated area of Cutaneous Burns)

REGION	INFANT AND TODDLER Age 0 - 2 years		YOUNG CHILD Age 2 - 8 years		OLDER CHILD Age 8 - 13 years		ADOLESCENT Age over 13 years	
HEAD AND NECK	19		15		11		9	
RIGHT UPPER LIMB	5		7		8		9	
LEFT UPPER LIMB	5		7		8		9	
TRUNK ANTERIOR	25		20		20		18	
TRUNK POSTERIOR	25		20		20		18	
RIGHT LOWER LIMB	10		15		16		18	
LEFT LOWER LIMB	10		15		16		18	
PERINIUM	1		1		1		1	
TOTAL	100%		100%		100%		100%	

FIGURE 17.15 Chart of burn surface area at different ages.

dextran are effective alternatives but half of the fluid given in the first 24 hours should be plasma. When deep burns involve more than 20%, whole blood is substituted for part of the plasma; 1% of the blood volume (75 ml/kg) is given for each 1% of deep burn. By the time cross-matching has been done blood can be safely substituted for the plasma that is being infused. Blood samples are therefore taken at the outset of treatment for compatibility tests and to estimate haemoconcentration by the assessment of haemoglobin and haemocrit.

The colour and temperature of the undamaged skin returns to normal as the patient recovers from shock. Peripheral/core temperature difference is a useful indicator of the adequacy of resuscitation. Blood pressure rises to normal levels for the patient's age and the pulse slows to a normal rate. Serial estimations of the haemoglobin and haematocrit will show a fall towards normal (when uncomplicated by previous anaemia) and the excretion of urine (judged by the output from an indwelling catheter in burns over 35%) will start and increase. Intravenous therapy is not usually required for more than 36–48 hours.

The normal requirements for water are given by mouth but the amount is curtailed during the first 24 hours because of the antidiuretic and catabolic effects of injury. Some elevation of the blood urea can be anticipated due to haemoconcentration and catabolism but a rising blood urea with persistent anuria indicate acute renal failure and may justify haemodialysis. After extensive deep burning, haemoglobinuria is often evident at first but it clears rapidly. It is evidence for blood destruction rather than renal damage.

Pethidine hydrochloride depresses respiration less than other narcotics and is given as a sedative and to relieve pain. The vasoconstriction of shock renders intramuscular injection less effective so that the drug is given cautiously in divided doses by the intravenous route in a dilution of 5 mg/ml. The total intravenous dose should not exceed 0.5 mg/kg body weight given in a period of 15 minutes; less is given if respiratory depression develops during administration.

Inhalation of oxygen has no effect on peripheral cyanosis due to stasis, but it can be helpful if the lungs are oligaemic or have been irritated by hot air or smoke. There is no evidence that corticosteroids have any beneficial effect in the early treatment of burns, but epithelialisation is accelerated by small doses of prednisolone (5–10 mg daily) in the late stages.

Local treatment of the burn wound

The object of treatment is to restore the integrity of the skin, meanwhile preventing infection. In the absence of infection and dermal necrosis, cutaneous burns and scalds heal in 14–21 days irrespective of the method of local treatment. Bacterial infection can delay healing and may add to the damage by causing dermal necrosis in a burn of less than full thickness.

The first practical step is to attempt to prevent contamination of the wound. This is done after any danger from shock has passed. The pain of cleansing is eased by intramuscular injection of pethidine (1 mg/kg body weight) and the wound is gently cleansed with cotton-wool soaked in 1% warm aqueous cetrimide. Loose epidermis is removed and large blisters snipped but small blisters are not opened. Further treatment may be by exposure which alleviates the distress of further dressings. Excision of slough and skin grafting for areas of full thickness damage are performed.

Burns of specific areas

Eyes

The cornea is rarely burned but conjunctivitis is common. Conjunctivitis is treated by 4-hourly irrigation with isotonic saline followed by instillation of drops containing 1% hydrocortisone and 0.5% neomycin. For iritis 1% atropine sulphate eye drops are instilled. Aqueous sodium bicarbonate 3.5% helps to remove crusts from the edges of the eyelids; sterile liquid paraffin will lubricate and soften scabs. Deeply burnt eyelids retract and expose the cornea, thus endangering the eye. Contraction may progress despite skin grafting and a second skin graft may be required.

Upper airway

Crusting of the nostrils is relieved by applications of lubricant jelly. Hot air and smoke may cause oedema of the upper airway, tracheitis and bronchitis with copious secretions. Tracheostomy aids ventilation and facilitates repeated tracheo-bronchial suction toilet to remove secretions and avoid damage to the burned cords by an endotracheal tube. The danger of pyogenic infection is reduced by appropriate antibiotic treatment.

Hands

Circumferential burns of the digits are decompressed by longitudinal mid-lateral incisions to prevent ischaemic gangrene. Contact burns of the palms (which do not involve tendons) may be excised early and the defect repaired with thick free grafts. The hand is splinted to hold the interphalangeal joints extended and the metacarpophalangeal joints flexed with thumb abducted. Oedema is reduced by elevation. Silver sulphadiazine (Flamazine) cream is applied and the hand burns are treated by "closed" method rather than exposure.

Perineum

Under the age of 5 years, gallows traction is applied and the perineum exposed. In older children the area is dressed and precautions are taken to avoid urinary infection while using an indwelling balloon catheter.

Legs

In older children the legs are elevated until healing is complete; thereafter elastic bandages are applied for about a month to counteract gravitational oedema.

Electric and chemical burns

The heat created in the tissues by the passage of a large electric current produces burns which are deep rather than extensive. Excision and pedicle grafting is often the best treatment. Infants and toddlers may suck "live" electric plug connectors and sustain "socket" burns of the lips and mouth which fortunately heal well with expectant treatment. Serious injury by chemical burns can be prevented by immediate rinsing of the affected part in running water. Baking powder and washing soda are good domestic antidotes for acids, vinegar is an antidote for alkalis.

Nutritional and long-term supervision

Tissue catabolism increases after a burn injury and causes loss of weight, elevation of blood urea and a deficit in nitrogen balance. Further loss of protein occurs in the exudate from the burn – just when it is most needed to promote healing. Despite the increased metabolic rate due to pyrexia, the appetite is often impaired. If the patient is reluctant to take a diet based on reinforced milk drinks which are rich in protein and have a high calorie content, supplementary tube feeding may be required. Burns will not heal unless the haemoglobin concentration is maintained over 8 g/100 ml. Anaemia may prove a persistent problem until the burn has healed unless prevented by transfusion of whole blood – best given when the patient is anaesthetised for dressing of skin grafting. High-protein/high-calorie feeds are given as raspberry, chocolate, etc. milkshakes of Casilan or

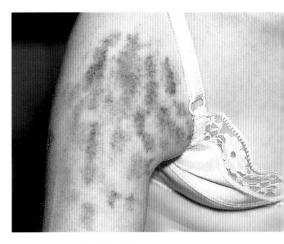

FIGURE 17.16 Self-inflicted injury.

Complan mixtures – over and above the normal diet (High-protein feeding may cause diarrhoea and can be dangerous if the kidneys are failing.) Iron and vitamin therapy – ferrous gluconate and thiamine riboflavin, nicotinamide and ascorbic acid – is routine from the end of the shock phase until healing is complete.

Late care

Following epithelialisation of the burned area there is a tendency for keloid formation and contraction of scars. These can be minimised by pressure dressings and contracted scars may require later excision and grafting.

Self-inflicted trauma

Trauma when self-inflicted may be very difficult to diagnose and treat. Bruises over the face or sides of the body may be self-inflicted by mentally disturbed children or those who have a serious underlying psychological problem and seek attention in these ways. Such children often have many medical investigations and are seen by medical specialists before a diagnosis is made (Fig. 17.16).

18

Accidental Poisoning in Childhood

INTRODUCTION

The peak incidence of poisoning in paediatric practice is between the ages of 1 and 4 years. Certain children with strong oral tendencies can be identified as especially likely to poison themselves by ingesting tablets or liquids, particularly if these have a pleasing colour or are held in an attractively labelled bottle or container. Patterns of accidental poisoning have been changing in recent years and while the number of children poisoned remains high, the incidence has shown a fall. There were nine deaths from accidental poisoning in children aged less than 15 years in Scotland during 1991 and 391 deaths (254 boys) from road traffic accidents in that same age group. This is related to a number of factors including changes in prescribing practices, educational programmes directed towards prevention and safer packaging of dangerous drugs. In a recent survey the rank order of poisons, drugs and chemicals which have most often led to hospital admission was: petroleum distillates; antihistamines; benzodiazepines; bleach and detergents; and aspirin. However, when the ratios of fatalities to ingestion were analysed to give an index of the practical danger of the substances to which children are exposed the rank order became: cardiotoxic drugs (digoxin, quinidine); tricyclic antidepressants; sympath-

omimetic drugs; caustic soda; and aspirin. In the United Kingdom the tricyclic antidepressants and cardiac drugs are now the biggest killers of very young children, while the rates of both fatality and morbidity for aspirin have declined considerably over the past 10 years. While noxious plants such as laburnum, foxglove and deadly nightshade continue to be ingested, a fatal outcome is exceedingly rare. Ingestions of petroleum distillates, insecticides such as chlorinated hydrocarbons and organic phosphates, and weedkillers particularly of the dipyridyl group (e.g. paraquat, diquat) are commoner in rural areas. Clearly, first aid management before referral to a paediatric unit is important. Lead poisoning is in a different category as it usually involves ingestion over a fairly prolonged period. Faced with a poisoned child the doctor should also be aware that intentional poisoning of children is a form of child abuse which is, regrettably, not unknown and not infrequently fatal. Poisoning from self-administration by the depressed older child is not very rare and the self-administration of drugs of addiction by adolescents is on the increase. Also on the increase is "glue sniffing", i.e. inhalation of various solvent vapours and ingestion of "ecstasy" and alcohol. All cases of possible poisoning should be taken seriously and it is to be preferred that a symptomless child be kept in hospital overnight than that a child be admitted gravely ill from the delayed effects of a poison some hours later. In this chapter it is proposed to describe the general therapeutic measures applicable to acute poisoning and then to consider some of the more common individual poisonings. The possibility of poisoning should always be entertained in an acute illness of sudden onset if no cause is immediately discoverable, particularly if it is associated with vomiting and diarrhoea or if there are marked disturbances of consciousness or behaviour. An emergency drug screen should be carried out to identify and quantify poisons amenable to specific treatment in children who are desperately ill and in whom the exact nature of the poison is uncertain. For drug screening samples of gastric aspirate, urine and blood should be obtained. Drugs and their metabolites are usually present in aspirate and urine in much higher concentrations than in blood.

In the United Kingdom and the Republic of Ireland the physician confronted with a patient suffering from a form of poisoning about which he lacks information can obtain assistance, day or night, by telephoning one of the poison centres. Most accident and emergency departments have access to a poisons centre database for management advice.

General therapeutic measures

Unless the child has swallowed kerosene, corrosive acid or strong alkali, vomiting should be induced with paediatric ipecacuanha emetic mixture (BP), 10 ml for children aged 6 months to 2 years and 15 ml for older children, followed immediately by a tumblerful of water. The dose of ipecacuanha can be repeated after 20 minutes if necessary. In the hospital gastric lavage can be carried out in the unconscious child with half-strength physiological saline or in the case of iron poisoning with 1% sodium bicarbonate. It is important to employ a stomach tube of adequate size and the airway must be assured with a cuffed endotracheal tube.

Oxygen should be administered if there is respiratory depression, cyanosis or shock. It is only rarely in children that mechanical ventilation is required and then the services of a skilled anaesthetist are invaluable. Severe shock and hypotension are also uncommon in children and may be combated with intravenous plasma according to age and blood pressure response. In severe poisonings intravenous fluids such as 5% dextrose in quarter strength saline will usually be necessary and it is important that periodic measurements be made of the serum electrolytes and of the acid–base status. In corrosive poisonings, which are not very common in children, milk is the best oral fluid because the poison is likely to react with the protein. In poisoning with alkaloids or glycosides of plants the poison can be absorbed by

activated medicinal charcoal (activated charcoal BNF). This can be placed in the stomach, 8–12 g in 300 ml after ipecacuanha-induced vomiting or after gastric lavage has been completed. When convulsions occur, as in poisoning by strychnine, picrotoxin or nicotine, intravenous diazepam 2–10 mg may be sufficient but intravenous thiopentone and intermittent positive-pressure ventilation is sometimes required. The restlessness and excitement of amphetamine poisoning is best treated with chlorpromazine (Largactil) or promazine (Sparine) in intramuscular doses of 0.7 mg/kg; they antagonise both the central and peripheral effects of the poison. One of the few true antidotes is to be found in naloxone, a competitive antagonist of the narcotic analgesics such as morphine, pethidine and related substances. It is best given intravenously in a dose of 10 µg/kg and can be repeated every 2–3 minutes as necessary.

SALICYLATE POISONING

Accidental poisoning in children due to salicylate has recently declined in incidence following the packaging of salicylates in child-resistant containers and also because aspirin is being superseded by paracetamol as the standard domestic analgesic. Salicylate is usually ingested in the form of aspirin (acetyl salicylate). This is often accidental but sometimes it has been given with therapeutic intent by the parents and even by the doctor. On occasion the source of the salicylate has been swallowed oil of wintergreen (methyl salicylate), one teaspoonful of which contains the equivalent of 4 g aspirin.

Prognosis in the individual case is determined much more by the interval of time which has elapsed between the ingestion of the poison and the start of treatment than by the level of the serum salicylate. Indeed, the toddler can show signs of severe poisoning with a salicylate level as low as 2.9 mmol/l (40 mg/100 ml). "Therapeutic" cases tend to be of longer duration and more often fatal because the deterioration in the child's condition is at first attributed to the disease for which the aspirin was initially prescribed. "Accidental" cases are promptly recognised by the parents who seek treatment and usually give a clear history that aspirin has been taken so that a fatal outcome is much less likely. With the exceptions of rheumatic fever, rheumatoid arthritis and Kawasaki disease, aspirin should not be prescribed for infants or children. A raised body temperature can be more effectively lowered by tepid sponging and/or paracetamol.

Clinical features

Rapid, deep, regular, acyanotic breathing or air hunger is almost diagnostic in salicylate poisoning.

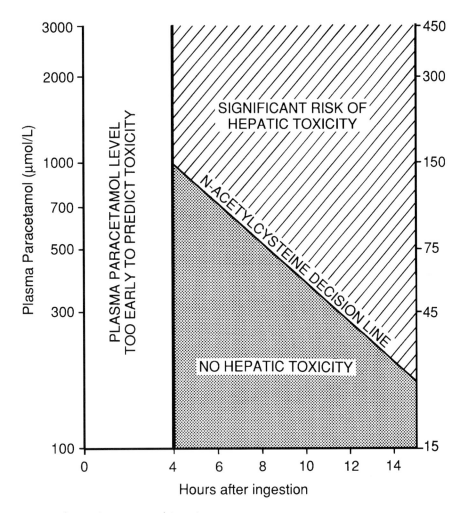

FIGURE 18.1 Nomogram for use in paracetamol ingestion.

Cases may be misdiagnosed as "pneumonia" but the hyperpnoea of salicylate poisoning is quite different from the short, grunting respirations of pneumonia. Other early manifestations of salicylate poisoning such as nausea and vomiting are difficult to evaluate in infants and toddlers and they cannot often describe tinnitus.

The hyperpnoea has a double aetiology. It is due initially to the direct stimulation by salicylate of the respiratory centre of the brain. The resultant overbreathing washes out CO_2 from the lungs and causes a respiratory alkalosis with a raised blood pH (> 7.42) and a lowered P_{CO_2} (< 33 mmHg; 4.4 kPa). This alkalotic phase is commonly seen in adults with salicylate poisoning, but in young children an accelerated fatty-acid catabolism with excess production of ketones results in the early establishment of a metabolic acidosis. By the time the poisoned toddler reaches hospital the blood pH is usually reduced (< 7.35). The compensatory hyperventilation of metabolic acidosis adds to the stimulant effect of salicylate on the respiratory centre so that the overbreathing of the poisoned child is often extreme.

A side effect of salicylate overdosage is fever. There is also a disturbance of carbohydrate metabolism and the blood glucose may rise above 11.1 mmol/l (200 mg/100 ml) although not above 16.7 mmol/l (300 mg/100 ml). Hypoglycaemia has been recorded but it is uncommon.

The child with salicylate poisoning shows peripheral vasodilatation until near to death. Death is preceded by cyanosis, twitching, rigidity and coma.

Treatment

The immediate treatment in the child's home is to induce vomiting. On arrival at hospital blood is taken for estimation of the plasma salicylate level and acid–base state. If there is marked air hunger and dehydration an intravenous infusion of 5% dextrose in quarter strength saline should be set up to deliver 200 ml/kg in 24 hours. Metabolic acidosis, which is usually severe in the toddler can be safely corrected using the formula: base deficit $\times$ 0.3 $\times$ body weight (kg) = mmol sodium bicarbonate given over 30 minutes intravenously. This treatment is repeated until the acid–base status is corrected and stable. In older children and adults the initial respiratory alkalosis is frequently more marked than metabolic acidosis and bicarbonate must be used more cautiously.

It is important to avoid hypernatraemia and if hypokalaemia develops, potassium chloride 10–20 mmol, should be added to each litre of infusion fluid. Haemorrhagic manifestations are uncommon and should be treated with 10 mg of intramuscular vitamin K (phytomenadione). In severe cases, haemodialysis is the method of choice for rapid removal of salicylate because it has the additional advantages of permitting removal of fluid and correction of acid–base and electrolyte disturbances. Exchange transfusion is another effective method of treatment for the worst cases but it is not free from risk and should not be lightly undertaken.

PARACETAMOL POISONING

While paracetamol (acetaminophen) accounts for a large number of attempted suicides in adults (either alone or in combination with dextropropoxyphene as "Distalgesic"), cases of serious poisoning are rare in children. None the less, as it can lead to irreversible liver and renal failure any child who may have ingested an excess should be admitted to hospital without delay.

Clinical features

The first symptoms are nausea, vomiting and abdominal pain. Evidence of severe liver damage may be revealed by elevated levels of aspartate aminotransferace (AST) and alanine aminotransferase (ALT) over 1000 IU/l and of renal impairment by a plasma creatinine concentration over 300 µmol/l (3.4 mg/100 ml). The child may become comatose and die from respiratory arrest.

Treatment

The immediate treatment is to induce vomiting. At hospital gastric lavage should be performed and blood taken for estimation of the plasma paracetamol concentration. Complete protection against liver failure can be achieved with N-acetylcysteine provided it is given within 8 hours of the ingestion of paracetamol but protection is virtually nil if treatment is delayed for over 15 hours. Side effects are rare, and fewer than with cysteamine or methionine. A clear indication for the administration of N-acetylcysteine is a plasma paracetamol level above 150 mg/l at 4 hours as shown in the nomogram (Fig. 18.1). It should be given intravenously in an initial dose of 150 mg/kg in 200 ml of 5% dextrose solution over 15 minutes. This is followed by 50 mg/kg in 500 ml of 5% dextrose solution over 4 hours and 100 mg/kg in l litre over the next 16 hours (total 300 mg in 20 hours).

IRON POISONING

The most common source of iron poisoning is ferrous sulphate tablets which the young child mistakes for sweets. Other ferrous salts such as gluconate or succinate are less dangerous. A child of 2 years can be fatally poisoned by taking only 3 g of ferrous sulphate.

Clinical features

Four phases can be distinguished in iron poisoning. The first begins 0.5–1 hour after ingestion of the tablets with severe vomiting, diarrhoea, haematemesis, melaena, pallor, metabolic acidosis and in fatal cases pre-terminal coma. In the child who survives, the second phase is associated with a misleading abatement of symptoms which may persist for a period of 8–16 hours. The highly dangerous third phase is then likely to ensue. Iron encephalopathy may cause convulsions and unconsciousness; liver parenchymal damage may result in jaundice and other metabolic derangements; progressive circulatory collapse may end in death. Finally, for the survivors, the fourth phase of recovery follows. Later severe fibrosis and cicatricial scarring of the pyloric end of the stomach may develop and so severely interfere with nutrition that surgical intervention is required. We have seen this late sequela lead to profound emaciation before its existence was suspected.

Treatment

Vomiting should be induced as soon as possible after ingestion of the tablets. On arrival in hospital gastric lavage should be performed with a 1% solution of sodium bicarbonate. Blood should be taken for estimation of the serum iron; values above 16 mmol/l at 4 hours indicate significant poisoning. A straight X-ray of the abdomen may help substantiate the number of tablets ingested and a repeat X-ray will demonstrate whether or not gastric emptying has been complete. Immediately after completion of the gastric lavage 5 g desferrioxamine should be left in the stomach in 50–100 ml of water. At this time 2 g of the drug should be given intramuscularly. If the child is severely ill and vomiting persistently, an intravenous infusion should be set up and desferrioxamine should be added to the solution to give not more than 15 mg/kg per hour to a maximum of 80 mg/kg in 24 hours. The intramuscular dose of desferrioxamine 2 g should be repeated every 12 hours until the serum iron level falls to normal. There is evidence that desferrioxamine must be started before the third phase is established to prove effective. If convulsions develop, treatment should include intravenous diazepam 2–10 mg.

BARBITURATE POISONING

Barbiturates are now much less commonly prescribed and are rarely encountered as a cause of poisoning in children.

Clinical features

In most cases the child is only extremely drowsy. Infrequently he/she may be flushed, excited, restless and may vomit. In severe cases the child is comatose, unresponsive to stimuli and may show respiratory depression with cyanosis, absence of the deep reflexes and circulatory failure with hypotension.

Treatment

Emesis should be induced with ipecacuanha and on admission to hospital, if the child is unconscious, gastric lavage should be performed and activated charcoal given. Blood should be withdrawn for estimation of the blood barbiturate concentration. In most children no further measures are required. In severe cases where response to painful stimuli is minimal or absent, a patent airway must be assured.

POISONING BY PHENOTHIAZINE DERIVATIVES AND ANTIHISTAMINES

The common prescribing of "tranquillizers" of many kinds has, unfortunately increased the opportunity for young children to ingest them accidentally. There is sometimes a fairly long period between ingestion and the appearance of symptoms. These include anorexia, progressive drowsiness, stupor and extrapyramidal signs such as inco-ordinated movements, rigidity or tremor. This form of poisoning is, however, rarely fatal in children.

Treatment

This should be along the lines already recommended for barbiturate poisoning.

POISONING BY THE TRICYCLIC ANTIDEPRESSANTS

Imipramine (Tofranil) and amitriptyline (Tryptizol) have a similar chemical structure and pharmacological activity. Their frequent use as antidepressants for adults has resulted in a rapidly increasing incidence of their accidental ingestion by children. Moreover these drugs are prescribed for enuresis in children and the fact that overdosage can produce dangerous toxic effects in a young child is not sufficiently stressed to the parents.

Clinical features

Mildly affected children develop drowsiness, ataxia, abnormal postures, agitation when stimulated, dilated pupils and tachycardia. Thirst and nystagmus have been present in some cases. In severely affected children convulsions may be followed by coma and severe respiratory depression. Cardiac arrhythmias such as ventricular tachycardia and various degrees of heart block with profound hypotension in children are prominent and dangerous.

Treatment

Because there is no known antidote the management of poisoning with the tricyclics is mainly symptomatic. Emesis is induced with ipecacuanha and gastric lavage and activated charcoal are used with the usual precautions. The amount of tricyclic drugs and their metabolites recovered by forced diuresis, peritoneal dialysis and haemodialysis is so small that these procedures are of little value. Convulsions are controlled with intravenous diazepam 2–10 mg. The cardiac rhythm should be continuously monitored by electrocardiography. If cardiac arrhythmias develop they can be combated with anti-arrhythmic measures. Propranolol and phenytoin have been used in cardiac arrhythmias associated with tricyclic antidepressant poisoning but digoxin is not recommended. Some of the cardiac effects respond to infusions of sodium bicarbonate or to the cautious administration of physostigmine salicylate but the routine use of the latter is not recommended. Continuous intravenous infusion of 5% dextrose in quarter strength saline is required for severely poisoned children but it must be given slowly to avoid cerebral oedema. Severe respiratory depression may require ventilation. There have been several reports of the successful use of prolonged cardiac massage in tricyclic depressant poisoning where the patient had severe hypotension or asystole unresponsive to all the inotropic agents.

ATROPINE POISONING

This type of poisoning may arise from ingestion of the plant deadly nightshade. It may also occur when drugs such as tincture of belladonna, atropine or hyoscine are taken accidentally or prescribed in excessive doses. We have seen severe poisoning develop in a child who drank about 4 ml (40 mg) of his own 1% atropine eye drops.

Clinical features

The onset of symptoms is soon after ingestion with thirst, dryness of the mouth, blurring of vision and photophobia. The child is markedly flushed with widely dilated pupils. Tachycardia is severe and there may be a high fever. Extreme restlessness, confusion, delirium and inco-ordination are characteristic. Indeed, the picture may be mistaken for an acute psychosis. In babies there may be gross gaseous abdominal distension. In fatal cases circulatory collapse and respiratory failure precede death.

Treatment

This can only by symptomatic and supportive. Induced emesis or gastric lavage is essential. They can be followed by the instillation of activated charcoal. Fever should be reduced by tepid sponging. Severe restlessness is best treated with intravenous diazepam 0.2 mg/kg.

AMPHETAMINE POISONING

Acute poisoning can arise from accidental ingestion or inhalation. Symptoms include nausea and vomiting, excitement and delirium, blurred vision, fever and convulsions. Death is preceded by coma and respiratory depression.

Treatment

This is along the lines advised for atropine poisoning but the sedation required is best obtained with intramuscular chlorpromazine or promazine 25–50 mg.

POISONING BY DIGITALIS

The increasing number of older adults taking digitalis preparations in our community is resulting in accidental ingestion by children (often grandchildren) of cardiac glycosides. The most commonly involved preparation is digoxin. The toxic effects may not become marked for some hours and it is important to treat every case as potentially dangerous.

Clinical features

The most striking presenting feature is severe and intractable vomiting which is largely due to the action of digoxin on the central nervous system. Other neurological manifestations include visual disturbances, drowsiness, and convulsions which are usually delayed for several hours in their appearance. Indeed, even if the cardiac effects of the drug can be obviated, death may occur due to depression of the central nervous system. The cardiac manifestations of digoxin intoxication in a previously healthy child are somewhat different from those seen in diseased hearts, e.g. prolonged P-R, short Q-T and S-T segment changes are frequently absent. Exaggeration of normal sinus arrhythmia is a common early finding; sinus pauses with nodal escape beats may occur. Other findings include sinus bradycardia, nodal rhythm, coupled-idioventricular rhythm and complete heart block. Ventricular extrasystoles, common in adults, appear to be an unknown consequence of digitalis poisoning in children.

Treatment

The stomach should be emptied as rapidly as possible by inducing vomiting or by gastric lavage. The most important measure is the administration of potassium chloride intravenously, e.g. 10–20 mmol/l by slow intravenous infusion. The electrocardiograph should be continuously monitored and the serum electrolytes frequently measured because excessive potassium and hyperkalaemia may also aggravate digoxin toxicity. Calcium must not be given intravenously under any circumstances because it acts synergistically with digoxin but a 1% solution of magnesium sulphate given intravenously at a slow rate may be beneficial. Cardiac arrhythmias may respond to practolol intravenously 2.5–5 mg followed by a similar dose every 2 hours to a total of 25 mg; lignocaine 1 mg/kg followed by 1 mg by intravenous infusion every 1 to 2 minutes; procainamide intravenously 50 mg followed by 50 mg every 2 hours; or an external cardiac pacemaker. Exchange transfusion, peritoneal dialysis and haemodialysis are of no value because most of the drug is tissue-bound and plasma concentrations are low. The most promising therapeutic approach to severe digoxin poisoning involves giving Fab fragments of digoxin-specific antibodies (Digibind, Wellcome).

POISONING BY PETROLEUM DISTILLATES, INSECTICIDES AND WEEDKILLERS

Ingestion of petroleum distillates is a common childhood problem because they are readily available in most households, including developing countries where kerosene in particular is used for heating, cooking and lighting. Petroleum distillates (petrol, paraffin, turpentine, turps substitute, white spirit and kerosene) cause irritation of mucous membranes, vomiting and diarrhoea when ingested and respiratory distress, cyanosis, tachycardia and pyrexia when inhaled. Ingestion of more than 1 mg/kg body weight will cause drowsiness and depression of the central nervous system. Emetics and gastric lavage are contraindicated because they increase the risk of hydrocarbon pneumonia in which there may be pulmonary oedema and haemorrhage. Respiratory symptoms usually occur within 6 hours and after this time complications are unlikely. There is no evidence to support the use of steroids in the treatment of lipid aspiration pneumonitis. Antibiotics should be reserved for those who develop proven secondary bacterial infection.

Chlorinated hydrocarbon insecticides such as DDT, dieldrin, aldrin and lindane can be absorbed through the skin and respiratory tract as well as from the gastrointestinal tract and can cause salivation, abdominal pain with vomiting and diarrhoea, and central nervous system depression with convulsions. Contaminated clothing should be removed, the child washed with soap and water, emesis induced and convulsions treated with diazepam.

Organic phosphate insecticides such as malathion, chlorthion, parathion, phosdrin and TEPP are cholinesterase inhibitors which can also be absorbed from skin, lungs and intestines. The accumulation of acetylcholine in tissues causes nausea, vomiting, diarrhoea, blurred vision, miosis, headache, muscle weakness and twitching, loss of reflexes and sphincter control and finally loss of consciousness. Treatment is as for chlorinated hydrocarbons with, in addition, atropine sulphate 0.05 mg/kg given intramuscularly and then pralidoxime, the specific cholinesterase reactivator, in a dose of 25 mg/kg in 10% solution by intravenous infusion at a rate not exceeding 5 mg/min. Pralidoxime is only of use if administered within 12 hours of exposure; after this the enzyme inactivation becomes increasingly irreversible. During transfer to a paediatric unit provision for intubation and assisted ventilation must be available.

Weedkillers of the paraquat type may also be absorbed through skin and respiratory and intestinal tracts. Particularly when concentrated solutions of paraquat have been swallowed, children can experience a burning sensation in the mouth, nausea, vomiting, abdominal pain and diarrhoea which may be bloody. Hours later, ulceration of the mouth, throat and gastrointestinal tract may occur. The absence of initial symptoms does not exclude a diagnosis of paraquat poisoning.

When low to moderate doses of paraquat have been ingested the signs of kidney and liver damage may occur after 2–3 days. Both types of damage are irreversible. After 5–10 days, or very occasionally up to 14 days after poisoning, the child may develop signs of lung damage, which is almost always irreversible. When relatively large doses of paraquat are ingested multi-organ damage and failure occur quickly and death usually occurs within a few hours or days. Tissue damage is probably caused by local hydrogen peroxide and this might be aggravated by giving oxygen to breathe. Quantitative analysis of paraquat in the plasma can be used as a measure of the severity of paraquat poisoning.

Treatment

Treatment consists of emptying the stomach by gastric lavage (if no more than 4 hours have elapsed after ingestion, and there is no suggestion of severe oesophageal damage) and the administration of Fuller's earth (250 ml of a 30% solution) or 50 g activated charcoal together with a purgative (250 ml of 5% magnesium sulphate solution) 4-hourly until diarrhoea occurs.

ACUTE ALCOHOL POISONING

Episodes of acute alcohol (ethanol) poisoning occur predominantly in infancy and pre-adolescence with peaks at ages 3 and 12 years and is commoner in boys. In the younger age group ease of access to spirits and fortified wines allied with poor parental surveillance in the home are important factors. In the older children the episodes are more likely to occur outside the home, thus increasing the risks of physical danger from accidents and hypothermia. The younger infants are at risk of significant hypoglycaemia especially if they drink alcohol in the early morning after an obligate overnight fasting.

Clinical features

Nausea, accompanied by vomiting, ataxia and progressive loss of consciousness are the usual features. Aspiration pneumonia, hypoxic and alcoholic brain damage with cerebral oedema, hypothermia, hypoglycaemia and convulsions are not uncommon complications.

Diagnosis

This is based predominantly on history and on the finding of an elevated blood alcohol concentration. In one series of 17 children with blood alcohol concentrations greater than 200 mg/dl all required intensive care. The blood glucose concentrations must be measured.

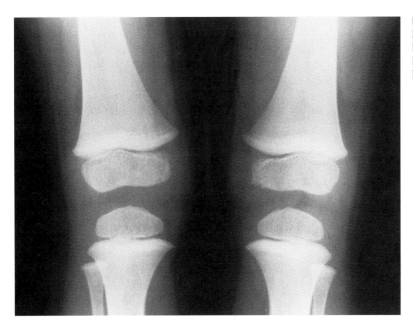

FIGURE 18.2 Radiograph of lowe limbs in chronic lead poisoning. Note bands of increased density ("lead lines") at metaphyseal ends of the long bones.

Treatment

Many children will have vomited but if not should be given gastric lavage (with respiratory support and ventilation when there is significant respiratory depression). Hypoglycaemia should be managed with intravenous infusion of 10% dextrose solution. Glucagon may be ineffective if hepatic glycogen stores are depleted. Intravenous naloxone may be tried in deeply unconscious children and peritoneal dialysis may be required.

After the resolution of the acute problem it is important to make sure that the conditions which predisposed to the episode are examined and corrected where possible. In the younger age group the problem can be resolved by locking up the supply. In the older children there are occasions when they have been plied with alcohol by adults sometimes as a prelude to sexual abuse. Other adolescents continue "heavy" drinking and quickly become alcohol and drug dependent if help is not given.

LEAD POISONING

Lead is usually ingested in small quantities over a long period and the manifestations of poisoning develop insidiously. There are various possible sources of lead such as lead-containing paint which may be used on a child's cot, flakes or paint from plasterwork or woodwork in old Victorian houses, burnt out lead batteries or swallowed pieces of yellow crayon. Pica is common in children suffering from lead poisoning and is a valuable clue to the diagnosis. It is more common in children from the poorest homes. Surma which contains lead sulphide is applied to the eyelids and conjunctivae of infants and children by Asian mothers, mainly for cosmetic reasons. It seems that an appreciable absorption of lead in these children occurs from drainage down the tear duct, or from rubbing the eyes and then licking the fingers. An early diagnosis is extremely important in lead poisoning because if it is left untreated lead encephalopathy may result in death or permanent brain damage.

Clinical features

The earliest signs, such as lethargy, anorexia, vomiting and abdominal pain, are too common to arouse suspicion in themselves, but their persistence without other discoverable cause should do so. The pallor of anaemia is a frequent and characteristic sign. Insomnia and headache frequently precede the onset of lead encephalopathy with convulsions, papilloedema and a cracked-pot sound on percussion of the skull. Radiographs of the skull may then reveal separation of the sutures. Peripheral neuropathy is uncommon in the young child but may develop with paralysis of the dorsiflexors of the wrist or feet. Radiographs of the bones may show characteristic bands of increased density at the metaphyses (Fig. 18.2) but this is a relatively late sign and, therefore, of limited diagnostic value. Excess aminoaciduria is a common manifestation of renal tubular damage and glycosuria may also occur. Renal hypertension has also been reported.

The most dangerous development, both in regard to life and future mental health, is lead encephalopathy. Depending upon the amount of lead ingested this dreaded complication may develop quite quickly, or only following a long period of relatively mild ill health.

Diagnosis

The diagnosis of lead poisoning can be justified in the presence of two or more of the following findings:

1 microcytic hypochromic anaemia with punctate basophilia;
2 radio-opaque foreign bodies in the bowel lumen and lines of increased density at the growing ends of the long bones;
3 coproporphyrinuria;
4 renal glycosuria and aminoaciduria;
5 raised intracranial pressure and protein in the cerebrospinal fluid.

However, the most sensitive test is a marked increase in the urinary excretion of lead after an oral dose of D-penicillamine, 20 mg/kg/day. Increased excretion of δ-aminolaevulinic acid is less commonly found in the child than in the adult with chronic lead poisoning.

Interpretation of the blood lead concentration is, unfortunately, much more difficult. While levels below 1.9 µmol/l (40 µg/100 ml) exclude lead poisoning and levels in the region of 2.9 µmol/l (60 µg/100 ml) are associated with clinical signs, it is possible that behaviour and learning difficulties occur at values between these levels.

Treatment

It is essential that the child be immediately removed from all sources of lead. Deposition of lead in the bones should be encouraged by giving a diet rich in calcium (2 pints of milk daily), phosphorus and vitamin D, thereby lowering the level of lead in the blood. The most important measure is to increase the excretion of lead in the urine. In chronic lead poisoning the chelating agent of choice is probably D-penicillamine. It has the advantage of being extremely effective when given orally. A suitable dose is 20 mg/kg/day for 7 days. Further courses may be required if the blood lead level rises again or if symptoms recur.

In lead encephalopathy combination of lead with sulphydryl groups leads to inhibition of intracellular enzyme systems. The resultant cellular injury is followed by oedema which adds further injury to the brain. The most effective and rapid method of removing lead from the brain is by the parenteral administration of sodium calcium edetate (calcium disodium versenate; CaEDTA). This therapy is combined with measures to diminish cerebral oedema. As soon as the diagnosis has been made CaEDTA 80 mg/kg/day (0.4 ml/kg/day) is given intravenously in four divided doses per 24 hours for 5–7 days. The CaEDTA

should be given by adding each dose to 250 ml of 5% dextrose solution which is given by intravenous infusion. A second course of CaEDTA should be given some 1–10 days after the end of the first course. Subsequent courses may be required if the blood level remains elevated, or at this stage oral D-penicillamine might be employed as described above.

The dangers of cerebral oedema are sufficiently great to demand palliative measures while CaEDTA is being used. Various measures, including surgical decompression, have been tried in this emergency. Mannitol is the safest and most effective agent. It can be given in a dosage of 2.5 g/kg by intravenous infusion of a 20% solution. Dexamethasone has also been advised by the intravenous route in doses of 1 mg/kg/day given in four equal 6-hourly injections for 48 hours. Once lead encephalopathy has been allowed to develop, the risks to life and subsequent mental development are very great.

CAUSTIC INGESTION

Accidental ingestion of caustic substances by inquisitive toddlers may result in serious injury to the mouth, oropharynx, oesophagus or stomach. The most corrosive and commonly ingested caustics are the liquid form of sodium or potassium hydroxide drain cleaners. Other less caustic alkalis which may be ingested are bleach (sodium hypochlorite), laundry and dishwasher detergents and disinfectants usually kept in the kitchen. Ingestion of these substances is most likely to result in injury to the oesophagus, but if ingested in large amounts they can produce extensive damage to the upper gastrointestinal tract. If the hydroxide concentration is high it may lead to perforation of the oesophagus and thus penetration into the peri-oesophageal tissues which may cause mediastinitis. The presence of oral burns confirms that ingestion of a caustic substance has taken place but it does not suggest the degree of oesophageal damage. Dyspnoea, stridor or hoarseness suggest laryngeal injury.

Treatment

All children with caustic ingestion should be admitted for observation of at least 24 hours. No emetics should be given because regurgitation of the caustic substance will aggravate the injury. Milk or water should be given as they will dilute the caustic. After hospital admission a decision, based on the severity of clinical findings and the history, will be made whether endoscopic assessment of the extent of the damage should be made. Antibiotic prophylaxis for infection of the severely burned tissue should be given for 10 days and prednisolone 2 mg/kg/day must be

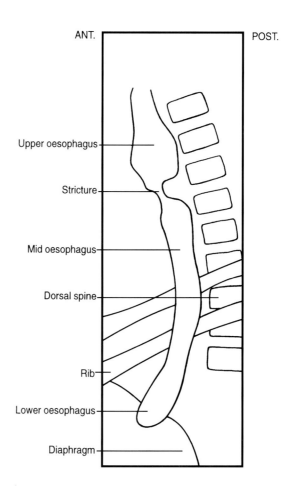

ANT.   POST.

Upper oesophagus

Stricture

Mid oesophagus

Dorsal spine

Rib

Lower oesophagus

Diaphragm

FIGURE 18.3 Oesophageal stricture: barium swallow showing short smooth stricture secondary to caustic ingestion.

given for 3 weeks early in the course of the injury to minimise the formation of scar tissue and stricture (Fig. 18.3). Oesophagoscopy should be carried out 12–24 hours after ingestion to determine whether or not there has been an oesophageal burn. If a burn is discovered both antibiotics and prednisolone should be given as above; otherwise, they should be stopped.

Children with oesophageal stricture usually respond to repeated dilatations but some require oesophageal replacement surgery.

SWALLOWED FOREIGN BODIES

Foreign body ingestion is common in children because they have a tendency to explore and to taste new objects and thus they swallow bizarre and multiple objects. Most foreign bodies swallowed pass through the alimentary tract without symptoms. However, if the foreign body is lodged in the oesophagus it should be removed immediately through an

endoscope to avoid the serious complications of oesophageal obstruction, asphyxia or mediastinitis. In the absence of symptoms the management simply consists of an X-ray of the abdomen to confirm the presence of a radio-opaque object and a careful watch kept on the stools until the foreign body is recovered.

Disc batteries (button batteries) are often ingested in young children these days due to their widespread use in electrical products in the home. These batteries contain alkalies in sufficient concentration to cause caustic injuries and mercury in sufficient quantities to create problems. However, the highly toxic mercuric oxide is converted to essentially nontoxic elemental mercury on leakage or complete disintegration of the battery (Fig. 18.4). In addition, mercuric oxide is poorly soluble and not well absorbed and this may account for the very low incidence of mercury poisoning and therefore children may not need chelation therapy. The vast majority of battery ingestions are benign and can be managed without endoscopic or surgical intervention. Evaluation and treatment of the burns caused by the

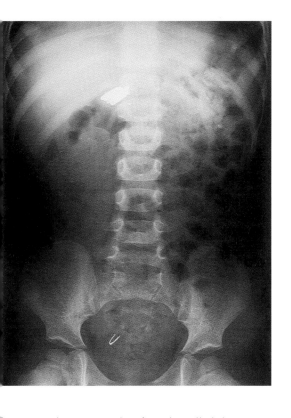

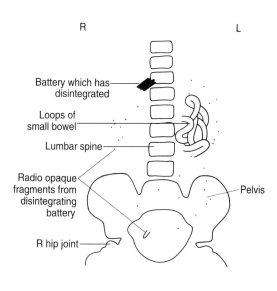

FIGURE 18.4 X-ray of abdomen showing disintegrating battery.

battery is the same as that for other alkali burns (see caustic ingestions). Batteries lodged in the oesophagus must be removed by endoscopic means. If they have recently passed into the stomach, purgation can speed their passage; if, however, they have been in the stomach for more than 3 hours their removal by endoscopy is essential.

SNAKE BITE

Snake bite is a major medical problem in many parts of the world. The snakes of medical importance are the vipers (e.g. carpet viper, Russell viper, adder, etc.) and the elapids (cobra, mamba, krait, etc.) Local effects of the venom in both groups may result in severe swelling and local necrosis which can cause severe permanent scarring and deformity, occasionally necessitating amputation of the bitten limb. Clinical effects of systemic viperine envenoming usually involve haemorrhage and coagulation defects resulting in incoagulable blood. Systemic elapid poisoning usually causes neurotoxic effects which, in untreated cases, results in ptosis and paralysis of the respiratory muscles.

Antivenom is virtually ineffective in reducing or eliminating the local effects of envenoming which should be treated symptomatically, whereas administration of antivenom via the intravenous route is the only proven effective therapeutic treatment of systemic envenoming. The dose of antivenom should be the same in children as in adults. The only antivenom of value is the Zagreb antivenom. Two ampoules of the antivenom should be added to 100 ml normal saline and administered at a rate of 15 drops per minute. The benefits of antivenom should be weighed against the risk of hypersensitivity reaction to the serum. A history of an allergic condition is a relative contraindication to its use.

PLANT POISONING

Plants found in the home, garden and field now constitute the most common source of ingested poison in children. Fortunately, poisonous plants are rarely ingested in quantities sufficient to cause serious illness. Deliberate ingestion of magic mushroom is also a potential source of poisoning. Identification of the plant must be attempted early and a computerised database can be accessed through the poisons centres. Caution should be used in accepting common names of plants or in identifying a plant from a verbal description of its fruit or foliage. If substantial doubt exists, a portion of the plant should be brought for identification. However, each plant ingestion in a child must be viewed as potentially toxic until the plant has been positively identified or sufficient time has passed for a conclusion on non-toxicity.

19

Childhood Tumours

INTRODUCTION

Malignancy in childhood is rare. It has been estimated that in 20 years of a busy family doctor's practice, he might see one or two new patients with tumours. Malignant disease in infancy and childhood is the third commonest cause of death in this age group, following deaths from accidents and deaths from congenital malformation. Indeed, because they are so rare and yet so malignant for most tumours there is an average delay of 3 months from the time that suspicion is aroused to the time when surgery is performed. This delay is very often due to the fact that both parents and clinicians do not have a high index of suspicion of malignancy in childhood. The malignancies of infants and children are very different from those seen in adults. A lot of unnecessary anxiety on the part of the parents can be relieved by reassurance that children who have *lumps* in the breast or rectal bleeding are most unlikely to have malignancies. These physical signs which are so often ominous in adults, heralding a cancer of the breast or a cancer of the bowel, are pathologies virtually non-existent in this particular age group. Congenital malformation such as lipomata and hamartoma may easily be confused in developing children with a malignant growth. These benign lumps which can appear on any part of the body in a child may confuse the parents since they grow disproportionately and give rise to a lot of concern. Surgery for these lesions is rarely necessary because of the potential risk of malignant change but may be indicated for cosmetic reasons.

Epithelial cancers in infancy and childhood are extremely rare and for practical purposes, lung, breast and gastrointestinal cancers, which are common in adults, never occur in children. The tumours that are encountered in infancy and childhood are tumours of mesodermal origin and can be classified as the leukaemias, brain tumours and the solid tumours (Fig. 19.l). Many of these tumours are dealt with in regional centres, e.g. approximately 20 new patients a year with solid tumours attend RHSC Glasgow from a population of approximately 3 million.

Whereas survival figures for adult tumours have not changed all that much over the past 20 years, the same cannot be said for tumours of infancy and childhood. The percentage survival illustrated in Fig. 19.2 shows a 15% survival for Wilms tumours in the 1950s compared with an 85% 5 year survival in

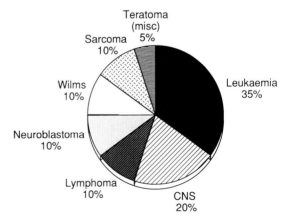

FIGURE 19.1 Chart illustrating frequency of malignancy in childhood.

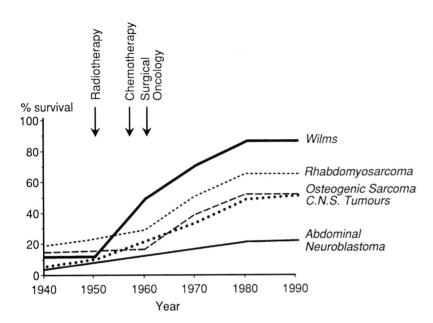

FIGURE 19.2 Percentage survival of the common malignancies in childhood.

the 1990s. Abdominal neuroblastoma, which carries the worst prognosis, still has only a 30% survival.

Hospital admission

Admission to hospital is a traumatic experience for both child and family especially when dealing with a suspected malignancy. The child requires explanation of his surroundings, who people are, and what is happening to him. This must be given at a level which the child understands. Accommodation should be available for a parent, as should unrestricted visiting; both are known to reduce anxiety. The parents also need time spent with them explaining the situation and orientating them to the ward whether resident or not. Nursing and medical staff should work together and if at all possible a senior nurse should accompany the doctor when the diagnosis is being discussed with the parents. Privacy should then be possible for the parents. Admission procedures will vary but the same basic information about the child, the family and their normal life is necessary to allow the staff to have a clearer picture. This also helps to maintain as near normal life as is possible in hospital. Certain clinical information is essential and includes vital signs including blood pressure. Height and weight are essential measurements required to assess the child and also to calculate drug dosages on the basis of the surface area. Parents often help with filling in fluid balance charts and should be encouraged to participate in the nursing care as much as they want. This makes the child more relaxed and helps the parent(s) to feel more useful and needed.

A child with a suspected malignancy is not always obviously ill on admission. Often the child does not understand why he is in hospital because he does not feel ill. In such situations the ward school teacher and playleader are very useful because they help to maintain a certain degree of normality and also relieve boredom. On the other hand, the ill child on admission will require more detailed care, e.g. IV fluids and pain relief. In some ways this is easier to deal with because the child feels unwell and illness can be more readily discussed.

Regardless of whether the child is "well" or ill on admission a social worker experienced in the problems facing these families should be available. Once the malignancy is confirmed the social worker will have more contact to offer services including financial help when needed.

Assessment

An accurate diagnosis involves many tests or procedures some of which may be painful and frightening. The child requires explanation of what will happen, how it will happen and reassurance that he will not be left alone. If his mother or father cannot be there, a nurse will be, preferably one whom he knows. Sedation may be used prior to certain procedures such as bone marrow puncture or lumbar puncture. Hypnosis is a possible alternative to sedation in the older child. This enables the procedure to be carried out as efficiently and quickly as possible and minimises the stress for the child. Other tests such as X-rays and ultrasounds are less frightening and can be made out to be games but a CT or MRI scan can be very frightening for a child.

Once the assessment is complete and the diagnosis made the parents are interviewed by the consultant and told the most recent news. A senior nurse again should be present because often the parents do not absorb what they are being told or do not understand but do not want to seem ignorant by saying so. They will often ask the nurse to repeat the information once the doctor is away. Ideally, both parents should be present so that they are both given the same information. All parents react differently but no matter how they appear to be they are all devastated by the news.

The child or siblings are not often present at this interview and one question which often arises is what will we tell our son/daughter. No-one can decide that for parents – they know their child best. They can be advised that it is better to be honest with all children regardless of their age, although it does not necessarily mean that every last detail should be given. The parents at this stage must be given opportunities to be alone together or to contact their families and to try to begin to come to terms with their temporarily shattered lives. One important point to advise parents is that to the best of their ability they should treat the child as before, i.e. if he misbehaves disciplining will continue. This helps to minimise potential jealousy in other siblings. It is impossible for a nurse not to become involved and she will find that empathy, listening and communication by touch provide comfort and support. It is important that a nurse's personal feelings do not affect her care.

Pre- and post-operative care

Pre-operative care is the same as for any major operation, remembering again to explain to the child that although the operation is going to help to make him better, he will still be sore afterwards but will be given pain relief. Explanation of the expected postoperative condition has been shown to reduce anxiety and the amount of pain experienced. Orientation to the intensive care unit at this stage is recommended to reduce anxiety increased by the environment of an intensive care unit.

Post-operatively the normal basic care involves regular observation of vital signs including BP, replacement of fluid, relief of pain and reassurance. Malignancy and chemotherapy can result in delayed wound healing. Sutures are normally dissolving and it is important to remember to tell the child and his parents of this – many people worry about removal of sutures. Visiting in the ward can be restricted to immediate family only in the first 24–48 hours postoperatively and only once the child is feeling better should free visiting be restored. As soon as possible after the operation the parents are seen by the consultant to explain the findings and the proposed treatment. Once again both parents and a senior nurse should be present.

Nutrition

In the immediate post-operative period and for some time afterwards the child may either not be allowed food orally or may not want it. This may be due to anorexia post-operatively, emotional upset or simply the presence of disease. It is vital to have a maximum nutritional state to promote wound healing. Adding extra calories in the form of snacks, flavoured milk shakes or disguised calories in the form of drink additives may help. Paediatric dietitians perform a valuable service here. Overnight continuous high calorie nasogastric feeds may be necessary. This enables the child to be free during the day to attempt to eat attractive foods at normal times and make up the losses overnight. The nasogastric tube may be replaced daily or left *in situ*.

Chemotherapy

If chemotherapy is decided upon the parents should be interviewed again, this time to explain the drugs, how they are given, how often and their potential side effects (Chapter 13). Depending on which drugs are involved and the child's reaction to them, the treatment may be given as a day patient, therefore reducing the number of admissions. Side effects in children are similar to those in adults, the most common being alopecia, nausea/vomiting/diarrhoea and weight loss. Children tend to adapt well to the side effects, e.g. may put up with continued nausea and vomiting during and after their treatment despite the use of IV anti-emetics. Often as soon as an IV is established (even just for hydration prior to treatment) the child stops eating and drinking and as soon as the infusion is removed his appetite gradually returns. For this reason there is no point in insisting that a child eats or drinks while the IV is in progress because it will simply be refused. A child will ask for what he wants when he wants it. Hair loss causes great upset to adults and adolescents but not so with children. A boy will wear a cap or a woolly hat and a girl a head scarf – most children will not entertain wigs. Repeated injections are a source of stress to children but despite this the child is actively involved, i.e. he wears a face mask like the staff. Praise for the child who has coped well with a painful procedure improves relationships as does being honest in saying that a procedure will hurt rather then denying the inevitable pain.

Neutropenia less than 100 neutrophils per mm^3 secondary to chemotherapy requires protective isolation in which the child is nursed in a cubicle and has restricted visiting from both staff and visitors to reduce the risk of infection. Various antiseptics including nasal cream and mouthwashes, dental gel (no toothbrushing) and an antiseptic soap are used by the child to minimise risk. This is continued until the WBC returns to normal. Most children adapt well to isolation providing they do not feel ill and boredom is relieved by having plenty to do. An essential item is a TV set!

Radiotherapy

The care of the child and the side effects are the same as with adults but with the added problems that irradiation interferes with the growth of tissues in the young and can result in long-term deformity and short stature. It is important that the same area is irradiated at each treatment and involves the child being absolutely still for the minutes that the treatment takes. This can be accomplished by making the procedure into a game, i.e. wearing "starwars helmet"! With very young or uncooperative children sedation or occasionally general anaesthesia may be used. It is important to observe for radiation burns. Should one occur, ensuring that the area is kept dry will promote healing. Constant explanation and emotional support must be continued for both child and family. Having radiotherapy does not necessarily require the child to be an inpatient.

Discharge

A diagnosis of malignancy is likely to involve many hospital admissions or at least visits to outpatient clinics or day bed facilities. Regardless of where the child is seen it must always be stressed to the parents that they can contact staff at the hospital 24 hours a day if they have a problem. It can be reassuring to know that advice is not far away even for an apparently trivial query. This particularly applies when the child goes home for the first time after diagnosis, after the first treatment or after relapse when the family do not know what to expect or whether they will cope at home. A return appointment should always be given at discharge. Drug prescriptions must be fully explained to the parents and the importance of continuing treatment for the full course emphasised. The hospital should be informed immediately of any *contact with infectious diseases* such as measles or chicken pox so that a gammaglobulin injection can be given within 24 hours. Infectious diseases in such children can prove fatal.

Many parents are taught in hospital how to cope with nasogastric feeds and this is continued by them at home. A visit from a community nurse, a doctor or a hospital liaison nurse is reassuring and they should be informed before the child's discharge from hospital.

LEUKAEMIAS

Leukaemia is the one malignancy that the public most closely associate with childhood malignancies. Thirty-five per cent of children with malignancies fall into this category, most of them presenting with acute illnesses. The incidence of leukaemias has received much publicity over the past few years showing clusters occurring in various parts of the country especially near certain nuclear installations. There is no conclusive evidence that links nuclear waste disposal with a higher incidence of leukaemias in these areas. Chromosomal abnormalities such as Down syndrome with the Philadelphia chromosome 21 is associated with a higher incidence of leukaemia and there is good genetic evidence for this aetiology. The clinical presentation of children with leukaemia is very often an acute haematological crisis with anaemia, sepsis, bleeding and petechial haemorrhages. Diagnosis is made by blood film, lumbar puncture as well as bone marrow aspirations and trephine. There are various therapeutic schedules for children with leukaemia and a majority of these children are now cured by intensive chemotherapy and, when necessary, bone marrow transplantation (Chapter 13).

BRAIN TUMOURS

Brain tumours encountered in children are of unknown aetiology and present usually with signs of raised intracranial pressure which can be mistaken for meningitis. The clinical signs are those of neck rigidity and limited straight leg lifting, occasionally opisthotonos and papilloedema. Lumbar puncture in these cases should never be carried out as it might produce coning and sudden death. Diagnosis can be made by ultrasound examination if the anterior fontanelle is open, or by CT scanning with or without contrast to outline the tumour (Fig. 19.3). Most brain tumours in children are in the posterior fossa. They arise from the medulla or cerebellum and are commonly medulloblastomas. A histological diagnosis is essential. Combination chemotherapy and radiotherapy after excisional biopsy when possible have increased the 2-year survival in this malignancy to 40%. In the acute situation when children present with raised intracranial pressure the pressure may have to be relieved by making a burr hole and putting an external drain into the ventricles. These procedures should be carried out by a neurosurgeon competent to deal with adequate biopsy and excision of the tumour when possible.

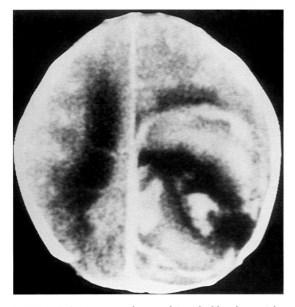

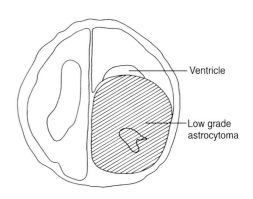

FIGURE 19.3 Astrocytoma (low-grade) with dilated ventricles.

LYMPHOMAS

This group constitutes approximately 10% of patients with malignant disease. The aetiology of lymphoma is unknown, although a number of children with lymphoma are now presenting as a result of previous anti-tumour chemotherapy. Treatment received for leukaemia might have a role to play in the induction of the lymphoma. Lymphomas may present as masses wherever lymph nodes are present in the body. Enlarged cervical lymph nodes are a very common manifestation of inflammatory disease in children and at times it may be extremely difficult to decide whether cervical lymphadenopathy is secondary to infection or to lymphoma. This issue may have to be decided by biopsy and membrane markers must be performed on biopsy material in order to type the lymphoma. It must be remembered that matted lymph nodes in the neck, secondary to infection, may take several months to resolve once the infection is under control and

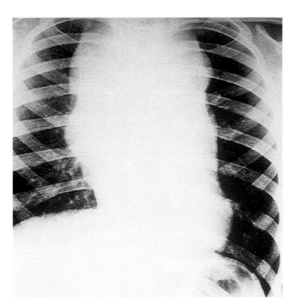

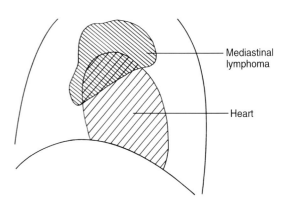

FIGURE 19.4 Lymphoma of mediastinum.

could easily be mistaken for a lymphoma. Mediastinal lymphomas are notorious since their clinical presentations may be acute with dyspnoea and pleural effusions (Fig. 19.4). There is a real danger that when biopsying these mediastinal masses acute extrinsic compression of the trachea can result from bleeding and oedema. It is recommended that these patients be intubated and ventilated for 24–48 hours post-surgery in order to avoid catastrophe. Abdominal lymphomata usually present as large abdominal masses, the origin of which is very often unclear. These may arise from abdominal mesenteric nodes, the spleen, or Peyer patches within the small bowel. Most of these abdominal lymphomata are B-cell lymphomas and carry a poor prognosis. Surgery in lymphomata should be of a limited nature and should be just sufficient to obtain histological confirmation of the type of lymphoma present. If a pleural effusion or bone marrow involvement is present, then surgery might be avoided by simply taking pleural fluid or bone marrow aspirates and cytospinning them to obtain a diagnosis. Most patients with lymphoma are put on regimens of chemotherapy which include complicated protocols. Once patients with lymphoma have started treatment the tumour resolves within 24 hours, hence it is very often unnecessary to carry out major surgery to excise all the tumour in these patients. Patients with B-cell lymphoma carry the worst prognosis, a third of them dying from the disease no matter what their treatment. One of the precautions one has to take when commencing a patient with a large lymphoma on chemotherapy is hydrating the patient and alkalinising the urine as there is a real risk of uric acid nephropathy from tumour lysis.

NEPHROBLASTOMA

Wilms tumour, also known as nephroblastoma, is one of the commonest solid tumours encountered in childhood and the peak incidence is at approximately 2 years of age (Fig. 19.5). They hardly ever occur in the neonatal age group. On review of the pathology nephroblastomas that in the past were described in the neonatal age group have turned out to be congenital mesoblastic nephromas which are not malignant tumours but are hamartomas. These benign tumours of the kidney in the newborn are treated by surgical excision.

A review of 100 children presenting at Yorkhill with nephroblastoma between 1950 and 1985 revealed that 85% of them were below the age of 5 years. On clinical presentation, 56% had an abdominal mass which had been present for 3 months before surgical excision (Fig. 19.6). Abdominal pain, very often non-specific, was the presenting complaint in

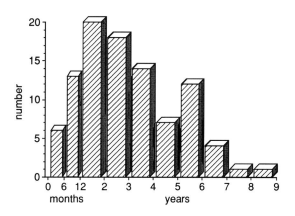
FIGURE 19.5 Incidence of nephroblastoma.

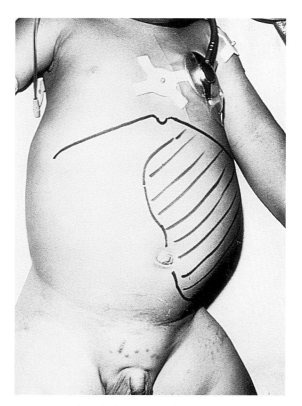
FIGURE 19.6 Clinical photograph of nephroblastoma.

31%, 29% had nausea and vomiting, 19% complained of malaise and weight loss and 18% had haematuria. Patients who had haematuria presented to the hospital within 2 weeks and had their tumour dealt with early. The intravenous urogram or CT scan (Fig. 19.7) which shows a distorted calyceal system and ultrasound confirmation of a solid tumour rather than a hydronephrosis usually confirm the diagnosis. Invasive angiography has been of limited use in the past and does not help in the management. The histopathology of nephroblastoma allows classifica-

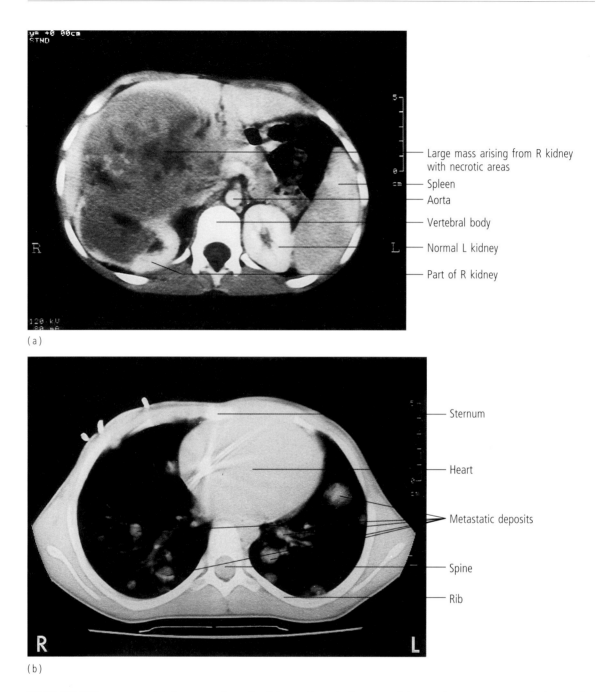

(a)

Large mass arising from R kidney with necrotic areas
Spleen
Aorta
Vertebral body
Normal L kidney
Part of R kidney

(b)

Sternum
Heart
Metastatic deposits
Spine
Rib

FIGURE 19.7 Wilms tumour. (a) Contrast-enhanced axial scan through the upper abdomen showing an extremely large right-sided Wilms tumour which contains areas of necrosis. (b) Unenhanced axial scan of the lungs showing numerous metastatic deposits of varying sizes.

tion into three major groups, the favourable pathology, the unfavourable pathology and pathology which shows the presence of bone metastasising renal tumour of childhood. Patients with a favourable histology, i.e. differentiation of tubular structures, have a good prognosis with greater than 80% 5-year survival rate. Those patients having a non-favourable

pathology with evidence of embryonal undifferentiated structures and the more specialised bone metastasising renal tumour of childhood have a worse prognosis with a 40% 5-year survival rate. The role of the surgeon in nephroblastoma is not only one of surgical excision but also tumour staging (Fig. 19.8; Table 19.1).

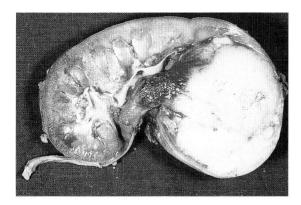

FIGURE 19.8 Gross specimen of kidney. Stage I nephroblastoma.

TABLE 19.1 Nephroblastoma staging

STAGE	DESCRIPTION OF TUMOUR
I	Limited to renal capsule
II	Extended beyond capsule or into renal vein
III	In regional lymph nodes or if gross spillage at operation
IV	Distant spread to lung or brain
V	Both kidneys involved – rare

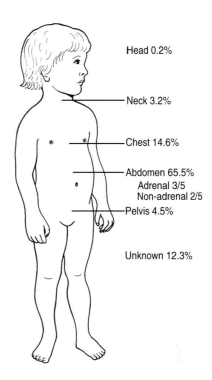

FIGURE 19.9 Sites of neuroblastoma.

With the current chemotherapy/radiology schedules the overall 5-year survival rate is now more than 85%. Even in patients with metastatic disease with unfavourable pathology there is a 40% 5-year survival rate.

NEUROBLASTOMA

These are tumours arising from neural crest tissue. They vary from the most aggressive type of tumour which is a primitive neuroblastoma also known as a primitive neuroectodermal tumour (PNET), to a ganglioneuroblastoma which is better differentiated and more mature, to the most mature tumour, a ganglioneuroma. More than 65% of these tumours present as abdominal masses, three-fifths of them arise from the adrenal medulla and two-fifths from a non-adrenal site (Fig. 19.9). They account for roughly 10% of childhood tumours and usually present as an abdominal mass in a child who is under the age of 2 years. Diagnosis of a neuroblastoma can be made on clinical grounds and investigations usually include a plain X-ray of the abdomen which may show calcification in the tumour. An intravenous urogram very often shows a kidney displaced by a suprarenal mass (Fig. 19.10). CT scanning with contrast gives more detailed information on the involvement and displacement of other structures by the tumour (Fig. 19.11).

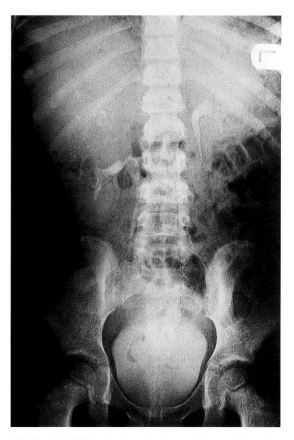

FIGURE 19.10 IVU showing displaced kidney right side. Speckled calcification in neuroblastoma.

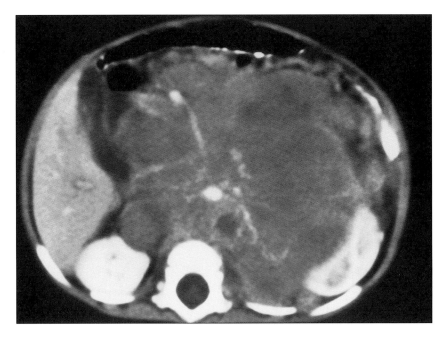

FIGURE 19.11 CT of a suprarenal calcified mass displacing the kidney.

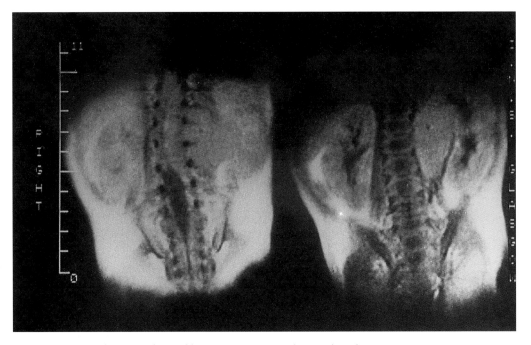

FIGURE 19.12 MRI of congenital neuroblastoma compressing the spinal cord.

More recently imaging by MRI (magnetic resonance imaging) shows greater detail (Fig. 19.12). Biochemical investigations should include a 24-hour urine collection for measurement of homovanillic acid. Excretion of these catecholamine breakdown products is increased in up to 90% of patients with neuroblastomas. Neuroblasts have malignant charac-teristics and spread very rapidly so that the neuro-blastoma is usually diagnosed when it has reached stage III or IV, i.e. with metastatic disease (Fig. 19.13). Very rarely are neuroblastomas found at stage I and stage II. A very specialised stage IV-S neuro-blastoma can occur in the infant in which neuroblas-toma cells invade soft tissues, e.g. the liver with gross

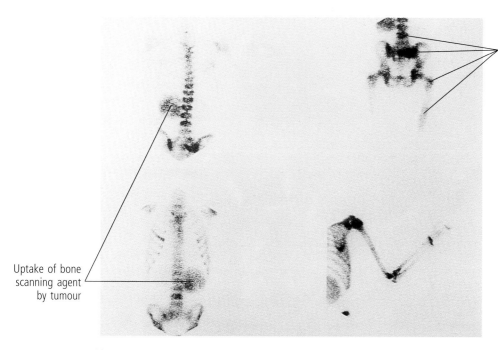

Uptake of scanning agent by bone metastases

Uptake of bone scanning agent by tumour

FIGURE 19.13 Neuroblastoma bone scan. ^{99m}Tc methylene diphosphonate bone scan in a 6-year-old boy with recurrence of an abdominal mass in the left hypochondrium and a normal skeletal survey. The bone scanning agent has been taken up by the tumour mass. There is increased uptake of the scanning agent in a lower lumbar vertebral body, in the sacroiliac joints, in the right femur and in the anterior end of a right rib due to bony metastatic disease.

hepatomegaly, skin lumps and bone marrow involvement but no spread to bone. More than 50% of these patients survive without treatment since the neuroblastoma matures to a ganglioneuroma. Most deaths from this special type of tumour occur because of respiratory failure induced by the very large abdominal masses (Fig. 19.14). Localised radiotherapy can help shrinkage of the tumour and allow these patients to "outgrow and outlive their tumour". The prognosis of a neuroblastoma is related to:

1   The age at presentation – a neonate has a 60–70% survival rate, a child under the age of 1 has a 56–70% survival rate, over the age of 1 up to 2 years of age the survival is between 19 and 28%, whereas over the age of 2 the chances of survival are 15–20%.
2   The site of origin – a child who has abdominal neuroblastoma has the worst prognosis, whereas a child presenting with a pelvic or a thoracic neuroblastoma has a very good chance of survival since most of the tumours in this site will mature to a ganglioneuroblastoma or even ganglioneuroma.

Treatment schedules have increased the survival rate for less favourable tumours using chemotherapy and radiotherapy and, when indicated, autologous bone marrow transplantation after high dose methotrexate and total body radiation. More recent forms of therapy involve "targeted therapy" using MIBG (meta-iodobenzylguanidine) selectively taken up by

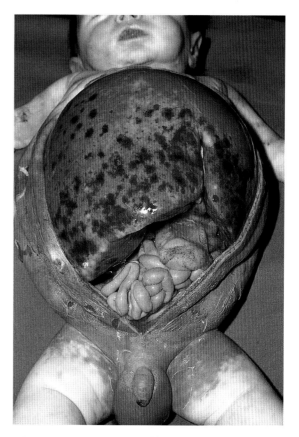

FIGURE 19.14 Stage IV-S neuroblastoma.

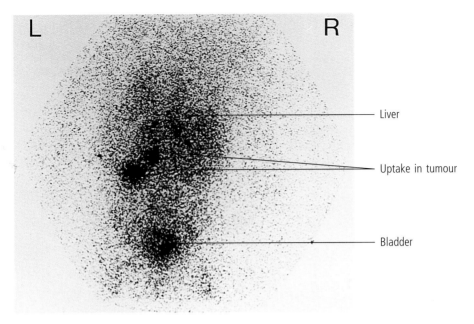

L R

— Liver

— Uptake in tumour

— Bladder

FIGURE 19.15 MIBG scan. 48-hour scan of the abdomen showing two areas of uptake of ^{131}I-meta-iodobenzylgunaidine in the left hypochondrium at the site of neuroblastoma deposits. There is normal uptake of the radionuclide in the liver and in the bladder.

neuroblastomas (Fig. 19.15). Radioactive iodine is used to demonstrate and at higher doses kill neuroblast cells. This form of therapy is still under review.

SARCOMAS

Sarcomas constitute 10% of all malignancies in children. Three areas in the body are affected by sarcomas. These are the limbs, the genitourinary system and the head and neck. The clinical presentation in the limb is usually one of a mass appearing after minor trauma (Fig. 19.16). A diagnosis can be extremely difficult since the lesion is often mistaken for a traumatic haematoma and an underlying tumour is not suspected. In children the commonest pathology is rhabdomyosarcoma whereas osteogenic sarcomas are more common in teenagers. Investigations usually include soft tissue X-rays, skeletal surveys and chest X-rays. CT scanning and MRI help determine the extent of the disease and whether metastatic disease is present. These tumours tend to spread by haematogenous as well as lymphatic routes. The diagnosis is usually established by biopsy and when attempting a curative resection the regional lymph nodes must be dissected and removed for staging purposes. Treatment schedules for rhabdomyosarcomas are complicated and various schedules by the Inter-state Rhabdomyosarcoma Study Group in the United States, and the European

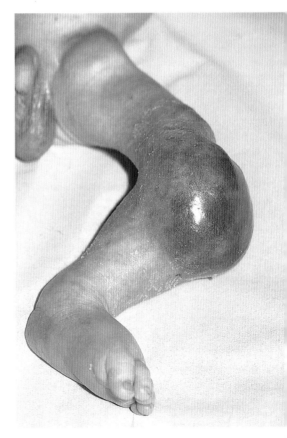

FIGURE 19.16 Rhabdomyosarcoma of the left leg with enlarged inguinal lymph nodes.

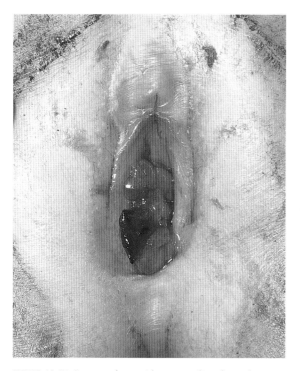
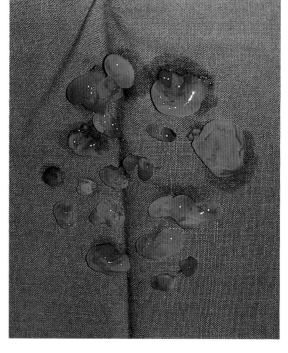

FIGURE 19.17 Sarcoma botryoides protruding from the vagina.

group (SIOP) are used for therapy by the UK Cancer Children's Study Group. The prognosis for children with limb rhabdomyosarcomas is approximately 40% 5-year survival rate which is not as good as for tumours in other sites. Rhabdomyosarcoma of the genitourinary system usually presents as a pelvic mass causing extrinsic or intrinsic urinary tract obstruction. The tumour is palpable on digital rectal examination. Occasionally in little girls uterine rhabdomyosarcoma polyps, also known as sarcoma botryoides, can extrude as grape-like structures from the vulval orifice (Fig. 19.17). Earlier treatments required extensive surgical exenterations with mutilation and gave poor results. With the current regimen of chemotherapy and radiotherapy it is possible to shrink these tumours and perform minimal excisional surgery and achieve good survival rates. Head and neck rhabdomyosarcomas usually present as malignant masses which may extend into the brain and meninges. If the meninges are involved there is a poor prognosis but if not, after limited surgery and extensive radiotherapy, the prognosis is good.

TERATOMA

Teratomas may arise in germ cells of ovaries in older girls and testes in younger boys. However, the commonest tumour found in the ovary is a benign

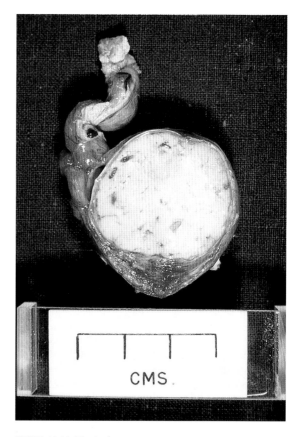

FIGURE 19.18 Testicular tumour.

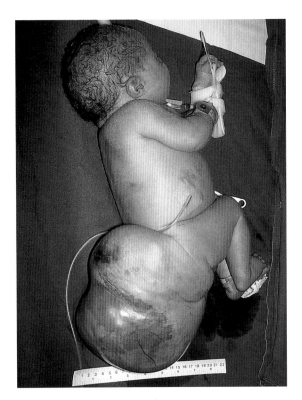

FIGURE 19.19 Benign sacrococal teratoma.

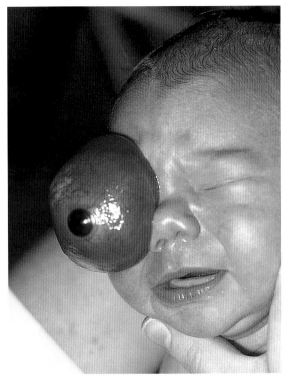

FIGURE 19.20 Orbital teratoma benign.

teratoma which is rarely malignant. Ovarian tumours in older girls are more solid and not as cystic as those found in younger girls. The solid parts in ovarian teratomata usually have epithelial components which secrete high concentrations of α-fetoprotein as well as carcinoembryonic antigen. Testicular tumours encountered in children are usually orchidoblastomas (Fig. 19.18). These are easily confused with inguinal herniae, tense hydroceles and haematomas of the scrotum following trauma. Complete surgical removal with meticulous surgical technique can achieve cure in most instances when the tumour is localised to the testes. Careful follow-up is indicated using serial measurements of α-fetoprotein which is a very good tumour marker and routine chest X-rays to exclude metastatic disease. Should there be evidence of spread of tumour, intensive chemotherapy is indicated.

The overall survival rate of metastatic disease is poor. The commonest sites of teratomata are sacrococcygeal tumours in the newborn (Fig. 19.19). A rare site can occur in the orbit (Fig. 19.20). More than 85% of these are benign and are being detected by antenatal ultrasound. Simple surgical excision is curative in these early diagnosed tumours but some have an intrapelvic dumb-bell component which could become malignant if left beyond 3 months of age. Malignant change occurs in 10–30% and contains epithelial or endodermal sinus components, also known as yolk sac tumours, which secrete high

levels of α-fetoprotein. This is a useful marker to check for residual disease, recurrence or metastatic disease (Table 19.2).

RETINOBLASTOMA

Retinoblastoma is the commonest primary tumour of the eye in children. It accounts for 1% or less of all childhood malignancies. Its genetic features are of interest as well as of importance in the management and counselling of families with this malignancy. Ninety per cent of retinoblastomas develop as an apparently spontaneous event. Less than 10% are affected by the autosomal dominant type of disease. Most of these children have bilateral disease. A deletion of the long arm of chromosome 13 (13q) has been noted in some patients.

Most children are detected after leukocoria (white or cat's eye reflex) is observed. Other signs are unexplained strabismus or squint. In some underdeveloped countries exophthalmos is the most common presenting sign. The mean age of diagnosis is 17 months. Any child with a positive family history of retinoblastoma should be examined at birth and at regular intervals thereafter. Careful complete examination of both retinae by direct and indirect ophthalmoscopy under anaesthesia must be performed (see Fig. 3.2). Bone marrow and lumbar puncture as well as a CT scan of the orbit should be

TABLE 19.2 Comparison of nephroblastoma, neuroblastoma and sarcoma

	NEPHROBLASTOMA	NEUROBLASTOMA	SARCOMA
Mean age	2 years	4 years	6 years
Organ	Kidney	Adrenal or sympathetic chain	Mesodermal tissues
Presentation	Abdominal mass (unilateral)	"Great mimic"	Mass – variable site
	Abdominal distension	Abdominal mass (crosses midline)	Urinary tract signs & symptoms
	pain	Malaise, anaemia, bone pain, others	
	vomiting		
Abdominal X-ray – calcification	Seldom	10–20%	–
Distant spread	Lungs	Bone	Lungs
Tumour marker	Prorenin (blood)	VMA/HVA (urine)	–
Prognosis	Good	Poor	Variable – good

obtained prior to undertaking surgery. Ultrasound is also of value. A skeletal survey is necessary to exclude distant metastasis.

The cell of origin is a cell of the outer layer of the retina and is composed of small round cells with scarcity of cytoplasm. The cells aggregate around blood vessels to form true Flexner–Wintersteiner rosettes.

Most children have multifocal disease at the time of presentation. Children with unilateral early or intermediate disease have a 70% likelihood of tumour eradication with visual preservation and radiotherapy should be seriously considered. Loss of vision in an eye should be treated by enucleation with as much of the optic nerve required to remove any infiltrated tumour. Chemotherapy has little to offer but therapeutic trials are in progress. Patients with hereditary retinoblastomas have an increased risk of second tumours unrelated to the radiation therapy they receive. These include osteosarcomas and Wilms tumours.

LIVER TUMOUR

Liver tumours in childhood are extremely rare. The benign mesenchymal hamartoma which presents as a tumour mass in the liver is of very low malignant potential (Fig. 19.21). These tumours are simply excised and no further chemotherapy or radiotherapy is indicated. The tumour arises from the mesenchymal tissue and causes problems by simple compression of liver tissue. The hepatoblastoma secretes α-fetoprotein in high quantities. This tumour usually presents with an abdominal mass in a child under the age of 2 years. The diagnosis can be made by ultrasound and CT scan (Fig. 19.22). Plasma α-fetoprotein concentrations can help differentiate a malignant from a benign liver tumour. It is important always to remember the possibility of liver metastatic disease from a hidden primary such as a neuroblastoma. The tumour usually is multifocal and the prognosis is related to the extent of the disease. The best prognosis is for patients whose disease is limited to one lobe and where complete surgical removal will achieve a cure. Chemotherapeutic agents which have most effect on hepatoblastoma are Doxorubicin Rapid Dissolution and cisplatin. Measurement of plasma α-fetoprotein will enable determination of the total tumour mass before surgical excision and subsequent monitoring of the plasma values will help determine whether any tumour remains.

Hepatocellular carcinoma is found in children over the age of 3 years and is even rarer than hepatoblastoma; many are α-fetoprotein secreting. The role of liver transplantation in liver tumour management in childhood is still under discussion but where the malignant disease is limited to the liver then there is a real potential for cure if the affected liver can be excised and a transplant performed.

CARE OF THE CHILD WITH CANCER

Nursing care of a child with cancer

Nursing a child with malignant disease involves specialised care. This should be given by trained

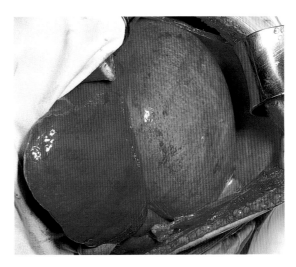

FIGURE 19.21 Benign mesenchymal hamartoma of the liver.

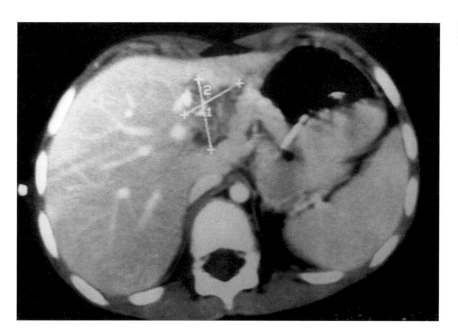

FIGURE 19.22 CT scan of hepatoblastoma.

paediatric nurses who are experienced in looking after children with tumours as well as dealing with emotive illnesses. The whole family is involved and should be treated together as a group. Children are individuals. Their care should include coping with their physical and emotional problems, taking account of their social circumstances.

Verbal communication is an acquired skill in paediatric nursing and requires an understanding of children's development. It is important to gain a child's trust and confidence by being honest at a level which each child understands. Listening to the child and the mother is a skill which the nurse develops and which plays an important role in communications since the nurse is often the co-ordinator of the different specialists.

Care of the terminally ill child

A dying child may be cared for in hospital but many parents prefer to take their child home to die in familiar surroundings and with the family. When in hospital all basic care is given, always ensuring that the child is as pain free as possible. A terminally ill child should be allowed to do as he wishes; children are good judges of their limitations. A single room provides privacy for the family who should be allowed to come and go as they please – residential accommodation should be available for both parents. Parents can have many questions at this time, e.g. "What is a dead child like? Does the child know that he is dying?" These families (including the siblings)

require a lot of emotional support from each other, from their family and from the staff – they must never feel that the staff are too busy to be approached. Religious support may also be of help at this time and should be offered if appropriate. The child must not be forgotten. It is too easy to detach oneself deliberately from a dying child so that awkward questions are not asked. This alters relationships at a crucial time when the child also needs support from the people he knows and trusts. Children are very perceptive and quickly realise that they are being avoided.

Caring for the terminally ill child at home, in a hospice or in the hospital demands the full support of both community and hospital staff. Parents must understand that if they have difficulty in coping and change their minds they will be welcomed back to the hospice or hospital day or night.

Staff support

Finally, it should be remembered that it is a minority of children who develop cancer and an even smaller minority who die from their disease. Despite this, nursing children with such conditions causes stress amongst the carers involved. The permanent ward staff who have known the child and family and the learners who are often young, inexperienced and vulnerable, especially in emotive situations, all need support to help them to cope. Possible methods of support include regular ward meetings and having a psychologist or psychiatrist attached to the ward for both the child and his family and the staff.

20

Tropical Paediatrics

The tropical paediatric diseases which have been chosen for consideration are of common occurrence in some parts of the world. Untreated they carry a high morbidity and mortality and with some exceptions they can all be treated effectively. In developing countries a quarter, or in some rural areas even one-half, of all children born, die during the first 5 years of life. Usually "tropical" diseases other than malaria account for only a small proportion of childhood disease. The diseases encountered are more related to the material poverty and the ignorance of the people, leading to malnutrition, which may or may not be preventable, and to preventable infections. Mortality could be significantly reduced by investing in preventive measures. Not only is a knowledge of the diseases themselves necessary for the western-trained paediatrician but also there is a need to realise that the whole cultural background against which they must study these diseases will be very different from anything with which they have been previously familiar.

THE PATTERN OF DISEASE IN THE TROPICS

Diseases confined to the tropics which are an important cause of mortality are, in fact, relatively few in number. Over 90% of the problems are related to infections. In the late stages, which are very often complicated due to delay in children reaching medical care, infections of the lower respiratory tract, gastrointestinal, urinary tract infections together with meningitis and osteomyelitis have a high mortality rate. Diseases such as measles and pertussis have an appalling mortality amongst the underprivileged children of developing countries. This is related to prolonged malnutrition and lack of "herd" immunity. Similar mortality rates were common in the slums of our large British cities around the turn of the century. Some diseases of the developing countries, such as poliomyelitis, diphtheria, rheumatic fever, tuberculosis, congenital syphilis, gonococcal ophthalmia and pemphigus neonatorum have become relative strangers to the younger paediatrician in developed countries. Hyperbilirubinaemia of a degree requiring replacement transfusion and due to glucose-6-phosphate dehydrogenase deficiency is common in parts of Africa and Asia but also occurs in immigrants to the developed countries.

In some tropical countries children will die simply because their relatives do not have the money to pay for the drugs which would assuredly save their children's lives. This high child mortality which is common to all developing countries could be radically and rapidly reduced by widespread programmes of active immunisation, e.g. against tuberculosis, measles, pertussis, tetanus, poliomyelitis and diphtheria. None the less, successful if restricted immunisation campaigns have been achieved in several areas of Africa and Asia. Even the least sensitive of visitors from the western world must appreciate what a huge economic and emotional drain high maternal and child mortality and morbidity rates create in a community. At the same time, their rapid reduction by methods of modern preventive and curative medicine will only lead to an increase in the size of the population without any improvement in the quality of life unless the concept of family planning can be introduced simultaneously and on a widespread scale. There is, however, some concern that use of the contraceptive pill may reduce the duration and frequency of breast feeding. In women who cannot be assured of a regular and constant supply of the contraceptive pill there may be increased risks of pregnancy by removing the powerful anti-ovulatory influence of prolonged and frequent suckling.

CULTURAL AND ECONOMIC INFLUENCES

The practice of paediatrics in the tropical countries, as in the western world, is greatly influenced by cultural heritage and economic circumstances. Thus, low standards of personal hygiene, the lack of safe water supplies and sewage disposal and overcrowded primitive dwellings all add to the toll of preventable infections. Extreme poverty of the mass of the people, their ignorance and illiteracy, the constant childbearing suffered by the women, correlate with malnutrition, tuberculosis and the attitude that not more than half the children born are expected to survive to maturity. Different cultural or tribal customs have their effects, usually bad but occasionally good, upon the health of their children. The custom of prolonged breast feeding tends to protect the infant from the most severe degrees of malnutrition until the second or third years of life, although iron deficiency anaemia is common. Other good customs are the early feeding with "fish tea" in parts of Jamaica and the "chicken a day" diet recommended for mothers after delivery in many Chinese communities. On the other hand, the results of female circumcision, taboos such as belief that eggs should not be fed to children lest they grow into thieves, the custom of burning the soles of the feet of the convulsing child or of forcing cow's urine down his throat are entirely bad and likely to make a considerable emotional impact upon the western paediatrician. The use of cow dung as a dressing for the cord is a bad custom as it easily leads to tetanus of the newborn. The paediatrician will find, however, that the useful practice of mothers staying in the hospital with their children was established in some developing countries long before it made a hesitant start in the sophisticated west.

Artificial feeding with dried milks can be a death sentence for infants in tropical countries, because mothers have no understanding of units of measurement, sterility or even simple cleanliness. Indeed, by advertising such products the manufacturers of the proprietary infant milks may even add to the toll of child ill-health by encouraging illiterate mothers to copy their "educated" sisters in the western countries, and the privileged few in their own, and to abandon breast feeding, which is safe and cheap, for proprietary milks which they cannot afford and do not know how to prepare. In most tropical countries the paediatrician faced with a mother who has given up breast feeding for one reason or another advises positively against the use of bottle and teat. This is a certain way of causing marasmus, gastroenteritis or hypernatraemia from feeding a contaminated milk mixture which is too dilute or too concentrated from a bottle which may have been "washed" in contaminated water. He will, instead, supply from the "young child clinic" skimmed milk powder which can be made into a gruel with local sources of fat and carbohydrate and fed from a cup or from a bowl and spoon. He knows, too, that the illiterate mother must be shown how to prepare her infant's food, preferably by a nurse who understands the local people and their customs. Thus investment in nurses who can teach the principles of hygiene to mothers in third world countries is more rewarding than the development of high technology.

Finally, the point must be made that, while the treatment of acute organic disease such as cerebral malaria or pyogenic meningitis will be the same everywhere in the world, irrespective of race, the western-trained paediatrician will be unable to function adequately, especially in the field of health education and prevention, unless they have an understanding of the cultural customs, the beliefs and the taboos, the attitudes to disease and nutrition of the people among whom they are to work. In this chapter, only the most common and serious tropical diseases of children together with common nutritional problems are described. Many other diseases of common occurrence in developing countries have been considered in earlier chapters.

MARASMUS AND KWASHIORKOR (PROTEIN-ENERGY MALNUTRITION)

Aetiology

The terms protein-calorie and protein-energy malnutrition embrace several clinical entities which are interrelated and occur in the same communities. Mixed forms are common. Marasmus affects the

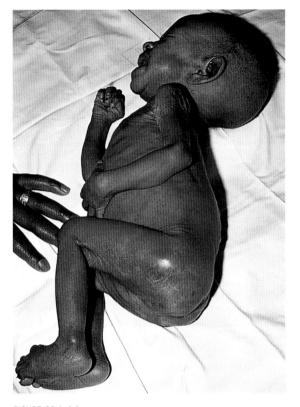
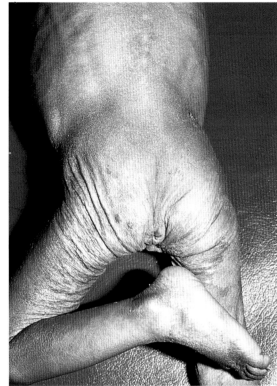

FIGURE 20.1 Marasmus.

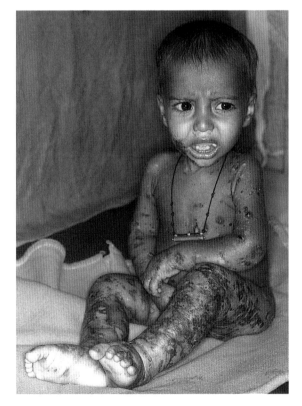
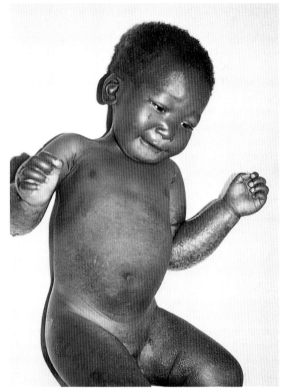

FIGURE 20.2 Kwashiorkor.

young infant who has been fed a diet lacking in total calories. Pure calorie starvation resulting in marasmus is commonly encountered among the underprivileged who form a vast majority of the population of many tropical countries. It is uncommon in breast fed infants, save where extreme maternal malnutrition causes reduction in the amount of breast milk. Unfortunately, failure to breast feed is now not uncommon in developing countries, especially in areas of rapid urbanisation and where uneducated women may try to copy their more sophisticated and educated sisters. Too often they lack the money, kitchen facilities and training to prepare safe artificial milk formulae; the result may be a disastrous combination of underfeeding and infantile diarrhoea. Marasmus may also be secondary to various types of disease and this possibility should not be overlooked in the case of the marasmic infant from a primitive community.

In contrast to marasmus, *kwashiorkor* is a disease which most often develops during the second or third years of life. It is related to a diet which may be reasonably adequate in total calorie value but is severely deficient in protein. The infant is protected from malnutrition while breast fed and kwashiorkor develops when breast feeding stops and a diet lacking in animal or vegetable protein is substituted. This is often due to taboos against the use of certain foods, such as eggs, fish or milk, as much as to local shortage of suitable foods or poverty. It is frequently complicated by other and variable dietary deficiencies such as folic acid, vitamin B, iron or vitamin A which modify the clinical features in different parts of the world. Further variations in clinical presentations may be occasioned by intercurrent diseases like hookworm infestation, ascariasis, tuberculosis or post-measles debility. Indeed, the features of kwashiorkor may be precipitated in a child already the victim of mild protein malnutrition by an attack of measles, malaria, diarrhoea or bronchitis; or by the extra protein loss from burns (a common accident in primitive communities), or by the failure of protein synthesis which occurs in cirrhosis of the liver or bilharziasis.

Clinical features

Children with marasmus are shrunken and wizened (Fig. 20.1). Loss of subcutaneous fat causes their skin to hang in folds over their shrunken buttocks. Typically they are wide eyed, irritable, hungry and active. There are no distinctive or constant biochemical derangements and pathological findings are those produced by wasting and are non-specific. In contrast to marasmus, kwashiorkor occurs mainly in the recently weaned child, with age incidence tending to reflect weaning practices. There is still no satisfactory definition of kwashiorkor but the features of fully

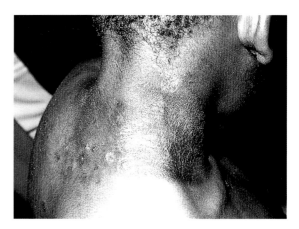

FIGURE 20.3 Pellagra – "Casal's necklace" on the neck.

established kwashiorkor are fairly characteristic (Fig. 20.2). Generalised oedema from hypoproteinaemia is an important sign. This may mask gross tissue wasting although the amount of subcutaneous fat is variable, depending upon the total calorie intake. The hair shows characteristic changes: dry and coarse, depigmented to reddish or brown, loss of curliness, and it can often be pulled out painlessly. The skin shows areas of darkening, especially at the groins, elbows, knees and outer aspects of the thighs and trunk (in contrast to pellagra, in which only the exposed areas are affected) (Fig. 20.3). Later there is desquamation and scaling leaving areas of depigmentation. Dermatitis is also common, and deep fissures may develop in the flexures and behind the ears. In advanced cases diarrhoea is severe with foul smelling, watery stools, dehydration and severe electrolyte loss. The child who smiles does not have kwashiorkor. Anorexia is severe and vomiting is common. Anaemia is always present but its aetiology is multifactorial and varies in different parts of the world, e.g. deficiencies of iron, folic acid, protein or vitamin E; haemolysis from malaria; blood loss from ankylostomiasis. The blood picture may be normocytic, microcytic or macrocytic. Mental changes invariably occur, including apathy, whining fretfulness and intellectual deterioration. In some children the liver is enlarged and it always shows extensive fatty infiltration. Cirrhosis is uncommon. Additional deficiencies may be superimposed, e.g. angular stomatitis due to B complex deficiency, xerophthalmia due to vitamin A deficiency, rarely scurvy or beriberi.

Biochemical abnormalities include severe hypoproteinaemia, a decreased urinary excretion of hydroxyproline relative to creatinine, and aminoaciduria. The plasma concentrations of essential amino acids are reduced as is the total plasma free amino-acid concentration. Blood urea is low. Several serum enzyme activities are reduced, e.g. transaminases, amylase, cholinesterase, alkaline phosphatase. Likewise the pancreatic enzymes are reduced. Serum cholesterol and triglycerides are low in the fasting state. Hypokalaemia, hypomagnesaemia and hypogly-caemia are common and can be dangerous.

Once the picture of kwashiorkor has developed, death is almost certain without treatment. Even in hospital the mortality rate may reach 20%.

Simple dietary instruction to mothers is becoming increasingly available in the developing countries in the "young child clinics" or "under-fives clinics" which serve a dual preventive and curative role. Health care workers and nurses rather than doctors give mothers advice and practical demonstrations on diet, in addition to offering immunisations, anti-malarials, etc. Supplements such as dried skimmed milk (to be mixed into the diet, never reconstituted in liquid form), iron, and vitamins are usually supplied free and mothers are encouraged to attend clinics. In most tropical countries protein foods are comparatively costly and a satisfactory diet for the young child should consist of the local carbohydrate staple (e.g. cereal, tuber or plantain), vegetable protein (e.g. beans, groundnuts, lentils or peas) and a little animal protein to supply essential amino acids (e.g. milk, fish, eggs or meat). It is a good plan for the paediatrician working in an area where protein-calorie malnutrition is prevalent to make up a "protein sources list" of the various kinds of protein locally available, their cost and seasonal variations.

Treatment

Protein malnutrition at the "pre-kwashiorkor" stage can be treated on an outpatient basis. Several hospitals in Africa have developed special nutritional rehabilitation units for this specific purpose. A child with oedema and other manifestations of fully developed kwashiorkor is dangerously ill and should be admitted to hospital. Hypothermia is common in these cases, even in warm weather, and must be prevented or corrected. Dehydration may demand intravenous fluid therapy, and severe anaemia may require slow blood transfusion and haematinics.

Hypokalaemia must always be corrected by adding potassium 10–20 mmol/litre to the maintenance infusion fluids. Severe hypoglycaemia can be corrected with intravenous 20% dextrose, 10–15 ml. The tendency to hypothermia may mask malaria and other infections. The basic requirement of treatment for kwashiorkor is an adequate protein intake (3–4 g/kg/day), best achieved with dried skimmed milk, dried full-cream milk or calcium caseinate. The cheapest of these is dried skimmed milk which can be obtained free from UNICEF in some of the developing countries. None of these high protein foods can supply sufficient total calories by itself and they should be "enriched" in one of the variety of ways. One formula is

TABLE 20.1 Electrolyte mixture

Sodium chloride	106 g
Potassium chloride	106 g
Magnesium hydroxide	10 g
Water (flavoured and coloured to taste) to 1 litre	

composed of dried skimmed milk, cane sugar, and a locally available vegetable oil (e.g. palm oil or cotton seed oil) which can be mixed with water (150 g dried skimmed milk, 40 g vegetable oil, 40 g sugar, providing over 1000 calories and 54 g protein).

Alternatively, full-cream dried milk and cane sugar may be used, although this is more expensive. Severely ill children may suffer from an intolerance to lactose due to deficient production of intestinal lactase, and milk may greatly aggravate their diarrhoea. The lactose content of the diet can be reduced by using a formula of calcium caseinate (which is lactose-free), some dried skimmed milk, cane sugar and vegetable oil. A suitable mixture which supplies over 1000 calories and 65 g protein is calcium caseinate 50 g, dried skimmed milk 50 g, vegetable oil 50 g and sugar 50 g. In the early stages of treatment marked anorexia may necessitate feeding continuously by gastric feeding. It is also important to supplement the diet with extra electrolytes and a useful mixture is shown in Table 20.1. A volume of 15 ml to each 600 ml of dried milk formula, and the mixture is shaken well before use. This must be preceded by correction of dehydration and hypoten-sion. A multivitamin preparation and folic acid should also be prescribed.

When recovery is well under way the child should be fed the calcium caseinate, dried skimmed milk, cane sugar and vegetable oil diet and the progress carefully supervised by regular attendances at the Nutrition Rehabilitation Unit. No opportunity should be lost, in or out of hospital, for teaching the mother the principles and methods of preparation of a good diet.

Vitamins and minerals

Although deficiencies of vitamins and minerals are not restricted to developing countries or to tropical countries they are often found in association with severe malnutrition states which are common in these parts of the world. Even vitamin D deficiency which should not occur in sun-blessed countries does occur and is largely caused by "sheltering" infants from the beneficial effects of sunlight. Many of the deficiency states arise subsequent to weaning. In western countries weaning is usually recommended about the age of 6 months. In primitive communities breast feeding is often continued well into the second year of life. By then, however, milk alone is not an adequate diet and iron deficiency anaemia is a major problem. Between 4 and 6 months sources of first class protein such as cereals, vegetables, egg yolk, potato, minced meat and fish are recommended. Such foods should ensure adequate intakes of minerals and vitamins.

Supplements of vitamins and iron

The normal infant during the first year of life requires daily intakes of 1500 units vitamin A, 400 units (10 µg) vitamin D, 15–30 mg vitamin C (ascorbic acid) and 5–7 mg of iron. All proprietary dried milks are sufficiently fortified with vitamins D, C and iron to meet the infant's requirements. The practice of feeding unfortified fresh cows' milk will ensure that infants receive inadequate amounts of vitamins D, C and of iron. In areas where there is no fluoridation of the water supply a valuable measure to combat dental caries is the administration of fluoride in liquid form. A suitable preparation is Fluodrops (En-De-Kay), 5 drops daily until the age of 18 months when the dose can be increased to 15 drops daily. Fluotabs are available for older children and fluoride-containing toothpaste is also of value.

Underfeeding

The underfed infant fails to gain weight satisfactorily and if the problem is uncorrected a state of marasmus develops. The infant becomes irritable, sleepless and cries long before feeds are due. When introduced to breast or bottle he feeds eagerly and often swallows air so that colic aggravates the misery and restlessness. Constipation is an early sign. Later the infant may pass small amounts of dark green stained mucus – "starvation stools". These must not be mistaken for the large, watery grass-green stool of gastroenteritis. The underfed infant requires more food and not the starvation regimen employed in gastoenteritis.

INFANTILE RICKETS

Rickets is a metabolic disturbance of growth which affects bone, skeletal muscles and sometimes the nervous system. The disorder is due primarily to an insufficiency of vitamin D_3 (cholecalciferol) which is a naturally occurring steroid. It can be formed in the skin from 7-dehydrocholesterol by irradiation with ultra-violet light in the wavelengths 280–305 nm; or it can be ingested in the form of fish-liver oils, eggs, butter, margarine and meat. The most important natural source of vitamin D is that formed from solar irradiation of the skin. Ultra-violet irradiation of ergosterol produces vitamin D_2 (ergocalciferol) which,

in humans, is a potent antirachitic substance. It is however, not a natural animal vitamin and may have some adverse effects.

Vitamin D metabolism

Cholecalficerol (D_3) is converted in the liver to 25–hydroxyvitamin D_3 (25–OHD_3) by means of enzymatic hydroxylation in the C25 position. This metabolite circulates in the plasma with a transport protein which migrates with the alphaglobulins. It is then 1α-hydroxylated in the kidney to 1,25-dihydroxyvitamin D_3 ($1,25(OH)_2D_3$) by the action of 25-hydroxyvitamin D hydroxylase. Its production appears to be regulated by several factors, including the phosphate concentration in the plasma, the renal intracellular calcium and phosphate concentrations and parathyroid hormone. It acts on the cells of the gastrointestinal tract to increase calcium absorption and on bone to increase calcium resorption. In the kidney it improves the reabsorption of calcium whilst causing a phosphate diuresis. It also acts on muscle with the ability to correct the muscle weakness often associated with rickets.

Vitamin D deficiency causes a fall in the concentration of calcium in extracellular fluid which in turn stimulates parathormone production. The phosphate diuresis effect of a raised parathyroid hormone level results in lowering of the plasma phosphate. This produces the low (Ca) × (P) product which is such a characteristic feature of active rickets. This stage is quickly followed by an increase in the plasma alkaline phosphatase concentration and then by radiological and clinical features of rickets.

Aetiology

Deficiency of vitamin D which once resulted in so much infantile rickets, with its toll of permanent deformities and death during childbirth, arose principally because of the limited amount of sunshine and skyshine in northern latitudes. Furthermore, in large industrial cities the skyshine contained very little ultra-violet light after filtering through dust, smoke and fog. The need in a cold climate for heat-retaining clothing and the tendency to remain indoors in inclement weather further deprived infants of ultra-violet radiation. The natural diet of the human infant contains little vitamin D, especially if fed artificially on cows' milk. Cereals which are commonly used have a rachitogenic effect because the phosphorus in cereals is in an unavailable form, phytic acid (inositol-hexaphosphoric acid) which combines with calcium and magnesium in the gut to form the complex compound, phytin. It is essential to fortify the infant's diet with vitamin D if rickets is to be avoided. This would not be necessary in the wholly breast fed infant living in a sunny land. A high incidence of rickets and osteomalacia was noted in Asian immigrants to the United Kingdom, particularly those from Pakistan. Up to 45% of Asians living in the northern English town of Bradford at one time showed evidence of the disease and 5% of Asian children attending Glasgow schools had florid rickets with a further 7.5% showing subclinical rickets. Since the introduction of vitamin D supplementation to these population subgroups the problem has virtually resolved.

Another important causative factor, necessary for the development of rickets, is growth. The marasmic infant does not develop rickets when vitamin D deficient until re-fed and growth commences. The preterm low birthweight infant who grows rapidly is particularly prone to develop rickets. There is evidence that hydroxylation of vitamin D in the liver of preterm infants is impaired and this together with dietary phosphate deficiency is an important factor in the osteopenia of preterm infants.

Pathology

In the normal infant there is a zone of cartilage between the diaphysis and the epiphysis – the epiphyseal plate. At the epiphyseal end this cartilage is actively growing (proliferative zone), whereas at the diaphyseal end, where mature cartilage cells are arranged in orderly columns, osteoblasts lay down calcium phosphate to form new bone. In rickets the cartilage near the diaphysis (resting zone) shows a disordered arrangement of capillaries and although osteoblasts are numerous normal calcification does not take place. This is called osteoid tissue. In the meantime active growth of the proliferative zone continues so that the epiphyseal plate is enlarged and swollen. Osteoid tissue instead of normal bone is also formed under the periosteum. There is also, in severe cases, a general decalcification of the skeleton so that curvatures and deformities readily develop.

The diagnosis of infantile rickets is not difficult but its rarity in developed countries has resulted in its being unfamiliar to many doctors. A careful dietary history with especial reference to the ingestion of vitamin D fortified milks and cereals and of vitamin supplements will reveal the child who is at risk. In the era before the Second World War rickets usually had its onset about the age of 6 months and even earlier in preterm infants. In recent years most cases of rickets have had a later onset because most white infants in the United Kingdom are fed on vitamin D fortified dried milks during the early months of life. In the case of mothers with osteomalacia from their own malnutrition, rickets has been present in their infants at birth, as the fetal requirements of 25-OHD$_3$ are obtained directly from the maternal pool. In congenital rickets the presenting feature is usually a hypocalcaemic convulsion although typical bone

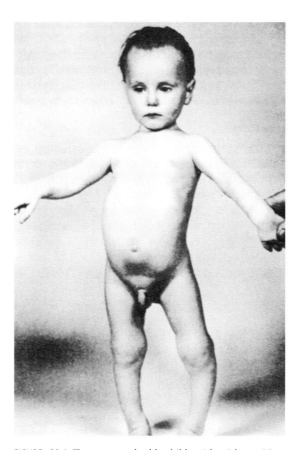

FIGURE 20.4 Twenty-month-old child with rickets. Note swollen radial epiphyses, enlarged costochondral junctions, bowing of tibiae and lumbar lordosis.

changes are to be expected in radiographs. Subclinical maternal and fetal vitamin D deficiency has also been found in white mothers and infants, particularly in infants born in early spring. It causes compensatory maternal hyperparathyroidism, and dental enamel defects in the infant's primary dentition. Such infants are predisposed to neonatal tetany if fed on unmodified cows' milk.

There are few subjective signs of rickets. Head sweating is probably one. General muscular hypotonia encourages abdominal protuberance; this can be increased by flaring out of the rib margins and by fermentation of the excess carbohydrate so commonly included in the diets of nutritionally ignorant people. The rachitic child commonly suffers from a concomitant iron deficiency anaemia. His frequent susceptibility to respiratory infections is related more to the poor environment and overcrowding rather than to the rickets. The same applies to the unhappy irritable behaviour which rachitic children sometimes exhibit.

The objective signs of rickets are found in the skeleton. The earliest physical sign is craniotabes. This is due to softening of the occipital bones where the head

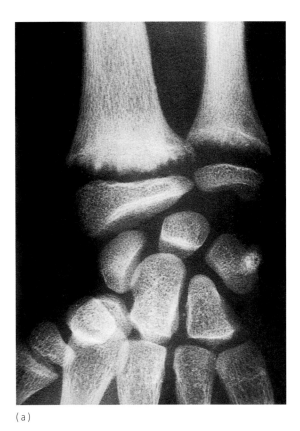 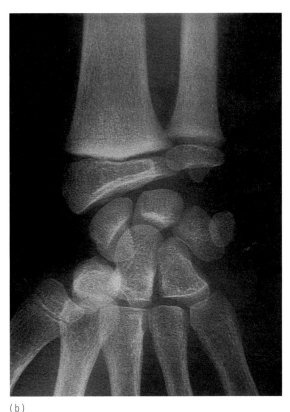

(a)   (b)

FIGURE 20.5 (a) Florid rickets showing splaying and fraying of ends of the long bones. (b) Radiograph of the same case as in (a). Rickets has healed.

rubs on the pillow. When the examiner's fingers press upon the occipital area the bone can be depressed in and out like a piece of old parchment or table tennis ball. Another common early sign is the "rachitic rosary" or "beading of the ribs" due to swelling of the costochondral junctions. The appearance is of a row of swellings, both visible and palpable, passing downwards and backwards on both sides of the thorax in the situation of the rib ends (Fig. 20.4). Swelling of the epiphyses is also seen at an early stage, especially at the wrists, knees and ankles.

In severe cases the shafts of the long bones may develop various curvatures leading to genu varum, genu valgum and coxa vara. A particularly common deformity, shown in Fig. 20.4, is curvature at the junction of the middle and lower thirds of the tibiae. This is often due to the child, who may have "gone off his feet", being sat on a chair with his feet project-ing over the edge in such a fashion that their weight bends the softened tibial shafts. Bossing over the frontal and parietal bones, due to the subperiosteal deposition of osteoid, gives the child a broad square forehead, or the "hot-cross-bun head". The anterior fontanelle may not close until well past the age of 18 months, although this delay can also occur in

hypothyroidism, hydrocephalus, and even in some healthy children. Another deformity affecting the bony thorax results in Harrison grooves. These are seen as depressions or sulci on each side of the chest running parallel to but above the diaphragmatic attachment. This sign, however, may also develop in cases of congenital heart disease, asthma and chronic respiratory infections. Laxity of the spinal ligaments can also allow the development of various spinal deformities such as dorsolumbar kyphoscoliosis. In children who have learned to stand there may be an exaggerated lumbar lordosis. The severely rachitic child will also be considerably dwarfed. Pelvic defor-mities are not readily appreciated in young children but in the case of girls can lead to severe difficulty during childbirth in later years. The pelvic inlet may be narrowed by forward displacement of the sacral promontory, or the outlet may be narrowed by forward movement of the lower parts of the sacrum and of the coccyx.

Radiological features

The normally smooth and slightly convex ends of the long bones become splayed out with the appearance of fraying or "cupping" of the edges. The distance between the diaphysis and the epiphysis is increased because the metaphysis consists largely of non-radio-opaque osteoid tissue. Periosteum may be raised because of the laying down of osteoid tissue, and the shafts may appear decalcified and curved. In the worst cases greenstick fractures with poor callus formation may occur. The earliest sign of healing is a thin line of preparatory calcification near the diaphysis (Fig. 20.5) followed by calcification in the osteoid just distal to the frayed ends of the diaphysis. In time both the ends and shafts of the bone usually return to normal.

Biochemical findings

Typical findings are a normal plasma calcium concentration (2.25–2.75 mmol/l; 9–11 mg/100 ml) whereas the plasma phosphate (normally 1.6–2.26 mmol/l; 5–7 mg/l00 ml) is markedly reduced to between 0.64 and 1 mmol/l (2–3 mg/100 ml). The normal plasma calcium in the presence of diminished intestinal absorption of calcium is best explained on the basis of increased parathyroid activity which mobilises calcium from the bones. Plasma phosphate diminishes due to the phosphaturia which results from the effects of parathyroid hormone on the renal tubules. A plasma calcium $\times$ phosphorus product (mg/100 ml) above 40 excludes rickets, while a figure below 30 indicates active rickets. This formula is useful in clinical practice but it has no real meaning in terms of physical chemistry. The plasma alkaline phosphatase activity (normal 56–190 IU/litre) is markedly increased in rickets and only returns to normal with effective treatment. It is, in fact, a very sensitive and early reflection of rachitic activity but can be raised in a variety of unrelated disease states such as hyperparathyroidism, obstructive jaundice, fractures, malignant disease of bone and the "battered baby" syndrome. The mean 25-OHD$_3$ level in healthy British children is 30 nmol/l (12.5 µg/l), although considerably greater concentrations are reported from the USA. In children with active rickets or osteomalacia, the level of 25-OHD$_3$ may fall below 7.5 nmol/l (3 µg/l). However, it is not possible to equate the presence of rickets with particular absolute values for 25-OHD$_3$, although its measurement can provide the most sensitive index of the vitamin D status of a population.

Differential diagnosis

Few diseases can simulate infantile rickets. In hypophosphatasia some of the clinical and radiological features resemble those seen in rickets, but their presence in the early weeks of life exclude vitamin D deficiency. Other features such as defective calcification of the membranous bones of the skull, low

plasma alkaline phosphatase and hypercalcaemia are never found in rickets. The characteristic features of achondroplasia – short upper limb segments, large head with relatively small face and retroussé nose, trident arrangement of the fingers, lordosis, waddling gait, and X-ray evidence of endochondral ossification – are unmistakenly different from anything seen in rickets. The globular enlargement of the hydrocephalic skull is quite distinct from the square bossed head of severe rickets. The bone lesions of congenital syphilis are present in the early months of life and are associated with other characteristic clinical signs such as rashes, bloody snuffles, hepatosplenomegaly and lymphadenopathy. In later childhood the sabre-blade tibia of syphilis shows anterior bowing and thickening which is different from rachitic bowing. Some healthy toddlers show an apparent bowing of the legs due to the normal deposition of fat over the outer aspects; this is unimportant and temporary, and there are no other signs of skeletal abnormality. Other normal young children have a mild, and physiological, degree of genu valgum due to a mild valgus position of the feet; in rachitic genu valgum there will be other rickety deformities. Other types of rickets due to coeliac disease and renal disease must be excluded by appropriate investigations. Their existence is almost always indicated in a carefully taken history.

Prevention

It is important to keep a degree of awareness of the problem of rickets as the feeding pattern of many adolescents in inner city areas would indicate that they are unaware and/or unconcerned of the need to ensure an adequate vitamin D status for themselves and for their children. Departments of health are striving hard to maintain a public awareness of the importance of nutrition to health and through the supply of vitamin D fortified foods are endeavouring to prevent the recrudescence of this preventable disorder.

Treatment

Although rickets can be healed by exposure to ultraviolet light it is more practicable and reliable to administer vitamin D in adequate dosage by mouth. A suitable dose is 1600–2000 International Units (IU) orally (1 mg calciferol = 40 000 IU). This can be achieved using the BP or a proprietary concentrated preparation. Although calcium deficiency *per se* very rarely has caused rickets there should be an adequate amount of calcium in the infant's diet (approx 600 mg/day). This is contained in l pint (600 ml) of milk per day. An alternative method of treatment, especially useful where it is suspected that the parents are unreliable and unlikely to administer a daily dose of vitamin D, is the oral or intramuscular administration of a massive dose of vitamin D ("Stoss therapy") (300 000–600 000 IU). It is, however, uncertain how much of such a large dose the body can utilise although rapid healing of rickets can be confidently expected.

Even major deformities will disappear with adequate treatment in the young child and surgical correction is rarely required. The child should be kept from weight-bearing until X-rays show advanced healing, to prevent aggravation of the deformities. The parent of a rachitic child requires education in nutrition and child care. They should be urged to take the child, after treatment, for regular supervision by their family doctor or at a local child health clinic.

Hereditary vitamin D dependent rickets ("pseudo-deficiency" rickets)

Vitamin D resistant rickets due to a renal tubular defect in the reabsorption of phosphate is described in Chapter 6. It has to be differentiated from the "pseudo-deficiency" rickets in which there appears to be an inherited deficiency of 1α-hydroxylase in the kidney with a failure in the production of $1\alpha,25(OH)_2D_3$. The mode of inheritance is autosomal recessive. "Pseudo-deficiency" rickets is characterised by the onset in early infancy of the clinical, radiological and biochemical features of severe rickets but which fails to respond to treatment with vitamin D in daily doses of up to 4000 IU. The major abnormality in the blood chemistry is hypocalcaemia, whereas the plasma phosphate may be low or normal. Other findings include a generalised aminoaciduria, raised plasma alkaline phosphatase and increased serum immunoreactive parathyroid hormone (iPTH).

Treatment

While this form of rickets can be cured by long-term massive doses of calciferol, it is best treated by oral administration of 1α-hydroxyvitamin $D_3(1\alpha$-OHD_3). This is an analogue of $1,25(OH)_2D_3$. Most or all of its biological activity depends on conversion in the liver to $1\alpha,25(OH)_2D_3$, but since it possesses a 1α-hydroxyl group the need for renal hydroxylation is bypassed. In "pseudo-deficiency" rickets, 1α-hydroxyvitamin $D_3(1\alpha$-OHD_3) corrects the intestinal malabsorption of calcium and phosphorus, normalises the serum calcium and phosphate concentrations and promotes healing of the skeletal lesions. 1α-OHD_3 dosage varies according to growth velocity, the degree of secondary hyperparathyroidism and familial sensitivity and may range from 0.5 to 2 μg daily. It is important to avoid hypercalcaemia but this can rapidly be reversed when 1α-OHD_3 is discontinued due to its short half-life, in contrast to calciferol

overdosage. Alternatively $1,25(OH)_2D_3$ or calcitriol may be given in similar dosage. It may have a greater tendency to induce hypercalcaemia.

INFANTILE TETANY (SPASMOPHILIA)

Aetiology

Tetany can occur in a variety of situations such as hypoparathyroidism, respiratory alkalosis due to hysterical overbreathing, metabolic acidosis due to pyloric stenosis, high intestinal obstruction or the excessive administration of sodium bicarbonate and in hypokalaemic alkalosis. In infancy, however, the common types of tetany are seen in the neonatal period in some infants fed on cows' milk preparations and in older infants or children with rickets often in association with a mild febrile illness.

Pathogenesis

The manifestation of tetany depends upon a decrease in the ionisable fraction of plasma calcium. Provided the non-ionisable protein-bound calcium is normal, tetany is likely to occur when the total plasma calcium concentration falls below 2 mmol/l (8 mg/100 ml). The cause of the marked diminution in plasma calcium in some cases of rickets is unknown. In a few, the administration of vitamin D has this effect, possibly by increasing un-ionised calcium at the expense of the ionised fraction. Alkalotic tetany, on the other hand, may exist with a normal plasma calcium because the ionised calcium fraction alone is decreased. Conversely, a low total plasma calcium concentration is not necessarily associated with tetany. In the nephrotic syndrome the low protein-bound calcium value is accompanied by a normal amount of ionised and diffusible calcium.

Clinical features

The increased neuromuscular irritability of hypocalcaemia may produce overt clinical manifestations (active tetany) or it may be detected by means of certain specific tests (latent tetany).

Active tetany most often presents in infancy as multifocal myoclonic seizures. In the period when infantile rickets was common in Glasgow, convulsions during the first 2 years of life were more often due to hypocalcaemia than to any other cause. In some infants tetany may produce laryngismus stridulus in which laryngeal spasm causes apnoea and cyanosis, each followed by a deep inspiration and crowing noise. A fatal outcome can result from such an attack. A third manifestation of active tetany is carpopedal spasm; the hands and metacarpophalangeal joints are strongly flexed, the fingers are extended with the thumbs adducted across the palms (main d'accoucheur), while the feet are inverted and the toes flexed.

Latent tetany should be looked for in every child with rickets. The most useful test is the facial phenomenon (Chvostek sign) in which a twitch of the facial muscles on one side can be elicited by tapping over the facial nerve where it crosses the ramus of the mandible. The Trousseau sign is elicited by compressing the arm with the hand or sphygmomanometer cuff when overt carpal spasm is produced within 1–3 minutes. The ECG may show a prolonged Q-T interval in hypocalcaemia.

Treatment

Active tetany complicating infantile rickets may be effectively treated with an intravenous injection of 10–20 ml of 10% calcium gluconate, repeated every 8 hours as required. Vitamin D treatment should be started and close biochemical control maintained.

IDIOPATHIC HYPERCALCAEMIA OF INFANCY

The disease was first reported in the United Kingdom in 1952 and has been reported at a varying rate in different developed countries since that time.

Aetiology

The resemblance of the features of idiopathic hypercalcaemia to those of vitamin D poisoning was quickly recognised. All affected infants had been wholly or partially fed on cows' milk formulae and some had received from various sources (dried milk, vitamin supplements, fortified cereals) unnecessarily large doses of calciferol, e.g. 4000 units/day. Some, however, had received quite small amounts of vitamin D but none the less there was a natural suspicion that the individuals had an undue susceptibility to the increased vitamin D intake. Some of these infants are now recognised to have a syndrome known as William syndrome, in which there is an unusual facial appearance, mental handicap and hypercalcaemia, together with supravalvular aortic stenosis. The incidence of idiopathic hypercalcaemia in the UK has been reduced since the calciferol content of infant formulae and fortified cereals was reduced in 1958.

Pathology

The only constant finding is medullary nephrocalcinosis but occasionally metastatic calcification is found in other tissues such as the mitral valve ring.

Clinical features

The relationship of neonatal hypercalcaemia with William syndrome is still uncertain. The first form of the disease described by Lightwood is now referred to as the "benign" type but there is a more serious form described by Fanconi in 1952 and is known as the "severe type".

Benign type

The onset is between the age of 6 weeks and 8 months with anorexia, frequent vomiting, failure to thrive and severe constipation. The infant becomes marasmic and exhibits severe generalised hypotonia. Numerous hard faecal masses are palpable in the abdomen. Thirst and polyuria may have been noted. The urine is acid and contains moderate amounts of protein. There may be a low grade pyuria. The diagnostic finding is an increased plasma calcium (above 3 mmol/l; 12 mg/100 ml). In many instances the blood urea and plasma cholesterol concentrations are increased. The electrocardiographic changes include a broad T wave, usually of high voltage, and a short S-T interval. The clinical picture resembles that seen in hyperchloraemic renal acidosis.

Severe type

In addition to the features found in the benign type there is mental retardation and many of these infants have a characteristically "elf-like" face with low-set ears, depressed nasal bridge, long, thick upper lip and prominent epicanthic folds (Fig. 20.6). Hypertension and a loud systolic murmur are commonly present. Hyperostosis of marked degree is found on X-ray, affecting predominantly the base of the skull, orbits, vertebrae and epiphyses. Marked azotaemia and hypercholesterolaemia accompany the hypercalcaemia. Death may occur from renal failure and the survivors are poorly grown and have mental retardation. It is likely that this group of infants with supravalvular stenosis and sometimes constrictions along the major branches of the pulmonary artery are those now described as William syndrome. In some instances the possibility of the disease commencing during intrauterine life has been raised.

Treatment

Vitamin D containing foods and preparations must be withdrawn and the infant fed a low calcium milk. In severe cases of marked hypercalcaemia, prednisolone 5 mg is given four times daily for 7–10 days followed by a gradual reduction.

INFANTILE SCURVY

Aetiology

The primary cause is an inadequate intake of vitamin C (ascorbic acid), a vitamin which the human, unlike

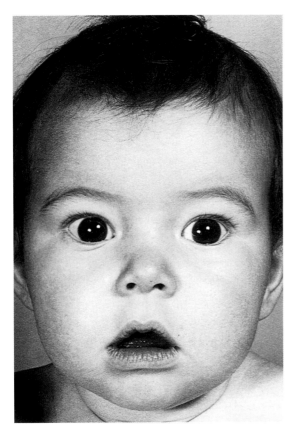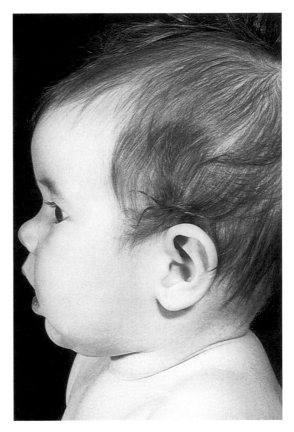

FIGURE 20.6 Typical facial appearance in severe type of idiopathic hypercalcaemia.

most other animals, is unable to synthesise within his own body. It is rare in the breast fed infant unless the mother has subclinical avitaminosis C. Cows' milk contains only about a quarter of the vitamin C content of human milk and this is further reduced by boiling, drying or evaporating. Scurvy is particularly common in infants who receive a high carbohydrate diet.

Pathology

Vitamin C deficiency results in faulty collagen which affects many tissues including bone, cartilage and teeth. The intercellular substance of the capillaries is also defective. This results in spontaneous haemorrhages and defective ossification affecting both the shafts and the metaphyseo-epiphyseal junctions. The periosteum becomes detached from the cortex and extensive subperiosteal haemorrhages occur; these explain the intense pain and tenderness, especially of the lower extremities.

Clinical features

Increasing irritibility, anorexia, malaise and low-grade fever develop between the ages of 7 and 15 months. A most striking feature is the obvious pain and tenderness which the infant exhibits when handled, e.g. during napkin changing. The legs are most severely affected and they characteristically assume a position ("frog-position") in which the hips and knees are flexed and the feet are rotated outwards. Gums become swollen and discoloured and may bleed; this is seen only after teeth have erupted and the teeth may become loose in the jaws. Periorbital ecchymosis ("black eye") or proptosis due to retro-orbital haemorrhage is common but haemorrhages into the skin, epistaxis or gastrointestinal haemorrhages are not commonly seen in infantile scurvy. The anterior ends of the ribs frequently become visibly and palpably swollen but this does not affect the costal cartilages as in rickets; the sternum has the appearance of having been displaced backwards. Microscopic haematuria is frequently present. A mild orthochromic anaemia is characteristic.

Radiological features

The diagnosis is most reliably confirmed by X-rays. The shafts of the long bones have a "ground glass" appearance due to loss of normal trabeculation. A

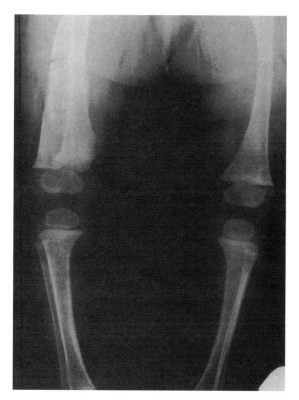

FIGURE 20.7 Radiograph from a case of infantile scurvy in the healing stage with calcified subperiosteal haematoma. Note also "ringing" of epiphyses, Fraenkels' white lines and proximal zone of translucency.

dense white line of calcification (Fraenkel's line) forms proximal to the epiphyseal plate and there is often a zone of translucency due to an incomplete transverse fracture immediately proximal to Fraenkel's line. A small spur of bone may project from the end of the shaft at this point ("the corner sign"). The epiphyses, especially at the knees, have the appearance of being "ringed" by white ink. Subperiosteal haemorrhages only become visible when they are undergoing calcification but a striking X-ray appearance is then seen (Fig. 20.7).

Differential diagnosis

The clinical picture of scurvy rarely presents difficulties in interpretation. Pseudoparesis of the limb due to the pain of subperiosteal haemorrhage might be confused with poliomyelitis but the other features of scurvy should quickly define the position. Similarly the generalised nature of the bone changes in scurvy should avoid any confusion with osteitis. Blood diseases which cause bone pain such as leukaemia can be excluded by examination of the peripheral blood. The easiest mistake is to overlook the existence of mild scurvy in the child suffering from florid rickets;

the radiological appearances of both diseases will be present.

Treatment and prevention

The most rapid recovery can be obtained with oral ascorbic acid, 200 mg/day. There is no advantage in parenteral administration. Excess vitamin C is excreted in the urine and there is no evidence that vitamin C is in any way poisonous. In developed countries the usual cause of vitamin C deficiency is ignorance of the parents of the need to supply adequate amounts of vitamin C or alternatively some obsessive parents boil fruit juices which would normally supply adequate vitamin C to the child but the act of boiling destroys the ascorbic acid.

AVITAMINOSIS A

Vitamin A deficiency remains the most widespread and serious nutritional disorder causing blindness in India, Africa, South-east Asia and in Central and South America.

Aetiology

While vitamin A is present in milk, butter, egg yolk and fish livers, in countries where its deficiency is common most vitamin A is derived from the provitamin A carotenoids (e.g. β-carotene) of dark green leafy vegetables, carrots and some fruits. After absorption vitamin A is stored in the liver as retinyl esters. These esters are then hydrolysed to retinol which binds to a carrier, retinol-binding protein (RBP) before its release from the liver. In the circulation RBP forms a complex with thyroxine-binding prealbumin. Protein deficiency inhibits the release of RBP which may relate to the frequent association of xerophthalmia with protein-energy malnutrition. Before entering the target cells the retinol leaves the plasma RBP to be picked up by a cellular RBP. It is essential for the maintenance of the body's epithelial tissues and important for glycosylation but clinical manifestations of deficiency will only appear when a child has been fed for a long period on a grossly substandard diet, e.g. cereals, skimmed milk and flour.

Pathology

Avitaminosis A affects vision because vitamin A is necessary for light appreciation in the eye. The photosensitive pigments opsin and iodopsin are bound to retinal (oxidised retinol) which retains the *cis*-form in the dark and the *trans*-form in the light. The change from the *cis*- to the *trans*-form releases energy and stimulates nerve endings. The earliest sign of vitamin A deficiency is impaired dark adaptation. Retinols are also necessary in the control of free radical generation and the maintenance of membrane stability throughout the body. Deficiency results in the rupture of lysosomal membranes and release of the contained enzymes. Children on diets low in animal fats and vegetable oils are at risk of vitamin A deficiency particularly if born preterm. Deficiency of retinols can cause squamous metaplasia at epithelial surfaces including the skin, bronchial tree and urinary tract. The skin changes also increase the susceptibility of the child to infection. Avitaminosis A leads to arrest of growth and to increased susceptibility to infection because various types of epithelium undergo atrophy or change to stratified squamous epithelium, e.g. skin, bronchial tree, urinary tract.

Clinical features

The first objective sign is night blindness. This is followed by xerosis: the conjunctiva and later the cornea become dry and injected. Bitot spots may be seen on the bulbar conjunctiva as small, yellowish-white triangular patches. Photophobia is marked. In advanced cases of xerophthalmia the cornea may become opaque and necrotic (keratomalacia), leading to blindness. The skin may become dry and roughened – follicular hyperkeratosis. Intercurrent infections such as pneumonia and pyelonephritis may prove fatal. Plasma carotene concentrations are reduced and in severe instances the plasma vitamin A levels are also very low. The age group most affected is from 6 months to 4 years.

Prevention

The global occurrence of xerophthalmia and its association with malnutrition, infections such as measles and diarrhoea, and poor sanitation presents a formidable problem to which the WHO addressed itself in a report published in 1982. Strategies proposed for its control included the distribution of vitamin A capsules to communities with low vitamin A status, education on local sources of vitamin or carotenoids, fortification of staple foods, programmes to encourage breast feeding, and the increased consumption of dark green leafy vegetables. Anyone with experience in developing countries will appreciate the political and social obstructions which such strategies are likely to encounter.

Treatment

The schedule recommended in the WHO report consists in the oral administration of retinyl palmitate (110 mg) or retinyl acetate (60 mg) on two successive days with a third dose to be given 2–4 weeks later. Intramuscular administration is only necessary if there is severe vomiting or diarrhoea. The eye lesions are completely reversible at the stage of conjunctival or corneal xerosis, but once keratomalacia develops, and this can proceed unsuspected behind the photophobic child's closed eyelids, blindness is inevitable.

Chronic vitamin A poisoning

There are increasing reports of vitamin A poisoning in situations where mothers greatly overdose their infants (over 20 000 µg daily) with foods containing vitamin A. Only some infants seem susceptible to develop clinical manifestations which include malaise, failure to thrive, anorexia and pruritus. The most characteristic change is found radiologically to be a hyperostosis, particularly of the middle portion of the shafts of the long bones. This is associated with tender swelling of the limbs. The jaw is not affected as it is in infantile cortical hyperostosis (Chapter 4). The liver may be enlarged. Skin manifestations are alopecia, seborrhoeic-type dermatitis and angular stomatitis.

VITAMIN B DEFICIENCIES

The B vitamins are widely distributed in animal and vegetable foods. Deficiency of one of the B group vitamins is commonly associated with deficiencies of the others. The main functions of B vitamins are as cofactors for metabolic processes or as precursors of essential metabolites. Deficiencies occur when there is severe famine, where there are dietary fads, where diets are severely restricted or where there has been inappropriate preparation of the food. Many B vitamins are destroyed by cooking.

Thiamine (vitamin B$_1$) deficiency

Thiamine, as are all the B vitamins, is water soluble and readily destroyed by heat and alkali. It is necessary for mitochondrial function and for the synthesis of acetylcholine. It is present in a wide variety of foods but deficiency states have been particulary common in communities where polishing rice and refining flour has removed the vitamin B containing husks.

Clinical features

Deficiency of thiamine (beriberi) causes clinical manifestations in the nervous and cardiovascular systems predominantly although all tissues are affected. There is degeneration of peripheral nerve fibres and haemorrhage and vascular dilatation in the brain (Wernicke encephalopathy). There can be high output cardiac failure and erythemas. Signs of the disease develop in infants born to thiamine deficient mothers at the age of 2–3 months. They appear restless with vasodilatation, anorexia, vomiting and constipation and pale with a waxy skin, hypertonia and dyspnoea. There is peripheral vasodilatation and bounding pulses with later development of oedema, hepatomegaly and evidence of cardiac failure. The oedema is due to a combination of the peripheral vasodilatation and decreased renal flow. This is known as the "wet" form of beriberi. There is reduction of the phasic reflexes at knee and ankle.

In older children "dry" beriberi or the neurological complication of thiamine deficiency results in paraesthesia and burning sensations particularly affecting the feet. There is generalised muscle weakness and calf muscles are tender. Tendon reflexes may be absent, a stocking and glove peripheral neuritis develops and sensory loss accompanies the motor weakness. Increased intracranial pressure, meningism and coma may follow.

Diagnosis

There are few useful laboratory tests although in severe deficiency states the red blood cell transketolase is reduced and lactate and pyruvate may be increased in the blood, particularly after exercise.

Treatment

The usual thiamine requirement is 0.5 mg/day during infancy and 0.7–1 mg daily for older children. Pregnant and lactating women should have a minimal intake of 1 mg/day. Treatment of B_1 deficiency is 10 mg/day for infants and young children increasing to 50 mg/day for adults. In the infant with cardiac failure intravenous or intramuscular thiamine (100 mg daily) can be given. The response can at times be dramatic.

Riboflavine (vitamin B_2) deficiency

Clinical features

Deficiency is usually secondary to inadequate intake although in biliary atresia and chronic hepatitis there may be malabsorption. Clinical features are those common to a number of B group deficiency states namely cheilosis, glossitis, keratitis, conjunctivitis, photophobia and lacrimation. Cheilosis begins with pallor, thinning and maceration of the skin at the angles of the mouth and then extends laterally. The whole mouth may become reddened and swollen and there is loss of papillae of the tongue. A normochromic, normocytic anaemia is secondary to bone marrow hypoplasia. There may be associated seborrhoeic dermatitis involving the nasolabial folds and forehead. Conjunctival suffusion may proceed to proliferation of blood vessels onto the cornea.

Diagnosis

Urinary riboflavine excretion of less than 30 mg/day is characteristic of a deficiency state. There is reduction of red cell glutathione reductase.

Treatment

In childhood the daily requirement for riboflavine is 0.6 mg per 4.2 mJ (1000 kcal) and treatment of a deficiency state requires 10 mg oral riboflavine daily. In some circumstances riboflavine 2 mg three times per day can be given by intramuscular injection until there is clinical improvement.

Pellagra (niacin deficiency)

Niacin is the precursor of nicotinamide, adenine dinucleotide (NAD) and its reduced form NADP. It can be synthesised from tryptophan and pellagra tends to occur when maize, which is a poor source tryptophan and niacin, is the staple diet. Niacin is lost in the milling process. Communities where millet, which has a high leucine content, is consumed also have a high incidence of pellagra.

Clinical features

The classical triad for pellagra is diarrhoea, dermatitis and dementia although in children the diarrhoea and dementia are less obvious than in the adolescent and adult. There is light-sensitive dermatitis on exposed areas which can result in blistering and desquamation of the skin. On healing the skin becomes pigmented (see Fig. 20.3). The children are apathetic and disinterested and feed poorly because of an associated glossitis and stomatitis.

Diagnosis

There are no diagnostic tests and diagnosis is usually by therapeutic trial with niacin. N-Methyl nicotinamide excretion in the urine, when it can be measured, is found to be low.

Treatment

The normal requirement for niacin in infancy and childhood is 8–10 mg/day when the tryptophan intake is adequate. Deficiency states can be treated with up to 300 mg/day given orally but care must be taken as large doses will produce flushing and burning sensations in the skin. There is almost always other associated vitamin B deficiencies and these should be supplied during the treatment of pellagra. Because of the intimate involvement of the three major B vitamins described in intermediary metabolism the requirement is best determined in relation to energy intake. Recommended intakes on this basis are: thiamine 0.4 mg per 4.2 mJ (1000 kcal); riboflavin 0.55 mg per 4.2 mJ; niacin 6.6 mg per 4.2 mJ.

Vitamin B$_6$ (pyridoxine deficiency)

There may be inadequate intake of dietary pyridoxine when there is prolonged heat processing of milk and cereals or when unsupplemented milk formulae or elemental diets are used. There can be inadequate absorption in coeliac disease and drug treatment with izoniazid, penicillamine and oral contraceptives will aggravate deficiency states.

The disorder has to be differentiated from pyridoxine dependency in which pyridoxine dependent convulsions and anaemia are secondary to a genetic disorder of the apoenzyme.

Clinical features

Pyridoxine deficiency states result in convulsions, peripheral neuritis, cheilosis, glossitis, seborrhoea and anaemia. The anaemia is microcytic and is aggravated when intercurrent infections complicate the clinical picture. There may be oxaluria with bladder stones, hyperglycinaemia, lymphopenia and decreased antibody production.

Diagnosis

There is increased xanthurenic acid in the urine after an oral dose of tryptophan. Glutamine-oxaloacetic acid transaminase is reduced in the red cells.

Treatment

The usual requirements for non-pyridoxine dependent individuals is 0.5 mg/day in infancy and 1 mg/day in children.

Vitamin B$_{12}$

If maternal vitamin B$_{12}$ status is satisfactory the reserves of B$_{12}$ in the term newborn infant should last throughout the first year of life especially if the infant is breast fed. Dietary deficiency of vitamin B$_{12}$ is unusual except amongst the strict vegans who consume neither milk nor eggs. Absorption of B$_{12}$ requires a gastric intrinsic factor which promotes absorption in the terminal ileum. Deficiency of intrinsic factor, secondary to gastric achlorhydria is rare in childhood. It has been reported secondarily to the development of gastric parietal cell antibody but this is extremely rare. Familial pernicious anaemia is secondary to a series of autosomal recessively inherited defects in B$_{12}$ metabolism or in the function of B$_{12}$ binding proteins. Resection of the terminal ileum or Crohn disease will predispose children to B$_{12}$ deficiency unless B$_{12}$ supplementation is given.

Clinical features

Pallor, anorexia and glossitis are common features. Paraesthesia with loss of position and vibration sense is a disorder of adolescence rather than childhood. There is a megaloblastic anaemia with neutropenia, thrombocytopenia and hypersegmentation of polymorphonuclear leucocytes. The bone marrow shows a megaloblastic, erythroid picture with giant metamyelocytes.

The neurological signs of subacute combined degeneration of the cord with peripheral neuritis, degeneration of the dorsal columns and corticospinal tract is a late phenomenon as is retrobulbar neuropathy.

Treatment

In the rare instance of dietary deficiency oral supplementation is satisfactory. Where there is inadequate absorption intramuscular injections, initially of 1 mg/day reducing to 1 mg at 3-monthly intervals in the light of clinical improvement is the usual management in older children and adolescents. Oral hydroxocobalamin is now available and may be used also in the treatment of the B$_{12}$ responsive methylmalonic acidaemias.

Folic acid deficiency

Deficiency of folic acid is widespread in many communities and is a known factor in the aetiology of neural tube defects. Although found widely in plant and animal tissues the vitamin is easily destroyed by cooking and storage processes. Requirements for growth during fetal and neonatal life and childhood are high. Deficiency states are likely to occur during childhood particularly when there is excessive cell turnover such as occurs in the haemolytic anaemias (sickle-cell disease) and in exfoliative skin conditions such as eczema. Folic acid is the precursor of tetrahydrofolate which is intimately involved in a series of enzyme reactions of amino acid, purine and intermediary metabolism.

Folate is absorbed in the duodenum and in malabsorptive states including coeliac disease folate deficiency is common. In some situations where the small intestine is colonised by bacteria (blind loop syndrome) folate is diverted into bacterial metabolism. Some anticonvulsants and antibacterial agents either increase the metabolism of folate or compete with folate.

Clinical features

Megaloblastic anaemia and pancytopenia together with poor growth are the result of the cessation of cell division which comes about when nucleoprotein formation is interrupted because of the lack of synthesis of purines and pyrimidines.

Diagnosis

The blood picture is one of a megalobastic anaemia with neutropenia and thrombocytopenia. The neutrophils contain large hypersegmented nuclei and bone marrow is hypercellular because of erythroid hyperplasia. Although the reticulocyte count is low nucleated red cells appear in the peripheral blood. Red cell folate measurements are <75 ng/ml. There is a close interaction of B_{12} and folic acid in the synthesis of tetrahydrofolate and formyltetrahydrofolate which are required for purine ring formation. With isolated folate deficiency there are none of the neuropathies associated with the megaloblastic anaemia of B_{12} deficiency.

Treatment

Response to treatment with oral or parenteral folic acid 2–5 mg/day is usually rapid. If there is a combined folate and B_{12} deficiency folic acid alone may cure the megaloblastic anaemia but the subacute combined degeneration of the cord will persist until B_{12} is given. In order to reduce the risk of neural tube defect it is recommended that all women should ensure an intake of 0.4 mg folic acid/day from before conception and throughout pregnancy. Any woman giving birth to an infant with a neural tube defect should have 4 mg folic acid from before conception and throughout pregnancy.

Vitamin E

Vitamin E deficiency except in the preterm infant is rare. In the preterm vitamin E deficiency is occasionally associated with haemolytic anaemia and may contribute to the membrane damage associated with intraventricular haemorrhage and bronchopulmonary dysplasia. Vitamin E is essential for the insertion and maintenance of long-chain polyunsaturated fatty acids in the phospholipid bilayer of cell membranes by counteracting the effect of free radicals on these fatty acids. When the essential fatty acid content of the diet is high, vitamin E is required in increased amounts. Natural sources of vitamin E are oily fish, milk, cereal, seed oils, peanuts and soya beans. Children with abetalipoproteinaemia have steatorrhoea and low circulating levels of vitamin E associated with neurological signs. More recently older children and adults with cystic fibrosis have developed neurological signs similar to those in abetalipoproteinaemia due to vitamin E deficiency. In any child with fat malabsorption it would be important to give supplementary vitamin E in addition to correcting the underlying fat malabsorption where possible.

MINERAL DEFICIENCIES

Iron deficiency

Reasons for iron deficiency in the weanling are given in Chapter 1. In older children infection and iron deficiency cause anorexia which is further aggravated by recurrent infection. This can cause a vicious cycle since iron deficiency lowers resistance to infection and the pyrexia and anorexia of infection aggravates the iron deficiency further. Early introduction of iron containing foods such as red meats, egg yolk and highly coloured vegetables such as spinach, tomatoes and peppers should be encouraged. Adequate vitamin C to augment iron absorption is important particularly in vegans. Phytates tend to bind iron in the gut and thus reduce iron absorption. Absorption takes place in the duodenum and upper jejunum and iron is transported in the blood bound to transferrin. Transferrin concentrations are low in infectious states but high in iron deficiency states. Ferritin is present in small amounts in the plasma and red cells but the red cell concentration directly parallels the tissue iron storage. Values below 10 mg/litre at any age indicate iron depletion states.

Clinical features

Iron deficient children are often irritable or apathetic and anorexic. Studies have shown a relationship between iron deficiency states and reduced attention span and learning ability. It may be that there is permanent intellectual impairment when the deficiency state is prolonged during the early learning period. Most parents, however, report considerable improvement in appetite, behaviour and well-being of their children after the onset of iron therapy, often before there is any significant change in haemoglobin

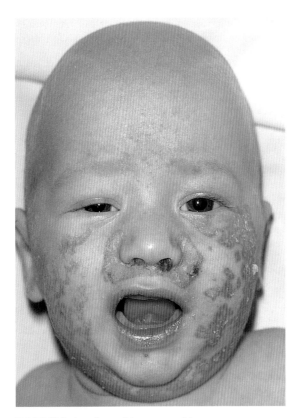

FIGURE 20.8 Acrodermatitis enteropathica.

concentration. It is unclear whether the poor performance, perceptual disturbance and conduct problems in anaemic children are the consequence of anaemia or of a general nutritional inadequacy. Iron repletion therapy tends to improve mental development scores in iron deficient children whether they are anaemic or non-anaemic. Treatment with iron also improves weight gain velocity.

Treatment

Most iron preparations are unpalatable and require to be given for several months in order to restore iron to the tissues. Ferrous sulphate by tablet or mixture to supply a total daily dose of 12 mg elemental iron for those under 6 months; 36 mg at one year; 72 mg for the 1–5-year-old; 120 mg for the 6–12-year-old; and 120–180 mg for adults is the usual recommended dosage. It must be remembered that iron is a dangerous poison for children when ingested in excess (Chapter 18).

Zinc deficiency

Zinc is involved in every enzyme system dealing with nucleoprotein as well as many other enzymes active in intermediary metabolism. Food sources are liver, shellfish, nuts, beans, cocoa and in some areas from the water supply.

Clinical features

There are two types of presentation. In acrodermatitis enteropathica a congenital abnormality of zinc absorption causes a severe and potentially lethal condition in which there is mucucutaneous ulceration, failure to thrive and susceptibility to infection (Fig. 20.8). In older children zinc deficiency may occur in malnutrition states particularly in vegans where there is a high phytate content in the diet. Growth retardation, anorexia and loss of taste (ageusia), glossitis, alopecia and nail dystrophy are reported and diarrhoea is common. Immunodeficiency and delayed puberty have been described in areas of zinc deficiency in the Middle East. There can be delayed wound healing and skin repair in infants maintained parenterally without adequate zinc supplies.

Treatment

The usual requirement for zinc in infancy is 1 mg/kg/day and in childhood 10 mg/day. Excess copper in the diet will interfere with zinc absorption. Treatment with additional zinc will result in rapid improvement in acrodermatitis enteropathica and to improved healing of skin and other lesions in zinc deficiency states.

Copper deficiency

Copper is also an important constituent of many enzyme systems such as cytochrome oxidase and dismutase yet clinical copper deficiency states are rare except in very low birthweight infants, in states of severe protein energy malnutrition and during prolonged parenteral nutrition. The term infant is born with substantial stores of liver copper largely laid down in the last trimester of pregnancy bound to metallothionein. Preterm infants will therefore be born with inadequate liver stores of copper and may develop deficiency in the newborn period unless fed foods supplemented with copper. It is thought that the daily requirement for copper in term infants is 0.2 mg/day increasing to 1 mg/day by the end of the first year of life. Thereafter the requirement for copper is between 1 and 3 mg/day. Human milk contains about 0.6 mmol (39 µg)/100 ml copper but cows' milk only contains 0.13 mmol (9 µg)/100 ml. Many infant formulae are supplemented with copper. In soya-based infant formulas, phytate binding prohibits absorption and additional copper supplementation is required. Percentage absorption of copper is increased in deficiency states although, like iron, absorption is partly dependent on the form in which copper is presented to the gut. Other trace elements such as iron, zinc, cadmium, calcium, sulphur and molybdenum interfere with copper absorption. After absorption the copper is bound to albumin in the portal circulation. Ceruloplasmin is formed in the liver and is the major transport protein for copper. It has been used as a measure of copper deficiency but ceruloplasmin also acts as an acute-phase reactant and will increase in stress situations particularly during infections. The normal plasma copper concentration is 11–25 mmol/l (0.7–1.6 mg/l) and ceruloplasmin 0.1–0.7 g/l. These values are decreased in deficiency states.

Clinical features

In preterm infants there may be severe osteoporosis with cupping and flaring of the bone ends with periosteal reaction and submetaphyseal fractures. Severe bone disease has been reported in older infants on bizarre diets. It has been argued that subclinical copper deficiency may account for some of the fractures in suspected non-accidental injury. It is most unlikely that copper deficiency in an otherwise healthy child could result in unexplained fracture. To suggest that copper deficiency develops without obvious cause and results in bone fractures without other evidence of copper deficiency is at best unwise.

Menkes steely-hair or kinky-hair syndrome is a rare X-linked disorder associated with disturbed copper metabolism. There is gross osteoporosis and progressive neurological impairment. Scalp hair is sparse and brittle with pili torti on microscopic examination. The disorder does not respond to copper therapy.

Selenium deficiency

Muscular dystrophy in lambs and calves has been reported in parts of the world where there is deficiency of selenium in the soil. In humans Keshan disease has been reported in China. Selenium is essential for glutathione peroxidase activity which catalyses the reduction of fatty acid hydroperoxides and protects tissues from peroxidation. Thus selenium is important in maintaining the fatty acid integrity of phospholipid membranes and reducing free radical damage. It is found in fish, meat and whole grain and reflects the soil selenium content of the region. Vitamin C improves the absorption of selenium.

Clinical features

In China an endemic cardiomyopathy known as Kesham disease, affecting women of childbearing age and children, has been reported. The condition responds to selenium supplementation. In New Zealand low selenium concentrations in the soil result in low plasma levels and in children with phenylketonuria on a low phenylalanine diet low plasma levels of selenium have been reported. There is no obvious clinical abnormality in the New Zealand population although poor growth and dry skin has been reported in the selenium deficient PKU children.

Chromium

Chromium may be involved in nucleic acid metabolism and is recognised as a cofactor for insulin. It is poorly absorbed and there is some evidence that in the elderly, glucose tolerance can be improved by chromium supplementation. Chromium deficiency has been reported in severely malnourished children and in children on prolonged parenteral nutrition. Weight gain and glucose tolerance in such children has been reported to improve after chromium supplementation. In long-term parenteral nutrition peripheral neuropathy and encephalopathy have also been reported to respond to chromium administration.

Iodine

Endemic goitre has been recognised for many centuries in mountainous regions of the world. The Andes, Himalayas, mountains of Central Africa and Papua, New Guinea, as well as Derbyshire in the UK, are areas where the condition has been recognised. Minimal requirements are probably less than 20 µg/day in infants and young children increasing to 50 µg/day during adolescence. Breast milk contains up to 90 µg/l. Goitre occurs when the iodine intake is less than 15 µg/day and results in a reduced serum thyroxine (T_4) but a decreased tri-iodothyronine (T_3). Thyroid stimulating hormone (TSH) values increase. The introduction of iodised salt to areas of endemic goitrous and cretinism have largely eradicated goitre cretinism in these regions. Some plants, including brassicas, act as goitrogens by inhibiting iodine uptake by the thyroid gland.

Fluorine

Fluorine has been recognised as an important factor in the prevention of caries. When drinking water contains 1 mg fluoride per litre, rates of caries are low.

Other trace minerals

Manganese, molybdenum and cadmium are known to be necessary for health in animals but no clear human evidence of deficiency states are known to man.

TUBERCULOSIS

The incidence of infection by human-type tubercle bacilli has fallen abruptly in Britain in the past 30 years. This has been due to earlier diagnosis of phthisis in adults, to the detection by mass radiography of previously unknown sources of infection, and to the efficiency of modern antituberculous drugs in rendering patients non-infective within a relatively short period. The routine vaccination with BCG of tuberculin-negative children aged 11–13 years with BCG has also played a part. It would, however, be a grave error to regard the disease as having been defeated, and cases still occur too frequently to permit complacency. In some of the underdeveloped countries of the world tuberculosis remains a major public health problem and is the commonest cause of death. On the other hand, bovine tuberculosis, which until about 50 years ago was very common in the form of abdominal tuberculosis, cervical tuberculosis and disease of bone and joints, has disappeared from Britain. Indeed, there is evidence to suggest that in indigenous British children cervical adenitis is nowadays more often due to infection by atypical or "anonymous" mycobacteria than by the "typical" *Mycobacterium tuberculosis*. However, intrathoracic tuberculosis is almost always due to the human type of *M. tuberculosis*, and must be regarded as a major problem deserving a close study and understanding by the physicians of all countries. In countries with significant numbers of the population affected by human immunodeficiency virus (HIV) there has been a marked resurgence of tuberculosis.

Intrathoracic tuberculosis

Sources of infection

By far the most usual source of tuberculous infection in infancy and childhood is the adult contact who suffers from "open" phthisis. In Britain the known case of adult tuberculosis is quickly rendered non-infectious by appropriate drug treatment and the danger is the undiagnosed or unsuspected adult. Infrequently, a child can be infected from a tuberculous animal such as a dog, and this possibility should not be overlooked.

Pathology

When a patient of any age inhales tubercle bacilli for the first time they produce a small caseous focus in the lung parenchyma. This is called "the primary focus" or Ghon focus. It is usually single, occasionally multiple, and most often situated subpleurally, in 45% of cases in the right upper lobe. From the primary focus, which is usually large enough to be visible to the naked eye, there is a peribronchial lymphangitis spreading towards the bronchopulmonary and tracheobronchial glands on the same side. These become enlarged and caseous, ultimately undergoing softening. Indeed, in primary tuberculosis the lung parenchyma lesion is small, almost trivial, while the regional lymph glands are heavily involved. This is in contrast to adult-type phthisis, in which the tissues have earlier been sensitised by primary tuberculosis, and where the lung parenchyma may show extensive infiltration, caseation, cavitation and fibrosis while the regional lymphadenitis is slight or absent. The primary focus, lymphangitis and hilar adenitis constitute "the primary tuberculous complex". In more severe examples the disease may spread upwards, involving the paratracheal and the supraclavicular glands.

In the majority of cases the primary complex heals by calcification in the primary focus and regional lymph nodes. These are visible on radiographs but ultimately the calcium is absorbed so that no trace of the infection may remain. In others, especially infants and young children, the caseous hilar nodes exert local effects upon the adjoining bronchi which are thin-walled and pliable. Most often the enlarged glands completely obstruct a primary or secondary bronchus and the distal lobe or segment becomes airless. Histologically it shows resorption atelectasis and possibly low-grade tuberculous inflammation. Whereas in some cases the bronchial occlusion is brought about by extrinsic compression, in many the caseous glands erode their way through the bronchial wall, so that the mucous membrane is perforated and tuberculous granulation tissue can then be seen to fill the lumen. The right middle lobe is most often affected. This type of atelectasis or absorption collapse may completely resolve, but not infrequently it leaves behind bronchial narrowing and distortion, or a "dry" bronchiectasis which may become the seat of severe pyogenic infection many years later.

Acute miliary tuberculosis

This classical form of the disease arises from erosion of some part of the primary complex into a blood vessel and the discharge into the circulation of a large dose of tubercle bacilli. Like tuberculous meningitis this is most likely to occur within the first 6 months after the primary infection. All the organs of the body are studded with small miliary tubercles which are usually visible to the naked eye. Erosion of a caseous gland into a branch of the pulmonary artery explains those uncommon cases where the miliary spread is confined to the lungs.

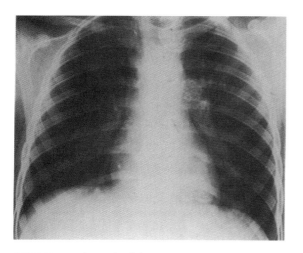

FIGURE 20.9 Radiograph of chest showing exceptionally large primary tuberculous focus in left upper lobe. Early calcification is present.

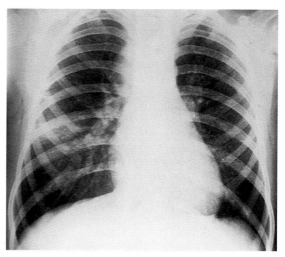

FIGURE 20.10 Chest radiograph showing tuberculous cavity in the right lower lobe.

Acute tuberculous pneumonia

This rapidly progressive form of pulmonary tuberculosis may be lobar or lobular in distribution. Once common as "galloping consumption", it has become rare and is almost confined to young children. Cavitation, spontaneous pneumothorax and tuberculous empyema were common complications, but they have virtually disappeared in Britain since the advent of the antituberculous drugs.

Clinical aspects of the primary tuberculous infection

The child with an intrathoracic primary infection may be symptomless or severely ill. When symptoms do appear they coincide with the development by the tissues of an allergic sensitivity towards tuberculoprotein. This takes about 6–8 weeks to develop and may be demonstrated by means of a tuberculin skin test. In some patients spontaneous manifestations of this allergic state appear in the form of phylctenular conjunctivitis or erythema nodosum, and these conditions should always be presumed to indicate tuberculous infection in children until they are proved to be otherwise caused. In some children, who are usually over the age of 5 years, the development of pleurisy with effusion makes the diagnosis easy.

In most cases, the symptomatology tends to be non-specific and of a type common in other non-tuberculous ailments, e.g. loss of energy, lethargy, undue irritability, anorexia and a general loss of well-being. An irregular fever (37–38°C) in the late afternoons is common. Less often there may be brisk sustained fever. Loss of weight or failure to gain are usual but not invariable. Local symptoms due to the effect on surrounding structures of pressure from caseous mediastinal glands are most severe in infants. Whereas in the school child cough may be relatively unimpressive, in the infant glandular pressure on the main bronchi frequently gives rise to spasmodic outbursts of coughing which closely simulate pertussis. In fact, the bronchi may be sufficiently narrowed by extrinsic pressure that a loud wheeze – "the asthmatoid wheeze" – may be heard. Physical examination of the chest is rarely helpful unless there is absorption collapse or obstructive emphysema. The diagnosis of primary intrathoracic tuberculosis must depend largely upon the ease with which the physician's suspicions are aroused. In some instances, of course, the child is brought to the doctor because of known recent contact with a tuberculous adult. The possibility of such contact, within or outside the family circle, should always be the subject of direct enquiry in the case of an unwell child in whom a satisfactory diagnosis has not been reached.

Diagnostic tests

Tuberculin skin tests are, of all tests, the most useful in the diagnosis of primary tuberculosis. A positive reaction before the age of 3 years is evidence of active infection. After this age a positive test may only indicate previous infection not now necessarily active, but in an ill child it obviously merits further investigation. The most reliable test is the Mantoux intradermal reaction using suitable dilutions of Old Tuberculin (OT) or purified protein derivative (PPD). The "tine" test is convenient in domicilliary practice although less reliable. When large numbers have to be tested, the Heaf test, which makes multiple

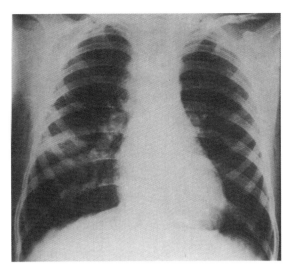

FIGURE 20.11 Primary tuberculous complex showing a Ghon's focus in right midzone with enlarged paratracheal glands.

punctures with a test-gun through undiluted OT or PPD, is useful. False negative results with all tests may be found in children who are overwhelmed by miliary tuberculosis and in those convalescent from measles. Apart from these exceptions a negative tuberculin test, properly performed with active material, excludes tuberculosis. It must be remembered, however, that these tests lose some of their value in children who have been immunised with BCG.

In the child with an active tuberculous infection the standard Mantoux test is likely to give an area of induration exceeding 6 mm in diameter with a larger area of erythema.

A chest radiograph may fail to reveal any abnormality in early primary tuberculosis. Most often, however, unilateral enlargement of the hilar glands is visible, but as this could be due to diseases other than tuberculosis the chest radiograph by itself cannot justify a diagnosis of primary tuberculosis. Only very rarely is the primary focus in the lung parenchyma visible, although it can be large enough to be seen (Fig. 20.9). It is quite exceptional for the primary focus to cavitate (Fig. 20.10). When the primary complex heals by calcification it will become radiologically obvious (Fig. 20.11) although no longer responsible for symptoms. It must be stressed that the diagnostic value of the radiograph is limited in primary tuberculosis, in marked contrast to adult-type phthisis where the lung parenchyma is heavily involved.

Gastric washings should be examined by direct staining, culture and guinea-pig inoculation. They are of limited usefulness in diagnosis in view of the time-lag usually involved, but successful isolation of tuber-

cle bacilli allows their sensitivities towards the antituberculous drugs to be tested and this information is valuable.

The erythrocyte sedimentation rate (ESR), preferably determined by the Westergren technique, is not of direct diagnostic value, but a raised ESR helps to confirm the presence of active disease, and serial estimations are valuable in assessing progress during treatment.

Enough has been said to make it clear that a diagnosis of active primary tuberculosis can rarely be established on the basis of a single test, and certainly not on the X-ray appearances. However, when all the findings are weighed together – clinical history, possible adult contact, results of tuberculin tests, radiographs and ESR – it is almost always possible to arrive at a correct diagnosis.

Extrathoracic tuberculosis

Sources of infection

Cervical and abdominal tuberculosis were once common in Britain as a consequence of the ingestion of milk from tuberculous cows, but as we have already pointed out bovine tuberculosis no longer exists in this country. However, bovine strains of tubercle bacilli are still isolated from immigrant patients of Asian and African origin, and it is, of course, not unknown for cervical tuberculosis to arise from the entry of human strains of tubercle bacilli. Primary infection of the skin, conjunctiva, or within the mouth following tooth extraction may also occur and in such cases there is frequently a history of contact with an adult case of phthisis. Presumably the organisms find entry through a minor break in the skin or mucous membrane.

Pathological course

The primary tuberculous complex behaves in the same basic fashion whatever its site. In cervical tuberculosis the primary focus is in the tonsil, although it can only be seen under the microscope. There has often been preceding chronic sepsis in the tonsils. The affected cervical lymph nodes become caseous. They may later liquefy and coalesce, at the same time becoming adherent to the skin and surrounding tissues. If rupture occurs the classical "collar stud" abscess extending through a fascial plane, or one or more sinuses discharging through the skin may develop (scrofula). In abdominal tuberculosis the primary focus is in the small intestine. This is a solitary microscopic lesion, not to be confused with the secondary tuberculous enteritis which may complicate advanced cases of adult-type phthisis.

Mesenteric lymph nodes are massively involved, and rupture into the peritoneal cavity leads to the once common picture of tuberculous peritonitis. The possibility of cutaneous, conjunctival or buccal primary tuberculosis should be considered when solitary but chronic enlargement of lymph nodes appears in unusual sites, e.g. pre-auricular, submandibular or inguinal. In all types of extrathoracic tuberculosis haematogenous spread may occur, although less acutely than in the intrathoracic disease. In the case of bovine infections, bone and joint lesions were at one time common complications which resulted in long periods of invalidism or crippling, even in death.

Clinical aspects

The general symptoms tend to be common to all types of primary tuberculosis. They vary from none at all to listlessness, anorexia, undue fatiguability, low-grade fever and loss of weight. When the cervical glands are involved the first sign is a painless, firm, mobile mass at the angle of the jaw. Later the glands become matted together, adherent to the skin and no longer freely movable. Liquefaction is indicated by palpable fluctuation. Healing is by fibrosis and calcification which become radiologically visible. The differential diagnosis from other causes of cervical adenitis can be made by tuberculin skin testing.

Treatment of primary tuberculosis

It is possible to achieve a cure in every type of tuberculosis provided that the disease is diagnosed at a reasonably early stage; and the tubercle bacilli in the lesions are sensitive to the drugs employed. In the economically developed countries "classic chemotherapy" using streptomycin, para-aminosalicylic acid and isoniazid has now been replaced by newer antituberculous drugs such as rifampicin, ethambutol, or pyrazinamide, along with isoniazid. However, in many developing countries problems of cost control still require the use of 3 "standard" drugs, each given once daily, in the following dosage:

- streptomycin (intramuscular) 40 mg/kg/day;
- isoniazid (oral) 10–20 mg/kg/day;
- para-aminosalicylic acid PAS (oral) 300 mg/kg/day.

Highly satisfactory results in active tuberculosis can be obtained with these drugs when given over periods of 1–1½ years in children and 1½ –2 years in adolescents and adults. With the newer drugs now available the course of treatment can be reduced to 6–9 months (with the exception of tuberculous meningitis). The use of two or more drugs in combination is to prevent the emergence of drug-resistant strains of M. tuberculosis, although this risk is less in cases of primary tuberculosis than in adult-type phthisis. Various chemotherapy regimens are available. For children over the age of 3 years a suitable regimen, each drug given once daily, is:

- rifampicin (oral) 10–15 mg/kg/day;
- isoniazid (oral) 10–20 mg/kg/day;
- ethambutol (oral) 15 mg/kg/day.

Rifampicin may cause gastric upset and a rise in liver transaminases but these side effects are rarely severe. Very rarely the development of thrombocytopenia necessitates withdrawal of the drug. The most serious toxic effect of ethambutol is optic neuritis, with loss of visual acuity, and colour blindness. While this is rare with doses below 25 mg/kg/day, the drug is best avoided in very young children for whom an alternative drug regimen is:

- rifampicin (oral) 10–15 mg/kg/day;
- isoniazid (oral) 10–29 mg/kg/day;
- pyrazinamide (oral) 20–30 mg/kg/day.

Side effects with isoniazid are rare. They include convulsions in young infants and peripheral neuropathy in older patients. They should be prevented by giving pyridoxine 50 mg daily by mouth.

It is no longer necessary to confine children suffering from tuberculosis to bed for long periods, nor to banish them to inaccessible sanatoria in the country. When the child is fevered or feels ill he should be in bed, but can safely be allowed up and outside in the fresh air as soon as he is afebrile and feeling well. Indeed, in many instances he can be permitted to live his normal life and to attend school, provided his parents can be relied upon to give him his drugs regularly. Inadequate compliance by the parents is sometimes the cause of therapeutic failure and it is important that supervision is in the hands of a physician who is familiar with the behaviour of primary tuberculosis. In developing countries it is frequently necessary to counter malnutrition in addition to prescribing antituberculous drugs.

MALARIA

Aetiology

Malaria is still one of the major causes of child mortality in many countries especially in tropical Africa. According to the statistical information reported to WHO, the overall world malaria situation has not improved over the past two decades. The mortality due to malaria is unknown in many parts of the world. This is due mainly to under-reporting of deaths in general and the inability to diagnose the

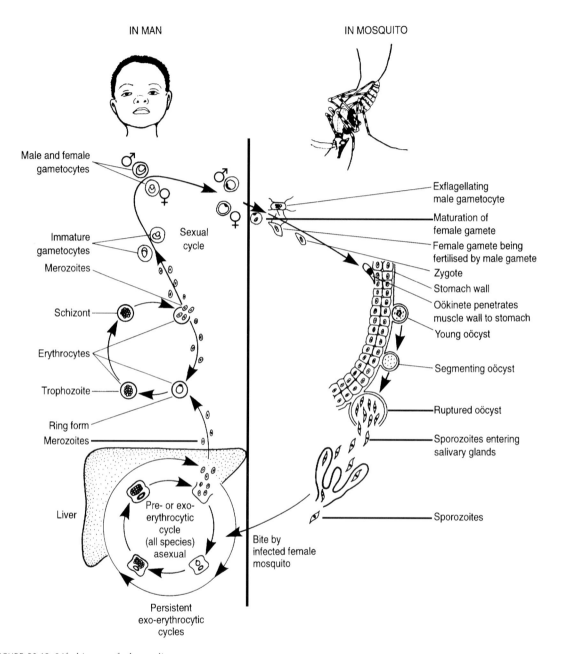

FIGURE 20.12 Life history of plasmodium.

cause of death accurately. There are four species of human malarial parasite. *Plasmodium falciparum* causes malignant tertian (MT) malaria; this is an extremely dangerous disease which should be regarded as different in kind from the other varieties of malaria because of the way in which the arterioles in vital organs may be blocked by parasitised erythro-

cytes. *P. vivax* causes benign tertian (BT) malaria. Quartan malaria is due to *P. malariae* and is a not uncommon cause of the nephrotic syndrome in children in malarial areas. *P. ovale* causes ovale malaria. The infection is acquired when the patient is bitten by an infected female mosquito of the genus *Anopheles* (Fig. 20.12). The parasites, in the form of sporozoites, quickly leave the blood stream and undergo a pre-erythrocytic stage of development which takes place in the liver parenchyma cells and is symptomless. In cases of *P. falciparum* the pre-erythrocytic schizont reaches maturity in 6 days when it ruptures to liberate merozoites into the circulation. These enter the erythrocytes but no parasites remain in the liver. The pre-erythrocytic stages of *P. vivax* and *P. ovale* last 8 days, that of *P. malariae* longer. In addition to the invasion of erythrocytes by merozoites there is a persisting exo-erythrocytic infection in the liver in these species of parasite and this is the explanation for later relapses. The attacks of malarial fever are due to the liberation of merozoites from the schizonts which develop in the erythrocytes. This erythrocytic cycle takes 48 hours in the case of *P. vivax* and *P. ovale* and 72 hours in *P. malariae* infections. In *P. falciparum* the fever is irregular. Some of the circulating parasites develop into sexual forms, gametocytes, which are infective for mosquitoes so that the disease is then spread to others. The development of a degree of immunity to malaria is an important factor but very complicated. In highly malarious areas young infants seem to escape infection for some months after birth, due presumably to the transplacental transfer of maternal antibodies. This is also associated with a tendency to relatively mild attacks when malaria does occur in early infancy, thus permitting the slow acquisition of an active immunity towards the disease. On the other hand, the parasites may themselves cross the placenta and congenital malaria results. This is much more likely in the case of a mother who lacks immunity than in one who has grown up in a malarious area and so acquired a degree of immunity. Most cases of congenital malaria are caused by *P. falciparum* and *P. vivax*; however, all four species that infect man can infect the newborn. Treatment of congenital malaria is aimed at the erythrocytic stages of the parasite, as no persistent liver phase exists in congenitally acquired infections.

Clinical features

Malaria presents a less "typical" picture in the child than in the adult; and it tends to be more severe in the expatriate child than in the partially immune indigenous child, who may have remarkably mild symptoms despite a heavy parasitaemia. Irritability, anorexia, listlessness and obvious pallor are usual whereas rigors are uncommon even when fever is high. Severe vomiting frequently accompanies the fever. Convulsions are not uncommon and in malignant tertian (MT) malaria it may be difficult to determine whether these indicate true cerebral malaria with its attendant risk of permanent brain damage. Hepatomegaly develops early but splenomegaly is often absent in the early stages of a primary attack

although in holo-endemic areas of malaria few other diseases produce such massive enlargement of the spleen. The urine may contain excess protein and urobilinogen. The fever tends to be irregular and remittent. There are no reliable distinctive clinical features of malaria in children except for periodic fever. Malaria may masquerade as many other illnesses and in young children and infants can mimic gastroenteritis, pneumonia, meningitis, encephalitis or hepatitis.

Most of the deaths from malaria in endemic areas occur in young children during the transition period from passive to acquired immunity and they are due to falciparum (MT) infections. The most dangerous complication is *cerebral malaria*, in which parasitised red cells block the smallest arterioles and convulsions with coma develop. Cerebrospinal fluid may be normal or show a mild increase in cells and globulin content. This dangerous emergency is uncommon in the indigenous child after the age of 5 years but is only too likely to complicate MT malaria in the expatriate child or adult. It is, of course, essential to exclude other possible causes of convulsions such as meningitis, encephalitis, or poisoning by indigenous "medicines". *Vomiting and diarrhoea* in MT malaria can result in rapid and severe dehydration infrequently associated with jaundice. *Hyperpyrexia* with failure of sweating may also occur, but *algid (cold) malaria* in which hypotension, cold clammy skin and "shock" develop, is rare in the child. This syndrome is felt to be a consequence of acute adrenal failure.

Severe anaemia may result from repeated attacks of malaria, often untreated, in holo-endemic areas. This is because parasitised red cells are destroyed. It is usually associated with stunting of growth, gross hepatosplenomegaly and is not uncommonly accompanied by iron deficiency, malnutrition, hookworm infestation, etc. Disseminated intravascular coagulation (DIC) is a rare complication of malaria associated with a high parasite load, pulmonary oedema, a rapidly developing anaemia and cerebral and renal complications.

Diagnosis

The indentification of malarial parasites in thick or thin blood films or bone marrow aspirate is the only basis for a certain diagnosis. Thick smears concentrate the parasites and are used for detecting their presence. Thin smears are used for morphological identification. In severe emergency it may be necessary to start treatment before the blood films have been examined but it is important that they always be taken before any antimalarial drug is administered. In an area where falciparum malaria is endemic *the report of a negative blood film in suspected cerebral malaria usually means that the diagnosis has been wrong*. It is worth pointing out, however, that the only trophozoite form of *P. falciparum* to occur in peripheral blood (the so-called ring) is easily missed by the inexperienced. On the other hand, in chronic malaria with gross hepatosplenomegaly in a partially immune indigenous child, repeated blood films may have to be examined before a few parasites, more often *P. vivax* or *malariae* are found. Serological techniques are not routinely available for the detection of malaria.

Treatment

The drug of choice is chloroquine and the dose should always be calculated in terms of the base content of the table or solution. When there is severe vomiting an initial intramuscular dose of 5 mg base/kg body weight can often be followed by oral treatment. In most cases effective treatment consists of a single daily dose of chloroquine for 3–5 consecutive days: the adult dose is 300 mg base/day. The appropriate dosage for children can be found in Table 20.2. When possible chloroquine should be given by the oral route which is safe. In a patient who is unable to take it orally, e.g. severe vomiting or in coma, then the drug should be administered parenterally. This route of administration is not without risks, e.g. hypotension, sudden death, chloroquine encephalopathy.

In emergency situations, such as cerebral malaria, chloroquine should be given intramuscularly in a dose of 5 mg base/kg. This may be repeated in 6 hours but the total dose in 24 hours must not exceed 10 mg base/kg. In the most dire emergency the initial dose can be given intravenously in dilute solution by slow drip although the risk in a young child is not negligible. Some physicians still prefer to use intravenous quinine in this situation, 10–15 mg/kg in dilute solution by intravenous infusion. A second dose may be given in 6 hours, but the total dosage must not exceed 20 mg/kg per 24 hours. Severe dehydration demands intravenous fluid therapy and severe anaemia is an indication for slow blood transfusion. In severe cerebral malaria replacement transfusion can be a valuable therapeutic measure.

Unfortunately chloroquine-resistant falciparum malaria has become a widespread phenomenon in many parts of South-east Asia, the Indian subcontinent, Africa and South America. In these areas two preparations have been effective. Fansidar (pyrimethamine + sulfadoxine) and Maloprim (pyrimethamine + dapsone), but resistance is now developing towards Fansidar and both drugs are less effective against vivax malaria than choloroquine. Mefloquine, a long-acting quinine analogue, was developed by the US Army Antimalarial Drug Research Programme. It is highly effective against falciparum and vivax infections in a single oral (adult) dose of 1.0–1.5 g. Qinghaosu is a crystalline

TABLE 20.2 Doses of antimalarial drugs for children (preferably based on weight when known)

WEIGHT (kg)	AGE (years)	PROPORTION OF ADULT DOSE
<5	<1	One-quarter
5–20	1–5	One-half
21–40	6–12	Three-quarters
>40	>12	Adult dose

extract of a medicinal herb (*Artemisia annua*) used in China for treating malaria for 2000 years. It is highly effective when given orally in (adult) doses of 1.0 g initially and 1.0 g 24 hours later. As qinghaosu has a short half-life of only a few hours it clears parasitaemia more rapidly than mefloquine, but it has a low radical cure rate in falciparum malaria in contrast to mefloquine (over 90%). This can be raised to 90% when qinghaosu is given intramuscularly on 3 successive days although at the cost of some inconvenience and pain.

None of the antimalarials affects the intrahepatic exo-erythrocytic stages of *P. vivax*, *oval* or *malariae* and primaquine must be given to effect a radical cure. It can be given in a dosage of 0.3 mg base/kg/day for 14 days following the course of chloroquine or other antimalarial drug. Care must be taken in administering primaquine to G-6-PD deficient children. Therapeutic doses do not usually precipitate haemolysis; however, the G-6-PD level should be checked before administration of the drug.

Chemoprophylaxis

The prevention of malarial attacks by continuous drug administration is impracticable for the scattered and rural indigenous populations of tropical countries on the grounds of cost and administrative difficulties. Mosquito control programmes remain the only practicable means of eradicating malaria and it is unfortunate that these have been poorly executed in some countries. Prophylactic drugs are, however, extremely effective in preventing malaria in expatriates when they are combined with measures to avoid mosquito bites, e.g. long sleeves and trousers after sunset, mosquito nets over beds and the use of mosquito repellents of various kinds including mosquito coils and vaporisers. Recently it has been shown that the use of impregnated curtains and bed nets is very effective. They can also be used effectively in certain indigenous groups such as those who have lost their immunity by long sojourn abroad, those in boarding schools, etc. The prophylactic drug should always be taken by expatriates 2 weeks before travelling to an endemic area and for 1 month after return home from a malarious area. In highly endemic areas pregnant women, especially primagravidae, should take full prophylaxis throughout pregnancy. The drug of choice is chloroquine, 300 mg base weekly. Although these drugs may be toxic, the risks of malaria are greater. Drugs containing pyrimethamine should not be taken by pregnant women.

In areas without chloroquine resistance the three standard prophylactic drugs with their appropriate adult doses are: chloroquine 300 mg base once or twice weekly, proguanil 100–200 mg daily; or pyrimethamine 50 mg once per week. In areas where falciparum malaria has become chloroquine resistant, drug prophylaxis may be effected with Fansidar (pyrimethamine 25 mg + sulfadoxine 500 mg), adult dose = one tablet weekly; or with Maloprim (pyrimethamine 12.5 mg + dapsone 100 mg), adult dose = one tablet once or twice weekly. Also mefloquine may be used for chemoprophylaxis for travellers to sub-Saharan Africa, where there is a high transmission rate of chloroquine-resistant *Plasmodium falciparum*. To prevent vivax malaria it may be wise to prescribe chloroquine at the usual dosage as well. Fansidar should be avoided during the third trimester of pregnancy and during the neonatal period as it can induce jaundice in the newborn. It is probable that mefloquine will prove to be an effective prophylactic drug but the role of qinghaosu in this respect has not yet been determined. Resistance patterns are still changing and prospective travellers would be well advised to seek advice from special centres such as the London or Liverpool Schools of Tropical Medicine or the Communicable Disease (Scotland) Unit in Glasgow.

BLACKWATER FEVER

This dread complication of MT malaria has become less common, possibly related to the less frequent use of quinine for treatment or prophylaxis. The name refers to the black colour of acidic urine with a high methaemoglobin content. It was always more common in non-immune adults whose malaria had been inadequately suppressed with quinine. The condition is one of severe intravascular haemolysis with haemoglobinuria. Renal tubular necrosis may result in anuria and uraemia. Haemolytic anaemia results in pallor rapidly followed by jaundice. Vomiting and hiccup may be severe. The disease tends to be less severe in children.

Treatment

Chloroquine (never quinine) should be given by the intramuscular route. Severe anaemia is treated by carefully matched blood transfusion. Intravenous fluids are advised but should be in the volume recommended for renal failure. Anuria may be an indication for peritoneal dialysis or haemodialysis. Intravenous dexamethasone may have the effect of stopping the haemolysis.

SCHISTOSOMIASIS (BILHARZIASIS)

This disease is one of the major causes of morbidity and mortality in many tropical countries, e.g. Egypt, Ethiopia, Sudan, Zimbabwe, Malawi, Indonesia, Brazil. The World Health Organization lists schistosomiasis amongst the six most important tropical diseases. Despite great world-wide activity against the disease the overall prevalence of schistosomiasis seems to be increasing due to intensive irrigation projects in the tropics. In endemic areas schistosomiasis is acquired mainly in childhood or adolescence and can thus be regarded as a common tropical paediatric disease. The incidence rises from the age of 5–6 years, but the disease, being of shorter duration, responds better to treatment in children than in adults. Unfortunately, children may leave hospital cured only to suffer reinfection and increasing visceral damage. While attempts may be made to kill the snails which harbour the worm by treating the irrigation canals with copper sulphate or more modern molluscicides, the long-term eradication of the disease must depend upon education of the people in personal hygiene and the safer disposal of human excreta. Furthermore, it requires only a few heavily infested children in a population to contaminate water in canals and drains and transmit the disease. In the European child living in Africa, bilharziasis may occur as the sole disease present, but in the indigenous African it is frequently accompanied by other disease such as malaria, ankylostomiasis, amoebiasis and iron deficiency.

Aetiology and pathology

In most areas of the tropical world this disease is due either to *Schistosoma haematobium* or *S. mansoni* which are trematodes (intestinal blood flukes). Their life cycle includes a sexual phase in man and an asexual phase in a variety of molluscs. In the Orient (China, Japan, Phillipines, Thailand) *S. japonicum* is responsible for many cases of the disease and this fluke has other mammalian hosts in addition to man.

The ova of the schistosomes are passed into water with human excreta. When they hatch, ciliated larvae (miracidia) are liberated to infect snails. Ultimately the snail discharges fork-tailed cercariae which swim about until they enter their definitive host (man); there they lose their tails and travel in the blood stream through the right side of the heart to the lungs. From the lungs they migrate to the liver where they attain sexual maturity and mate. They then migrate against the portal blood stream to the small veins of the colon or rectum and, in the case of *S. haematobium*, to the urinary bladder and ureters. Ova may be widely deposited throughout the viscera. Those from *S. mansoni* are usually excreted in the faeces, those from *S. haematobium* in the urine, although the converse can occur. Disease due to *S. haematobium* tends to be more severe because of widespread involvement and because of the frequency of urinary tract obstruction.

Clinical features

Shortly after the cercariae enter the skin after bathing in infected water, the child develops an itchy papular rash – kabure itch – which disappears in a few days. This stage is, in fact, rarely seen by the doctor. Some 6–12 weeks later the larval worms are passing through the lungs and the child reaches the stage of "bilharzial fever" which may be accompanied by malaise, urticaria, arthralgia, cough and eosinophilia. Diarrhoea may develop, also hepatic enlargement and tenderness. Chest radiographs show patchy opacities and infiltrations. This stage is more likely to be seen in the European child. The later stage of the disease is associated with chronic ill health – malaise, tiredness, loss of weight. In *S. haematobium* infections, haematuria and less commonly, dysuria may occur. In *S. mansoni* infections, diarrhoea with blood and mucus is not uncommon. Ultimately severe complications ensue such as ureteric stricture, hydronephrosis, fibrosis and thickening of the bladder with stone formation; or hepatic cirrhosis with gross hepatosplenomegaly, ascites and portal hypertension. Cor pulmonale due to bilharzial obliterative pulmonary arteriolitis may also hasten death in the child. The clinical picture may be further complicated by malnutrition and anaemia.

Diagnosis

Identification of the appropriate ova in faeces or urine is possible in most infected children. Double infections are not uncommon. In negative cases rectal biopsy in which two or three small snips of mucous membrane are made available for microscopy may reveal ova of both types of schistosome. Straight X-rays may show calcification in the bladder or lower ureters. Cystoscopy may reveal characteristic lesions. Less direct evidence may be found in the presence of eosinophilia, positive intradermal antigen test or positive fluorescent antibody test of ELISA are available but false positives and negatives occur.

Treatment

The long-established use of sodium antimony tartrate has now been displaced by the development of new, safe, and highly effective schistosomicides. These new drugs can also have an important role in controlling transmission of the disease by population based chemotherapy, in combination with control of the snails by molluscicides. Metriphonate (Bilarcil) is cheap but only effective against *S. haematobium*. It may be given in oral doses of 10 mg/kg on three occasions at intervals of 14 days. Oxamniquine (Mansil, Vansil) is extremely effective in all stages of infestation by *S. mansoni* only. To achieve good results in children it needs to be given in three oral doses, each of 20 mg/kg over 2 or 3 days. Praziquantel (Biltricide) is the most effective drug available and it is effective against all human schistosome species. For *S. haematobium* and *S. mansoni* a single oral dose of 40 mg/kg is usually sufficient. For *S. japonicum* the regimens recommended are either 2×30 mg at an interval of 4 hours in one day, or 3×20 mg in one day. While praziquantel is an ideal drug for mass chemotherapy programmes in the control of disease transmission, its cost may militate against its use in some countries. However, health education is a most important weapon in the control of bilharzial disease and its aim should be to elicit community participation in the protection of water and in improving environmental sanitation. No vaccine is yet available.

YAWS (FRAMBOESIA) NON-VENEREAL TREPONEMATOSES

This is a contagious disease of children in the tropics, especially the warm, humid areas of Africa, Southeast Asia, the Pacific, Caribbean and Central and South America. There has been a marked fall in the incidence of the disease but constant surveillance is required to detect resurgence and institute prompt treatment. It is related to overcrowding, lack of elementary hygiene and the ease with which children collect sores and abrasions. The lesions of impetigo and scabies also offer portals of entry for the causal spirochaete, *Treponema pertunue*. This organism is indistinguishable from the spirochaete of syphilis (*Treponema pallidum*) on microscopy (light or electron). In certain areas of the world, which are usually dry, non-venereal endemic syphilis occurs and its relationship to yaws has been much debated. A third spirochaetal disease of similar behaviour but less severity and due to the *Treponema carateum* is called "pinta". It occurs predominantly in the dark skinned people of Mexico, Central and South America, North Africa, Middle East, India and some areas of the Pacific. The control of pinta is as for yaws.

Clinical features

Yaws, like syphilis, can be divided into three stages. The incubation period varies from 2 weeks to 2 months.

Primary

This is rarely seen by the doctor. The primary lesion starts as an erythematous papule which grows into a granulomatous framboesial lesion of 2–5 cm diameter ("the mother yaw"). It may become ulcerated and secondarily infected and is usually painful. Healing leaves behind a depigmented scar.

Secondary

Most children are first seen in the secondary stage about 1–3 months after full development of the primary lesion mainly affecting the skin and bones. By then there are multiple granulomata, particularly in areas such as the groin, perineum, perianal region and axilla. In moist areas they may take the form of condylomata, e.g. at mucocutaneous junctions of lips, nose, vagina and anus. On the trunk the lesions often assume a circinate shape as partial healing takes place. Unlike syphilis the lesions of yaws rarely affect the mucous membranes. A common feature is dactylitis and osteitis with periostitis may develop in other bones, e.g. causing sable-blade tibiae. A patchy plantar and palmar hyperkeratosis is frequently seen in the secondary stage. This has to be differentiated from the much more extensive fissured and painful hyperkeratosis of the tertiary stage and which is, in fact, uncommon in children.

Tertiary

The tertiary lesions of yaws take 5 years or more for their development. Gummata of skin and bone can result in unsightly ulcers and scarring. The bone lesions may be very destructive, involve joints, and lead to crippling and mutilation. A characteristic bony thickening of the maxilla on each side of the nose is known as "goundou". Extensive gummatous destruction of the nose and palate may cause horrible disfiguration and is called "gangosa". Tertiary syphilis and cutaneous leishmaniasis must be excluded as they can cause similar ulcerating lesions of the face and palate.

Diagnosis

In many countries where yaws is prevalent, laboratory facilities are meagre and diagnosis must rest upon clinical findings. The Wassermann, Kahn and VDRL tests are positive as in syphilis and also the treponemal immobilisation and fluorescent antibody tests.

Treatment

Yaws responds well to penicillin. The most commonly used preparation is penicillin aluminium monostearate (PAM) 1.2 megaunits intramuscularly on three successive days. In yaws eradication campaigns a house-to-house search is made for active and latent cases, also contracts, all of whom are given a single dose of PAM.

LEISHMANIASIS

Visceral leishmaniasis (kala-azar)

This disease is caused by a protozoon called *Leishmania donovani* and its vector is the sandfly genus (*Phlebotomus*). It has been transmitted by blood transfusion and transplacentally. It is prevalent in North Africa, Sudan, East Africa, India and South America. It is particularly common in children and infants living along the coast of the Mediterranean seem to be frequently infected. The sandfly does not survive in the colder climates north of the Mediterranean and leishmaniasis is virtually unknown in these countries. It has a long incubation period (6 weeks to 3 years) and it is possible for kala-azar acquired in an endemic area to present in a country where the disease is not endemic.

Clinical features

Infantile kala-azar has an acute onset as in the enteric group of fevers. The temperature rises to the fastigium in the first week. After a further week or two of remittent fever it may settle by lysis. In the older child, as in the adult, the onset is often insidious with lethargy, headache, and general malaise. The fever is irregular and may be continuous, remittent or intermittent. A double rise in 24 hours is characteristic of kala-azar. Splenomegaly develops early and may reach enormous proportions, usually in association with hepatomegaly. Common manifestations include loss of weight, intercurrent infections, purpura, oedema, ascites and severe anaemia. Neutropenia and thrombocytopenia are also common. Agranulocytosis may lead to cancrum oris, or death may be due to bronchopneumonia. A characteristic pigmentation may occasionally develop over the forehead, nose, temples, hands and feet. The hair becomes brittle and falls out. On the other hand the appetite usually stays remarkably good. Death is inevitable in the absence of treatment.

Diagnosis

The serum albumin level is markedly reduced and the gammaglobulin is raised. Indirect diagnostic tests include the Napier formol-gel (aldehyde) test and Chopra antimony test. Fluorescent antibody tests and

ELISA techniques are now also available to assist in diagnosis but may give cross-reactions with other protozoal infections such as malaria and toxoplasmosis. Direct diagnosis rests upon indentification of the Leishman–Donovan bodies (amastigotes) in material obtained by needle puncture of the spleen, liver or bone marrow. The leishmanin skin test for delayed hypersensitivity is usually negative in active infection.

Treatment

Most cases respond to one of the pentavalent antimonials although this seems to differ in degree in different parts of the world. The drug commonly recommended and which is generally well tolerated is sodium stibogluconate (Pentostam). It contains 100 mg pentavalent antimony per ml. One of the main objectives of treatment is to prevent relapse which is demoralising for the patients and may make them unresponsive to antimony. It is not known whether parasites need to be completely eradicated to effect a cure and, indeed, there is no reliable method to determine whether parasites have been completely eradicated apart from repeat splenic aspirates. The recommended dosage of sodium stibogluconate is 20 mg/kg given daily by intramuscular or intravenous injection for 4 weeks. The infrequent relapse may be cured by a second, longer course of the drug. True unresponsiveness to antimony is an indication for treatment with one of the potentially toxic aromatic diamidines, e.g. pentamidine in 15 intramuscular doses of 4 mg/kg on alternate days.

Cutaneous leishmaniasis

Ulcerating and destructive lesions occur on the skin, especially of the face, and contrasts with kala-azar in not usually causing systemic illness. While they tend towards self-healing, disfiguring scarring may be left behind. They are due to protozoa from the genus *Leishmania*, but of different strains in the *oriental sore* of Africa, India and the Sudan and in the nasopharyngeal *espundia* of South America and *Chiclero's ear ulcer* of Mexico and Central Africa. It is important to identify the protozoon in material from the ulcer to distinguish it from other diseases such as yaws, syphilis, leprosy and lupus vulgaris. Treatment is with antimonials in cases of multiple sores. In solitary lesions local infiltrations with 5% mepacrine methosulphonate or 2% berberine sulphate are now considered to be of doubtful value. Single lesions may respond to removal of crusts by moist dressings and applications of a topical antibiotic to discourage secondary bacterial infection.

TRYPANOSOMIASIS (AFRICAN SLEEPING SICKNESS)

This serious disease is transmitted from cattle by the tsetse fly (*Glossina morsitans*), and has a fairly localised incidence in the African continent, e.g. Tanzania, Uganda, South West Ethiopia, Senegal, Angola, Mozambique. Two varieties of trypanosome are involved: *T. rhodesiense* which is highly virulent (resistant to tryparasamide), and the less virulent *T. gambiense*. The disease affects adult males who are hunters or fisherman more often than women or children who are usually tied to their villages. (Chagas disease of South America due to *T. cruzi* is different from African trypanosomiasis and will not be discussed here.)

Clinical features

The bite of the tsetse fly results in an oval, inflamed, indurated and tender lump. Parasitaemia develops 7–14 days later and the child becomes ill with fever, headache and muscular tenderness. Lymph node enlargement, splenomegaly, hepatomegaly, weakness and loss of weight follow. Oedema is common, and in the less severe infection with *T. gambiense*, facial puffiness may be striking although the other manifestations are less severe. Involvement of the central nervous system is reflected in unsteadiness of gait, tremors and a typical vacant "fishy stare". The typical lethargy and trance-like sleep is more common in *T. gambiense* infections, although cases associated with *T. rhodesiense* have a more rapid course and may, in fact, end fatally before signs of CNS involvement have become apparent. Cardiac involvement can cause fatal arrhythmias and pleural and pericardial effusions occur.

Diagnosis

Trypanosomes should be sought in Giemsa-stained thick blood films, in lymph node lymph fluid obtained by needle puncture and examined as a wet preparation and in the CSF after centrifugation. Animal inoculation may also yield trypanosomes but the monkey is the only animal susceptible to *T. gambiense*. Serological tests are helpful but not specific, which limits their value in patients continually exposed. There is commonly a normochromic anaemia, raised ESR, and a very high serum IgM level.

Treatment

Several drugs are available, none free from toxic effects. In early cases with normal CSF, the drug choice is suramin (antrypol; Bayer-205). It is given intravenously in doses of 20 mg/kg on days 1, 3, 7, 14 and 21. Suramin does not penetrate into the central nervous system and in cases with CNS involvement and with increased protein and cells in the CSF the most favoured drug is melarsoprol (Arsobal; melarsen oxide-BAL; mel B). It is given by slow intravenous injection as a 3.6% solution in propylene glycol, the dose unit being 1.8 mg/kg. The first few doses should be smaller. The drug may be given daily in three to four courses each for 3 days at intervals of 7–10 days. In advanced cases the dose unit of the last course may be raised to 3.6 mg/kg. Herxheimer reactions and arsenical encephalopathy may occur. The treated child should be followed up for 2 years because relapses may require further courses of melarsoprol.

BURKITT LYMPHOMA

It is associated with a herpes-like virus called Epstein–Barr (EB) virus and to which antibodies can always be demonstrated in these unfortunate children. The distribution of the tumour across Africa from Nigeria to Uganda and Tanzania suggests that the causal virus might be transmitted by insects. This type of lymphoma, which is histologically quite distinguishable from other lymphomas, is a much more common cause of death in the countries mentioned than is acute leukaemia. It is now known that Burkitt lymphoma is a B-lymphocyte malignancy.

Clinical features

The tumour most commonly arises in the maxilla or the mandible producing gross swelling and deformity of the face. Loosening of the teeth, proptosis of an eye, encroachment with the mouth or pharynx occur. Other sites for this tumour include the ovaries or kidneys with gross abdominal masses, the vertebral column with paraplegia, cervical lymph nodes, testes, salivary glands and bones other than the maxilla and mandible. The peak age incidence is 2–5 years with a 2:1 male preponderance.

Treatment

The tumour responds dramatically to cyclophosphamide given orally each day (2.5 mg/kg) or preferably intravenously in a weekly dose of 300 mg/m² body surface. In developing countries, adequate follow-up is extremely difficult, and accurate information as to the incidence of relapses, permanent cures, etc., is not available. Indeed, single drug treatment should have no place in the modern management of any lymphoma. There is a need for trials of protocols which in addition to high dose cyclophosphamide include drugs such as vincristine, doxorubicin, methotrexate and prednisolone. These are not easy to implement in most parts of Africa.

ONCHOCERCIASIS

This infection is caused by the nematode *Onchocerca volvulus* and is characterised by skin changes, subcutaneous nodules and ocular lesions. It is spread by a small black fly (*Simulium damnosum*) which breeds in swiftly flowing rivers.

The estimated and the actual number of affected patients in the world has increased considerably in the last 40 years. The actual increase is a consequence of population growth in the affected areas and also due to the development of greatly improved diagnostic procedures. It is a disabling disease and is regarded as a major public health problem especially in many west and central African countries.

It presents with skin nodules which vary in number but in most endemic areas there are seldom more than five or six in one individual. An allergic dermatitis may occur and patients complain of intense itching. The most severe lesions are those of the eye, mainly punctate keratitis, chorioretinitis, optic atrophy, progressive visual impairment and finally complete blindness. Onchocerciasis is responsible for 50% of all cases of blindness in West Africa.

Diagnosis

Eosinophilia is usual and the microfilariae of *Onchocerca volvulus* are identified by examination of skin or conjunctival snips. They are most easily found in samples of skin taken from the region of the nodule. Serological tests are available but cross-reactions with other nematode infections make interpretation difficult.

Treatment

Treatment is with diethylcarbamazine. Also removal of the subcutaneous nodules reduces the incidence of eye lesions and mass treatment with diethylcarbamazine of all infected persons in the community kills the microfilariae and reduces transmission.

ENDOMYOCARDIAL FIBROSIS

This is a disease of unknown aetiology which is largely confined to Africa. It is most common in the third and fourth decades of life, but is not uncommon in children in contrast to the rarity of the cardiomyopathies in the children of Europe and the USA. It is, however, quite rare in expatriate children living in Africa. The characteristic pathology is fibrous thickening of the endocardium and subendocardial myocardium. There is no excess of elastic tissue as in the endocardial fibro-elastosis of infancy. The disease starts at the apex of one or both ventricles and spreads upwards to involve the mitral or the tricuspid valves, which are often rendered incompetent. The aortic and pulmonary valves are not involved but the capacity of the right ventricle may be severely reduced so that the situation is not dissimilar to that in constrictive pericarditis. Thrombus formation may occur over the grossly thickened endocardium and lead to embolic episodes.

Various workers have suggested that endomyocardial fibrosis is but one end of the spectrum of "idiopathic hypereosinophilic syndrome". This is a heterogeneous group of disorders sharing the common features of prolonged eosinophilia and damage to various tissues. While the other end of the spectrum may be represented by patients with a relatively benign disorder such as tropical eosinophilia, the major source of morbidity and mortality is cardiac disease. In endomyocardial fibrosis as seen in Africa, however, eosinophilia is mild or absent, in contrast to the endocardial fibrosis seen in the USA and Europe where eosinophils are present in abundance.

Clinical features

Variations depend upon whether the left or the right side of the heart is more severely involved. In disease of the left ventricle with mitral regurgitation, the patient becomes increasingly breathless on exertion and may have haemoptysis. Nocturnal attacks of acute dyspnoea occur. There is cardiomegaly due to left atrial and ventricular enlargement, and the right ventricle may also be enlarged. Gallop rhythm is common, and where there is mitral involvement, a loud apical pansystolic murmur. Congestive cardiac failure ultimately supervenes. When the right ventricle and atrium are severely involved with tricuspid regurgitation the physical signs include overfilling and systolic pulsation of the external jugular veins, hepatomegaly with expansile pulsation over the liver, ascites, gallop rhythm and a pansystolic murmur at the left lower sternal border. In cases involving an obliterative process in the right ventricle, there is distension of the jugular veins, hepatomegaly and gross ascites, but the typical venous and hepatic pulsation of tricuspid incompetence will be absent.

The ECG shows marked abnormalities. In left heart disease the P wave is large and flat and the P-R interval may be prolonged. In right heart disease the P waves are often tall and peaked. T wave changes include flattening or inversion. There may be low-voltage QRS complexes. Varying degrees of right or left bundle-branch block occur. Radiographs show marked cardiomegaly due to enlargements of various chambers and intracardiac calcifications may be visible. Pulmonary congestion is often marked in left heart disease and strikingly absent in obliterative disease of the right ventricle. Pleural transudates may be present.

Treatment

The treatment of congestive cardiac failure is described in Chapter 5 and correction of anaemia or nutritional deficiencies may prolong life, but death usually follows within a few years of diagnosis.

TROPICAL PYOMOSITIS

This clinical condition is very common in tropical countries particularly in Africa, areas of South America and Japan. It mainly affects the indigenous population. Tropical pyomyositis can occur at any age but it usually affects adolescents and young adults. The commonest site of the abscesses is the lower limb (thighs, calves and buttocks) although upper limbs, chest wall and abdominal wall may be affected. There is usually only one abscess. In most cases the pus contains *Staphylococcus aureus* or streptococci.

Treatment is adequate surgical drainage and a course of antibiotic therapy.

NEONATAL TETANUS

In spite of the fact that effective immunisation is available against tetanus it remains a major cause of death in many developing countries. In the newborn, the portal of entry is the umbilicus. Neonatal tetanus is usually generalised. Most commonly it occurs following infections of the umbilical cord after an unattended home delivery or a delivery attended by an untrained midwife. Unclean objects, such as old glass, razor blades or sharpened pieces of wood used to cut the cord following delivery may cause contamination with *Clostridium tetani*. The newborn infant may be infected following delivery if the umbilical stump is covered with materials such as dirty rags, or cow dung, or if unsterile methods are used for the postpartum care of the cord. Neonatal tetanus has a short incubation period with signs occurring as early as 3 days after exposure. The first sign is a sudden inability to suck. The infant rapidly develops stiffness of the body, followed by generalised spasms and opisthotonus. Persistent risus sardonicus is common. Due to spasms of the larynx the child is unable to swallow. Spasms of the respiratory muscles can lead to episodes of apnoea. Most deaths occur between 4 and 14 days after birth.

The prevention of neonatal tetanus lies in the improvement of obstetrical and neonatal care. Cleanliness in cutting, tying and dressing the umbilical cord at birth will prevent tetanus in the newborn. In populations with a high incidence of neonatal tetanus active immunisation of pregnant women using tetanus toxoid should be routine and, in fact, may be the only practical way to decrease the incidence of the disease. Passive immunisation of newborns who are likely to have exposure to tetanus spores with 750 IU of tetanus antiserum will afford protection from tetanus and is recommended.

Treatment of established tetanus whether neonatal or in older children includes therapy with specific anti-tetanus human immunoglobulin, use of penicillin in a dose of 100 000 units/kg daily for 5 days and supportive measures such as parenteral nutrition and ventilatory support of the paralysed patient are often needed. In older children surgical care of wounds and the use of other antibiotics for wound infections may be necessary.

IMPORTED DISEASES

Movement of people by air, land or sea to and from tropical and subtropical countries is increasing every year and thus mode of travel is mainly responsible for spreading diseases across the world (Table 20.3). The impact which increased travel has made on the incidence of certain types of diseases in tropical and non-tropical countries cannot be ignored. Diseases are not imported only by immigrants to developed countries. Measles imported into tropical countries by travellers can be the cause of major childhood mortality in the host country. Many members of the immigrant communities in developed countries now take regular holidays in their countries of origin and have considerably increased the number and variety of tropical diseases imported to temperate countries. Therefore the movement of human population is responsible for the introduction of exotic diseases into non-endemic areas. This occurs regardless of whether the country of origin of the displaced population is in a tropical or a temperate region. Of particular importance in this respect is paediatric HIV infection which has become a major health problem in sub-Saharan Africa and parts of South-east Asia. The dangers of import/export of disease will not be relieved until the diseases themselves are eradicated in the endemic regions as with smallpox.

In today's world of global travel with the export/import of diseases any medical practitioner who is approached for medical advice should be familiar with the wide spectrum of "imported diseases" and be able to recognise their diverse clinical manifestations. An enquiry into a child's country of origin and travel abroad remains an important part of the medical history. The reply must be comprehensive enough to include not only the ports of departure and destination but also mention must be made of all ports at which the plane touched down or the ship anchored. Most of the "imported diseases" are mentioned in Table 20.3 but only a few commonly encountered imported diseases are briefly discussed.

Protection in the form of immunisation and chemoprophylaxis is now offered to individuals travelling to countries where the imported infections are endemic. Unfortunately at present these two measures are not available for the vast majority of imported diseases.

TABLE 20.3 Imported diseases

Commonly imported diseases
Parasitic diseases
  Malaria
  Giardiasis
  Amoebiasis
  Schistosomiasis
  Helminthiasis
Bacterial diseases
  Salmonellosis
  Shigellosis
  Vibrio infections
  Tuberculosis
Viral diseases
  Influenza

Less commonly imported diseases
Parasitic diseases
  Leishmaniasis
  Trypanosomiasis
  Roundworms
  Filarial infections
  Larva migrans
Bacterial and chlamydial diseases
  Diphtheria
  Leprosy
  Trachoma
Virus diseases
  Viral hepatitis
  Poliomyelitis

Less commonly imported "high risk" virus infections
  Rabies
  Lassa fever

Miscellaneous disorders
  Burkitt lymphoma
  Endomyocardial fibrosis
  Tropical sprue
  Legionnaire disease

For the tourist or short-term visitor the immunisations usually recommended to ensure some degree of immunity are those against typhoid, paratyphoid, diphtheria, tetanus, poliomyelitis and measles. For long-term visitors, in addition to these prophylactic measures, immunisation against rabies and hepatitis A and BCG vaccination for those who are tuberculin negative should be advised.

Chemoprophylaxis has a role in the prevention of a limited number of exotic diseases seen in temperate countries. These include malaria, trypanosomiasis, traveller's diarrhoea and onchocerciasis.

Advice should be given to potential travellers to tropical and subtropical countries on protective measures to avoid insect bites and contaminated foods and drinking water.

Appendix

A GUIDE TO CLINICAL CHEMISTRY VALUES

The values given are a guide to the normal range but local laboratories may because of differing methodologies and nomenclature vary from these. If in any doubt, check with the laboratory.

Blood

Acid–base [H^+]		38–45 nmol/l	pH 7.35–7.42	
P_{CO_2}		4.5–6.0 kPa	(32–45 mmHg)	
P_{O_2}		11–14 kPa	(78–105 mmHg)	
Bicarbonate [HCO_3^-]		18–25 mmol/l		
Base excess		−4 to +3 mmol/l		

Plasma: electrolytes and minerals

Sodium		135–145	mmol/l
Potassium	0–2 weeks	3.7–6.0	mmol/l
	2 weeks–2 months	3.7–5.8	mmol/l
	>2 months	3.5–5.0	mmol/l
Chloride		95–105	mmol/l
Calcium	Preterm	1.5–2.5	mmol/l
	First year	2.25–2.75	mmol/l
	Children	2.25–2.60	mmol/l
Phosphate (lower in breast fed)	Preterm	1.4–3.4	mmol/l
	First year	1.2–2.5	mmol/l
	Children	0.8–1.8	mmol/l
Magnesium	First year	0.7–1.2	mmol/l
	Children	0.7–1.0	mmol/l
Copper		12.0–29.0	µmol/l
Zinc		9.0–29.0	µmol/l
Iron		11.0–31.0	µmol/l
Ceruloplasmin	Newborn	0.3–1.3	µmol/l
	Children	1.3–2.7	µmol/l
Ferritin	Infant	20–200	ng/ml
	Children	10–100	ng/ml

Plasma: other analytes

Acetoacetate (incl acetone)		< 30	mg/l
Acid phosphatase		5.0–12.6	U/l
Alkaline phosphatase	Newborn	<1000	U/l
	Children	100–800	U/l
Alanine aminotransferase (ALT)	Infants	10–70	U/l
	Children	10–40	U/l
Ammonia	Newborn	50–80	µmol/l
	Infants and children	20–50	µmol/l
Amylase		50–400	U/l
Ascorbic acid		30–80	µmol/l

Aspartate aminotransferase (AST)		10–50	U/l
Bilirubin total	Cord blood	< 50	μmol/l
(preterm greater) {	Term day 1	< 100	μmol/l
	Term days 2–5	< 200	μmol/l
	> 1 month	< 20	μmol/l
Cholesterol	Cord blood	0.5–3.5	mmol/l
	Newborn	2.5–5.5	mmol/l
	Infants and children	3.0–6.5	mmol/l
Cortisol	Newborn	100–600	nmol/l
	Infants and children 08:00	200–700	nmol/l
	22:00	< 200	nmol/l
Creatine kinase (CK)	Newborn	< 600	U/l
	Infants	< 300	U/l
	Children	< 200	U/l
Creatinine	Newborn	20–100	μmol/l
	Infants and children	20–80	μmol/l
Creatinine clearance	0–3 months	15–50	ml/min/m^2
	3–12 months	25–75	ml/min/m^2
	12–24 months	35–95	ml/min/m^2
	Older children	50–85	ml/min/m^2
C-reactive protein (CRP)		< 20	mg/l
Fibrinogen	Newborn	4.5–10	μmol/l
	Children	5.5–11.5	μmol/l
Fibrin degradation products (FDPs)		12–20	mg/l
Folic acid		10–30	nmol/l
Follicle-stimulating hormone (FSH)		< 3	U/l
Gammaglutamyltransferase (γGT)	Newborn	< 200	U/l
	Infants	< 120	U/l
	Children	< 30	U/l
Glucose	Newborn (< 48 h)	2.2–5.0	mmol/l
	Infants and children	3.0–5.0	mmol/l
Glycosylated haemoglobin		4.5–7.5	%
Insulin	fasting	5–40	mU/l
Lactate (blood)	Newborn	< 3.0	mmol/l
	Infants and children	1.0–1.8	mmol/l
Lactate dehydrogenase (LDH)		60–200	U/l
Lipids – total	Newborn	1.5–4.0	g/l
	Infants and children	4–10	g/l
– phospholipids	Newborn	0.75–2.5	g/l
	Infants and children	1.5–3.0	g/l
– triglycerides (fasting)		0.6–1.7	mmol/l
Luteinising hormone (LH)		< 1.9	U/l
Osmolality		275–295	mmol/kg
Protein – total	Newborn	45–75	g/l
	Infants	55–75	g/l
	Children	60–80	g/l
– albumin	Newborn	25–50	g/l
	Infants and children	35–50	g/l
– immunoglobulins (g/l)			

	IgG	IgA	IgM
Newborn	6.5–14.5	0–0.1	0–0.3
Infants	1.5–10.0	0.1–0.8	0.1–2.0
Children > 3 years	5.0–15.0	0.3–3.0	0.4–2.0

Pyruvate (blood)		50–80	μmol/l
Thyroxine (T$_4$)	Newborn	140–440	nmol/l
	Infants	90–195	nmol/l
	Children	70–180	nmol/l

Thyroid-stimulating hormone (TSH)	Newborn	< 25	mU/l
	Infants and children	0.3–5.0	mU/l
Tri-iodothyronine (T$_3$)	Newborn	0.5–6.0	nmol/l
	Infants and children	1.5–3.8	nmol/l
Urea		2.5–6.5	mmol/l
Uric acid		0.12–0.42	mmol/l
Vitamin A		0.7–3.5	µmol/l
25-Hydroxyvitamin D		> 25	nmol/l
Vitamin E (α-tocopherol)		10–28	µmol/l

A GUIDE TO HAEMATOLOGICAL VALUES*

Red blood cell values at various stages: mean and lower limit of normal (–2 SD)

Age	HAEMOGLOBIN (g/dl)		HAEMATOCRIT (%)		RED CELL COUNT (×10^{12}/litre)		MCV (fl)		MCH (pg)		MCHC (g/dl)	
	mean	–2 SD	mean	–2 SD	mean	–2 SD	mean	–2 SD	mean	–2 SD	mean	–2 SD
Birth	16.5	13.5	51	42	4.7	3.9	108	98	34	31	33	30
1 month	14.0	10.0	43	31	4.2	3.0	104	85	34	28	33	29
1 year	12.0	10.5	36	33	4.5	3.7	78	70	27	23	33	30
8 years	13.5	11.5	40	35	4.6	4.0	86	77	29	25	34	31

Normal leucocyte counts

Age	TOTAL LEUCOCYTES (×10^9/litre)		NEUTROPHILS (×10^9/litre)			LYMPHOCYTES (×10^9/litre)			MONOCYTES (×10^9/litre)		EOSINOPHILS (×10^9/litre)	
	mean	(range)	mean	(range)	%	mean	(range)	%	mean	%	mean	%
Birth	18.1	(9.0–30.0)	11.0	(6.0–26.0)	61	5.5	(2.0–11.0)	31	1.1	6	0.4	2
1 month	10.8	(5.0–19.5)	3.8	(1.0–9.0)	35	6.0	(2.5–16.5)	56	0.7	7	0.3	3
1 year	11.4	(6.0–17.5)	3.5	(1.5–8.5)	31	7.0	(4.0–10.5)	61	0.6	5	0.3	3
8 years	8.3	(4.5–13.5)	4.4	(1.5–8.0)	53	3.3	(1.5–6.8)	39	0.4	4	0.2	2

*Dallman, P.R. *Pediatrics*. 16th ed. Rudolph, A. (ed.) New York, Appleton-Century-Crofts, 1977, p1111.

REFERENCE RANGES

TEST	UNITS	RANGE
Activated partial thromboplasmin time	seconds	26–40
Bleeding time (template)	minutes	2–9.25
D-dimer	mg/l	< 0.25
Erythrocyte sedimentation rate	mm/h	1–5
Fibrinogen: functional	g/l	1.5–4
Folate: red cell	µg/l	125–600
Folate: serum	µg/l	3–14
Haemoglobin A$_2$ (adult value by 4 months)	%	1.5–3.2
Haemoglobin F (adult value by 6–12 months)	%	< 2.0
Platelet count	×10^9/l	150–400
Prothrombin time	seconds	11.8–15.2
Reptilase time	seconds	13–17
Thrombin time	seconds	10–13
Vitamin B$_{12}$	ng/l	170–960

Index

Note: page numbers in **bold** refer to major discussions in the text, and usually include discussions on aetiology, clinical features, diagnosis and treatment.

4.